A Model of Human Occupation: Theory and Application

Third Edition

A Model of Human Occupation: Theory and Application

Third Edition

Gary Kielhofner, DrPH, OTR, FAOTA
Wade/Meyer Chair, Professor and Head,
Department of Occupational Therapy,
College of Applied Health Sciences
University of Illinois at Chicago
Chicago, Illinois

Foreign Adjunct Professor
Division of Occupational Therapy
Karolinska Institutet
Stockholm, Sweden

Visiting Professor
School of Occupational Therapy
University of London
London, England, United Kingdom

Editor: Tim Julet
Managing Editor: Ulita Lushnycky
Marketing Manager: Debby Hartman
Production Editor: Jennifer D. Weir
Designer: Risa Clow
Compositor: Maryland Composition

Library of Congress Cataloging-in-Publication Data
Kielhofner, Gary, 1949–
   A model of human occupation : theory and application / Gary Kielhofner.—3rd ed.
      p. cm.
   Includes bibliographical references and index.
   ISBN 0-7817-2800-2
   1. Occupational therapy. I. Title.

   RM735 .M55 2002
   615.8'515—dc21   2001050627

02 03 04 05 06
1 2 3 4 5 6 7 8 9 10

To those whose lives are chronicled herein.

Acknowledgments

This third edition of A Model of Human Occupation goes to press over a quarter century after work on the model first began. The idea that took shape in my graduate work in the early 1970s has become more than I could have imagined then. This is due to literally hundreds of persons who have contributed to the development of various aspects of the model. It is simply impossible to recount all of them. Nonetheless, I am grateful for each of them.

Putting together a book like this one takes a great deal of time and effort from many people. Each time I have undertaken to write an edition of A Model of Human Occupation, I have had the uncommon good fortune of working with an outstanding team of people. The reader will recognize that authors from many corners of the world have directly contributed to the contents of this book. It has been a pleasure to work with each of them and to see the ways in which therapists have expanded and applied the model's concepts. This time around, Dr. Kirsty Forsyth made the work all the more exciting and the end-product so much better. Her imprint on this text is clear in the chapters she has co-authored with others and myself. Her keen mind and good humor have influenced me in bringing the volume together in ways that only I will ultimately appreciate. Lynn Summerfield Mann had the vision to institutionalize an effort in London to engage this model more deeply in a dialogue with practice. Her feedback, encouragement, and support have nourished and nudged our efforts to articulate herein a clearer connection between concepts and practice.

My research assistants, Judith Abelenda, Semonti Basu, Meghan Crisp, Monique Carson, Colleen Gauntner, Anita Iyenger, Lisa Jacobsen, Yanling Li, and Lisa Neiman, spent untold hours toiling over details, chasing down references, copy-editing, word-processing, and everything else that goes into bringing a book like this into being. They have also been a source of input and feedback that has shaped the contents. They all have my deepest gratitude.

Lippincott Williams & Wilkins engaged a number of blind reviewers to provide feedback on drafts of this text. Although their identities remain unknown to me, I am deeply indebted to them for their thoughtful and helpful input and hope that all can find ways that they have shaped the final product. I am indebted to Fran Oakley, Theresa Plummer, Renee Moore, and Trudy Mallinson, who provided some of the case materials and anecdotes shared in this book.

In addition, the book benefited much from solicited feedback from Marcia Finlayson, Gail Fisher, Christine Helfrich, Sue Parkinson, Liz Peterson, and Renee Taylor. Michael O'Malley graciously provided some emergency translation. David Mitchell examined the visual representations of disability in this text and provided thoughtful feedback. I can only hope we have been able in some small way to approximate the standard he recommended. Members of the MOHOC listserv have constantly raised issues and questions that led me and others to try to develop more thorough answers and arguments that have found their way into this book.

I owe a debt of gratitude to thank Ulita Lushnycky and Jennifer Weir for superb editorial support. The persistence and creative talents of Risa Clow has made this volume a visual delight. Anne Rains possesses not only an impressive artistic talent, but also an even more remarkable ability to render concepts visually. In sum, Lippincott Williams & Wilkins provided me with a remarkable editorial and artistic team.

In so many ways, disabled people have lent their stories and voices to this volume. Since A Model of Human Occupation grows out of a professional and personal desire to positively impact the lives of those who experience disability, I hope the book is worthy of what they have lent us of themselves. I also hope each rendering of a part of someone's life herein is both faithful and a tribute to them.

My wife, Nancy, tolerated my long hours of work and recognized the importance of this project to me. My children, Kim and Kris, each in their own unique ways and through their life journeys, have taught me more than I can ever say. What must be said is that much in this book reflects what I have learned from them.

Contributors

Susan Anderson, MS, OTR/L
Staff Occupational Therapist
Marklund Learning Campus
Des Plaines, Illinois

Marianne Masako Ankersjö, OT (reg.)
Master of Science Student
Division of Occupational Therapy
Department of Clinical Neuroscience
Occupational Therapy and Elderly Care Research
Karolinska Institutet
Stockholm, Sweden

Ana Laura Auzmendia, TO
Instructor
Department of Occupational Therapy
Universidad Nacional de Mar del Plata
Mar del Plata, Argentina

Kathi Brenneman Baron, MS, OTR/L
Project Coordinator
Center for Outcomes Research and Education
Department of Occupational Therapy
College of Applied Health Sciences
University of Illinois at Chicago
Chicago, Illinois

Tal Baz, MS, OTR/L
President
Attune, Inc.
Chicago, Illinois

René Bélanger, OT, M.B.A.
Chief Occupational Therapist
Specialized Young Psychotic Program
Hotel-Dieu de Levis Hospital
Levis, Quebec, Canada

Melinda Blondis, MS, OTR/L
Occupational Therapist
Proviso Area for Exceptional Children
Brookfield, Illinois

Lena Borell, PhD, OT (reg.)
Professor and Chair
Division of Occupational Therapy
Department of Clinical Neuroscience
Occupational Therapy and Elderly Care Research
Karolinska Institutet
Stockholm, Sweden

Brent Braveman, MEd, OTR/L
Clinical Assistant Professor
Department of Occupational Therapy
College of Applied Health Sciences
University of Illinois at Chicago
Chicago, Illinois

Kim Bryze, MS, OTR/L
Occupational Therapist
Child and Family Development Center, and
Clinical Instructor
Department of Occupational Therapy
College of Applied Health Sciences
University of Illinois at Chicago
Chicago, Illinois

Christine Clay, A.A.
Teacher Assistant
Chicago Lighthouse for the Blind
Chicago, Illinois

Laurie Rockwell-Dylla, MS, OTR/L
Project Coordinator
Department of Occupational Therapy
College of Applied Health Sciences
University of Illinois at Chicago
Chicago, Illinois

Elin Ekbladh, MSc, OT (reg.)
Department of Neuroscience and Locomotion
Section of Occupational Therapy
Faculty of Health Sciences
Linköpings Universitet
Linköping, Sweden

Jeanne Federico, BS, OTR/L
Occupational Therapist
La Grange Area Department of Special Education
La Grange, Illinois

Kirsty Forsyth, PhD, SROT, OTR
Post Doctoral Fellow
Department of Occupational Therapy
College of Applied Health Sciences
University of Illinois at Chicago
Chicago, Illinois
Lecturer
Queen Margaret University College
Edinburgh, Scotland, United Kingdom
Director
UK MOHO Center for Research and Education
University of London
London, England, United Kingdom

Ladonna Freidheim, MS, OTR/L
Chicago, Illinois

Gloria Furst, OTR/L, MPH
Occupational Therapy Consultant
Rehabilitation Medicine Department
National Institutes of Health
Bethesda, Maryland

Lauren Goldbaum, MS, OTR/L
Staff Occupational Therapist
Department of Occupational Therapy
College of Applied Health Sciences
University of Illinois at Chicago
Chicago, Illinois

Victoria Goldhammer, MS, OTR/L
Assistive Technology Specialist
Easter Seals of Massachusetts
Roslindale, Massachusetts

Karen Goldstein, MS, OTR/L
Staff Occupational Therapist
Department of Occupational Therapy
College of Applied Health Sciences
University of Illinois at Chicago
Chicago, Illinois

Lena Haglund, PhD, OT (reg.)
Department of Neuroscience and Locomotion
Section of Occupational Therapy
Faculty of Health Sciences
Linköpings Universitet
Linköping, Sweden

Junko Hayashi, MS, OTR
Occupational Therapist
Tamagawa Nursing Home
Tokyo, Japan

Christine Helfrich, PhD, OTR/L
Assistant Professor
Department of Occupational Therapy
College of Applied Health Sciences
University of Illinois at Chicago
Chicago, Illinois

Helena Hemmingsson, OT (reg.)
Doctoral Student
Division of Occupational Therapy
Department of Clinical Neuroscience
Occupational Therapy and Elderly Care Research
Karolinska Institutet
Stockholm, Sweden

Alexis Henry, ScD, OTR/L, FAOTA
Assistant Professor
Occupational Therapy Department
Sargent College of Health and Rehabilitation
  Sciences
Boston University
Boston, Massachusetts
Research Assistant Professor of Psychiatry
Center for Mental Health Services Research
University of Massachusetts Medical School
Worcester, Massachusetts

Carmen Gloria de las Heras, MS, OTR
Director
Reencuentros Rehabilitation Center
Santiago, Chile

Renee Hinson-Smith, MSOT, OTR/L
Director
Generations Adult and Child Daycare
Fort Lauderdale, Florida

Jennifer Hutson, MS, OTR/L, ATP
Clinical Occupational Therapist
Evanston Northwestern Hospital
Evanston, Illinois

Anita Iyenger, MS, OTR
Research Assistant
Model of Human Occupation Clearinghouse
Department of Occupational Therapy
College of Applied Health Sciences
University of Illinois at Chicago
Chicago, Illinois

Hans Jonsson, PhD, OT (reg.)
Associate Professor
Director of Master Program in Occupational Therapy
Division of Occupational Therapy
Department of Clinical Neuroscience
Occupational Therapy and Elderly Care Research
Karolinska Institutet
Stockholm, Sweden

Staffan Josephsson, PhD, OT (reg.)
Associate Professor
Division of Occupational Therapy
Department of Clinical Neuroscience
Occupational Therapy and Elderly Care Research
Karolinska Institutet
Stockholm, Sweden

Riitta Keponen, OT
Lecturer
Occupational Therapy Program
STADIA Helsinki Polytechnic
Helsinki, Finland

Dalleen Last, Dip.COT., SROT
Senior 1 Occupational Therapist
Oxfordshire Learning Disability
National Health Service Trust
Oxford, England, United Kingdom

Veronica Llerena, MS, OTR/L
Occupational Therapy Services Manager
Bonaventure House
Chicago, Illinois

Trudy Mallinson, PhD, OTR/L, NZROT
Postdoctoral Fellow
Institute for Health Services Research and Policy
    Studies
Northwestern University
Chicago, Illinois

Jane Melton, MSc, Dip.COT., SROT
Mental Health Directorate
East Gloucestershire National Health Service Trust
Cheltenham, England, United Kingdom

Christiane Mentrup, OT
Head
Occupational Therapy Program
Voelker-Schule College
Osnabrueck, Germany

Claudia Miranda, Lic. TO
Instructor
Department of Occupational Therapy
Researcher
Department of Psychology
Universidad Nacional de Mar del Plata
Mar del Plata, Argentina

Louise Nygård, PhD, OT (reg.)
Associate Professor
Division of Occupational Therapy
Department of Clinical Neuroscience
Occupational Therapy and Elderly Care Research
Karolinska Institutet
Stockholm, Sweden

Frances Oakley, MS, OTR, BCN, BCG, FAOTA
Clinical and Research Occupational Therapist
Occupational Therapy Section
Rehabilitation Medicine Department
National Institutes of Health
Bethesda, Maryland

Linda Olson, MS, OTR/L
Assistant Professor
Department of Occupational Therapy
College of Health Sciences
Rush University
Chicago, Illinois

Ay Woan Pan, PhD, OTR/L
Associate Professor
Department of Occupational Therapy
College of Medicine
National Taiwan University
Adjunct Occupational Therapist
Department of Psychiatry
National Taiwan University Hospital
Taipei, Taiwan

Sue Parkinson, Dip. COT
Acting Head Occupational Therapist
Acute Day Therapy Services
Chesterfield Royal Hospital
Derbyshire, England, United Kingdom

Laurie Raymond, MS, OTR/L
Staff Occupational Therapist
Beth Osten & Associates and Private Practice
Skokie, Illinois

Dommie Rey, Dip.COT, SROT
Professional Lead in Occupational Therapy
Oxfordshire Learning Disability
National Health Service Trust
Oxford, England, United Kingdom

Deborah M. Roitman, MS, OTR
Head of Occupational Therapy Services
Day Center for the Aged
Yehud, Israel
Director of Special Projects
The Israel Center for Technology and Accessibility
Ramat Gan, Israel

Marian K. Scheinholtz, MS, OTR/L
Practice Associate
American Occupational Therapy Association
Bethesda, Maryland

Daniela Schulte, OT
Staff Occupational Therapist
Psychiatrische Tagesklinik
St. Vinzenz Hospital
Osnabruck, Germany

Jayne Shepherd, MS, OTR/L
Associate Professor
Department of Occupational Therapy
School of Allied Health Professions
Virginia Commonwealth University
Richmond, Virginia

Camille Skubik-Peplaski, MS, OTR/L, BCP
Program Coordinator
Cardinal Hill Rehabilitation Hospital
Center for Outpatient Services
Lexington, Kentucky

Cynthia Stabenow, MS, OTR/L
Occupational Therapist
Martha Jefferson Hospital
Charlottesville, Virginia

Kerstin Tham, PhD, OT (reg.)
Associate Professor
Division of Occupational Therapy
Department of Clinical Neuroscience
Occupational Therapy and Elderly Care Research
Karolinska Institutet
Stockholm, Sweden

Luc Vercruysse, OT
Head and Supervisor
Occupational Therapy Department
University Center St. Jozef
Kortenberg, Belgium
Lecturer
Section Occupational Therapy
Department Parnas
Iris Hogeschool Brussel
Dilbeek, Belgium

Noga Ziv, MSc, OTR
Instructor
Department of Occupational Therapy
School of Health Professions
Tel Aviv University
Head of Occupational Therapy Services
Community Mental Health Center Ramat Chen
Tel Aviv, Israel

CONTENTS

Case Illustrations   357

IV   **Program Development, Research, and Further Resources   489**

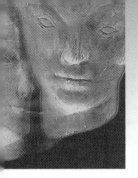

Introduction to the Model of Human Occupation

● Gary Kielhofner

The title of this text should raise, in any reader's mind, two questions: What is human occupation? What is a model? To a large extent these questions are answered throughout this volume. Nonetheless, initial responses are given here to provide an introduction to the model of human occupation.

Human Occupation

Importantly, the term "human occupation" connotes that occupation is part of the human condition. Whatever else characterizes being human—our spiritual yearnings, our capacity for love—we also share an innate occupational nature. **Human occupation** refers to the doing of work, play, or activities of daily living within a temporal, physical, and sociocultural context that characterizes much of human life. Let us consider what each of the elements of this definition means.

Doing

In the broadest sense, occupation denotes the action or doing (Fidler & Fidler, 1983; Nelson, 1988; Reilly, 1962; Rogers, 1983). Whereas all living species engage in some form of action, humans are unique in the extent to which they have evolved a pervasive and complex array of things to do. Moreover, human doing is often

> *Whatever else characterizes being human—our spiritual yearnings, our capacity for love—we also share an innate occupational nature.*

pursued for its own sake (Florey, 1969). The intense need to do things is uniquely human.

Understanding occupation requires that we characterize the rich diversity of human doing. Occupation is most typically portrayed as comprising three broad areas of doing: activities of daily living, play, and work. **Activities of daily living** are the typical life tasks required for self-care and self-maintenance, such as grooming, bathing, eating, cleaning the house, and doing laundry (Christiansen & Baum, 1997). **Play** refers to activities undertaken for their own sake (Shannon, 1970; Reilly, 1974). Examples of play are exploring, pretending, celebrating, engaging in games or sports, and pursuing hobbies. Play is the earliest occupation, persisting throughout life (Reilly, 1974; Robinson, 1977; Vandenberg & Kielhofner, 1982). **Work** refers to activities (both paid and unpaid) that provide services or commodities to others such as ideas, knowledge, help, information-sharing, entertainment, utilitarian or artistic objects, and protection (Chapple, 1970; Shannon, 1970). Activities such as studying, practicing, and apprenticing improve abilities for productive performance. Thus, work includes activities engaged in as a student, employee, volunteer, parent, serious hobbyist, and amateur. Activities of daily living, play, and work interweave and sometimes overlap in the course of everyday life. The delineation as areas of doing should serve to highlight the range of occupations in which persons engage, not to rigidly categorize what people do.

Occupying Time and Space

All that humans do exists in the framework of time (Hall, 1969; Kerby, 1991; Young, 1988). Time reveals itself as a vacuum, inviting us to fill it with doing (Meyer,

1922). Without action, time weighs heavily upon us. Consequently, we are moved to fill or occupy time with the things we do. Doing unfolds in the stream of time, carrying us forth, marking time's passing, and shaping the nature of things in the next moment. Consequently, our doing fills the present and anticipates the temporal horizon just beyond us.

Time also comes to us in cycles that shape the recurring patterns of what we do (Young, 1988). What we do consistently parallels what time it is. We mark the passage of temporal cycles by what we do. To a large extent we know what we should be doing by the measure of time. Such terms as mealtime, playtime, and workweek illustrate how the patterns of time and doing are intertwined.

Knowledge of the past and future gives human awareness a particular character (Kerby, 1991). We know our lives to be unfolding in the course of time. Much of what we do in the present is aimed toward some state of affairs we wish for at a distant future point. Therefore, our occupations not only fill and mark time, but also shape the course of our lives over time.

Occupying a Physical World

From the early struggle to move against gravity to the mastery of a complex world of places and objects, humans always do what they do in a physical world (Ayres, 1979; Reilly, 1962). They occupy this world of space and things by traversing, manipulating, and transforming it. Acting in, on, and with our physical surroundings is fundamental to human existence.

The many and varied ways that humans have evolved for interacting with the physical environment shape the kind of doing in which we engage. For example, over the course of evolution, making things has extended from the primitive tool-using and tool-fashioning activities of our ancestors to the contemporary manufacture and use of the complex instruments of modern technology.

Occupying Social and Cultural Worlds

Humans are sociocultural creatures who coordinate their behavior together and share common worlds of action and meaning. Occupation of the social world means that we do things among and with others (Rogers, 1983). It also means that we do things directed at the expression and maintenance of the social fabric that surrounds us. The way we interact with others, the rules we follow in going about work and play, or even the ways we dress and groom ourselves are expressions of our social nature. These behaviors not only follow social ways of doing things, but also serve to perpetuate those same social patterns they reflect.

We make places for ourselves in the social world by what we do. Our actions shape how others view us and who they take us to be. In turn, our social positions influence what we are expected to do and how we go about it. The places we occupy in various social groups require us to do certain things.

Culture is the medium through which humans make sense of their doing. Culture generates a whole range of things to do and gives them shape and significance. Members of a culture engage in things to do that are part of that culture. Moreover, they realize the significance of what they are doing by virtue of how their culture views and makes sense of it (Yerxa et al., 1989). The things that a culture provides for doing are given a place and a meaning within the larger cultural fabric. Indeed, culture reveals itself as an integrated continuum of ordinary to ritualistic things that people do and the meanings attached to them.

Occupation and Human Nature

As the previous discussion highlighted, occupation is complex and multifaceted. Occupation encompasses a wide range of doing that occurs in the context of time, space, society, and culture. Temporal, physical, social, and cultural contexts pose conditions that invite, shape, and inform our doing. The temporal and physi-

> *The kinds of things we do, why and how we do them, and what we think and feel about them all derive from the intersecting conditions and influences of time, space, society, and culture. The uniquely human occupation, which characterizes our species, is a function of these conditions and influences.*

cal worlds provide conditions that give doing its fundamental character. Society and culture provide and assign us things to do. They define how we should go about doing them. They give us instructions, reasons, and meanings for our doing.

The kinds of things we do, why and how we do them, and what we think and feel about them all derive from the intersecting conditions and influences of time, space, society, and culture. The uniquely human occupation, which characterizes our species, is a function of these conditions and influences.

Human occupation, as briefly discussed here, is the focus of the model of human occupation and of much of this book. As will be noted below, a good part of the aim of this model is to provide explanation of human occupation as it is manifest in individual lives.

The Nature of Conceptual Practice Models

Conceptual practice models are bodies of knowledge developed in occupational therapy for its practice (Kielhofner, 1997). Each conceptual practice model aims to:

- Generate and test theory about some phenomena of concern to the profession
- Develop and test related strategies, tools, and techniques for use in therapy.

Above all, models are dynamic bodies of knowledge that change and improve over time. Therefore, a **conceptual practice model** can be defined as a set of evolving theoretical arguments that are translated into a specific technology for practice and are refined and tested through research.

At any point in time, occupational therapy will have a number of models that guide different aspects of practice. Consequently, it is important to remember that the model of human occupation (MOHO) is only one of several conceptual practice models in occupational therapy. Each of these models addresses some specific phenomena. In the next chapter, we will identify the phenomena addressed by MOHO. Other occupational therapy models address such phenomena as the biomechanics of movement, motor control processes, organization of sensory information, perceptual and cognitive processes, and group dynamics that are involved in occupational performance (Allen & Earhart, 1992; Fisher,

> **A model must provide some insight into the nature and workings of some phenomena.**

Murray, & Bundy, 1991; Howe & Schwartzberg, 1995; Katz, 1992; Kielhofner, 1997; Mathiowetz & Haugen, 1994; Trombly, 1995).

Because each model has a specific focus, a single model ordinarily does not address all the multiple factors involved in the occupational functioning of any patient or client. Therefore, therapists will ordinarily use two or more models in combination. This means that therapists must understand both what MOHO offers for practice and what its limits are. In the vast majority of circumstances, it will not address all the problems faced by a client, requiring the therapist to actively use other models along with it.

Theory in Models

A conceptual practice model offers theory to guide practice and research in the field. The theoretical arguments of models ordinarily address three practical concerns. The first concern is to explain the organization and function of those aspects of occupation on which the model focuses. So, for example, we will attempt to explain how people are ordinarily motivated to choose their behavior.

The second concern is to conceptualize what happens when problems arise. Because occupational therapists work with persons who experience disabilities, there is a need to understand the kinds of problems that can be associated with disability. Throughout this text, discussions that attempt to explain processes such as motivation, the patterning of behavior, performance, and environmental influences, also include related discussions of the challenges or difficulties that may be encountered by persons who become disabled.

The third concern is to provide theoretical explanations of how therapy enables people to engage in occupations that provide meaning and satisfaction and that support their physical and emotional well-being. As with any model, it is important that the theoretical arguments of MOHO must give logic and coherence to the practical applications that emanate from it. The extent to which the model is successful in doing this depends both on the clarity with which the theory is explicated and the thoroughness with which the therapist understands the theory

As I have already indicated, the central purpose of theory is to explain some phenomena. But, of what are theories made? Every theory is composed of concepts and propositions (i.e., statements concerning the relationships between those concepts) (Mosey, 1992).

Concepts describe and define some entity, quality, or process. For example, intelligence and cognition are psychological concepts that refer to the relative ability of a person to think and to the process of thinking itself. Concepts provide a specific way of seeing and thinking about the phenomena they address. Consequently, theoretical definitions and discussions give us more insight into that which is being explained by a concept. In any theory it is important that concepts are clearly and thoroughly defined and explained.

Sometimes several subconcepts, referring to more specific qualities or processes, will be combined together within a larger concept referring to a more general quality or process. For example, many cognitive theorists have provided specific concepts describing and explaining aspects of cognition such as memory, problem-solving, and planning. Often, then, theories will be composed of more general concepts, which refer to larger chunks of reality, and more specific concepts, which refer to the elements of which they are composed.

Beyond identifying concepts, the second role of theory is to make statements about the relationships between concepts and the phenomena to which they refer. These statements are called theoretical propositions, and their purpose is to explain how the various qualities and processes described by concepts are linked together. So, **propositions** are statements about relationships between concepts. They assert how the characteristics or processes to which concepts refer are organized or put together. An example of such a proposition is that intelligence is associated with academic performance, since the extent of ability for thinking is a resource enabling students with more ability to more readily accomplish the thinking-oriented tasks of education.

When several concepts and propositions are linked together, they constitute a whole network of explanation. For example, consider the proposition that genetic inheritance and environmental nurturance directly affect a person's level of intelligence. This proposition, combined with the earlier proposition concerning the relationship between intelligence and school performance, creates an explanation of how the four variables are interrelated. Of course, in a theory whose aim was to explain school performance, further concepts such as motivation, learning style, and so forth would need to be added and their relationships to other variables specified. In the end, the aim of any theory should be to provide as comprehensive an explanation as possible of the phenomena with which the theory is concerned.

Theory then is a network of explanations that provides concepts that label and describe phenomena and propositions that specify relationships between concepts. It is important to differentiate theoretical explanations that give a plausible account for how something works from mere description or statements of beliefs or values. A model should do more than describe. It should go beyond statements of what is important, or how practice ought to be conducted. A model must provide some insight into the nature and workings of some phenomena.

> *The dialectic between theory and practice is important for development of better theory and more effective practice.*

Technology for Application

Theory can never tell therapists exactly what should be done in therapy. Nevertheless, theory is all-important in helping a therapist decide what to do. As noted above, the theory in a conceptual practice model provides an explanation of how some aspect of a human being works, about how things can go wrong, and about how therapy can alter the problem. Theory is abstract and therefore refers to people in general. When therapists use theory, they must establish a link between the general concepts and postulates made by the theory and the specific client or client group to whom they are providing services. This process of linking the general or more abstract concepts and postulates of theory to the specific and concrete realities of a person or group of persons is aided by a technology for application.

This technology aids therapists to make the link between theory and practice by providing specific tools, procedures, and examples. It may consist of such things as methods of gathering data, principles to follow in practice, and case examples showing how the model can be applied. This book will provide an overview of the technology for practice that has been developed for MOHO. However, over the past quarter century there has been an accumulation of resources for application that are far too vast to include in a volume such as this. A variety of very helpful resources beyond this volume are available to those wishing to use MOHO in practice. This text will provide information about these resources and how to obtain them.

Another important aspect of the process of applying theory in practice is that a great deal can be learned about the theory itself. Applying a model in practice can:

- Reveal which parts of its theory are more or less clear and useful
- Illuminate important things that the theory does not sufficiently address
- Show the limits of the theory in application.

Over the years, the attempts of many people to apply MOHO in practice have provided invaluable feedback, leading to changes in the theory.

Therefore, in a conceptual practice model, theory and practice mutually inform and influence each other. The dialectic between theory and practice is important for development of better theory and more effective practice.

Research

Models offer theory as a means of explaining things. However, these explanations must always remain a work in progress. By testing these explanations against the real world, we can develop increasing confidence in the explanations. More importantly, we can correct, change, and refine them so that they become better explanations. Consequently, therapists should always judge and place their confidence in the explanations provided by models in relation to the extent to which they have been tested and developed by research.

MOHO has generated a growing body of research in the past few decades. Although certainly not all aspects have been thoroughly tested, studies have provided some indication of the validity of the concepts and arguments offered in the model. Just as importantly, these investigations have provided examples of how it can be further tested and refined through research in the future. It is important that research not only test and elaborate the theory of a model, but also examine the usefulness of its technology for application. Such applied research includes studies that test the reliability and validity of assessments derived from a model and determine the outcomes of interventions based on the model. Moreover, studies that examine the process of applying a model in practice (e.g., how therapists use the theory or how interventions based on the theory work) are also very useful.

This volume contains a chapter on research that provides an overview of the range of studies completed and indicates what we have learned from them. It points toward what things need to be studied further in MOHO and provides students and therapists with a basic orientation to the research base of MOHO. It also serves as a resource to researchers who wish to test this model or use it as a conceptual framework for their research questions.

Dynamic Process of Developing a Model

As illustrated in *Figure 1-1*, developing a conceptual practice model is a dynamic process in which theory is continuously generated, used, tested, and refined. The theoretical arguments provide the central core of any model. However, the practical worth of this theory is dependent on the development of a technology for application. The process of translating theory into practice and informing theory from the experiences of practice enhances both theory and practice. Finally, research is used to test and refine the theoretical arguments and the practical applications of MOHO.

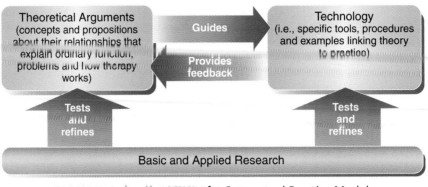

FIGURE 1-1   Dynamics of a Conceptual Practice Model.

Development of MOHO

As should be obvious, models are not developed overnight. Indeed, one of the most important ingredients in any model is the sustained work required to refine its theory, expand its application, and test its validity and utility. Above all else, models must change or they will become obsolete and irrelevant.

MOHO grew out of a particular moment in the history of occupational therapy. When I entered the field in the early 1970s, occupational therapy was in the midst of a crisis of professional identity (Kielhofner, 1997; Shannon, 1977). During the two previous decades, the field had aligned itself with a set of mechanistic ideas largely derived from medicine and, at the same time, had lost sight of its original occupationally based concepts. Reilly (1962) recognized this problem and began work with her students and colleagues to develop a new body of knowledge centered on occupation. This tradition of scholarship was referred to as occupational behavior (Kielhofner & Barrett, 1997). As a graduate student working in the occupational behavior tradition, I sought to synthesize a number of its diverse ideas into a coherent model that could be used in practice (Kielhofner, 1975). We (two of my former fellow graduate students and I) first published the model five years later after incorporating concepts from their theses, refining the concepts, and experimenting with them in practice (Kielhofner, 1980a, 1980b; Kielhofner & Burke, 1980; Kielhofner, Burke, & Heard, 1980). Five years later the text, *A Model of Human Occupation: Theory and Application*, introduced an expanded theory and a wide range of clinical appli-

cations, both of which reflected work from a growing circle of collaborators (Kielhofner, 1985). A decade later the second edition of that text was published (Kielhofner, 1995). It represented the cumulative contributions of colleagues from throughout the world.

This third edition of *A Model of Human Occupation: Theory and Application* presents the most recent theory and application of MOHO. It has benefited from the ideas, research, and practice efforts of a large number of people.

As a consequence of the contributions of so many persons, MOHO has developed significantly in the span represented by these three editions. Over that period, we have sought to make the theoretical concepts and postulates more clear, precise, and empirically valid. We have also sought to make assessments, treatment principles, and programs more specific and empirically grounded.

This text is, in large measure, a progress report that tells what we have learned in more than a quarter century since MOHO first began to take shape. Some of these advances in knowledge reflect research findings. Others draw on theoretical changes in related fields from which we import ideas. Some new concepts are the result of colleagues' work on the theory. Still other changes reflect the work of clinicians who have critiqued the model's utility and developed creative ways of applying the model in practice. Much of great value has been gained from each of these contributions.

Certain influences will stand out with each new rendering of the model in print. Two themes characterize the most important influences on the current volume. The first is a growing literature in the interdisciplinary field of disability studies (e.g., Albrecht, Seelman, & Bury 2001; Longmore, 1995; Oliver, 1994; Scotch, 1988; Shapiro, 1994). Although there are many perspectives within the field of disability studies, the following two themes from disability scholars have most influenced the current text. The first theme is that therapy designed for and theory that seeks to explain aspects of disability need to be informed more fully by the perspectives of those with disabilities. MOHO has always asserted that therapists should pay careful attention to the values, desires, interests, and self-concepts of their clients. Therefore, the aim of MOHO has been consistent with the idea of informing theory and practice with client's viewpoints. Nonetheless, in this edition, a special effort has been made to have the text resonate with the voices of disabled persons. We have sought to extend the reach of the text in more clearly articulating and helping the reader appreciate the experience of disability.

A second theme in disability studies literature is that current medical and rehabilitation practices still tend to locate disability primarily in the limitations or impairments of persons with a disability. However, many of the problems faced by persons with disabilities can more properly be located in the environment—in everything from physical barriers to stigmatizing attitudes to outright discrimination. A growing theme is that disability occurs because of a mis-fit between person and environment. This implies, of course, that change must include altering the environment.

Accordingly, this text pays much more attention to the environment as both an enabler of and a barrier to occupation. Throughout, an effort has been made to call attention to circumstances both within the person and within the environment that contribute to a person's motivation, patterns of behavior, and performance.

A second influence on MOHO reflected in this book is that of international scholars, leading to an increasingly multicultural focus. MOHO has its most immediate origins in the work of North American occupational therapists, especially the tradition of ideas developed in the mid-20th century by Reilly and her colleagues, as noted above. Nonetheless, the ideas of occupational therapy in the 20th century can be linked, as I have described elsewhere (Kielhofner, 1997), to an earlier, 18th and 19th century tradition of moral treat-

ment in Europe. Reilly's efforts were aimed at returning to many of the foundational ideas that North American occupational therapy inherited from European moral treatment. Thus, at its inception, MOHO already had been influenced by ideas that had crossed the Atlantic much earlier.

After its initial publication, MOHO has received much attention, including criticism, elaboration, application, and empirical testing by occupational therapists throughout the world. Attempts to apply and test MOHO in different cultures and under different national conditions have provided priceless feedback about how its theoretical arguments and technology for application can best be developed to transcend cultural differences and national boundaries.

By measure of the range of occupational therapists who make use of and are contributing to the development of MOHO, it has become an international conceptual practice model. The diversity of voices and perspectives reflected in this volume underscore the extent to which this model belongs to and is being developed by the multinational and multicultural community.

Approaching this Book

A quarter century of trying to better comprehend and explain human occupation has taught me that no one way of thinking about something is ever complete. In fact, the more one seeks to fit a single explanation to a phenomenon as complex as occupation, the more exceptions to the rule one finds. Consequently, in trying to develop theory for occupational therapy, I am increasingly compelled to approach a problem and explain it from many perspectives. That is the tack taken in this book. Consequently, readers will encounter a wide range of ideas, each one contributing to the total picture. The theoretical and practical arguments should become progressively clearer, like a picture coming into focus over time. However, this book alone cannot guarantee the reader will learn MOHO. Rather, such learning involves reflection, active use of the concepts, and discourse with others who use the same concepts. I am, for example, always drawn to more deeply understand the concepts of this model and am increasingly struck with how much others teach me about them. Therefore, understanding MOHO and knowing how to use it will only emerge gradually as one studies this text and other publications on the model, actively reflects on the theory, experiments in practice, and shares ideas with others. This text will have done its job if it encourages in the reader an ongoing process of learning and experimentation.

This book is divided into four sections. The first section covers MOHO theory. Section II discusses the technology for application covering such topics as therapeutic reasoning, assessments, and planning and documenting therapy. Section III illustrates the application of MOHO in therapy by providing a series of in-depth cases. Section IV contains resources for program development, research, and further exploration of MOHO.

I hope the reader will enjoy this book. In addition to the several contributing authors, there are many implicit and explicit voices here. They include those of theoreticians from many fields, those of colleagues who have helped to conceptualize MOHO, those of persons who have told their stories of living with disabilities, and those of therapists who have created practical means of applying MOHO. In the end, it is my hope that these voices have come together in an interesting, instructive, and instrumentally useful way.

Key Terms

Activities of daily living: The typical life tasks required for self-care and self-maintenance, such as grooming, bathing, eating, cleaning the house and doing laundry.

Concepts: Ideas that describe and define some entity, quality, or process.

Conceptual practice model: A set of evolving theoretical arguments that are translated into a specific technology for practice and are refined and tested through research.

Human occupation: The doing of work, play, or activities of daily living within a temporal, physical, and sociocultural context that characterizes much of human life.

Play: Activities undertaken for their own sake.

Propositions: Statements about relationships between concepts.

Theory: A network of explanations that provides concepts that label and describe phenomena and postulates that specify relationships between concepts.

Work: Activities (both paid and unpaid) that provide services or commodities to others such as ideas, knowledge, help, information-sharing, entertainment, utilitarian or artistic objects, and protection.

References

Albrecht, G. L., Seelman, K. D., & Bury, M. (2001). *Handbook of disability studies*. Thousand Oaks, CA: Sage Publications.

Allen, C. K., & Earhart, C. A. (1992). *Occupational therapy treatment goals for the physically and cognitively disabled*. Rockville, MD: American Occupational Therapy Association.

Ayres, A. J. (1979). *Sensory integration and the child*. Los Angeles: Western Psychological Services.

Chapple, E. (1970). *Rehabilitation: Dynamic of change*. Ithaca, NY: Center for Research in Education, Cornell University.

Christiansen, C., & Baum, C. (1997). *Occupational therapy—Enabling function and well-being* (2nd ed.). Thorofare, NJ: Slack.

Fidler, G., & Fidler, J. (1983). Doing and becoming: The occupational therapy experience. In G. Kielhofner (Ed.), *Health through occupation: Theory and practice in occupational therapy*. Philadelphia: FA Davis.

Fisher, A. G., Murray, E. A., & Bundy, A. C. (1991). *Sensory integration: Theory and practice* (1st ed.). Philadelphia: FA Davis.

Florey, L. L. (1969). Intrinsic motivation: The dynamics of occupational therapy theory. *American Journal of Occupational Therapy, 23*, 319–322.

Hall, E. T. (1969). *The silent language*. Greenwich, CT: Fawcett Publications.

Howe, M., & Schwartzberg, S. (1995). *A functional approach to group work in occupational therapy*. (2nd ed.). Philadelphia: JB Lippincott.

Katz, N. (1992). *Cognitive rehabilitation: Models for intervention in occupational therapy*. Boston: Andover Medical Publishers.

Kerby, A. P. (1991). *Narrative and the self*. Bloomington, IN: Indiana University Press.

Kielhofner, G. (1975). *The evolution of knowledge in occupational therapy: Understanding adaptation of the chronically disabled*. Unpublished master's thesis, University of Southern California at Los Angeles.

Kielhofner, G. (1980a). A model of human occupation, part

two. Ontogenesis from the perspective of temporal adaptation. *American Journal of Occupational Therapy, 34*, 657–663.

Kielhofner, G. (1980b). A model of human occupation, part three. Benign and vicious cycles. *American Journal of Occupational Therapy, 34*, 731–737.

Kielhofner, G. (1985). *A model of human occupation: Theory and application.* Baltimore: Williams & Wilkins.

Kielhofner, G. (1995). *A model of human occupation: Theory and application* (2nd ed.). Baltimore: Williams & Wilkins.

Kielhofner, G. (1997). *Conceptual foundations of occupational therapy* (2nd ed.). Philadelphia: FA Davis.

Kielhofner, G., & Barrett, L. (1997). An overview of occupational behavior. In H. Hopkins & H. Smith (Eds.), *Willard & Spackman's Occupational Therapy.* Philadelphia: JB Lippincott.

Kielhofner, G., & Burke, J. (1980). A model of human occupation, part one. Conceptual framework and content. *American Journal of Occupational Therapy, 34*, 572–581.

Kielhofner, G., Burke, J., & Heard, I. C. (1980). A model of human occupation, part four. Assessment and intervention. *American Journal of Occupational Therapy, 34*, 777–788.

Longmore, P.K. (1995). The second phase: From disability rights to disability culture. *The Disability Rag & Resource, Sept/Oct, 4*–11.

Mathiowetz, V., & Haugen, J. B. (1994). Motor behavior research: Implications for therapeutic approaches to central nervous system dysfunction. *American Journal of Occupational Therapy, 48*, 733–745.

Meyer, A. (1922). The philosophy of occupational therapy. *Archives of Occupational Therapy, 1*: 1.

Mosey, A. C. (1992). *Applied scientific inquiry in the health professions: An epistemological orientation.* Rockville, MD: The American Occupational Therapy Association.

Nelson, D. (1988). Occupation: Form and performance. *American Journal of Occupational Therapy, 38*, 777–788.

Oliver, M. (1994). The social model in context. In *Understanding Disability: From theory to practice.* London: Macmillan.

Reilly, M. (1962). Occupational therapy can be one of the great ideas of 20th century medicine. *American Journal of Occupational Therapy, 16*, 1–9.

Reilly, M. (1974). *Play as exploratory learning.* Beverly Hills, CA: Sage Publications.

Robinson, A. (1977). Play: The arena for acquisition of rules for competent behavior. *American Journal of Occupational Therapy, 31*, 248–253.

Rogers, J. (1983). The study of human occupation. In G. Kielhofner (Ed.), *Health through occupation: Theory and practice in occupational therapy.* Philadelphia: FA Davis.

Scotch, R. (1988). Disability as a basis for a social movement: Advocacy and the politics of definition. *Journal of Social Issues, 44*(1), 159–172.

Shannon, P. (1970). The work-play model: A basis for occupational therapy programming. *American Journal of Occupational Therapy, 24*, 215–218.

Shannon, P. (1977). Derailment of occupational therapy. *American Journal of Occupational Therapy, 31*(4), 229–234.

Shapiro, J. (1994). *No pity: People with disabilities forging a new civil rights movement.* New York: Times Books.

Trombly, C. (1995). *Occupational therapy for physical dysfunction* (4th ed.). Philadelphia: FA Davis.

Vandenberg, B., & Kielhofner, G. (1982). Play in evolution, culture, and individual adaptation: Implications for therapy. *American Journal of Occupational Therapy, 36*, 20–28.

Yerxa, E. J., Clark, F., Frank, G., Jackson, J., Parham, D., Pierce, D., Stein, C., & Zemke, R. (1989). An introduction to occupation science: A foundation for occupational therapy in the 21st century. *Occupational Therapy in Health Care, 6*(4), 1–17.

Young, M. (1988). *The metronomic society: Natural rhythms and human timetables.* Cambridge, MA: Harvard University Press.

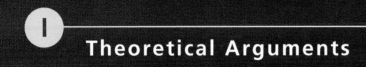

I

Theoretical Arguments

Introduction to Section I

Chapters 2 through 9 present the theory behind MOHO. The chapters are organized to present a cumulative argument. Consequently, successive chapters provide more detailed discussions of concepts introduced earlier or synthesize them into a larger whole. Reading the chapters should provide an increasingly detailed and integrated understanding of the theory.

Chapter 2 introduces concepts aimed at explaining how occupation is motivated, patterned, and performed. Chapter 3 provides a framework for integrating the concepts of the previous chapter into coherent understanding of human occupation. Chapters 4 through 6 expand on the Chapter 2 discussions of how occupation is motivated, patterned, and performed. Each of these three themes is discussed in depth in one of the chapters.

Chapter 7 discusses the environmental context of occupational behavior, explaining what aspects of the environment influence occupation and how they exert this influence. Chapter 8 examines occupation in detail, offering ways to examine it cross-sectionally (by identifying levels at which we can examine what a person does) and longitudinally (how doing shapes a person's identity and competence over time). Chapter 9 builds on Chapter 8 by focusing on how we narratively construct our occupational lives over time. Chapter 10 examines how occupation changes and overviews typical occupational changes through the life course.

Although the discussions in this section are theoretical and necessarily involve a level of abstraction, the chapters make extensive use of concrete examples that should both ground and clarify theoretical concepts. Each chapter includes key terms at the end to enable the reader to readily identify and review important concepts. These terms are set in bold when they first occur and are defined in the chapter.

Finally, mention must be made of terminology. Throughout this theoretical discussion, the authors have sought to simplify terminology by using only what are necessary terms to set apart important concepts. One of the conventions used in this section and throughout the book is to refer to the model of human occupation as MOHO. This is partly done to make the discussions more readable and partly because it reflects the popular usage of MOHO. In that spirit, the reader is invited to commence the chapters of this section that contain the latest theory of MOHO.

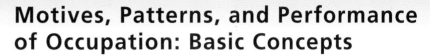

2

Motives, Patterns, and Performance of Occupation: Basic Concepts

● Gary Kielhofner

As noted in Chapter 1, each conceptual practice model is concerned with and seeks to explain specific phenomena. The current chapter identifies three primary phenomena addressed by MOHO and then overviews concepts and propositions that address them.

The first concern of MOHO is to understand how persons are motivated toward and choose to do the things that fill their lives. To explain these motives and choices a number of questions must be answered. Why are humans generally so active? What accounts for the individual differences in what persons want and choose to do? Why do different people experience doing the same thing in different ways? MOHO seeks to achieve a coherent explanation of the motivation for occupation by attempting to answer such questions.

The second phenomenon addressed by MOHO is the recurrent pattern of doing that makes up everyday life. People behave in a given way day after day. They follow similar patterns of time use. They do things much as they did them before. Moreover, different people act similarly when they occupy the same social position, while the same person acts differently when occupying different social positions. In sum, a great deal of human life follows routines and exhibits patterns reflective of a larger social order.

Therefore, questions can be raised as to how persons learn and sustain these patterns of everyday life. What holds all this regularity in life together? How do people, without consciously thinking, find their way through the course of the day and through familiar locales? How do persons manage to behave consistently as students, workers, family members, friends, and so on? To respond to such questions, MOHO offers concepts and propositions aimed at explaining regularity and pattern in occupation.

The third phenomenon addressed by MOHO is that when human beings do things, they exhibit an extraordinary range of capacity for performance. Occupational performance requires finely coordinated bodily movements. It requires that people anticipate, plan, and observe what happens; make adjustments; and decide what to do next. Finally, it requires that they participate and communicate, coordinating action and sharing information with others.

The question that naturally arises is how are people able to engage in such a wide range of physical, cognitive, and social actions? In occupational therapy, a number of models address aspects of performance and the capacities that underlie it. Therefore, MOHO offers an approach to thinking about the capacity for occupational performance that complements existing theory.

In summary, MOHO seeks to explain how occupation is motivated, patterned, and performed. By offering explanations of such diverse phenomena, MOHO offers a broad and integrative view of human occupation. Consequently, it incorporates a wide range of phenomena and corresponding concepts. For example, two of the phenomena addressed in MOHO, motivation and performance, are not typically considered together in the same theoretical framework. That is, occupational therapy theories that concentrate on physical performance have generally attended to the bodily components (brain and musculoskeletal system) involved in physical doing, while motives have been seen as part of a separate, mental domain.

There is growing recognition of the importance of considering body and mind together in explaining phenomena (Kielhofner, 1995; Trombly, 1995). After all, motivation for a task can influence the extent of physical effort directed to that task (Riccio, Nelson, & Bush, 1990), while physical impairments can weigh down the desire to do things (Murphy, 1987; Toombs, 1992). MOHO concepts seek to avoid dividing humans into separate physical and mental components. Rather, body and mind are viewed as integrated aspects of the total human being. Consequently, both body and mind are implicated in each of the major concepts that are introduced in the following sections.

Within MOHO, humans are conceptualized as being made up of three interrelated components: volition, habituation, and performance capacity. Volition refers to the motivation for occupation. Habituation refers to the process by which occupation is organized into patterns or routines. Performance capacity refers to the physical and mental abilities that underlie skilled occupational performance. Although the following sections discuss these components separately, it is important to keep in mind that they are three different aspects of the total person. Moreover, the discussions that follow are only introductory. They will provide only a broad outline of the theoretical arguments of MOHO. Later chapters explain each concept in more detail.

Volition

The motivational question will first be approached by asking why people occupy themselves with so much doing. This leads to the consideration of human biology.

Biological Need for Action

Humans are the product of an evolutionary process that has given them a biological mandate to be active. Spontaneous action is the most fundamental characteristic of all living things (Boulding, 1968; von Bertalanffy, 1968a, 1968b, 1969). Even the simplest organ-

> *That we can look at, touch, step into, reach toward, hold, and shape the world is an irresistible invitation to act.*

isms engage in some form of activity. Over the course of evolution, as more complex organisms emerged, the extent and range of action in which they engage has multiplied. Humans are at the apex of an evolutionary pathway that has produced in them a complex nervous system coupled with an intense and pervasive need to act (Berlyne, 1960; DeCharms, 1968; Florey, 1969; McClelland, 1961; Reilly, 1962, Shibutani, 1968, Smith, 1969; White, 1959).

Beyond the nervous system, the fact that humans are physical bodies with awareness of their potential is also part of the need to act. Having bodies with the potential for acting on the world bestows on us the wish to do things. As Reilly (1962, p. 6) observed, "the power to act creates a need to use the power, and the failure to use power results in dysfunction and unhappiness." That we can look at, touch, step into, reach toward, hold, and shape the world is an irresistible invitation to act.

Thus, the discussion of the concept of volition begins with the assertion that human beings have a fundamental, neurologically based, and embodied need for action that provides the foundation for motivation toward occupation. This need is pushed by a nervous system wired for action and pulled by the existential opening that our bodies provide for doing things.

The universal need for action manifests itself in each person's felt desire to encounter and be effective in interacting with the world. Moreover, because volition has its origins in the body, the volitional need for action is also mediated through other physically influenced phenomena such as mood, energy level, fatigue, arousal, and so on. As Nelson (1988) points out, other motives are sometimes involved in an occupation. For example, the expectation for financial rewards may partly motivate work. Some daily living tasks (e.g., meal preparation) are in part at the service of basic drives such as hunger. Similarly, recreational activities such as dating and dancing may have a sexual dimension as well. Consequently, one cannot always properly assign a single motive to all human occupation. Nonetheless, a desire for action or activity manifests itself throughout occupation and is its dominant motive.

Volitional Thoughts and Feelings

The concept of a biological need for action offers an explanation for why humans persist in occupying themselves. However, it does not account for all the differences in what people are motivated to do. Additional concepts are needed to account for how persons are uniquely motivated. Indeed, each person has distinct feelings and thoughts about doing things that are essential to volition. These thoughts and feelings concern three fundamental issues:

- Personal effectiveness or ability
- Importance or worth attached to what one does
- Enjoyment or satisfaction one experiences in doing things.

In other words, volitional thoughts and feelings are responses to questions about doing. Am I good at this? Is this worth doing? Do I like this? Ultimately, our whole orientation to the possibility of doing different things, during each moment and throughout our lives, is predicated on answers that our own experience gives to those questions. Thus, while we are all energized by a universal drive toward action, each of us will want to do those things that we value, feel competent to do, and find satisfying.

Personal Causation, Values, and Interests

Based on the previous considerations, volition is conceptualized as being made up of personal causation, values, and interests *(Fig. 2-1)*. **Personal causation** refers to one's sense of competence and effectiveness. **Values** refer to what one finds important and meaningful to do. **Interests** refer to what one finds enjoyable or satisfying to do. Accordingly, personal causation, values, and interests are concepts that describe the content of volitional feelings and thoughts.

In everyday life, personal causation, values, and interests are interwoven into a single interrelated cognitive and emotive complex. For example, a child's volition can be seen in his attraction to an object just out of reach and in the unsteadiness and insecurity he feels

> *Volition is reflected in the wide range of thoughts and feelings people have about the things they have done, are doing, or might do.*

> *The self and the world in which one acts are interwoven.*

when trying to reach for it. A grandmother's afternoon reflection on events in her life is part of volition, as is her choice to call up an old, forgotten friend as a result of that reflection. Volition is manifest in an adolescent's nervous stomach on the first day of high school, and in the admixture of satisfaction and exhaustion that settles over parents after a hard day's work and finally putting the children to bed. Volition is reflected in the wide range of thoughts and feelings people have about the things they have done, are doing, or might do.

Volition as Self in Relation to the World

Volitional thoughts and feelings are about self in relationship to one's particular world. The self and the world in which one acts are interwoven. Each is implied in the other.

The external world that we come to know is always a response to something we have done (Engelbrecht, 1968; Sartre, 1970). For example, we perceive objects in the environment to have properties because they respond in certain ways to our actions. We know that something is heavy because of the effort it takes to lift it. Similarly, when we say that some object or event in the world is interesting, we are referring to our own experience of that object or event. What happens to us when we encounter the world gives the world the properties that we perceive in it.

On the other hand, the self we know is constructed out of how the world responds to our actions. We know ourselves to be coordinated because the ball goes where we throw it. We feel intelligent because the teacher gives us a good grade. We see ourselves as persuasive when others come to agree with us. Our worth is validated by how others approve or praise our behavior.

How we see ourselves reflects how the world has responded to us. Moreover, what the world is always implies what we have done and experienced in encountering it. When we say that a task we have been

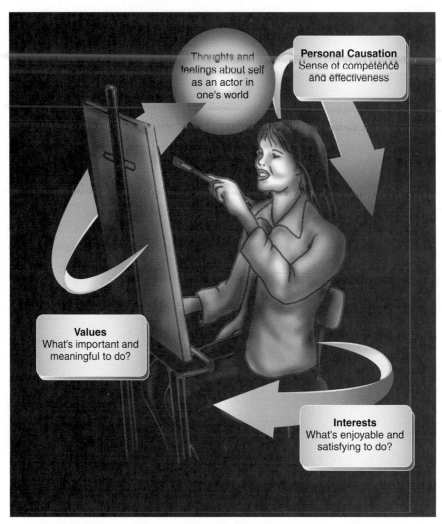

FIGURE 2-1   The Content of Volitional Thoughts and Feelings.

handed will be hard, we are saying something, not only about the task, but also about ourselves. That is, we are referring to a relationship between our inner capacities and the outer world.

Similarly, when we indicate that something is important to us or that we feel obligated to do something, we are implying a moral or social order in the world. For example, believing that one should be honest in taking an exam implies a view of the world. Honesty is important to persons who see their world as valuing, expecting, and rewarding honesty. The worth

of one's being honest derives from that perceived world. When high school students justify their own cheating as acceptable because everyone cheats, they are evoking a view of the world as the basis for their values.

Volitional Processes

Volition is an ongoing process. That is, volitional thoughts and feelings occur over time as people experience, interpret, anticipate, and choose occupations.

EXPERIENCE

Whenever we do something, a whole range of experiences are possible. We may, for example, feel pleasure, anxiety, comfort, challenge, or boredom. Moreover, we may have thoughts of self-doubt or confidence. We may proceed deliberately with solid convictions about why we are doing what we are doing or hesitantly, worrying that our actions are futile or meaningless. **Experience** refers, then, to such immediate thoughts and feelings that emerge in the midst of performance.

INTERPRETATION

Of course, we not only experience what we do, but also reflect on and interpret that experience. A person may do this in a variety of ways, and the following are some examples. One feels badly about an encounter with another person and recalls the incident to consider whether one should have behaved differently. Having felt serious pain several times when attempting an old hobby, one wonders if it's worth it. After receiving less than optimal feedback on some aspect of work performance, one resolves to try harder in the future. After spending a particularly boring evening engaged in some activity, one thinks, "I'll never do that again!" One joins teammates after a game to celebrate and discuss the victory.

Whenever we reflect on or discuss with others how we performed, what it was like to do something, and whether it is worth doing, we are engaged in the volitional process of interpretation. **Interpretation** is thus defined as recalling and reflecting on performance in terms of its significance for oneself and one's world. Through our interpretations of past performances, we also construct ideas about the future and its possibilities. These thoughts and feelings shape how we will anticipate opportunities or requirements for performing occupations in the future.

ANTICIPATION

We constantly encounter immediate and future possibilities for action. How we anticipate these possibilities for action is reflected in what we pay attention to in the world around us. It is also reflected in how we react to opportunities and expectations for action.

The following are some examples of volitional anticipation. A student walks into a classroom and dreads an upcoming exam. A child, baseball glove in hand, peers out the window to see if friends are gathered yet in the park. A homeowner notices that the lawn needs mowing. Two adolescents pour over the movie schedule in the newspaper while planning a Friday evening's events. A young worker looks over a college brochure and contemplates what it would be like to have a better education and a better job, wondering if it is really possible.

Anticipation always considers what we might be doing in the immediate or distant future. The world presents us possibilities and expectations for action, but which ones we notice and how we think and feel about them is influenced by what we like and feel competent and obligated to do. Consequently, **anticipation** is defined as the process of noticing and reacting to potentials or expectations for action.

ACTIVITY AND OCCUPATIONAL CHOICES

Anticipation naturally leads to decisions about what to do. Our hours, days, and weeks are shaped by myriad choices for what we will do next, later on, and tomorrow. These **activity choices** are defined as short-term, deliberate decisions to enter and exit occupational activities. Examples of activity choices include deciding to have lunch with a friend later in the day, to wash the car on Saturday morning, to mow the lawn after work, or to go for a walk before starting homework. Activity choices occur when we have the necessity or opportunity to make a decision about what to do. They may arise when we anticipate free time or when we have to choose between things to do. Whereas activity choices ordinarily require only brief deliberation, they are important because they determine a significant amount of what we actually do.

Individuals also make larger choices concerning occupations that will become an extended or permanent part of their lives. For example, most persons reading this book made a commitment at some point to become occupational therapists. This kind of resolution belongs to a class of decisions that have been called occupational choices (Heard, 1977; Matsutsuyu, 1971). Such decisions represent commitments to enter into a course of action or to sustain regular performance over time. We recognize these decisions when someone makes a commitment to enter an occupational role, such as becoming a student or a parent, or when taking a job. Moreover, occupational choices may involve making a commitment to establishing and sustaining a new activity as part of our permanent routine. Examples are the decisions to join a health club, exercise regularly, or to take up a new hobby. Finally, occupational choices may take the form of commitment to undertake personal projects that require an extended series of actions to complete. As I compose this chapter, I am engaged in the personal project of writing a book. Further examples of personal projects are learning a foreign language, building a new fence for the yard, making a dress, or taking a course for continuing education.

Ordinarily, occupational choices are the result of a process of deliberation over time. They may involve information gathering, reflection, imagining possibilities, and considering alternatives. In this way, commitment is established as a person considers the implications of a course of action over time and weighs its meaning. Occupational choices involve commitment since they require doing over time. Indeed, we may or may not realize the objectives of our occupational choices depending on whether we can sustain effort over time or establish new patterns of action. **Occupational choices are thus defined as deliberate commit-**

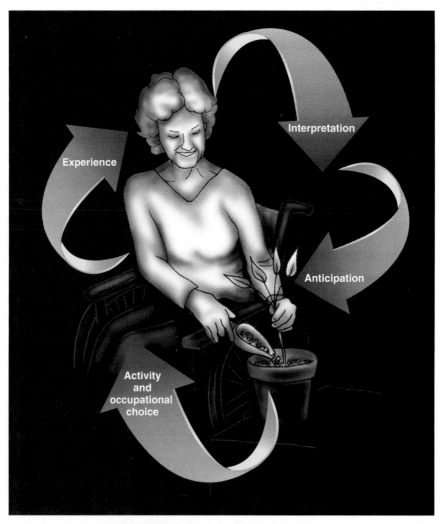

FIGURE 2-2   Volitional Processes.

ments to enter an occupational role, acquire a new habit, or undertake a personal project.

Together, activity choices and occupational choices influence, to a large extent, what kinds of occupational performance make up our daily lives. These choices are the function of volition, that is, they reflect our personal causation, our interests, and our values.

Summary and Definition of Volition

The cycle of experience, interpretation, anticipation, and choice is an integrated process. As shown in *Figure 2-2*, each process flows into the next. One chooses action, the doing of which stimulates experience. One recalls and reflects on experience to interpret what was done. Finally, the meanings generated from such reflections lead to the next choices.

Based on the previous discussion, **volition** can be defined as a pattern of thoughts and feelings about oneself as an actor in one's world which occur as one anticipates, chooses, experiences, and interprets what one does. Volitional thoughts and feelings include personal causation, values, and interests.

Through the cycle of anticipating, choosing, experiencing, and interpreting, volition tends to perpetuate itself. For example, once we experience ourselves as competent in an occupation, we will tend to anticipate that occupation with positive feelings and choose to do it again.

Volition is also an unfolding process in which changes take place. As we develop and age, and as we encounter new environments with new opportunities and demands for action, we may find new pleasures, lose old interests, discover new capabilities, or find that we are no longer so adept at a particular activity. In the end, there will be elements of both continuity and change in values, interests, and personal causation over the lifespan.

Habituation

Much of what we do belongs to a taken-for-granted round of daily life. Most of us repeat the same familiar weekday morning scenario of getting up, grooming, and heading to work or school. On the way, we drive

> *The world around us, our habitat, has a certain stability; we, in return, also have a tendency to act in consistent, patterned ways.*

the same route or take the same train, subway, or bus without having to consciously think about what we are doing. Once arrived, we set about doing tasks we previously have done multiple times, undertaking them in much the same way as before. We encounter others, saying and doing the same types of things with them that we have done in the past. We do these things unreflectively, and doing them feels familiar, locating us in our ordinary, taken-for-granted life. Moreover, by engaging in certain routine behaviors we reaffirm ourselves as having a certain identity. These aspects of routine daily life unfold automatically.

The term habituation is used here to refer to this semi-autonomous patterning of behavior. Habituation is a particularly appropriate term because, as shown in *Figure 2-3*, routine, automatic behavior is organized in concert with our familiar temporal, physical, and social habitats.

Habituation allows us to recognize and respond to repetitive temporal cues and time frames. That is, many automatic routines correspond to cyclical time wherein things are repeated and known sequences are experienced. Cyclical time is provided by the rhythms of nature (e.g., day and night and the seasons) and complemented by social convention (e.g., the recurring pattern of weeks with days for work, leisure, and worship).

The body also contributes much toward the patterning of behavior. Circadian rhythms biologically shape the sleep and waking cycles of night and day. Physiologic processes that result in fatigue after exertion or concentration also demand certain temporal rhythms of activity and rest.

Habituated behavior also involves using and traversing our familiar physical worlds. The constancy of our physical environments allows us to encounter them pretty much as we have before. In the morning, when one gets out of bed, the world will be arranged pretty much as it always has been. The road on the way

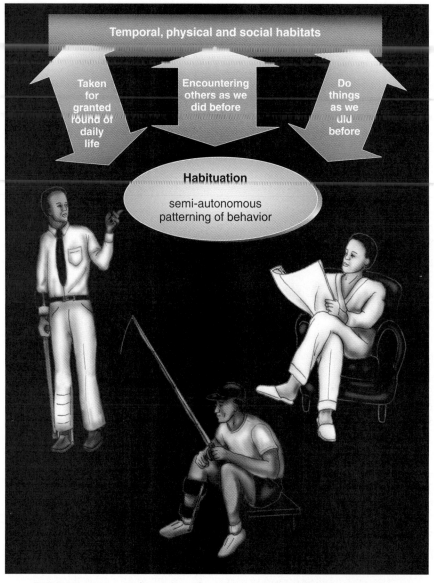

FIGURE 2-3   Habituation Shapes Interaction With Our Habitats.

to work will look similar and lead to the same destination as it has in the past. When we arrive at work or school, the buildings (and outdoors) and their contents will be as they have been before. Indeed, we recognize that on those unusual occasions when this is not the case—when there is a detour in the road, a change of meeting place, or even a minor rearrangement of furniture or other objects—our familiar routine is disrupted and cannot unfold automatically. On these occasions, we have to think about what to do.

The patterns of acting in the physical world that we establish are also a feature of our embodiment. Our physical characteristics and capabilities both enable and constrain the ways in which we can establish patterns of acting in a physical world. This becomes apparent whenever we experience a limitation of capacity. Suddenly, many of our ways of doings things no longer work.

Similarly, social custom and the stability of social patterns also facilitate the consistency with which we interact with others. Neighbors greet us in much the same way they always have. Riders line up in familiar ways to board the bus. At work our colleagues come to us with the same kinds of concerns, questions, and requests. Social life is characterized by the repetition of patterns of interpersonal behavior and events that resemble previous ones.

Given these familiar temporal, physical, and social environmental conditions, we behave in ways that closely resemble what we have done before. The world around us, our habitat, has a certain stability; we, in return, also have a tendency to act in consistent, patterned ways. That we do so is a function of habits and roles.

Habits

Habits preserve ways of doing things that we have internalized through repeated performance. We generate habits by consistently doing the same thing in the same context. What once required attention and concentration eventually becomes automatic.

Consequently, acquired ways of doing things unfold without deliberation once a given context calls for them. Indeed, we will occasionally find ourselves doing a routine behavior that has been cued by our context even when it is not what we intended to do. Each of us can recall when we have, despite our knowing better, gone to the wrong door or taken the wrong route because that is where our destination used to be.

Habits are defined as acquired tendencies to respond and perform in certain consistent ways in familiar environments or situations. Consequently, for habits to exist:

- We must repeat action sufficiently to establish the pattern
- Consistent environmental circumstances must be present.

Much of what we do in the course of a day or week is guided by habits. Our daily routine, our manner of going about most anything we do, and the peculiar ways we always do a given task are all examples of habits.

Internalized Roles

Our patterns of action also reflect roles that we have internalized. That is, we identify with and behave in ways that we have learned to associate with a public status or private identity. For example, when people act as spouses, parents, workers, or students, they exhibit patterns of behavior that reflect those socially identified statuses. Moreover, their behavior will tend to be along the lines of what others expect them to do as part of that role.

Through a process of socialization, people acquire those roles that derive from a social status. Socialization involves interacting over time with explicit and implicit definitions and expectations for the role. As a result, one internalizes a sense of self, attitudes and behaviors that correspond to the social definition, and expectations of the role.

Roles shape our sense of self, provide us with an outlook or attitude, and evoke certain behaviors. For example, I think about and interact with my own children differently than with other children precisely because I am their father. Consequently, my role as father is manifest in how I appreciate and enact my relationship and responsibilities to my children. Being a professor provides me with another identity and related responsibilities that shape how I interact with colleagues and students. My roles lead me to automatically know how to differentially greet my boss in a meeting and my children at the end of the day.

As these examples illustrate, many of our roles come from socially defined positions. Nonetheless, each of us may have other roles, such as being a home maintainer, that are defined less by social status and more by the interrelated and ongoing nature of a set of tasks for which we feel responsibility. Such roles arise out of personal circumstances or necessity. They are established as one engages in a pattern of related actions and assumes an identity connected to them. Generally, people seek some kind of reference group whose members will recognize one as having the role, since identity implies not only an internal view of the self, but also a public recognition of one's status. Other examples of self-generated roles are the person who daily fetches the mail for less able elderly neighbors and checks on their well-being, and the person who starts and leads a local movement to resist unwanted changes in the community.

Given these considerations, the **internalized role** can be defined as incorporation of a socially and/or personally defined status and a related cluster of attitudes and behaviors. People ordinarily have several roles that occupy routine times and spaces. For example, people generally are in the worker role during the workweek and in the workplace. On the other hand, they are mostly in the role of a spouse or parent at home and outside work hours. Having a complement of roles gives one rhythm and change between different identities and modes of doing.

Summary and Definition of Habituation

Habituation comes about as a consequence of repeating patterns of behavior under certain temporal, physical, and sociocultural contexts (Bruner, 1973; Koestler, 1969). As we interact over and over again with the various characteristics of these contexts (e.g., physical arrangement, temporal patterns, social attitudes and expectations, behaviors of others), we internalize patterns of attitude and action.

Sometimes we acquire these patterns because we have made repeated volitional choices. Kerby (1991) refers to this process as a sedimenting of prior choices. Indeed, when we voluntarily seek to acquire a new habit or role, we ordinarily must make repeated choices to act or enter into situations until the pattern is established and active choice is no longer required.

A pervasive influence on habituation is the environment. As noted earlier, habituation is a way we have learned to be within our habitats. Be it the physical arrangement of the world or the social patterns and norms that surround us, the features of our environments shape us to develop certain habituated ways of doing things.

Habituation is defined as an internalized readiness to exhibit consistent patterns of behavior guided by our habits and roles and fitted to the characteristics of routine temporal, physical, and social environments. As shown in *Figure 2-4*, habituation shapes what we take to be ordinary and mundane in our lives. It is responsible for our daily routine of behavior; our usual way of going about doing things; the various routes we take in going about our homes, neighbor-

hoods, and larger community; and our patterns of involvement with others.

Performance Capacity

The capacity for performance depends on the status of a person's musculoskeletal, neurologic, cardiopulmonary, and other bodily systems that are used when acting on the world. The capacity to perform also depends on mental or cognitive abilities such as memory and planning. Performance requires persons to call on an objective set of underlying capacities. Theory and practice in occupational therapy have always recognized the importance of these underlying components for competent performance. Notably, other models of practice (e.g., biomechanical, cognitive-perceptual, sensory integration, motor control) provide specific explanations of physical and mental components and their contribution to performance (Fisher, Murray, & Bundy, 1991; Katz, 1992; Kielhofner, 1997; Mathiowetz & Haugen, 1994; Trombly, 1995). Because other models address performance capacity, therapists use these models as a means to understanding and addressing specific problems of performance capacity.

Within this model, performance capacity is approached from a different but complementary viewpoint. Our emphasis is on subjective experience and its role in shaping how people perform. In occupational therapy and related fields, people's performance and difficulty in performing is approached objectively. For example, consideration may be given to understanding losses or disturbances of ordinary movement capacity, sensory abilities such as sight or hearing, or cognitive capacities such as memory or judgment. Various objective ways of describing, categorizing, and measuring these limitations have been developed. Examples of such objective depictions of impairments are limited range of

All persons who have objectively describable abilities and limitations of ability also have corresponding experiences of those abilities or limitations.

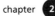

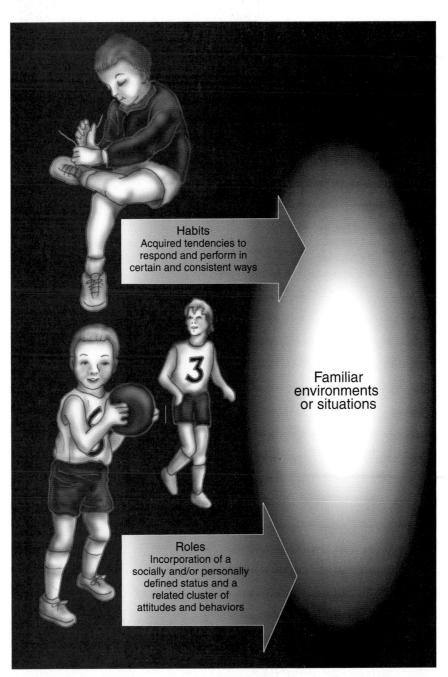

FIGURE 2-4 Habituation: Habits and Roles Influencing Behavior in Familiar Environments and Situations.

motion, decreased muscle strength, and limited attention span. Such depictions of impairments are important and helpful because they provide information that enables objective understanding of their nature and how they can be reversed, minimized, or compensated.

All persons who have objectively describable abilities and limitations of ability also have corresponding experiences of those abilities or limitations. Attention to the nature of these experiences and how they shape performance can complement and enhance the understanding we have from the objective approach to performance capacity.

Therefore, within MOHO, the concept of **performance capacity** is defined as the ability for doing things provided by the status of underlying objective physical and mental components and corresponding subjective experience. As shown in *Figure 2-5*, this definition calls attention to the objective approach to capacity, which is the focus of other models, and to the subjective, experiential focus on capacity that we emphasize.

In discussing the experiential aspect of performance capacity, we employ a concept referred to as the lived body. This concept derives from the work of philosophers who argue that the body must be

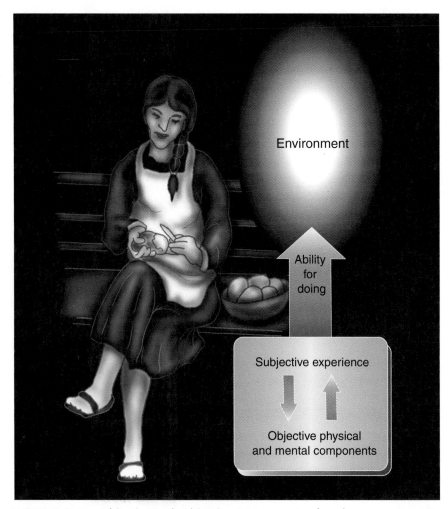

FIGURE 2-5   Objective and Subjective Components of Performance Capacity.

understood phenomenologically (Merleau-Ponty, 1945/1962). That is, in addition to understanding the body as a physical object that can be observed, measured, dissected, and experimented on, it is also important to understand the body from the point of view of lived experience. Such a view brings the concepts of mind and body together, demonstrating how they are dual aspects of the same thing.

We can examine this idea further by considering the human hand. The hand may be studied and understood as an object composed of muscle, bone, vein, artery, nerve, and connective tissue in a particular arrangement that shapes how it functions. However, this objective hand can be distinguished from our own hand, which we experience in everyday life. This lived hand "meets, perceives, touches, grasps, understands, receives, loves and declines the world" (Engelbrecht, 1968, p.3). In other words, we know our own hands to have intentions and experiences.

How we use our bodies is quite different from how we use other objects in the world. So while we can think of the hand as an object, its use in everyday in life is not objective. It is subjective. For example, when we initiate action requiring our hand, such as writing, we do not need to look for our hand in the way we must find our pen. The pen is only an object that we use, whereas we are our hands (Sartre, 1970). We know un-

reflectively where our hand is when we reach out for objects, because the hand is part of the self. When we move our hand in reaching for something, we simply go, with a part of ourselves, to where we need to go.

As this example illustrates, the concept of the lived body calls attention to the unique ways in which we experience ourselves as bodies and how our bodies are part of the self. This concept also offers new ways of understanding both how we are able to perform and how disease or impairment is experienced and affects performance.

Conclusion

At the beginning of this chapter, it was indicated that volition, habituation, and performance capacity are integrated parts of a whole person. As shown in *Figure 2-6*, they operate seamlessly, forming a coherent whole. Volition, habituation, and performance capacity each contribute different but complementary functions to what we do and how we experience our doing. We cannot fully understand occupation without reference to all three contributing factors. Taking this broader view presents a greater challenge for explanation and synthesis, but it nevertheless recognizes the complexity inherent in human occupation.

Key Terms

Activity choices: Short-term, deliberate decisions to enter and exit occupational activities.

Anticipation: Noticing and reacting to potentials or expectations for action.

Experience: Immediate thoughts and feelings that emerge in the midst of performance.

Habits: Acquired tendencies to respond and perform in certain consistent ways in familiar environments or situations.

Habituation: Internalized readiness to exhibit consistent patterns of behavior guided by our habits and roles and fitted to the characteristics of routine temporal, physical, and social environments.

Interests: What one finds enjoyable or satisfying to do.

Internalized role: Incorporation of a socially and/or personally defined status and a related cluster of attitudes and behaviors.

Interpretation: Recalling and reflecting on performance in terms of its significance for oneself and one's world.

Occupational choices: Deliberate commitments to enter an occupational role, acquire a new habit, or undertake a personal project.

Performance capacity: Ability for doing things provided by the status of underlying objective physical and mental components and corresponding subjective experience.

Personal causation: Sense of competence and effectiveness.

Values: What one finds important and meaningful to do.

Volition: Pattern of thoughts and feelings about oneself as an actor in one's world which occur as one anticipates, chooses, experiences, and interprets what one does.

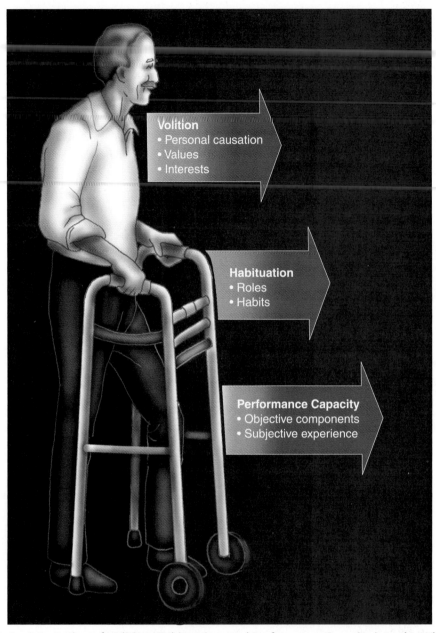

FIGURE 2-6   Integration of Volition, Habituation, and Performance Capacity into the Whole Person.

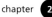

References

Berlyne, D. E. (1960). *Conflict, arousal, and curiosity.* New York: McGraw-Hill.

Boulding, K. (1968). General system theory: The skeleton of science. In W. Buckley (Ed.), *Modern systems research for the behavioral scientist.* Chicago: Aldine.

Bruner, J. (1973). Organization of early skilled action. *Child Development, 44,* 1–11.

DeCharms, R. E. (1968). *Personal causation: The internal affective determinants of behaviors.* New York: Academic Press.

Engelbrecht, F. J. (1968). The phenomenology of the human body. [Monograph], Series A, N. 8. Publications of the University College of the North: Sovenga, South Africa.

Fisher, A. G., Murray, E. A., & Bundy, A. C. (1991). *Sensory integration: Theory and practice.* Philadelphia: FA Davis.

Florey, L. L. (1969). Intrinsic motivation: The dynamics of occupational therapy theory. *American Journal of Occupational Therapy, 23,* 319–322.

Heard, C. (1977). Occupational role acquisition: A perspective on the chronically disabled. *American Journal of Occupational Therapy, 41,* 243–247.

Katz, N. (1992). *Cognitive rehabilitation: Models for intervention in occupational therapy.* Boston: Andover Medical Publishers.

Kerby, A. P. (1991). *Narrative and the self.* Bloomington, IN: Indiana University Press.

Kielhofner, G. (1995). A meditation on the use of hands. *Scandinavian Journal of Occupational Therapy, 2,* 153–166.

Kielhofner, G. (1997). *Conceptual foundations of occupational therapy* (2nd ed.). Philadelphia: FA Davis.

Koestler, A. (1969). Beyond atomism and holism: The concept of the holon. In A. Koestler & J. R. Smythies (Eds.), *Beyond reductionism.* Boston: Beacon Press.

Mathiowetz, V., & Haugen, J. B. (1994). Motor behavior research: Implications for therapeutic approaches to central nervous system dysfunction. *American Journal of Occupational Therapy, 48,* 733–745.

Matsutsuyu, J. (1971). Occupational behavior: A perspective on work and play. *American Journal of Occupational Therapy, 25,* 291–294.

McClelland, D. (1961). *The achieving society.* New York: Free Press.

Merleau-Ponty, M. (1962). *Phenomenology of perception* (C. Smith, Trans.). London: Routledge & Kegan Paul. (Original work published 1945)

Murphy, R. (1987). *The body silent.* New York: Henry Holt & Company.

Nelson, D. (1988). Occupation: Form and performance. *American Journal of Occupational Therapy, 34,* 777–788.

Reilly, M. (1962). Occupational therapy can be one of the great ideas of 20th century medicine. *American Journal of Occupational Therapy, 16,* 1–9.

Riccio, C. M., Nelson, D. L., & Bush, M. A.(1990). Adding purpose to the repetitive exercise of elderly women. *American Journal of Occupational Therapy, 44*: 714–719.

Sartre, J. P. (1970). The body. In S. F. Spricher (Ed.), *The philosophy of the body: Reflections on Cartesian dualism.* Chicago: Quadrangle Books.

Shibutani, T. (1968). A cybernetic approach to motivation. In W. Buckley (Ed.), *Modern systems research for the behavioral scientist.* Chicago: Aldine.

Smith, M. B. (1969). *Social psychology and human values.* Chicago: Aldine.

Toombs, K. (1992). *The meaning of illness: A phenomenological account of the different perspectives of physician and patient.* Boston: Kluwer Academic Publishers.

Trombly, C. (1995). Occupation: Purposefulness and meaningfulness as therapeutic mechanisms. *American Journal of Occupational Therapy, 49,* 960–972.

von Bertalanffy, L. (1968a). *General system theory: A critical review.* In W. Buckley (Ed.), *Modern systems research for the behavioral scientist.* Chicago: Aldine.

von Bertalanffy, L. (1968b). *General systems theory.* New York: George Braziller.

von Bertalanffy, L. (1969). General system theory and psychiatry. In S. Arieti (Ed.), *American handbook of psychiatry.* New York: Basic Books.

White, R. W. (1959). Excerpts from motivation reconsidered: The concept of competence. *Psychological Review, 66,* 126–134.

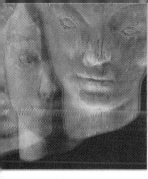

Dynamics of Human Occupation

• Gary Kielhofner

A Question of Order

In Chapter 2, the following conceptualization of how human occupation is motivated, patterned, and performed was introduced. Volitional thoughts and feelings (i.e., personal causation, values, and interests) are involved in anticipating, experiencing, interpreting, and choosing occupations. Habits and roles shape patterns of doing within routine environments. Physical and mental capacities are integrated in a lived body through which performance is achieved. But just how are these elements put together in the person we each take ourselves to be? Asked another way, what kind of order lies behind human beings and their thoughts, feelings, and actions? This is the question to which the present chapter is addressed.

Recall from Chapter 1 that all theories offer propositions and concepts. However, underlying these concepts and propositions are fundamental ideas that are assumed and unarticulated. These deeper ideas create a foundation on which most theories are based, determining what they say about us. This chapter examines these fundamental ideas and how they are changing. Significantly, the reader will come away with some important new ways of thinking about human occupation and about occupational therapy.

Mechanistic Reasoning

Biological, psychological, and social theories concerned with humans have been profoundly shaped by the insight that humans exhibit machine-like properties (Prigogine & Stengers, 1984; von Bertalanffy, 1968a, 1968b; Weiss, 1967). Scientists have created theories that explain human bodies and minds with underlying analogies borrowed from machines. This scientific viewpoint is often referred to as mechanistic reasoning. It has been tremendously successful in explaining many aspects of human beings.

Nonetheless, during the second half of the 20th century, scholars increasingly questioned the adequacy of mechanistic reasoning and began to offer an alternative. This new approach, usually referred to as systems theory, provided fresh insights into how humans are organized. Before one can fully appreciate what systems theory is saying about human beings, it is necessary to first understand mechanistic thought.

Workings of Machines

Machines are composed of parts in a fixed arrangement. They operate according to cause and effect principles in which one part acts on a subsequent part causing the latter to react in a very specific way. In this way, energy or action is transferred across parts, producing a linear, causal chain of events. A classic example is the mechanical clock as shown in *Figure 3-1*. In clockworks, energy is stored in a wound-up spring or suspended weight. This energy is transferred to a series of gears that convert the energy to movement of the clock's hands. The fixed way in which the parts of the clock are put together, and the causal pathway by which movement of each gear affects the next gear, makes the clock function as it does.

More sophisticated machines are arranged into hierarchies in which higher-level parts govern or control lower-level parts. Cruise control that maintains a car's travel at a preset speed is an example of such a hierarchy. As shown in *Figure 3-2*, a feedback mechanism at the top of this hierarchy detects deviations from the preset speed. Depending on whether the car's speed is too fast or slow, the cruise control either decreases or increases the flow of gas. This flow controls the

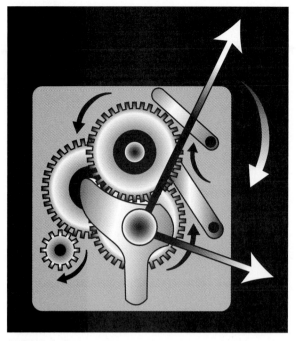

FIGURE 3-1   Clockworks: Linear Causation in a Fixed Mechanism With Each Part Directly Causing the Action of the Next Part.

amount of energy generated as the gas is burned and thus controls the speed of engine rotation. This rotation, in turn, transfers motion to the transmission and from it to the tires, which effect the speed at which the car moves. In this way, cruise control regulates a car's speed through a specific causal chain of events.

This and other types of hierarchical machines require a certain amount of built-in intelligence. In the example, the required intelligence is the ability to detect the car's speed, compare it against a standard, and select the right action to correct the car's speed toward that standard. Finally, it requires absolute control by the highest governing part. As can be seen in this example, a hierarchically organized machine works because it is made up of fixed mechanisms in which cause and effect is transferred from one part to the next, with causation flowing downward from the higher controlling part to the lower part(s).

A central idea in the design of traditional machines was that a machine's function could be totally explained by its structure (i.e., the parts of which it is composed and how they are put together). It follows, then, that any change in the machine's function can be brought on only by changes in the underlying structure

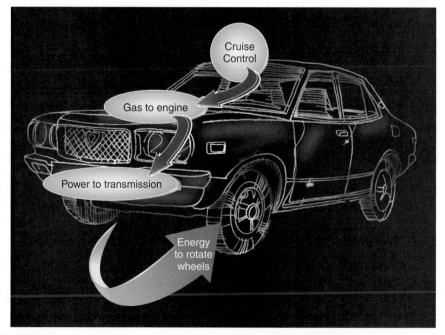

FIGURE 3-2   Cruise Control: An Example of Hierarchical Control in a Fixed Mechanism.

or mechanism of the machine. So, when engineers wanted to create a better functioning machine, they had to design a better configuration of inner parts.

The same principle also applies to machine repair. Because a machine's function is completely determined by the arrangement of its inner parts, failure of a machine to function always emanates from a problem in the inner mechanism. Repair requires locating, fixing, adjusting, or replacing the broken or maladjusted part(s).

Application of Mechanistic Thinking to Humans

As noted earlier, mechanistic reasoning came to be adopted by science as a way of comprehending humans (Koestler, 1969; Prigogine & Stengers, 1984; von Bertalanffy, 1969; Weiss, 1967). This means that those tenets that have provided the rationale for understanding machines are used to explain humans. The following tenets of mechanistic thought are applied to humans:

- Phenomena are composed of fixed structures organized in invariant causal chains
- Elements or components of any phenomena are hierarchically arranged with higher parts governing lower parts
- Action is directly caused by the inner arrangement of parts
- Any entity's function or behavior can be fully explained by how it is put together
- Faulty function is a direct consequence of a problem with the inner mechanism
- Problems of functioning can be repaired by fixing, adjusting, or replacing parts of the inner mechanism.

Part of the appeal of these tenets of mechanistic reasoning is that they constitute a coherent canon in which each of the ideas is connected logically to the other ideas. Together, they provide the logical foundation on which many concepts and propositions explaining humans are based.

This use of mechanistic reasoning is bolstered by the fact that many aspects of humans appear to operate in the same manner as machines. Take, for example, the regulation of body temperature. Similar to cruise control maintaining a constant speed, human

bodies maintain their temperatures by detecting deviations from the norm and stimulating physiologic events that help to correct the temperature (e.g., stimulating perspiration to evaporate on the skin and cool the body when it is too warm). Such instances of machine-like functions in the body reinforce the idea that people are very much like complex machines.

Over time, the entire logical structure of mechanistic thinking, reflected in the tenets noted above, became the way of framing theories about humans. A wide range of theories explained humans as if they were complex biological and psychological machines. Consequently, mechanistic thinking explained thoughts, emotions, and action as the direct consequence of how bodies and minds were put together. The study of humans was dominated by the search for underlying physical and mental structures, causal relationships between them, and the hierarchical architecture of their arrangement (Brent, 1978; Brody, 1973).

For example, mechanistic thought guides the classic explanation that human movement is determined by the arrangement of the neuromuscular system (Fogel & Thelen, 1987). Mechanistic thought also finds expression in the computer model of the mind that explains cognition as the consequence of neurologic hardware and software, and in psychological theories that view emotions as a function of those parts that make up the psyche (Allport, 1968; Bruner, 1990).

Mechanistic thought has also been applied to understanding human problems. Difficulties of thinking, feeling, and doing have been explained as disruptions of inner physical or mental mechanisms. In many cases, scientists have identified inner problems (e.g., infection by a foreign body, a genetic anomaly, or damage of a biological or psychological component due to physical or social trauma). Finally, mechanistic thought guides the search for ways to fix the faulty inner mechanisms of the human body and mind. Such mechanistic reasoning has been very successful! It has yielded a substantial medical and therapeutic technology for repairing human bodies and minds.

So we should ask: If mechanistic thinking is such a powerful tool, why would scientists be seeking to replace it? The answer is that mechanistic thought, for all its power, has important limitations. As a consequence, theories based on mechanistic thought offer incomplete and sometimes incorrect explanations of humans.

Limits of Mechanistic Reasoning

The main problem with mechanistic reasoning is that it only perceives part of the picture. As will be seen, some of the most important and interesting aspects of humans are beyond the grasp of mechanistic reasoning. One way to understand its limits is to examine how mechanistic reasoning answers a specific question about human behavior. Therefore, consider the following: When one is about to take a drink, how does one manage to reach out and grasp the glass in one's hand?

To answer this question, mechanistic thought assumes that this performance is caused, and therefore, can be explained by how the human organism is put together. Moreover it expects a fixed, hierarchical arrangement in which causation will flow from the highest level part down through the other parts that are involved in the action. As shown in *Figure 3-3*, the mechanistic explanation for how humans reach out and grasp a glass goes something like the following (Turvey, 1990).

Complex instructions for reaching and grasping are encoded in the brain. These instructions, containing all the necessary information about the finely tuned movements required to grasp a glass, are retrieved and used to send biochemical effector signals that travel down the spinal cord and through peripheral nerves to stimulate very specific muscle contractions. This precise stimulation of muscles to contract produces just the right amount and combinations of tension across the joints to effect the exact movements needed to reach for and grasp the glass. Therefore, a strict causal chain unfolds in which biochemical signals cause muscle contractions, and the latter cause movements of the bones that bring the body into the proper alignment.

This explanation makes a lot of sense. Nonetheless, it is not correct. To be sure, reaching out and grasping a glass involves information stored in the brain, biochemical signals flowing through nerves, and muscles exerting forces on bones. However, the way in which these parts and events are organized together is fundamentally different than envisioned by mechanistic thinking.

Let's first consider why this mechanistic explanation of movement cannot be right. If movement were organized as mechanistic reasoning suggests, different detailed instructions would be needed for tying shoes, handling forks or chopsticks, buttoning shirts, opening doors, flipping light switches, and so on. Consequently, an impossible amount of information would have to be stored in the brain (Turvey, 1990).

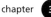

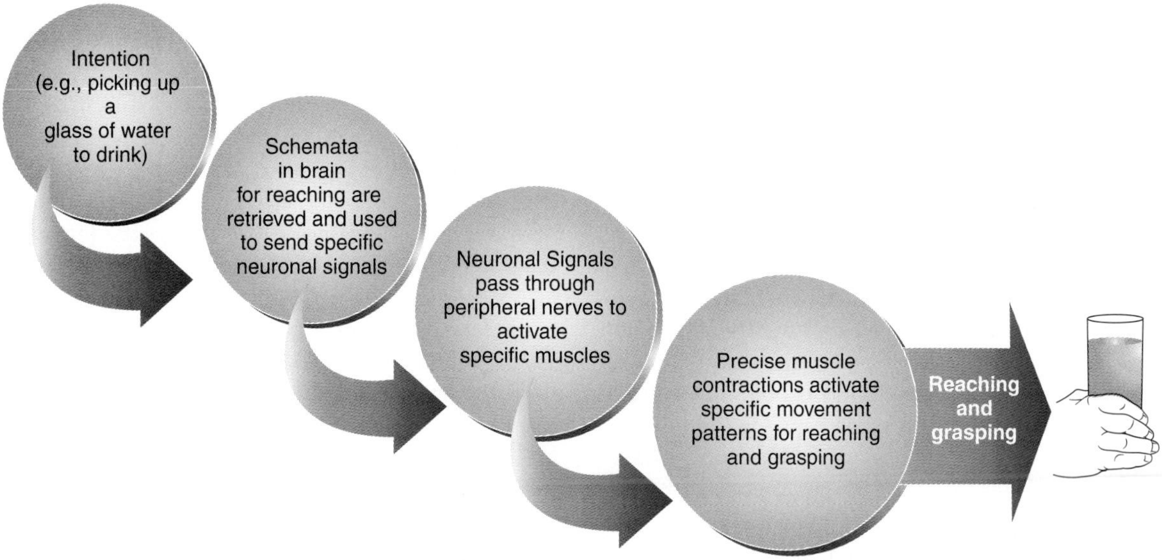

FIGURE 3-3 The Mechanistic Explanation of Reaching: A Hierarchical Model of Linear Causation.

Another problem with the mechanistic explanation is that human movement takes place in a variety of environments and circumstances. This contextual variation makes each and every performance unique. No two instances of doing the same thing are ever exactly the same (Fogel & Thelen, 1987; Turvey, 1990). The idea of preexisting instructions specifying all the details of movement fails to account for this variability in performance.

Beyond the problem of skilled movement, any theory of human occupation will also need to take into account other factors, such as thinking and emotions that influence how we choose, plan, and organize what we do. The sheer complexity of human occupation belies the impossibility of a hierarchically controlled process. The idea that the whole range of things we think, feel, and do are somehow caused by the inner workings of body and mind is untenable.

Toward a New Vision of Order

Mechanistic thought correctly recognized that the biological, cognitive, and emotional parts of which we are composed have much to do with how we function. Nevertheless, it faltered in explaining the nature of interactions between these parts and in painting an impossible picture of the order underlying them. In what follows, we will examine a new explanation for how the physical and mental parts of which we are composed interact and how what we think, feel, and do results from their interaction. Importantly, this new vision of order has some very practical implications for what we do in therapy.

Interactive Solutions to Behavior

If the mechanistic vision of a hierarchically organized process in which instructions from the brain are eventually translated into finely tuned movements is not plausible, how then does one manage to reach out and grasp a glass or cup? Surprisingly enough, part of our current understanding of what happens can be illustrated by how scientists designed the newest generation of machines—namely, robots. Designing robots turned the tables from consideration of how humans are machine-like to how machines can be made more human-like, generating some fascinating insights.

We will begin with how robots are designed to do movements requiring precision not unlike grasping a glass. Faced with the problem of getting a computer-controlled robot to assemble tight-fitting parts into a machine, engineers first followed design principles reflecting mechanistic reasoning (Clarke, 1997). That is, they designed a computer-driven robot with a detailed guidance program. This program used information about near misses to adjust the robot's movement so as to properly align the part for insertion into the machine. The robot was inefficient and clumsy as it made successive adjustments following near misses. Furthermore, it required too much computing power!

When engineers rethought the problem they found a much more effective and surprisingly simpler solution, illustrated in *Figure 3-4*. If the robot is given rubber joints that allow some freedom of movement in two axes, the robot arm will be guided to the right orientation by the contours of the mechanism into which the part is being fitted. To an observer unaware of the rubber joints, it would appear that the computer is making multiple tiny adjustments. In fact, the most intricate adjustments are done without the computer's control!

The human body achieves fine motor coordination in much the same way (Thelen & Ulrich, 1991; Turvey, 1990). Grasping a glass only appears to require a highly complex set of instructions for how to configure the fingers to effectively get hold of the glass. Configuring fingers to grasp the contours of a glass is, in part, accomplished when the fingers meet the glass. As shown in *Figure 3-5*, muscle tension makes the hand, in effect, a spring-loaded system. Once the hand is in position to grasp the object, the nervous system only needs to increase muscle tension. The fingers will flex until they reach the object's surface, which brakes the fingers in the appropriate spot. In fact, the most delicate adjustments are made in the rubber-like pads of the fingers, which take on the shape of the surface being held. All this fine-tuning of the grasp is accomplished without the brain having to specify all the details. Consequently, much less information is needed in the brain for functional grasp than was supposed by mechanistic thought.

Details of the action are worked out in the interaction between the person and the object being grasped (Clarke, 1997; Thelen & Ulrich, 1991; Turvey,

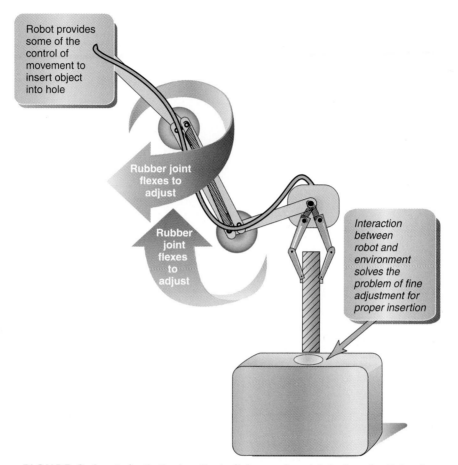

Robot provides some of the control of movement to insert object into hole

Rubber joint flexes to adjust

Rubber joint flexes to adjust

Interaction between robot and environment solves the problem of fine adjustment for proper insertion

FIGURE 3-4 Robotic Design Capitalizing on Local Solutions for Behavior.

1990). The fine-tuning of grasp depends on hand-glass interaction. Correct movements are generated in the midst of the interaction. This example points toward the system's **principle of interactive solutions**. According to this principle important aspects of any thought, emotion, or action are worked out in the actual dynamics of the person interacting with the environment.

We can recognize this principle in our interactions with others. Recall, for example, a time when you anticipated a particularly difficult encounter with someone. Perhaps it was a request you wanted to make of your boss or teacher, or a touchy problem you wanted to work out with a friend or family member. You may have thought about or even rehearsed what you were going say, but the words you actually spoke and the thoughts and emotions you expressed unfolded as a

function of the interaction. What you said and how you said it was certainly influenced by your intentions and plans, but it was also guided and shaped by how the other person acted and reacted.

Emergence and Heterarchy

We have only begun to address how humans manage complex performance without hierarchical control. Our discussion of how grasping is achieved has ignored other important factors involved in reaching for a glass. For instance, how do we make the coordinated movements required to move the hand into position to grasp the glass? If these movements also are not completely specified in the brain, what accounts for how the movement is done? The answer is found in the con-

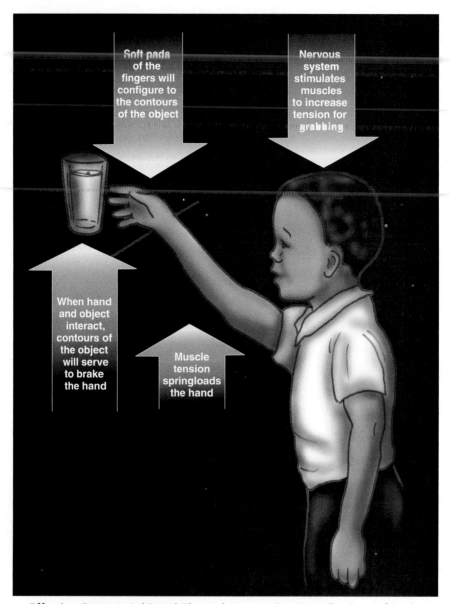

FIGURE 3-5   Effective Grasp Is Achieved Through Interactive Contributions of Brain, Musculoskeletal Components, Characteristics of the Hand Itself, and Object Being Grasped.

cept of emergence. As we will see, emergence explains how complex behavior action can occur in the absence of any prespecified or centrally orchestrated instructions (Capra, 1997).

Once again, the design of robots provides a telling model. When designing multiple-legged robots to tra-

verse complex terrain, engineers were faced with the impossibility of a central controller that could at once appraise the local terrain and give instructions to all six legs for how to move together so as to produce effective walking (Clarke, 1997). The solution they found was to give each leg a few rules for acting. These rules went something like, "push down with force sufficient to lift your load." Other rules had to do with how to behave with reference to the behavior of other legs, such as "push down when the leg next to you is up." With no more than these kinds of connections between the legs and a little capacity for adaptive learning, the robot walked! Notably, this six-legged robot ambulates with the same tripod pattern favored by six-legged insects, suggesting that nature solves the problem of walking in a similar way.

There is one all-important observation to make about the robot's walking. There are no instructions for this walking stored in any central program! The walking pattern materializes spontaneously out of the circumstances created when the legs have individual rules, interconnections with each other, and encounter the walking surface under conditions of gravity. The robot's walking exemplifies what is referred to as emergence. That is, **emergence** is the spontaneous occurrence of complex actions coming out of the interactions of several components without the benefit of a central controller (Clarke 1997; Haken, 1987).

As shown in *Figure 3-6* emergence envisions a very different order in humans from mechanistic thought. The latter assumed that everything was put together so that causation flowed in a neat, linear direction. Emergence recognizes that when components of a more complex entity are combined together, their collective interactions produce dynamics that yield more complex phenomena. Thought, emotion, and action emerge out of the total dynamics of the situation.

While working on this chapter, I observed an example of this kind of emergence in a flock of Canadian geese spied from my back porch. Geese fly in a V-shaped pattern. For a long time, ornithologists (and I) wondered what kind of flight instructions were encoded in a goose's brain so that it knew how to join other geese in this pattern. As it turns out, each goose needs only the inclination to fly in the most effortless way. The goose body type and aerodynamics take care of the rest. A goose flying diagonally to another goose exerts less effort in flying because of how wind resistance is deflected. Consequently, flying in a V-pattern is an emergent phenomenon coming out of the interacting dynamics of wings, wind, and wanting the path of least resistance.

Emergence is also found in the interaction of

bones, muscles, and nerves of the human body. The collective conditions created by these interactions generate complex motor actions without everything needing to be fixed or specified ahead of time (Clarke, 1997; Thelen & Ulrich, 1991; Turvey, 1990). Unlike the parts of a machine, which are rigidly fixed in a hierarchy, the parts of a living organism or groups of organisms cooperate together flexibly (Kelso & Tuller, 1984). This arrangement is referred to as heterarchy.

Heterarchy is the principle that parts of any system (e.g., parts of the body or different aspects of cognition and emotion) will interact with each other in ways that depend on the situation. In a heterarchy, each component contributes something to the total dynamic.

You can demonstrate this phenomenon to yourself. Begin with both hands at your side. Then, reach for two objects. Let the left hand reach for a nearer object and the right hand for a more distant object. When reaching, begin moving both hands at the same time and just do what feels natural.

You will observe that the two reaches become linked together in a specific way—that is, both hands terminate at their target objects at the same time. To accomplish this, the hand reaching for the more distant object travels at a higher speed than the other hand reaching for the nearer object. What feels most natural or effortless is to move your arms in such a way that the two different movements are functionally linked by a simple relationship. That is, the relative distance each must travel always defines the ratio of one hand's speed of travel to the other.

This bilateral reaching behavior emerges out of the heterarchy formed by the following elements. First, we intend to do a specific task (i.e., reach simultaneously with two hands toward two different objects). Second, there are specific environmental conditions (the two objects are situated at different distances). Third, the nervous system and musculoskeletal system have specific properties that unfold in the action of reaching. Each of these factors contributes to the heterarchy under which the bilateral reaching pattern takes place.

Heterarchy is manifest throughout human occupation. When we consider any thought, emotion, or action, the parts of the human being and environment cooperate together according to local conditions created by what each element brings to the total dynamic.

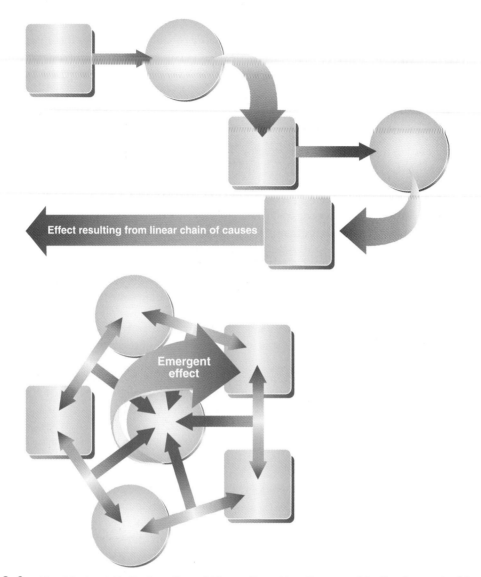

FIGURE 3-6   The Mechanistic Explanation of Linear Causation Compared to the Concept of Emergence.

So, let us apply the concepts of heterarchy and emergence to the problem of reaching and grasping a glass. Our new explanation is shown in *Figure 3-7*. Something is contributed by each of the following elements:

- Intention to pick up the glass for a drink of water
- Working instructions in the brain for moving groups of muscles
- Kinetic dynamics arising out of the biomechanical

organization of the shoulder and arm (i.e., how bones and muscles are connected and the movement possibilities they provide)

- Size, shape, weight, and texture of the glass.

Intention, neurologic organization, biomechanics, and the object to be grasped become a functional heterarchy, linked together in reaching and grasping. The actual movements for reaching and grasping

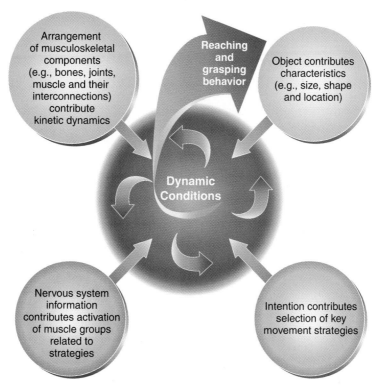

FIGURE 3-7   Dynamic Explanation of Reaching as an Emergent Behavior Arising out of Conditions to Which Components Make Contributions.

emerge out of their total dynamics. In this heterarchy, each element has some influence on both what gets done and how it gets done. No single element completely controls or determines what happens. Rather, the elements of the human being and environment cooperate together, each contributing something toward the total dynamics and the outcome (Kelso & Tuller, 1984).

Since the overall dynamics account for the emergent action, any difference in one of these elements that changes the total dynamics can alter the emergent action. For example, each of the following would change how one reaches and grasps a glass:

- One is reaching for a drink nervously at a formal reception versus having a relaxed glass of tea at home
- The glass is large, heavy, and full versus small, light, and nearly empty

- The glass is sitting on a table versus someone is handing it to you.

Whenever we think, feel, or do something, specific internal and external circumstances are combined in unique ways to guide what emerges.

Importance of Environmental Influences

As should be obvious from the previous discussions, the environment is always central to what we feel, think, and do (Clarke, 1997). When we do a physical move-

> *An eloquent cooperation of parts of the self with the environment underlies all human occupation.*

ment, the parts of which we are composed cooperate not only with each other but also with gravity, space, and objects. The influence of the environment is equally important in cognition and emotion. For example, memory may provide us with rough instructions for driving to a familiar destination. However, we rely on the physical environment to give us cues about when to speed up, slow down or stop, how to steer on the road, and when to turn at an intersection. Similarly, others' moods, statements, and deeds influence our own emotions, thoughts, and actions. An eloquent cooperation of parts of the self with the environment underlies all human occupation.

New Dynamic Features of Human Order

The systems perspective views thinking, feeling, and doing as arising out of a cooperative interaction between internal components and the environment. This means that the mix of factors behind any thought, emotion, or action will vary by circumstances. For example, one may be equally motivated to perform a task requiring concentration at two different times, but the outcome will be different if one is fresh and alert on the first attempt and tired and worried on the second occasion. Moreover, motivation may wax and wane or attenuate and be enhanced by conditions in the environment. Every instance of human occupation reflects a unique configuration of such elements that together determine what happens.

The systems view also offers different ways of thinking about functional problems. For example, if the arm with which I habitually reach for the glass in the bathroom is partially immobilized, placing the object out of my reach, I can reach with my other hand (modifying how I ordinarily do it) and still accomplish the task. Alternatively, I can change the position of the glass (modifying the environment) so that it is within reach. As the latter alternative illustrates, whether a dysfunction exists depends not only on the status of inner components, but also on the relationship between a person's inner circumstances and the external environment. Disruption of some element within a person does not necessarily result in functional limitations.

This same process underlies approaches that can be used to restore or enhance functioning in therapy. When a person experiences some limitation of capacity (e.g., mobility, strength, attention, or memory), we can seek to ameliorate the capacity, compensate for it with another capacity, alter the environment, or use some combination of these strategies. We are not limited to simply fixing the inner mechanism.

This understanding of human order offers a coherent framework, providing a foundation on which to generate further explanations of human occupation. These concepts and propositions are as follows:

- Humans are composed of flexible elements whose interaction with each other and with the environment depends on the situation
- Thinking, feeling, and doing emerge out of dynamic interactions between elements within the person and those in the environment
- Dysfunction is the result of the interaction of conditions internal and external to the person
- Function can be enhanced through remediation of a faulty element, compensation by another element within the person, and/or by environmental modification.

The following sections examine just how these ideas shape our thinking about human occupation.

Dynamic Perspective on Volition, Habituation, and Performance Capacity Contributions to Human Occupation

This morning I have parked my car at the train station and begin to insert four coins in the self-pay meter for my parking space. I am in a hurry to get to a newly opened coffee shop to purchase a cup of coffee for the train ride to work. As is my custom, I hold all four coins in the palm of my dominant, left hand. Next, I maneuver my hand so that the coins slide with gravity from the palm to a spot between my thumb and index finger. Having thus grasped one coin, I lift my hand to insert the coin into the slot. Just then, I intuitively sense that this process is not moving fast enough to accommodate the urgency to get in and out of the coffee shop on time to board the train and, thereby, arrive on time for my first meeting of the morning.

I am aware that this is an important meeting with the dean of our college. So although there is another train, just 5 minutes later, I don't want to risk being even a little late. On other days, when I am running behind and there is no early meeting, I take the later train.

Simultaneously, I can feel that it will move faster to place the coins in my left hand and take them with my right, nondominant hand to the slot. I don't think about it, it just occurs to me. I sense in my body both the inefficiency of my usual method of inserting coins and that it would be better to do it two-handed. What I feel reflects the objective fact that my left hand is in a splint following an injury, making the ordinary movements for putting coins into the slot clumsy.

> *Volition, habituation, performance capacity, and the environment always resonate together, creating conditions out of which our thoughts, feelings, and doing emerge.*

Notably, I've done it this way for the past few days—clumsy as it is—since it's my habitual way of doing it. I hadn't really noticed before how it slows me down. But today, with the urgency of time, my sluggish performance becomes suddenly problematic.

I catch myself in the midst of all this, noticing what I am doing and resolving to write it down once on the train. I notice what is happening because I've been trying to develop an explanation of just this kind of thing. Then the following thought occurs. Driving to the train station in the morning is part of my routine and I usually take, without thinking, the shortest route I have discovered. However, recently I have tried to make the drive more interesting by taking different routes through the countryside on the way to the station. It's part of a recent resolu-

tion to savor the small things in life, something one's 50th birthday makes you think about. I note that while I drove the shortest route to make time for getting coffee it wasn't quite enough, so I resolve to leave home a bit earlier tomorrow. Now that the coins are in the meter, I hurry off to the coffee shop. I take a dollar out of my wallet ahead of time to make the transaction quicker. I hope there's no one in line ahead of me.

The above vignette describes an episode of about 1 minute in duration. Yet, this tiny snapshot of daily life reveals a rich interplay of volition, habituation, performance capacity, and environmental conditions. They resonate with each other to contribute to what I think, feel, and do. How the episode unfolds reflects the convergence of:

- Values about being on time
- Activity choice to get a cup of coffee
- Felt obligations of my role
- Habitual way of doing this part of my morning routine
- My splinted hand and limited capacity (along with the lived experience of that limitation)
- The train schedule and the morning meeting.

Alter any part of volition, habituation, performance capacity, or the environment, and what happens will be different. If getting the coffee did not represent something larger about savoring life, if the hand was not in a splint, if American culture and my values did not put so much emphasis on being on time, or if the coffee shop were adjacent to the train station instead of a block away, I might have inserted the coins differently, caught the later train, or perhaps stopped to chat with the clerk while paying for the coffee.

Every moment is potentially infused with influences from and interactions of volition, habituation, performance capacity, and the environment. What emerges is not specifically caused by any single element. Instead, it reflects dynamic conditions created by their interactions. Consequently, the following is an important proposition for explaining human occupation. Volition, habituation, performance capacity, and the environment always resonate together, creating conditions out of which our thoughts, feelings, and doing emerge. Examples of such resonation are:

- Anxiety from a lack of belief in capacity interfering with performance
- The force of old habits resisting new volitional choices
- The pull of values to keep going despite pain and fatigue.

In these and endless other circumstances, values, interests, personal causation, role, habits, performance capacity, and the environment are always tethered together into a dynamic whole. What we do, think, and feel comes out of that dynamic whole.

Human Organization and Change

Machines are made and modified by external agents. Consequently, mechanistic thought has offered no real insight into how humans came to be organized as they are. Nor did it speak to the process of change. Systems theory views our ongoing actions, thoughts, and feelings as central to organization and change. To understand this view, we will need to divest ourselves of the mechanistic idea of structure.

In machines, structure is straightforward. It simply refers to parts and how they are arranged together. When we consider structure in human beings, a different picture emerges. What appear to be physical and mental structures are actually highly organized patterns. This organization is wholly dependent on an underlying, dynamic process (Brent, 1978; Sameroff, 1983).

The highly organized states of matter and mind of which we are composed are maintained and changed through what we do and what we think and feel about it. In large measure, the development, continued existence, and transformation of our characteristics depend on our ongoing acting, thinking, and feeling. This means that volition, habituation, and performance capacity are constituted, maintained, and changed through the very processes to which they are put to use.

Consider what happens to volition, habituation, and performance capacity in a person who takes up a new occupational form such as jogging. Repeated jogging reshapes existing physical, psychological, and social structures involved. Aerobic capacity is increased, muscles used to run are strengthened, the image of oneself as capable of jogging is reinforced, and one's public identity as a jogger may be affirmed when one swaps stories and tips about jogging with others or participates in an organized race.

In all these ways, when jogging and related behaviors are taken up, they serve to rearrange one's personal causation, role, and performance capacity into that of a jogger. A new organization of body and mind are created in the process. Moreover, as long as the behavior is sustained, the corresponding organization is maintained. However, if the jogger abandons the behavior for long enough, aerobic capacity diminishes, muscles weaken, and confidence and role identity wane. As this illustrates, we can also un-become what we cease to do.

Occupation is a dynamic process through which we maintain the organization of our bodies and minds. When we work, play, and perform the tasks of daily life, we are not merely engaging in occupation. We are organizing ourselves. In occupation, we use our bodies and minds, shaping them accordingly. We create our abilities, our thoughts and feelings about self, our social identities, and our habits through what we do.

As noted in the previous chapter, humans are endowed with a need to act. Consequently, from the time we enter this world, we set about doing things. Within the first weeks of life, we have begun a course of occupation that has already established some performance capacity, given us a rudimentary sense of ourselves and of the world around us, and created a basic daily routine. From then on, we persist in a process of doing that continually shapes and reshapes ourselves (Capra, 1997; Wolf 1987).

To consider how this process continues to unfold throughout life, we need to answer two questions. How do we maintain our organized patterns? How do we change? The remainder of this chapter attempts to provide some basic answers to these questions.

> *Occupation is a dynamic process through which we maintain the organization of our bodies and minds.*

Maintaining Organized Patterns

Across time, people do exhibit certain constancy in who they are and what they do. Maintaining these organized patterns of emotion, thought, choice, and behavior always involve the following elements:

- Our existing volition, habituation, and performance capacity (which we previously generated through our doing) provide certain resources, limitations, and tendencies for emoting, thinking, and behaving
- We encounter consistent environmental conditions, seek them out, or create them
- Given the interaction of internal resources, limitations, and tendencies with consistent environmental conditions, we repeat what we have done before, sustaining an organized pattern of behaving and of the thoughts and feelings that accompany behavior.

Importantly, this organized pattern represents a way of operating with its own internal coherence that resists perturbations. Once we have a way of feeling, thinking, and behaving, we tend to behave so as to preserve it.

Let us take as an example the maintenance of a volitional pattern. Consider an individual who receives feedback that he or she is not performing up to expectations at work. Such a circumstance may be responded to in different ways depending on the person's volition and how it is predisposed to interact with negative feedback.

A person's volition may be organized to be self-protective. This predisposition may be due to previous experiences, which have made one's personal causation fragile and criticism a particularly painful experience. Of course, another person may have this same self-protectiveness because of an extremely self-assured belief in his or her own capacity and efficacy combined with a value system that requires near self-perfection.

Let us say that negative feedback on performance has come from a certain coworker. If an individual's volition is organized so as to protect the self from criticism, the experience of receiving negative feedback will likely be interpreted in terms of attributing malice, bias, jealousy, or other motives, which explain away the criticism. In this way, thoughts and feelings about one's competence are protected from the negative feedback and one does not examine or revise the work-

ing version of one's efficacy on the job. This individual may also begin to actively seek out peers in the work environment to corroborate this version of things. Such modification of one's environment creates conditions that will tend to reinforce and sustain certain thoughts and feelings related to values and personal causation.

The individual may also begin to assign value to those aspects of work that allow public demonstration of competence, making activity choices to do those tasks that are more highly visible. Such actions may build up a more positive public image of the person. Such a volitional pattern can sustain itself indefinitely. As the example illustrates, each individual "actively constructs his or her view of self" (Gergen & Gergen, 1983, p. 255).

Note that no mention has been made about whether the person's actual performance is good or bad. Nonetheless, it is important to recognize that capacity for the job, habits that support or fail to support work competence, and worker role identity will all interact with this volitional pattern to influence what happens over time. Moreover, the nature of the work environment will also influence how things go.

We can readily imagine the scenario given above as pertaining to a good worker who has been unjustly criticized or a poor worker who is unable to accept feedback and improve. What is important to recognize in the example is how a pattern of thinking, behaving, and feeling resists disturbances and sustains itself over time through the person's ongoing action. Once a person's volition, habituation, or performance capacity has become organized in a particular way, it tends to stay that way. Nonetheless, change does occur. The next section considers how change occurs.

Change

Earlier in this chapter, it was noted that alteration of any single internal or external component in a heterarchy can contribute something new to the total dynamic out of which new thoughts, feelings, and actions may emerge. Therefore, a shift in volition, habituation, performance capacity, or the environment can alter the overall dynamics, leading to the emergence of something new. Thus, a key element in change is some alteration in internal or external circumstances that results in the emergence of novel thoughts, feelings, and behaviors.

The next requirement for change is that the novel thoughts, feelings, and behaviors must continue over time. Only by repetition do we begin to reshape ourselves. However, if the new pattern is repeated enough, then volition, habituation, and performance capacity will coalesce toward a new organization.

Therefore, we can specify that the process of change in occupation involves:

- An alteration in volition, habituation, performance capacity, or the environment creates dynamic conditions in which novel thoughts, feelings, and actions emerge
- Sufficient repetition of these conditions and the attendant thoughts, feelings, and actions allow volition, habituation, and/or performance capacity to coalesce toward a new internal organization
- Ongoing interaction of new internal organization with consistent environmental conditions maintains the new stable pattern of thinking, feeling, and acting.

These processes underlie all change.

Ordinarily, there is a natural history of new behaviors, thoughts, and emotions over time, in which volition, habituation, and performance capacity are being altered incrementally together along some trajectory. Throughout this natural history of change, these elements will resonate with each other, each taking turns in contributing something new to the mix of components that spur on the emergence of novel behavior.

These features of change will be illustrated by using the example of my children's transition from riding a tricycle to riding a bicycle. Wanting to ride a bicycle came about as they observed other children in the neighborhood beginning to do so. This change in external circumstances was coupled with their growing sense of being able to perform skilled motor behaviors. So, both personal causation and social influences contributed to the desire to ride a bicycle.

As a parent I altered an object in their environment, providing each child with a bicycle with training wheels. At first, my children were a bit unsteady and lacked confidence. However, a strong volitional desire enabled them to overcome initial uncertainty and continue to practice. Soon, each reached an increase in both performance capacity and personal causation

that led to their request that I further change their environment (i.e., take off the training wheels). Now, without the training wheels on the bicycle, each child requested yet another alteration in the environment. That is, they asked me to be alongside them to prevent them from falling. Over the course of the next few days, each child's skill developed and, correspondingly, the sense of efficacy in controlling the bicycle increased. Once each child reached a critical threshold in increased feelings of efficacy, they made an important request to change the environment further—namely, "I want to try it all by myself now."

In the transition from tricycling to bicycling, we can see that change occurs in an unfolding, dynamic process. Novel conditions leading to the emergence of something new may undergo several shifts before the new stable pattern is achieved. Chapter 10 examines this process of change in more depth.

Conclusion

At the outset, this chapter proposed to offer a response to the question of what kind of order lies behind our thoughts, feelings, and actions. We began with an examination of mechanistic thought and its vision of human organization, noting its limitations. Then, we identified systems thinking as an alternative, examining how it views the human being. The concepts of heterarchy and emergence painted a picture in which human order is substantially more dynamic than envisioned by mechanistic thought.

Next, we examined how systems ideas frame the way we think about volition, habituation, and performance capacity and their interaction with the environment. Finally, we examined how these ideas shape our understanding of the ways in which occupation influences who we are and what we become. We noted how our thoughts, feelings, and actions establish and maintain how we are organized. Finally, we examined how change takes place. These discussions have offered a way of thinking about humans that will be the foundation for the rest of the theoretical and applied discussions. The themes contained herein will be repeated and integrated throughout the text.

Key Terms

Emergence: Spontaneous occurrence of complex actions coming out of the interactions of several components without the benefit of a central controller.

Heterarchy: Principle that holds that parts of any system will interact with each other in ways that depend on the situation.

Interactive solutions: Principle that holds that important aspects of any thought, emotion, or action are worked out in the actual dynamics of the person interacting with the environment.

References

Allport, G. W. (1968). The open system in personality theory. In W. Buckley (Ed.), *Modern systems research for the behavioral scientist*. Chicago: Aldine.

Brent, S. B. (1978). Motivation, steady-state, and structural development. *Motivation and Emotion, 2*, 299–332.

Brody, H. (1973). The systems view of man: Implications for medicine, science and ethics. *Perspectives in Biology and Medicine, Autumn*, 71–92.

Bruner, J. (1990). *Acts of meaning*. Cambridge, MA: Harvard University Press.

Capra, F. (1997). *The web of life*. London: HarperCollins.

Clarke, A. (1997). *Being there: Putting brain, body and world together again*. Cambridge, MA: MIT Press

Fogel, A., & Thelen, E. (1987). Development of early expressive and communicative action: Reinterpreting the evidence from a dynamic systems perspective. *Developmental Psychology, 23*, 747–761.

Gergen, K. J., & Gergen, M. M. (1983). Narratives of the self. In T. R. Sarbin & K. E. Scheibe (Eds.), *Studies in social identity*. New York: Praeger.

Haken, H. (1987). Synergetics: An approach to self-organization. In F. E. Yates (Ed.), *Self-organizing systems: The emergence of order*. New York: Plenum.

Kelso, J. A. S., & Tuller, B. (1984). A dynamical basis for action systems. In M. S. Gazzaniga (Ed.), *Handbook of cognitive neuroscience*. New York: Plenum.

Koestler, A. (1969). Beyond atomism and holism: The concept of the holon. In A. Koestler & J. R. Smythies (Eds.), *Beyond reductionism*. Boston: Beacon Press.

Prigogine, I., & Stengers, I. (1984). *Order out of chaos*. New York: Bantam Books.

Sameroff, A. J. (1983). Developmental systems: Contexts and evolution. In P. H. Mussen (Ed.), *Handbook of child psychology*. New York: John Wiley & Sons.

Thelen, E., & Ulrich, B. D. (1991). Hidden skills: A dynamic systems analysis of treadmill stepping during the first year. *Monographs of the Society for Research in Child Development, 56* (1, Serial No. 223).

Turvey, M. T. (1990). Coordination. *American Psychologist, 45*, 938–953.

von Bertalanffy, L. (1968a). General system theory: A critical review. In W. Buckley (Ed.), *Modern systems research for the behavioral scientist*. Chicago: Aldine.

von Bertalanffy, L. (1968b). *General systems theory*. New York: George Braziller.

von Bertalanffy, L. (1969). General system theory and psychiatry. In S. Arieti (Ed.), *American handbook of psychiatry*. New York: Basic Books.

Weiss, P. S. (1967). One plus one does not equal two. In G. Quarton, T. Melnechuk, & F. Schmitt (Eds.), *The neurosciences: A study program*. New York: Rockefeller University Press.

Wolf, P. H. (1987). *The development of behavioral states and expression of emotion in early infancy*. Chicago: University of Chicago Press.

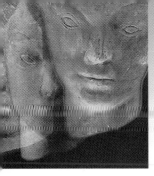

4

Volition

● Gary Kielhofner

Chapter 2 defined **volition** as a pattern of thoughts and feelings about oneself as an actor in one's world which occur as one anticipates, chooses, experiences, and interprets what one does. Volitional thoughts and feelings pertain to what one holds important (values), perceives as personal capacity and effectiveness (personal causation), and finds enjoyable (interests). Values, personal causation, and interests are universal themes in all persons' thoughts and feelings about what they do.

Across time, individuals tend to have similar patterns of volitional thoughts and feelings. The same hopes, fears, plans, and satisfaction in doing recur. Nonetheless, new circumstances, such as alterations in one's environment or in one's performance capacity, can change these thoughts and feelings. As shown in *Figure 4-1*, the ongoing cycle of anticipating, choosing, experiencing, and interpreting maintains or transforms one's values, personal causation, and interests. Consequently, volition is always a working version of self and the world.

Cultural Commonsense

Each person's volition is shaped by a commonsense perspective on self and the environment. This commonsense is acquired from one's culture through ongoing exchanges with others (Bruner, 1990; Gergen & Gergen, 1983, 1988; Markus, 1983). Since it is held in common with others, it is largely taken for granted.

We see our own actions and the world in which we act through the lens of our culture.

How culture shapes volitional thoughts and feelings can be appreciated by considering the following example. In groups in which hunting and gathering is a way of life, knowledge of the surrounding flora and fauna is essential to survival. In contrast, reading and writing are essential skills for white-collar workers in an industrialized society. Members of each of these cultures have volitional thoughts and feelings derived from their respective cultures. While one person is worried about whether he will find and kill dinner, another

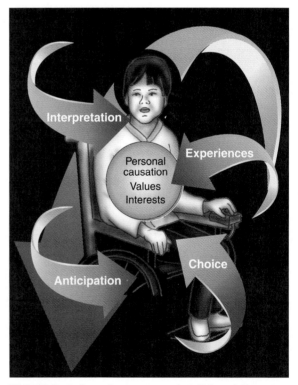

FIGURE 4-1 The Process of Volitional Change Over Time.

has anxiety about how well she will do at an upcoming business presentation. Moreover, the former views his work as mainly a matter of contributing to the welfare of the group, while the latter is mostly concerned over what it signifies about her individual achievement. Although values and personal causation are universal human concerns, how persons think and feel about personal effectiveness and assign significance to what they do will greatly depend on culture.

The influence of culture also includes local meanings shared by subgroups of persons within a society. Consequently, important cultural differences in persons' volition often exist in a single setting. For example, the custodial staff of a large university will differ significantly from faculty members in their perspectives about what they do in their lives. Within the same classroom a custodian and a professor will anticipate and choose very different things to do.

Culture, as it is broadly conceived here, infuses all aspects of volition. For instance, it shapes what kinds of abilities are of concern, what kinds of meanings are tied to actions, what pastimes are enjoyed, and what one should strive after in life. We see our own actions and the world in which we act through the lens of our culture.

Personal Circumstances and History

While sharing a cultural perspective with those around us, we each have unique volitional thoughts and feelings. These reflect characteristics emanating from our physical embodiment. They also reflect our accumulated personal history.

Volition begins with biological propensities such as our level of arousal, preferred sensory modes, and temperaments. These influence what we will develop capacity for, like, and consider important. The first things we do and our initial impact on the world around us involve the exercise of our physical capacities. As infants, we look around, move, touch, and so on. From these actions a sense of the world around us and of our own nature begins to emerge.

We learn that different kinds of doing produce particular results in the world and distinct thoughts and feelings in ourselves. In time, each of us discovers what we can and cannot do well, what kind of doing we enjoy, and what we find more or less worthy of do-

> *In time, each of us discovers what we can and cannot do well, what kind of doing we enjoy, and what we find more or less worthy of doing. Our volition reflects the unique personal history of such discoveries.*

ing. Our volition reflects the unique personal history of such discoveries.

Confluence of Personal Causation, Values, and Interests

We experience personal causation, values, and interests as a confluence of thinking and feeling about what we do well, what we enjoy, and the importance of what we do. We want to be competent at doing the things we value. We tend to find enjoyable those things that we do well and dislike those that overtax us. We suffer when we cannot perform well at the things about which we care deeply.

Themes of competence, enjoyment, and value are always interwoven. Consequently, a person's volition can only be understood fully by examining the dynamic relationship among personal causation, values, and interests. The following sections discuss each separately. However, the reader should be mindful that personal causation, values, and interests are each aspects of a larger volitional whole.

Personal Causation

One of the first discoveries of life is the connection between personal intention, action, and consequences (Bruner, 1973; Burke, 1977; DeCharms, 1968). Through-

> *The sense of capacity is not simply a catalogue of personal abilities. It is an active awareness of one's capabilities for carrying out the life one wants to live.*

out early development, individuals become increasingly aware that they can create effects in the environment. For example, infants come to realize that their movements and vocalizations influence what happens in the world around them. Soon, they choose to do things for their anticipated results.

This awareness that one can cause things to happen is the beginning of personal causation (DeCharms, 1968). Over time as we engage in a wider and wider range of action, we discover what we are capable of doing and what kinds of effects our doing can produce. As defined in Chapter 2, personal causation is one's sense of competence and effectiveness.

Two Dimensions of Personal Causation

One's thoughts and feelings about self as an actor can be distinguished into two dimensions. The first of these dimensions, **sense of personal capacity**, is a self-assessment of one's physical, intellectual, and social abilities (Harter, 1983, 1985; Harter & Connel, 1984). The second dimension, **self-efficacy**, is the thoughts and feelings one has concerning perceived effectiveness in using personal abilities to achieve desired outcomes in life (Lefcourt, 1981; Rotter, 1960). Self-efficacy is specific to different spheres of life (Connel, 1985; Fiske & Taylor, 1985; Lefcourt, 1981; Skinner, Chapman, & Baltes, 1988); that is, we feel more able to control outcomes in certain circumstances than in others.

Persons who feel capable and effective will seek out opportunities, use feedback to correct performance, and persevere to achieve goals. In contrast, individuals who feel incapable and lack a sense of efficacy will shy away from opportunity, avoid feedback, and have trouble persisting (Burke, 1977; DeCharms, 1968; Goodman, 1960). Consequently, personal causation influences how one is motivated toward doing things.

As shown in *Figure 4-2*, personal causation can be conceptualized as growing out of the original awareness of being a cause and developing over time— through a continuing cycle of anticipation, choice, experience, and interpretation—into the sense of personal capacity and self-efficacy. The following sections consider these two components of personal causation.

SENSE OF CAPACITY

We observe ourselves through the commonsense lens of our cultures, building up a store of knowledge about what kind of capacities we have for doing the things that matter. Moreover, as we proceed through life, new experiences can alter our views of our capabilities. Experience may happily show us that we have a hitherto hidden talent. It may instead remind us that our abilities are limited. It may confront us with a loss of capacity.

Concerns about capacity also change over the life course. To a 10-year-old boy, physical prowess may be more important than ability to perform in the classroom. However, if he attends college, intellectual ability will likely take a much more central place in his sense of capacity. Should he acquire an impairment, a whole new set of concerns about physical capacity would be created. In later life, when abilities wane, he may become much more concerned with physical capacity. The sense of capacity is not simply a catalogue of personal abilities. It is an active awareness of one's capabilities for carrying out the life one wants to live.

Challenges to a Sense of Capacity

Impairments challenge the view of self as capable (Molnar, 1989; Wright, 1960). Pain, fatigue, and limitations of sensation, cognition, or movement can constrain persons to achieve less than they desire or less than others (Werner-Beland, 1980). For example, Sienkiewicz-Mercer & Kaplan (1989, p. 64) write about their experience of cerebral palsy as being trapped in a body that "followed few directions of its mind and ignored the simple commands of speech and movement that nearly everyone takes for granted." Similarly, Deegan (1991) notes that due to schizophrenia facing everyday tasks was devastating:

> I remember being asked to come into the kitchen to help knead some bread dough. I got up, went into the kitchen, and looked at the dough for what seemed an eternity. Then I walked back to my chair and wept. The task seemed overwhelming to me. (p. 49)

> *. . . incapacity is experienced as difficulty doing the things that matter in one's life.*

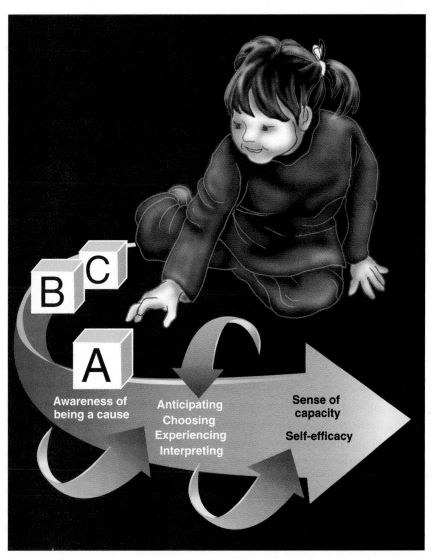

FIGURE 4-2   The Development of Personal Causation Over Time as One Encounters the World.

When one experiences a disability, issues of capacity become practical matters of whether and how one does the things that make up everyday life. For example, Diane, a woman with quadrilateral congenital amputation, describes the challenge of just managing doors:

> I can OPEN any door as long as I can get to the doorknob, which I turn with my arm and chin. I can not close a door behind me . . . (Frank, 1984, p. 641)

Another woman describes how chronic pain interferes with doing housework:

> Hanging the washing on the line. The arms ache. I might get about four things on the line, then it starts to ache. Washing up I can start. I can't do the saucepans, because of the scrubbing. Cooking—oh, I can do a bit of cooking, but I can't lift heavy saucepans. I have dropped them. I have burnt myself. (Ewan, Lowy, & Reid, 1991, p. 178)

Murphy (1987, p. 80), a professor, describes how his progressive paralysis made lecturing increasingly problematic as his voice "lost timbre and resonance, no longer projecting as well as it did." As the examples illustrate, incapacity is experienced as difficulty doing the things that matter in one's life.

The knowledge that one is less capable than others or than one once was can be a source of considerable emotional pain. For this reason some persons will go out of their way to avoid situations that provide occasions for failure (Cromwell, 1963; Moss, 1958). For example, emotionally disturbed adolescents indicate feelings of incompetence and often prefer solitary tasks whose results are not judged by others (American Psychiatric Association, 2000; Smyntek, 1983). Adults with developmental disabilities are often plagued with doubts about their abilities and go to great lengths to disguise their limitations (Edgerton, 1967; Kielhofner, 1983). For example, in the following episode, Doris (who spent much of her childhood and young adulthood in a state hospital) illustrates how she is haunted by concerns about her capacity:

> I heard Doris saying to Paula, "They discharged me from the state hospital and I wouldn't be on the outside if I wasn't okay." Then she asked rhetorically, "Isn't that right?" She talked on a while in that vein mentioning her [decade old] discharge papers in her wallet as 'proof' that she was okay. (Kielhofner, 1980, p. 172)

When shame or fear of failure governs a person's sense of capacity there is disincentive to take risks, to learn new skills, or to make the best use of what one has. A view of one's capacity plagued by negative comparisons to previous states or others can be as limiting as a person's actual impairments.

All things being equal, we are disposed to undertake that for which we feel capable and to avoid that which threatens us with failure. The close link between our sense of capacity and the desire to act accordingly is underscored by Murphy's (1987, p. 193) observation that, "With all bodily stimuli to movement muted and almost forgotten, one gradually loses the volition for physical activity." Our sense of capacity readies us to anticipate, choose, experience, and interpret behavior. When we know ourselves to be capable and effective, we are disposed to act and generate further evidence

of our talent. When we see ourselves to be incapable and ineffective, we feel compelled in the opposite direction.

SELF-EFFICACY

Self-efficacy is concerned with how one uses capacity to impact what happens in life. It includes the perception of self-control and being able to achieve what one desires. Through experience, we generate images of how effective we are in using our capacities and of how compliant or resistant life is to our efforts. Consequently, we develop a sense of how much we are able to bring about what we want.

Persons' beliefs about whether they can use their capacities to influence the course of events or circumstances in the external world are also powerful motivators. To be an effective agent, it is not enough to have capacity. It is also important that one is able to control and use that capacity toward desired outcomes.

Self-Control

Sense of efficacy hinges first on self-control. To use one's capacities effectively, one must be able to shape or contain emotions and thoughts and exercise control over one's actions. A strong sense of efficacy is impossible if one believes that one is at the mercy of overwhelming emotions or uncontrollable thoughts. Conversely, a strong sense of self-control can greatly enhance how persons adapt, as illustrated in the following passage from a young woman with quadriplegia:

> The ability to say my mind is in charge here. Not this environment. Not what's happening to me—it's not in charge. What determines what I will do and how I will handle things is right here (pointing to her head), and I do have control over it. That's the important thing, that events can't shake you, physical environments can't shake you as long as you are able to say, "my mind is in control here . . . " (Patsy & Kielhofner, 1989)

Impact of Efforts

Self-efficacy concerns whether one's efforts are sufficient to accomplish desired ends. The ability to achieve wanted outcomes in life is often challenged by disability. That disease and trauma arrive uninvited and with dire consequences readily engenders feelings of being controlled by outside factors (Burish & Bradley, 1983; Trieschmann, 1989).

Children who grow up with a disability learn that they cannot do what others do and are prone to develop feelings of ineffectiveness (Molnar, 1989). Such children may become unnecessarily dependent on others, because they do not see their own actions as the most effective route for achieving their desires (Wasserman, 1986).

Feeling helpless is concomitant with many forms of mental illness (American Psychiatric Association, 2000; Meissner, 1982). Persons with mental illness often lack a sense of control over life outcomes (Lovejoy, 1982; Wylie, 1979; Youkilis & Bootzin, 1979). Depression in particular is associated with the belief that one lacks control (Becker & Lesiak, 1977; Lefcourt, 1976; Leggett & Archer, 1979).

The loss of function significantly impacts self-efficacy. Hull (1990) gives a poignant description of how loss of sight took away personal control:

> I just sit here. The creatures emitting the noise have to engage in some activity. They have to scrape, bang, hit, club, strike surface upon surface, impact, make their vocal cords vibrate. They must take the initiative in announcing their presence to me. For my part, I have no power to explore them. I cannot penetrate them or discover them without their active cooperation. (p. 83)

Such constant reminders of one's inability to control the external world can result in feelings of powerlessness. Countering them requires extraordinary effort (Miller & Oertel, 1983; Murphy, 1987).

Dependence on medical personnel, family, or friends can exacerbate feelings of inefficacy. The patient role itself can contribute to a decreased sense of efficacy (Goffman, 1961). As persons are hospitalized and lose responsibility for their daily occupations, they may come to doubt whether they can manage their own lives. As Delaney-Naumoff (1980) notes:

> The patient feels he has lost power, direction, and goals—behaviors that characterize the mature adult in his interactions with others. Rather than feeling that he is in the center of activity, he feels pushed to the periphery. He becomes an outsider dependent upon the ministrations of others. (p. 87)

Disabled persons frequently note that the challenge of maintaining appropriate feelings of efficacy is complex and difficult. For example, Sienkiewicz-Mercer, who

has cerebral palsy, describes her own struggle with self-efficacy. After the disappointments of not being able to stand and feed herself, being able to talk was the one area in which she kept up hope since it was "something that was infinitely more important to me than anything else" (Sienkiewicz-Mercer & Kaplan, 1989, p.12). Although she had to go on to deal with not being able to speak, she found her voice in the autobiography, *I Raise My Eyes To Say Yes*.

Self-efficacy can be complicated by important and consequential factors that might take away personal control in the future. For example, Thelma, who has bipolar disorder, discusses the uncertainty surrounding her disease and social welfare:

> And if I ever got a job (then) I got to pay full fee for my (subsidized) apartment . . . I don't want to be making the wrong move and then I'll be stuck with nothing, you know . . . You see, you may get (a job) and then you may get sick again, or have a relapse. You're out in the cold again trying to get back on disability. (Helfrich, Kielhofner, & Mattingly, 1994, p. 316)

As Thelma illustrates, it is difficult to have a sense of self-efficacy when illness or the vagaries of a welfare system may foil one's efforts to achieve a better life.

Disabled persons must achieve a fine balance between necessary hope for the future and unrealistic expectations. The search for efficacy involves knowing disappointment, realizing what one cannot control, and finding and emphasizing what one is able to influence. Finding such a balanced view is not easy (Burish & Bradley, 1983).

APPRAISING THE SELF

How we judge our own ability and efficacy is a matter of great importance and consequence to each of us. Thoughts and feelings about personal capacity and control incur strong emotions. So just how accurately can we assess ourselves?

A number of factors impact our self-appraisals. Cognitive limitations may impair comprehension of one's capacity. The psychological pain of acknowledging limitations and failures invites denial, avoidance, and projection (Valient, 1994). On the other hand, secondary gains related to being incapacitated (e.g., freedom from unsatisfying work conditions) may bias persons toward overestimating their limitations.

Persons who exaggerate their limitations may unnecessarily limit their actions. Those who overestimate their capacities may make choices that can lead to injury, exacerbation of symptoms, and failure in performance. The view of personal capacity and efficacy can also impact therapy. For example, Krefting (1989) discusses a young man with a head injury that produced cognitive and communication deficits. He insisted that his only problem was walking and as a consequence "saw no need to compensate for his deficits" (p. 74).

Achieving an accurate view of one's capabilities and efficacy is not always easy. Persons with newly acquired impairments have not yet discovered what their capacities will be. Similarly, persons with progressive conditions or those who experience exacerbations and remissions cannot anticipate what abilities they will have in the future.

In the face of a disability, personal causation is a highly individualized process of discovering how impairment may curtail or complicate the things one must and wants to do. This discovery may be ongoing as one's impairment and life changes. Since personal causation involves self-control and effort, self-efficacy is not only a matter of accurate accounting. It is also a reflection of one's will. For example, some spinal-cord–injured individuals may claim they will walk again, but such views are an "assertion of will and strength" (Trieschmann, 1989). Such claims may reflect the substantial resources that a person will bring to coping with the disability.

Values

From earliest childhood, certain things matter to us. Long before we can articulate it, we act in accordance with matters of importance. Our first values have their roots in biological needs. We want to survive, to be safe, and to feel comfortable. We want to do things. Insecurity, pain, and boredom are negative values for young children.

> *Values commit us to a way of life and impart commonsense meaning to the lives we lead.*

Over the course of development, culture teaches us beliefs and commitments that signify what is good, right, and important to do (Grossack & Gardner, 1970; Kalish & Collier, 1981; Klavins, 1972; Lee, 1971; Smith, 1969). Cultures are "dramatic conversations about the things that matter" (Bellah, Madsen, Sullivan, Swidler, & Tipton, 1985, p. 27). They communicate how one ought to act to have merit, and what goals or aspirations deserve one's commitment. These messages are internalized and shape what one finds important and meaningful to do (i.e., one's **values**). Values commit us to a way of life and impart commonsense meaning to the lives we lead.

Each person's values belong to a coherent world view provided by culture. Thus, as Bruner (1990) notes:

> Values inhere in commitment to "ways of life," and ways of life in their complex interaction constitute a culture. We neither shoot our values from the hip, choice-situation by choice-situation, nor are they the product of isolated individuals with strong drives and compelling neuroses. Rather, they are communal and consequential in terms of our relations to a cultural community . . . (p. 29)

Values influence the sense of self-worth that one derives from doing certain things. For example, in a context in which academic achievement is highly valued, a student who does well in school is especially disposed to evaluate self positively. Since values involve commitments to performing in culturally meaningful and sanctioned ways, one experiences a sense of belonging and appropriateness when following values (Lee, 1971). Moreover, one does not act contrary to one's values without a feeling of shame, guilt, failure, or inadequacy.

We acquire our values as a coherent set of convictions. As we internalize these convictions, we acquire a strong disposition to act accordingly. As shown in *Figure 4-3*, the process of anticipating, choosing, experiencing, and interpreting in our cultural context generates personal convictions and the sense of obligation that goes with them.

Personal Convictions

The convictions we acquire both come from and imply a particular culturally defined world. Values are clustered together in ways that define a coherent lifestyle

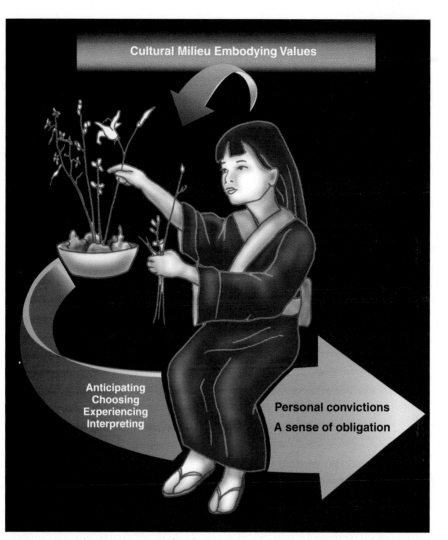

Cultural Milieu Embodying Values

Anticipating
Choosing
Experiencing
Interpreting

Personal convictions

A sense of obligation

FIGURE 4-3   The Emergence of Values From Interactions With the Cultural Milieu.

(Mitchell, 1983). Moreover, people do not simply hold these coherent views of life. They care deeply about the things they believe most matter (Gergen & Gergen, 1988).

A variety of themes may be the organizing medium for personal convictions. For example, personal convictions may be organized around a fundamental religious viewpoint of right and wrong that defines what is a good life. A very different set of convictions underlie a street-smart adolescent who

learns a code of gang solidarity, territoriality, and survival by aggression.

While these two sets of convictions are vastly different, each represents a way that someone views the world. Moreover, each expresses what matters to that person and his or her associates. These two elements, a view of how the world is and the identification of what matters, make up our convictions. Consequently, **personal convictions** are views of life that define what matters.

Sense of Obligation

To hold values is to commit our lives to their pursuit (Bruner, 1990). Thus, values bind us to action (Fein, 1990). Because values evoke powerful emotions such as feelings of importance, security, worthiness, belonging, and purpose, they create a sense of obligation to perform in ways consistent with those values.

This sense of obligation may include convictions about such things as how time should be spent, what aspects of performance are important, and what constitutes adequate effort or outcomes (Hall, 1959; Kluckholn, 1951). It may also be reflected in commitments to perform occupations in moral, excellent, efficient, or other ways made sense of by a coherent view of life. A sense of obligation often takes the form of goals (Cottle, 1971). In sum, the **sense of obligation** refers to strong emotional dispositions to follow what are perceived as right ways to act.

Values and Disability

The interface of disability and value is complex and multifaceted. Values shape how persons experience a disability. Values that conflict with what one is able to do can lead one to self-devaluation. Finally, experiencing a disability may challenge values.

Persons with disabilities often find that their very condition is in conflict with mainstream values. As Murphy (1987, pp. 116–117) notes, "The disabled, individually and as a group, contravene all the values of youth, virility, activity, and physical beauty." Similarly, DeLoach, Wilkins, and Walker (1983, p. 14) note that the American work ethic has "tended to discredit anyone who does not or cannot work." Indeed, persons with acquired disabilities often find themselves devalued by the very standards that they have held all their lives.

A discontinuity between one's capacity and what one values can lower self-esteem (Zane & Lowenthal, 1960). For example, a woman experiencing functional limitations imposed by repetitive strain injury, notes: "I got to the stage where you felt that you weren't worth anything, you were good for nothing. You couldn't do anything. What's the good of me? I can't do anything" (Ewan, Lowy, & Reid, 1991, p. 184). Loss of capacity can mean either rejecting old values or devaluing self as unable to live up to old values (Rabinowitz & Mitsos, 1964; Vash, 1981).

Values can commit one to impossible ideals (Fein, 1990). Persons with disabilities sometimes struggle futilely to achieve values inconsistent with their capacities. For example, Mike, throughout his adolescence and young adulthood, accepted his parents' vision that he would follow in the footsteps of his father, a successful surgeon. In college, he found the coursework overwhelming, failed his classes, became withdrawn and inactive, and finally required hospitalization for depression. Following this, he worked in a blue-collar position, which he enjoyed. Plagued with the idea that he was not living up to his parents' ideal, he returned to college only to experience the same pattern of failure, depression, and hospitalization. Twice more he repeated the same cycle, needing rehospitalization each time. Only after these repeated failures was he able to admit that the values he had pursued were not consistent with his abilities or his interests.

Like Mike, individuals may strive after certain values in the belief that their lives will not be fulfilled or that they will not have worth unless they somehow realize those values. In such instances, values can drive individuals toward choices that make life disappointing or difficult to bear.

Disability can radically challenge the whole view of life in which one's values are embedded. Consider, for example, persons who have made sense of their hard work as a means to a valued promotion and career development. In the face of a progressively disabling disease, their ideal of the progressive work career would no longer be viable.

As the previous example illustrates, the future as one imagined it may be partially or totally invalidated by disability. Without an image of what life will be like, it is more difficult to manage the taxing problems imposed by disability (Litman, 1972; Rogers & Figone, 1978, 1979). Without a sense of some valued future goal or state toward which one is striving, persons may question the worth of life and/or find themselves alienated and without a sense of purpose (Frankl, 1978; Korner, 1970; Menninger, 1962; Mitchell, 1975; Schiamberg, 1973).

DISABILITY VALUES

While preexisting values can have an important impact on what a disability means to an individual, the existence of a disability can also be the critical occasion for development of new values. This is not easy since most cultures devalue disability and persons with disabilities (Longmore, 1995; Oliver, 1996; Scotch, 1988; Shapiro, 1994). Indeed, one of the consistent messages that persons with disabilities receive is that the part of the self which is disabled is essentially "bad" and must be balanced or overcome with the parts which are still "good" or not disabled (Gill, 1997).

Because dominant societal values tend to denigrate persons with disabilities, a growing community of disabled persons emphasizes a different valuation of disability. They identify their disability as a positive value rather than an aberration from what is good or right. A disability culture is beginning to emerge that extols ideals such as disability pride and encourages exhibiting rather than hiding one's disability (Gill, 1994, 1997).

> *Because dominant societal values tend to denigrate persons with disabilities, a growing community of disabled persons emphasizes a different valuation of disability.*

Having a disability may serve as the impetus for a person to develop a new consciousness. For example, Mitchell and Snyder (in press) illustrate how many artists' visions were shaped by their experience of disability and how their art carried explicit messages aimed at questioning or contradicting societal values.

Exposure to others who share common experiences and positive disability values is important for disabled persons (Gill, 1994, 1997). Such exposure can be hampered by the fact that people with disabilities are a diverse group and a single disability culture does not yet exist (Hahn, 1985). Until a disability culture and the values it extols become more widespread, disabled persons will continue to carry the burden of mainstream cultural values that demean them.

Values, Disability, and Choice

By rendering many of the things one used to do as impossible, impairment may force persons to examine what is most important to them. For example, Roberts (1989) recalls of his own experience:

> One of my therapists insisted that I learn to feed myself. Meals took hours, and I was always exhausted. After, I realized then that I could either use my time to feed myself or have an attendant feed me, allowing me to spend the time saved to go to school. I went to school. (p. 234)

Another example is Melanie, who had arthritis. She routinely entertained her husband's business associates in their home, highly valuing her ability as a gourmet cook and expert hostess. However, after the onset of arthritis she found that her routine of shopping for products, preparing a complex meal, dressing appropriately, and then decorating the home for guests was no longer feasible. Her pain was so great by the time guests arrived that she could not enjoy the evening. Although she valued all components of the routine, she had to choose which aspects would be dropped or modified. She chose to have meals catered so that she would have the energy and relative freedom from pain to be a good hostess.

Disability can become a source of rethinking personal values and one's fundamental view of life. Wright (1960) argues that to adjust to disability persons may need to enlarge the scope of their values to incorporate behaviors for which they are still capable. In addition, persons may need to learn new values, which judge their performance given their capacities, and reject old values, which compare one's performance to that of others without disabilities. Since impairments typically invalidate some aspect of one's values, adjusting to disability almost invariably means a quest for new ways of viewing and valuing life.

Interests

As noted in Chapter 2, **interests** are what one finds enjoyable or satisfying to do. Interests are generated from the experience of pleasure and satisfaction in doing things (Matsutsuyu, 1969). As we accumulate expe-

> *The enjoyment of doing things ranges from the simple satisfaction derived from small daily rituals to the intense pleasure people feel in pursuing their driving passions.*

rience in doing things, we develop an attraction to particular occupations. Hence, as shown in *Figure 4-4*, interests reflect highly individual tastes generated from the cycle of anticipating, choosing, experiencing, and interpreting our actions. We view our interests both as enjoyment when we are doing things and as a preference for doing certain things over others.

Enjoyment

This refers to the feeling of pleasure or satisfaction that comes from doing things. The enjoyment of doing things ranges from the simple satisfaction derived from small

daily rituals to the intense pleasure people feel in pursuing their driving passions. The feeling of enjoyment may come from a wide range of factors. These include:

- Bodily pleasure associated with physical exertion
- Fulfillment of intellectual intrigue
- Aesthetic satisfaction from artistic production
- Fulfillment of using one's skill to face a challenge.

Those occupations that evoke the strongest feelings of attraction for us are generally those that evoke several sources of enjoyment.

Csikszentmihalyi (1990) describes a form of ultimate enjoyment in physical, intellectual, or social occu-

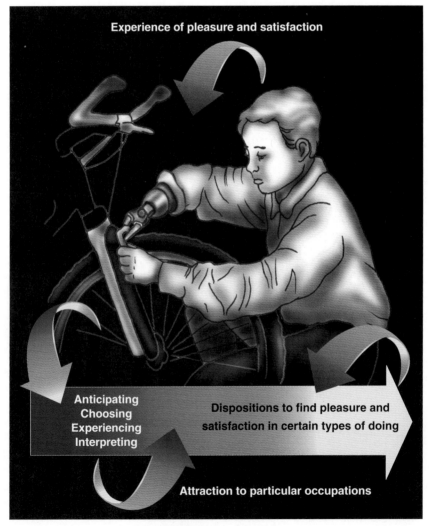

FIGURE 4-4 Interests.

pations, which he calls flow. The experience of flow is a complete saturation of one's awareness with the positive experience of performing the activity. According to his research, flow occurs when a person's capacities are optimally challenged.

Enjoyment from doing may emanate from sensory pleasures. For example, we may enjoy how tools feel in our hands, how our cooking smells, or the view of country scenery on a hike or bicycle ride. We may enjoy the muscular exertion and the vestibular pleasure associated with sports.

Since many occupations produce outcomes or products, satisfaction may emanate from what we have accomplished or produced. One may find a craft particularly satisfying because of the pleasing or useful object that results. Enjoyment may also come from the sense of association and fellowship experienced in occupations performed with others. Attraction to any particular occupation most likely represents a confluence of several of these factors.

Pattern

Since we do not experience all occupations with equal pleasure or satisfaction, we each develop a unique pattern of interests. One's **interest pattern** is the unique configuration of preferred things to do that one has accumulated from experience. In some cases, a pattern of interests will reflect an underlying theme such as athletic interest or cultural interests like theater and art. On the other hand, persons may have very diverse and seemingly unrelated preferences.

Preferring certain occupations to others allows one to choose. Feeling a preference for certain activities makes it easier to select what to do. Consequently, one's pattern of interests is usually paralleled by a routine in which one's interests are at least partially indulged.

Disability and Interests

Although commonly overlooked, one of the most pervasive effects of disability on occupation is its influence on the experience of satisfaction and pleasure in life. The daily pleasures, comforts, and enjoyments that enliven our existence and help maintain our energy and mood can be threatened or altered by disability.

> *The daily pleasures, comforts, and enjoyments that enliven our existence and help maintain our energy and mood can be threatened or altered by disability.*

Children with disabilities may have been given fewer opportunities to develop normal investment and satisfaction in occupational performance. Further, difficulties with performance and fear of being recognized as incompetent may lead a child to avoid opportunities to develop a sense of attraction to occupations.

Physical impairments and attendant fatigue, pain, and preoccupation with failure may reduce or eliminate the feeling of pleasure in occupations. Physical or procedural adaptations necessary to allow performance may negatively affect the ambiance and spirit of activities, making it difficult to experience the same sense of satisfaction as before. Many persons with acquired disabilities describe that it is no longer worth engaging in old pastimes. They are no longer enjoyable or do not warrant the additional effort required.

Further, persons may be prevented by limitations of capacity from participating in activities they previously enjoyed (Rogers & Figone, 1978; Trieschmann, 1989; Vash, 1981). For example, persons may have to give up activities involving excessive physical stress or requiring lost sensory, perceptual, or cognitive abilities. Consequently, the future may seem a bland and undesirable existence without the enjoyment and satisfaction that existed in the past.

Some psychiatric illnesses involve a loss of attraction to activities. For example, depressed persons frequently indicate few current interests even when their past interests were substantial (Neville, 1987). Many depressed persons speak about losing their enthusiasm for former interests and describe that they no longer enjoy doing things. Supporting such individual reports, research reveals that increases in depressed mood and decreases in enjoyment in activities go hand in hand (Neville, 1987; Turner, Ward, & Turner, 1979). Research also suggests that persons with psychiatric problems engage in few interests (Grob & Singer, 1974; Spivak, Siegel, Sklaver, Deuschle, & Garrett, 1982). Jack, who is psychiatrically disabled, represents the kind of limbo some people inhabit when they are neither able to establish nor be guided by interests:

> I don't have any drive. There's nothing I really feel like working for. I guess I wouldn't mind being a song-writer. But I never wrote anything worthwhile. No, I'd like to be an architect. I'd like to design bizarre houses. I'll never do it, because I'd lose interest. I'd like to do something with my life, but what I don't know. (Estroff, 1981, p. 142)

In discussing how persons with spinal cord injury may experience changes in interests, Trieschmann (1989) notes:

> Reduced access to satisfying activity can certainly lower mood, which tends to lower a person's interest in activity, which further lowers mood. Thus, a vicious circle evolves. (p. 242)

Her argument is supported by the finding that when persons increase their activities, their mood improves as well (Turner, Ward, & Turner, 1979). Thus, it appears that the reduction in interest and attraction associated with many forms of disability may reflect a complex process in which decreased feelings of attraction, decreases in activity, and demoralization interrelate in a downward spiral.

Thus, one of the challenges presented by disability is often to find new interests or new avenues for channeling one's interests. One of my earliest client encounters was a young man who had great promise as a swimmer and diver. He had won regional and national championships and was an Olympic hopeful. He broke his neck in a diving accident and was rendered a high-level quadriplegic. Fortunately, he discovered that he was also a talented writer and speaker and was able to channel his interest in sports toward the field of sports journalism.

Others do not so easily redirect their interests. Another client I knew at the same time had been an accomplished dancer in a nationally famous dance troupe. Following her spinal cord injury, she became despondent over her loss of ability. She slipped into chronic substance abuse.

When Interests Fail

Persons may develop preferences that lead to problematic activity choices. For example, there is evidence to suggest that some adolescents with psychosocial difficulties may be attracted to socially unacceptable interests (Lambert, Rothschild, Atland, & Green, 1978; Werthman, 1976). As another example, adults with developmental disabilities tend to have mainly solitary and sedentary interests (Cheseldine & Jeffree, 1981; Coyne, 1980; Matthews, 1980; Mitic & Stevenson, 1981). As a consequence of their interests, these persons made choices to do things that isolated themselves, led to chronic physical inactivity, or got them into trouble.

Other research has found that persons with alcoholism are less likely to pursue their stated interests (Scaffa, 1982). Some persons appear to substitute the pleasure induced by substance abuse for the enjoyment of doing things. Others feel they cannot enjoy themselves without the assistance of drugs or alcohol.

A prospective study of more than 3000 aircraft workers found that those who hardly ever enjoyed their job tasks were 2.5 times more likely to report a back injury than subjects who almost always enjoyed their job tasks (Bigos et al., 1991). Whereas there is some reason to suspect that many workers today may feel disaffected from their work (Kielhofner, 1993), this may be particularly true when one has a disability. For example, Alice, who has a psychiatric disability, notes:

> I hate my job. I just hate it. It takes the mind of a seven-year-old to work there. It's boring. My supervisor is like a slave driver. I tried so many Civil Service jobs you wouldn't believe it. Sometimes two to three job interviews a week. But no one would hire me. No one. They never did tell me why. I bet I'll be stuck at Goodwill forever . . . (Estroff, 1981, p. 136)

Since work is a fact of life for so many adults, the degree of interest persons find in their work is no small issue.

Interest as Inspiration

Interests can infuse life with meaning and energy, as illustrated in a story told by Christi Brown in his autobiography, *My Left Foot*. Brown, severely disabled with cerebral palsy, explains that as a 10-year-old boy he became depressed and despondent. With a set of watercolors bartered from his brother, he learned to paint with his foot. He explains:

I didn't know it then, but I had found a way to be happy. Slowly I begin to lose my early depression. I had a feeling of pure joy while I painted, a feeling I had never experienced before which seemed almost to lift me above myself. (Brown, 1990, pp. 57)

Brown's characterization of painting as a way to be happy underscores an important point about interests. The process of finding pleasure and satisfaction in doing things is a central component of adapting in occupational life. The contentment we find in doing things gives us positive emotional experiences. Even more importantly, we must find some enthusiasm for doing particular things that urges us to action and gives us something to which we can look forward. Interest gives life much of its appeal.

I remember vividly a conversation with my aged grandfather, an avid outdoorsman who was involved in hunting and fishing. Reflecting on his remaining days, he told me that each evening he expressed a private wish that went something like the following. He hoped there would be at least one more day when he could sit on the shore of some sparkling lake or stream and the fish would be biting. He wanted once more to sit in the dark woods while the morning light came slowly, serenaded by the emerging sounds of the forest. Having accompanied him as a boy on such outings and having seen the sparkle in his eye on those occasions, I knew exactly what he meant.

Volitional Processes

The previous sections examined personal causation, values, and interests independently. As noted at the outset of this chapter, these three elements are woven together in the thoughts and feelings we have about our actions and our world. Moreover, it was noted at the beginning of this chapter that volition is a dynamic process involving a cycle of anticipation, making choices, experience while doing, and subsequent evaluation or interpretation. This last section examines the dynamic process of volition. In doing so, it considers how personal causation, values, and interests are part of a coherent pattern of thoughts and feelings unfolding in everyday life.

Anticipation

Our interests, values, and personal causation influence what we notice and search out in the world. They also influence what we are likely to feel and think about prospects for involvement in the occupational opportunities we encounter. We need only observe how a person's interest (or lack thereof) in sports influences whether they pay attention to television sportscasts, perk up at conversations about sports, or know when upcoming home teams are scheduled to play. In a similar fashion, personal causation influences whether a potential involvement in an occupation evokes anxiety or excitement. Finally, values orient us to notice and seek out opportunities to realize our commitments and to pursue what we consider worth doing.

The world represents an invitation for action. We orient to those parts of the world that allow us to do things we value and like. We also tend to be unaware of that in which we have no volitional investment. Conversely, we notice what corresponds to our competence, interests, and commitments. What is out there in the world for us is very much a function of our volition.

Making Choices

We make choices for action that shape the texture of our everyday doing and influence the course of our lives. Chapter 2 distinguished two types of choices. Activity choices refer to the many decisions we make about doing things throughout each day. Occupational choices refer to the larger decisions that involve commitment to sustaining action over time.

Activity choices are made about our present or about our more or less immediate future. They involve decisions to begin or terminate activities as well as how to go about them. Consider, for example, activity choices one might make relative to studying for an exam. One may decide to get up early or stay up late to study. While studying, one loses concentration and then redoubles efforts to attend. After pausing to test oneself, one considers whether what has been learned suggests studying on or quitting.

As the example shows, activity choices commence, shape, and terminate what we do in the course of everyday life. Choosing whether and how to do something involves complex contributions from all components of volition. Let us return to the example of studying for an exam. The dual propositions of studying or joining friends on a Saturday afternoon create the opportunity for an activity choice. The choice of studying or socializing will emerge from feelings of efficacy and interest in the subject, combined with values pertaining to school performance and socializing with friends. One may simply feel the collective contributions of all these elements in making the decision or one may rationally deliberate the consequences of the decision. Nonetheless, personal causation, values, and interests will together exert an influence over the decision.

Occupational choices occur much less frequently than activity choices, but they have a much more far-reaching impact on our lives. In fact, what most characterizes an occupational choice is that it changes something fundamental about our lives. Consequently, most occupational choices are made over a period of deliberation as we consider what they mean for our lives.

As noted in Chapter 2, occupational choices involve decisions to begin or end roles, alter a habit pattern, or undertake a personal project. Sometimes we make occupational choices directly, as when we elect to attend college (e.g., student role) or to take a certain job (e.g., worker role). On other occasions we make decisions that indirectly assign roles to us. For example, in choosing to move into a house or apartment for which we have primary responsibility implies taking on the home-maintainer role.

In other cases, occupational choice evolves by degrees, as when we take up a new hobby or sport and find ourselves becoming increasingly involved and committed. At certain times developmental milestones may occasion occupational choices. For example, graduating from high school prompts the decision to begin working or further one's education. Similarly, as illustrated by Jonsson, Josephsson, and Kielhofner (2001), when people retire from their work roles they face the challenge of making occupational choices for how to regularly fill time left vacant by work. Those who succeed in identifying projects with which to become regularly involved are more likely to have a positive retirement.

The onset of an acquired disability is most often an occasion for new occupational choices. When a disability interferes with role performance, requires extra time to do things, or makes old habits or projects no longer viable, people must make a series of different occupational choices to find a new pattern of behavior. The success of such choices will have a great deal to do with how well a person adapts to the circumstance of having a disability.

Experience

Volition also influences how we experience what we do. When we engage in occupations our volition determines which we find more or less enjoyable or valuable. It also determines the extent of confidence or anxiety we feel. Volition leads each of us to experience action in our own unique way.

Our experience in performing is closely linked to our quality of life. After all, how we experience the things we do—be it enjoyment, boredom, fulfillment, angst, triumph, or disappointment—determines much of what we get out of life. Finding harmony between our volition and what we actually get to do in the course of daily life contributes to life satisfaction.

Finally, experience is also a critical dimension of therapy. The therapeutic transformation that comes from doing things depends on what we experience in the midst of performance. Research has shown that volition is an important determinant of how therapy is experienced (Barrett, Beer, & Kielhofner, 1999; Helfrich & Kielhofner, 1994; Kielhofner & Barrett, 1997).

Interpretation

Volition influences how we interpret our actions. Our values have an important influence on the significance we assign to what we have done. For example, the high school senior who is committed to going to college will interpret a poor grade differently from the one who envisions working as a carpenter in 3 months. Moreover, whether the student accepts responsibility for the grade or blames it on teacher bias will be a function of the student's personal causation. As the examples show, volition provides us with a framework for making sense of our actions.

Conclusion

Volition has a pervasive influence on occupational life. It shapes how we see the world and the opportunities and challenges it presents. It guides the activity and occupational choices that together determine much of what we do. It determines our experience. It shapes how we make sense of what we have done, including our effectiveness in achieving desired ends and our success in realizing important values. To a large extent, how we experience life and how we regard ourselves and our world has to do with volition.

Key Terms

Enjoyment: The feeling of pleasure or satisfaction that comes from doing things.

Interest pattern: The unique configuration of preferred things to do that one has accumulated from experience.

Interests: What one finds enjoyable or satisfying to do.

Personal causation: One's sense of competence and effectiveness.

Personal convictions: Views of life that define what matters.

Self-efficacy: Thoughts and feelings concerning perceived effectiveness in using personal abilities to achieve desired outcomes in life.

Sense of obligation: Strong emotional dispositions to follow what are perceived as right ways to act.

Sense of personal capacity: Self-assessment of one's physical, intellectual, and social abilities.

Values: What one finds important and meaningful to do.

Volition: Pattern of thoughts and feelings about oneself as an actor in one's world which occur as one anticipates, chooses, experiences, and interprets what one does.

References

American Psychiatric Association. (2000). *Diagnostic and statistical manual of mental disorders* (4th ed., text revision). Washington, DC: Author.

Barrett, L., Beer, D., & Kielhofner, G. (1999). The importance of volitional narrative in treatment: An ethnographic case study in a work program. *Work, 12,* 79–92.

Becker, E. W., & Lesiak, W. J. (1977). Feelings of hostility and personal control as related to depression. *Journal of Clinical Psychology, 33,* 654–657.

Bellah, R., Madsen, R., Sullivan, W., Swidler, A., & Tipton, S. (1985). *Habits of the heart.* Berkeley, CA: University of California Press.

Bigos, S. J., Battie, M. C., Spengler, M. D., Fisher, L. D., Fordyce, W. E., Hansson, T. H., Nachemson, A. L., & Wortley, M. D. (1991). A prospective study of work perceptions and psychosocial factors affecting the report of back injury. *Spine, 16,* 1–6.

Brown, C. (1990). *My left foot.* London: Minerva.

Bruner, J. (1973). Organization of early skilled action. *Child Development, 44,* 1–11.

Bruner, J. (1990). *Acts of meaning.* Cambridge, MA: Harvard University Press.

Burish, T. G., & Bradley, L. A. (1983). *Coping with chronic disease: Research and applications.* New York: Academic Press.

Burke, J. P. (1977). A clinical perspective on motivation: Pawn versus origin. *American Journal of Occupational Therapy, 31,* 254–258.

Cheseldine, S., & Jeffree, D. (1981). Mentally handicapped adolescents: Their use of leisure time. *Journal of Mental Health Deficiency Research, 25,* 49–59.

Connel, J. P. (1985). A new multidimensional measure of children's perceptions of control. *Child Development, 56,* 1018–1041.

Cottle, T. J. (1971). *Time's children: Impressions of youth.* Boston: Little, Brown & Co.

Coyne, P. (1980). Developing social skills in the developmentally disabled adolescent and young adult: A recreation and social/sexual approach. *Journal of Leisure, 7,* 70–76.

Cromwell, R. L. (1963). A social learning approach to mental retardation. In N. R. Ellis (Ed.), *Handbook of mental deficiency.* New York: McGraw-Hill.

Csikszentmihalyi, M. (1990). *Flow: The psychology of optimal experience.* New York: Harper & Row.

DeCharms, R.E. (1968). *Personal causation: The internal affective determinants of behaviors.* New York: Academic Press.

Deegan, P. (1991). Recovery: The lived experience of rehabilitation. In R. P. Marinelli & A. E. Dell Orto (Eds.), *The psychological and social impact of disability* (3rd ed.). New York: Springer-Verlag.

Delaney-Naumoff, M. (1980). Loss of heart. In J. A. Werner-Beland (Ed.), *Grief responses to long-term illness and disability*. Reston, VA: Reston Publishing.

DeLoach, C. P., Wilkins, R. D., & Walker, G. W. (1983). *Independent living: Philosophy, process, and services.* Baltimore: University Park Press.

Edgerton, R. B. (1967). *The cloak of competence: Stigma in the lives of the mentally retarded.* Berkeley, CA: University of California Press.

Estroff, S. E. (1981). *Making it crazy.* Berkeley, CA: University of California Press.

Ewan, C., Lowy, E., & Reid, J. (1991). `Falling out of culture: ' The effects of repetition strain injury on sufferers' roles and identity. *Sociology of Health and Illness, 13,* 168–192.

Fein, M. L. (1990). *Role change: A resocialization perspective.* New York: Praeger.

Fiske, S., & Taylor, S. E. (1985). *Social cognition.* New York: Random House.

Frank, G. (1984). Life history model of adaptation to disability: The case of a `congenital amputee.' *Social Science and Medicine, 19,* 639–645.

Frankl, V. E. (1978). *The unheard cry for meaning.* New York: Touchstone Books.

Gergen, K. J., & Gergen, M. M. (1983). Narratives of the self. In T. R. Sarbin & K. E. Scheibe (Eds.), *Studies in social identity.* New York: Praeger.

Gergen, K. J., & Gergen, M. M. (1988). Narrative and the self as relationship. In L. Berkowitz (Ed.), *Advances in experimental social psychology* (pp. 17–56). San Diego: Academic Press.

Gill, C. (1994). A bicultural framework for understanding disability. *The Family Psychologist, Fall,* 13–16.

Gill, C. (1997). Four types of integration in disability identity development. *Journal of Vocational Rehabilitation, 9,* 39–46.

Goffman, E. (1961). *Asylums.* New York: Doubleday.

Goodman, P. (1960). *Growing up absurd.* New York: Vintage Books.

Grob, M., & Singer, J. (1974). *Adolescent patients in transition: Impact and outcome of psychiatric hospitalization.* New York: Behavioral Publications.

Grossack, M., & Gardner, H. (1970). *Man and men: Social psychology as social science.* Scranton, PA: International Textbook.

Hahn, H. (1985). Disability policy and the problem of discrimination. *American Behavioral Scientist, 28,* 293–318.

Hall, E. T. (1959). *The silent language.* Greenwich, CT: Fawcett Publications.

Harter, S. (1983). The development of the self-system. In M. Hetherington (Ed.), *Handbook of child psychology: Social and personality development* (Vol. 4). New York: John Wiley & Sons.

Harter, S. (1985). Competence as a dimension of self-evaluation: Toward a comprehensive model of self-worth. In R. L. Leahy (Ed.), *The development of the self.* Orlando, FL: Academic Press.

Harter, S., & Connel, J. P. (1984). A model of relationships among children's academic achievement and self-perceptions of competence, control, and motivation. In J. Nicholls (Ed.), *The development of achievement motivation.* Greenwich, CT: JAI.

Helfrich, C., & Kielhofner, G. (1994). Volitional narratives and the meaning of therapy. *American Journal of Occupational Therapy, 48,* 318–326.

Helfrich, C., Kielhofner, G., & Mattingly, C. (1994). Volition as narrative: Understanding motivation in chronic illness. *American Journal of Occupational Therapy, 48,* 311–317.

Hull, J. M. (1990). *Touching the rock: An experience of blindness.* New York: Vintage Books.

Jonsson, H., Josephsson, S., & Kielhofner, G. (2001). Evolving narratives in the course of retirement: A longitudinal study. *American Journal of Occupational Therapy, 55,* 424–432.

Kalish, R. A., & Collier, K. W. (1981). *Exploring human values.* Monterey, CA: Brooks/Cole.

Kielhofner, G. (1980). *Evaluating deinstitutionalization: An ethnographic study of social policy.* Unpublished doctoral dissertation, University of California at Los Angeles.

Kielhofner, G. (1983). "Teaching" retarded adults: Paradoxical effects of a pedagogical enterprise. *Urban Life, 12,* 307–326.

Kielhofner, G. (1993). Functional assessment: Toward a dialectical view of person-environment relations. *American Journal of Occupational Therapy, 47,* 248–251.

Kielhofner, G., & Barrett, L. (1998). Meaning and misunderstanding in occupational forms: A study of therapeutic goal-setting. *American Journal of Occupational Therapy, 52,* 345–353.

Klavins, R. (1972). Work-play behavior: Cultural influences. *American Journal of Occupational Therapy, 26,* 176–179.

Kluckholn, C. (1951). Values and value orientations in the theory of action: An exploration in definition and classification. In T. Parsons & E. Shils (Eds.), *Toward a general theory of action.* Cambridge, MA: Harvard University Press.

Korner, I. (1970). Hope as a method of coping. *Journal of Consulting and Clinical Psychology, 34,* 134–139.

Krefting, L. (1989). Reintegration into the community after head injury: The results of an ethnographic study. *Occupational Therapy Journal of Research, 9,* 67–83.

Lambert, B. G., Rothschild, B. F., Atland, R., & Green, L. B. (1978). *Adolescence: Transition from childhood to maturity* (2nd ed.). Monterey, CA: Brooks/Cole.

Lee, D. (1971). Culture and the experience of value. In A. H. Maslow (Ed.), *Neural knowledge in human values.* Chicago: Henry Regnery.

Lefcourt, H. (1981). *Research with the locus of control construct, Vol. 1: Assessment and methods.* New York: Academic Press.

Lefcourt, H. M. (1976). *Locus of control: Current trends in theory and research.* Hillsdale, NJ: Erlbaum.

Leggett, J., & Archer, R. P. (1979). Locus of control and depression among psychiatric patients. *Psychology Report, 45,* 835–838.

Litman, T. J. (1972). Physical rehabilitation: A social-psychological approach. In E. G. Jaco (Ed.), *Patients, physicians and illness: A sourcebook in behavioral science and health* (2nd ed.). New York: Free Press.

Longmore, P. K. (1995). The second phase: From disability rights to disability culture. *The Disability Rag & Resource, Sept/Oct, 4*–11.

Lovejoy, M. (1982). Expectations and the recovery process. *Schizophrenia Bulletin, 8,* 605–609.

Markus, H. (1983). Self knowledge: An expanded view. *Journal of Personality, 51,* 543–562.

Matsutsuyu, J. (1969). The interest checklist. *American Journal of Occupational Therapy, 23,* 323–328.

Matthews, P. R. (1980). Why the mentally retarded do not participate in certain types of recreational activities. *Therapeutic Recreation Journal, 14,* 44–50.

Meissner, W. W. (1982). Notes on the potential differentiation of borderline conditions. *Psychoanalytic Review, 70,* 179–209.

Menninger, K. (1962). Hope. In S. Doniger (Ed.), *The nature of man in theological and psychological perspective.* New York: Harper Brothers.

Miller, J. F., & Oertel, C. B. (1983). Powerlessness in the elderly: Preventing hopelessness. In J. F. Miller (Ed.), *Coping with chronic illness: Overcoming powerlessness.* Philadelphia: FA Davis.

Mitchell, A. (1983). *The nine American lifestyles.* New York: Macmillan.

Mitchell, D., & Snyder, S. (in press). An 'infinity of forms: ' Figuring disability in the archives. In B. Brueggemann, S. Snyder, & R. Thompson (Eds.), *Enabling the humanities: A sourcebook in disability studies.* New York: Modern Languages Association.

Mitchell, J. J. (1975). *The adolescent predicament.* Toronto: Holt, Winston.

Mitic, T. D., & Stevenson, C. L. (1981). Mentally retarded people as a resource to the recreationist in planning for integrated community recreation. *Journal of Leisure Research, 8,* 30–34.

Molnar, G. E. (1989). The influence of psychosocial factors on personality development and emotional health in children with cerebral palsy and spina bifida. In B. W. Heller, L. M. Flohr, & L. S. Zegans (Eds.), *Psychosocial interventions with physically disabled persons.* New Brunswick, NJ: Rutgers University Press.

Moss, J. W. (1958). *Failure-avoiding and stress-striving behavior in mentally retarded and normal children.* Ann Arbor, MI: University Microfilms.

Murphy, R. (1987). *The body silent.* New York: WW Norton.

Neville, A. M. (1987). *The relationship of locus of control, future time perspective and interest to productivity among individuals with varying degrees of depression.* Unpublished doctoral dissertation, New York University.

Oliver, M. (1996). The social model in context. *Understanding disability from theory to practice.* New York: St. Martin's Press, pp. 30–42.

Patsy, D., & Kielhofner, G. (1989). *An exploratory study of psychosocial adaptation to spinal cord injury.* Unpublished manuscript.

Rabinowitz, H. S., & Mitsos, S. B. (1964). Rehabilitation as planned social change: A conceptual framework. *Journal of Health and Social Behavior, 5,* 2–13.

Roberts, E. V. (1989). A history of the independent living movement: A founder's perspective. In B. W. Heller, L. M. Flohr, & L. S. Zegans (Eds.), *Psychosocial interventions with physically disabled persons.* New Brunswick, NJ: Rutgers University Press.

Rogers, J. C., & Figone, J. J. (1978). The avocational pursuits of rehabilitants with traumatic quadriplegia. *American Journal of Occupational Therapy, 32,* 571–576.

Rogers, J. C., & Figone, J. J. (1979). Psychosocial parameters in treating the person with quadriplegia. *American Journal of Occupational Therapy, 33,* 432–439.

Rotter, J. B. (1960). Generalized expectancies for internal versus external control of reinforcement. *Psychological Monographs: General Applications, 80,* 1–28.

Scaffa, M. (1982). *Temporal adaptation and alcoholism.* Unpublished master's thesis, Virginia Commonwealth University, Richmond.

Schiamberg, L. B. (1973). *Adolescent alienation.* Columbus, OH: Merrill.

Scotch, R. (1988). Disability as a basis for a social movement: Advocacy and the politics of definition. *Journal of Social Issues, 44* (1), 159–172.

Shapiro, J. (1994). *No pity. People with disabilities forging a new civil rights movement.* New York. Times Books.

Sienkiewicz-Mercer, R., & Kaplan, S. B. (1989). *I raise my eyes to say yes.* New York: Avon Books.

Skinner, E. A., Chapman, M., & Baltes, P. B. (1988). Control, means-end, and agency beliefs: A new conceptualization and its measurement during childhood. *Journal of Personality and Social Psychology, 54,* 117–133.

Smith, M. B. (1969). *Social psychology and human values.* Chicago: Aldine.

Smyntek, L. E. (1983). *A comparison of occupationally functional and dysfunctional adolescents.* Unpublished master's project, Virginia Commonwealth University, Richmond.

Spivak, G., Siegel, J., Sklaver, D., Deuschle, L., & Garrett, L. (1982). The long-term patient in the community: Lifestyle patterns and treatment implications. *Hospital Community Psychiatry, 33,* 291–295.

Trieschmann, R. B. (1989). Psychosocial adjustment to spinal cord injury. In B. W. Heller, L. M. Flohr, & L. S. Zegans (Eds.), *Psychosocial interventions with physically disabled persons.* New Brunswick, NJ: Rutgers University Press.

Turner, R. W., Ward, M. F., & Turner, D. J. (1979). Behavioral treatment for depression: An evaluation of therapeutic components. *Journal of Clinical Psychology, 35,* 166–175.

Valient, G. E. (1994). Ego mechanisms of defense and personality psychopathology. *Journal of Abnormal Psychology, 103,* 44–50.

Vash, C. L. (1981). *The psychology of disability.* New York: Springer-Verlag.

Wasserman, G. A. (1986). Affective expression in normal and physically handicapped infants. Situational and developmental effects. *Journal of the American Academy of Child and Adolescent Psychiatry, 25,* 393–399.

Werner-Beland, J. A. (Ed.). (1980). *Grief responses to long-term illness and disability.* Reston, VA: Reston Publishing.

Werthman, C. (1976). The function of sociological definitions in the development of the gang boy's career. In R. Giallombardo (Ed.), *Juvenile delinquency: A book of readings* (3rd ed.). New York: John Wiley & Sons.

Wright, B. A. (1960). *Physical disability: A psychological approach.* New York: Harper & Row.

Wylie, R. (1979). *The self-concept: Theory and research* (2nd ed.). Lincoln, NE: University of Nebraska Press.

Youkilis, H., & Bootzin, R. (1979). The relationship between adjustment and perceived locus of control in female psychiatric in-patients. *Journal of Genetic Psychology, 135,* 297–299.

Zane, M. D., & Lowenthal, M. (1960). Motivation in rehabilitation of the physically handicapped. *Archive of Physical Medicine and Rehabilitation, 41,* 400–407.

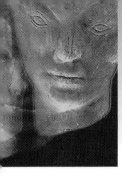

5

Habituation: Patterns of Daily Occupation

● Gary Kielhofner

Much of what we do everyday resembles what we have done before. We structure our days much as we have structured previous days. We traverse familiar routes. We carry out interactions with others that mimic previous encounters. We go about completing a range of tasks as before. We do these routine things automatically, without the necessity of planning or reflecting on what we are doing.

Chapter 2 proposed that these familiar and automatic aspects of daily life are a function of habituation. **Habituation** is an internalized readiness to exhibit consistent patterns of behavior guided by our habits and roles and fitted to the characteristics of routine temporal, physical, and social environments. As shown in *Figure 5-1,* habituation allows persons to appreciate their environments to cooperate with them in doing routine actions.

Appreciation refers to the routine way in which we recognize the action significance of certain aspects of the environment. For example, when encountering a familiar person we recognize an occasion for a greeting. When we come to a familiar intersection on our route to work we know it is where we should turn left. When the alarm sounds in the morning we know to rise from bed. Our habituated reading of such cues in the environment allows us to collaborate with the environment to accomplish routine actions. The tools, materials, events, and people of our environments have stable features that we have incorporated into how we do routine things. Habituation is orchestrated to fit with, take advantage of, and accommodate those various environmental characteristics.

Whereas it is recurrent and stable, habituated action is not predetermined and rigid. Rather, habituation involves a strategy of action. These strategies for doing things are preserved as habits and roles. They shape much of what we do in our temporal, physical, and social contexts.

Interdependency of Habituation and Habitat

The regularity in our habituated behavior depends on the reliability of our habitats. A degree of sameness in the physical environment provides a stable arena for performance. The recurring temporal patterns—such as day and night, workweek and weekend—provide a stable structure within which routines unfold. Similarly, the social order has sufficient stability to furnish us known situations for which we have ways of responding. Because of the regularity of our environments, we are mostly grounded in the familiar, not having to calculate our moves consciously. As Young (1988, p. 79) notes, habituated performances are "generated and locked into place by recurrences."

Habituation involves the internalization of action-oriented representations that, in the words of Clarke (1997, p. 49), "simultaneously describe aspects of the world and prescribe possible actions." When we repeat behavior in a constant context, we learn to filter out a whole array of things about the environment that are irrelevant to what we are doing and to selectively attend to those that are relevant. We learn to attend to aspects of the environment that will help sculpt the action that is part of any habit or role.

Habits

Habits are curiously elusive. What exactly do we mean by habits? Young (1988) notes that a defining characteristic of habits is that they are automatic. Camic

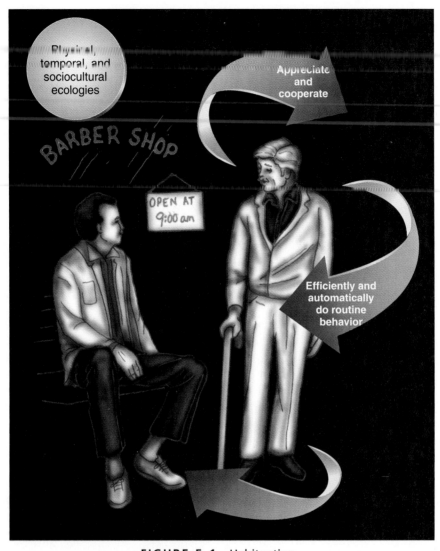

FIGURE 5-1 Habituation.

(1986, p. 1044) describes a habit as "a more or less self-actuating disposition or tendency to engage in a previously adopted or acquired form of action." Dewey (1922, p. 40) also recognizes habits as involving "a certain ordering . . . of action." He proposes that habits organize the smallest elements of action into a pattern or way of doing things. Clarke (1997) emphasizes that habits are dependent on familiar contexts for their execution. Based on these ideas, **habits** can be defined as acquired tendencies to automatically respond and perform in certain, consistent ways in familiar environments or situations.

> *We incorporate features of the environment into how we go about doing habitual things.*

Habit as a Grammar of Action

The idea of habits as automatic might suggest that they consist of prepackaged strings of actions that simply unfold. However, habits regulate behavior not by fixed instructions for behavior, but by providing a regulated manner of dealing with environmental contingencies. In this regard, Dewey (1922, p. 42) notes, "the essence of habit is an acquired disposition to ways or modes of response, not to particular acts." Camic (1986) echoes this idea, noting that while habitual behavior may be automatic, it is no more mechanical than action that is guided by conscious reflection. Young (1988, p. 91) points out that habits have rules that guide automatic behavior, but goes on to explain that "these rules are flexible, more like the grammar than a particular sentence." Similarly, Koestler (1969) refers to habits as operating much like the rules of a game, which keep order among players by letting them know how to play the game without dictating in advance everything they will do.

Bourdieu (1977, p. 82) refers to habits as "a system of lasting, transposable dispositions which, integrating past experiences, functions at every moment as a matrix of perceptions, appreciations and actions." He underscores that when one learns a habit, one learns a set of rules for how to simultaneously appreciate and act in the world. Appreciating the environment means that we automatically locate ourselves in the midst of familiar environmental features, apprehending their action implications for a habitual behavior we are doing. For example, in the routine of getting dressed, people automatically recognize which piece of clothing goes where and which pieces of clothing need to be donned before others. Even when we find ourselves in somewhat novel but recognizable environments such as a hotel room, we can appreciate where to hang our clothes, where our toiletries should go, where we will bathe, and so on. We attend to and comprehend our environments in terms of their implications for our routine doing. We incorporate features of the environment into how we go about doing habitual things. Therefore, a large component of any habitual action will be strategies for incorporating the things, people, and events around us into what we do.

So long as we experience the world as familiar, habits operate smoothly and without need of attention. It is the unfamiliar (i.e., that for which we do not have internalized rules) that extricates us from our habitual way of doing things. Consequently, habits operate as internalized, appreciative capacities for recognizing familiar events and contexts and for guiding action. Habits give us a way to appreciate and construct action appropriate to what is going on in the world around us.

Effectiveness and Efficiency of Habits

Habits preserve a way we have learned to do something from earlier performance in a given environment. Only after action proves effective in some way, and is therefore repeated over and over, does it become habituated. For instance, we may take the wrong turn on a journey, but over time such ineffective or inefficient action is weeded out. Repeated journeys incorporate and eventually put into place a series of turns that allow us to reach the destination. In a whole range of tasks, persons settle into ways of performing actions that are realized over time and that incorporate successful ways of doing something. This is not to say that all habits are the most efficient ways to accomplish tasks or undertake a process, but habits will incorporate ways of doing things that have a certain value within the environment in which they are performed. As Camic (1986) notes, the habitual organization of routine activities allows us to perform them in a consistent and effective manner. As a consequence of habits, we are able to go about much of our everyday lives depending on ways of doing things that consistently accomplish our intentions.

> *Habits hold together the patterns of ordinary action that give life its familiar and relatively effortless character.*

Habits hold together the patterns of ordinary action that give life its familiar and relatively effortless character. Young (1988) argues that habits serve as a kind of self-perpetuating flywheel conserving patterns of action. Once launched, habits provide a momentum that allows action to unfold on its own. This frees up conscious attention for other purposes. In this regard James (1950) notes:

The more of the details of our daily life we can hand over to the effortless custody of automatism, the more our higher powers of mind will be set free for their own proper work. There is no more miserable human being than one in whom nothing is habitual. (p. 122)

As James alludes, habits can allow two or more behaviors to occur simultaneously. While one is performing habituated behaviors (e.g., getting dressed in the morning, driving home after work) it is possible to engage in other thoughts and behaviors (e.g., making a phone call, planning a meeting, or listening to the radio). Therefore, habits decrease the effort required for occupational performance not only by reducing the amount of conscious attention required, but also freeing up persons for other simultaneous activity. In sum, habits produce patterns of behavior that are both effective and efficient.

Social Relevance of Habits

Habits also serve a purpose for society. Young (1988) notes that habits shared by a group of people constitute social customs. Thus, by acquiring habits humans become carriers and messengers of the customs that make up the way of life of a particular group. Moreover, in a social group one person's habitual behavior may be part of the environmental context necessary for another's habits. For example, Rowles (1991) provided the following description of a group of elderly men engaging in the habit of gathering at the post office:

Every morning, shortly before 10:00 a.m., Walter takes a leisurely 400-yard stroll down the hill from his house to the trailer that serves as the post office to "pick up the mail." He traces exactly the same path each day. Several male age peers from different locations within Colton embark on the same trip at about the same time . . . picking up the mail provides a rationale for an informal gathering of the elderly men of the community at the bench outside the Colton Store, which is located adjacent to the post office. The men generally linger throughout the morning. They watch the passing traffic, converse with patrons of the store, and discuss events of the day. Then, around lunchtime, the group disperses and Walter wends his way home again. (p. 268)

Walter's habit of getting the mail and meeting with other older residents illustrates how habits guide us to take advantage of, and be in harmony with, others' behavior (Cardwell, 1971).

Our typical behaviors are to a large extent those recognized, expected, and depended on by others in the environment. For example, the habits of punctuality and industriousness reflect typical expectations of Western society. One is to be at work, meetings, and appointments at scheduled times and to focus on the task at hand during periods so designated. A person who is not punctual or attentive to work tasks will not be in synchrony with such an environment. Consequently, habits also allow a person to be integrated into the smooth functioning of society.

Three Influences of Habits in Daily Occupations

The influence of habits on everyday behavior is pervasive (Camic, 1986). What we do, when we do it, and how we go about it reflect our habits. As shown in *Figure 5-2*, we can recognize three influences of habits:

- Habits impact how routine activity is performed
- Habits regulate how time is typically used
- Habits generate styles of behavior that characterize a range of occupational performances.

HABITS OF OCCUPATIONAL PERFORMANCE

Each person has his or her own way of performing routine activities such as grooming and dressing, making the bed, preparing morning coffee, taking out the dog, paying bills, and going to work or school. Habits may fit with our ideas about proper etiquette or form. They may reflect the way a parent or mentor taught us. They may simply emanate from what is simplest and most efficient. Whatever the reasons, people tend to be firmly entrenched in their particular ways of doing familiar activities.

> *Although the habitual ways of doing almost everything we do go largely unnoticed, getting through the day without them would be unbearably cumbersome.*

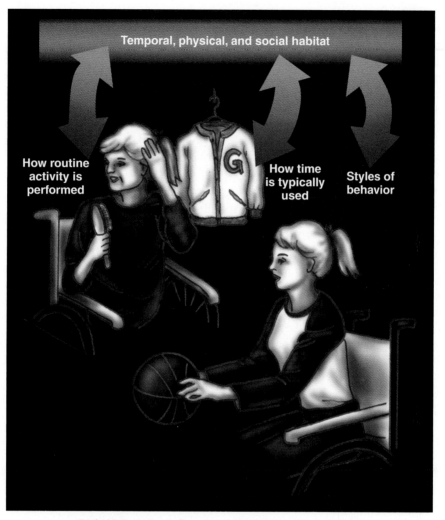

FIGURE 5-2 Influences of Habits on Occupation.

Seamon (1980) noted that habits ordinarily involve a sequence of physical movements. He refers to them as body ballets, noting that they are "a set of integrated behaviors which sustain a particular task or aim" (p. 157). Habitual ways of performing ordinary activities organize actions together to accomplish a goal under routine conditions. For example, in driving to the train station on workdays, my morning routine includes transporting my briefcase and coffee to the car while opening and then closing the garage door. There are a variety of minor variations in my environment that might slightly alter the routine (e.g., my wife has

already opened the garage door, our dog is begging for a treat in the garage, or I am carrying an umbrella in addition to my briefcase). However, almost every morning, without thinking about it, my briefcase ends up in the back seat and my coffee mug next to me in its holder. For this to happen, I have to manipulate not only the briefcase and mug, but also a doorknob, garage door button, keys, and car door handle. My keys are already in my pocket as part of my dressing routine and I ordinarily carry my briefcase to the kitchen so it is handy to take out with the coffee to the car in one trip. On careful examination this routine could be accomplished in any number of ways. Nonetheless, there is a way in which I generally do it that has evolved out of my repeated forays to the car in the morning in my familiar home environment.

I depend on this routine performance as an essential part of my workday. Moreover, much of my day consists of similar routine ways of doing things. Each of these will reflect both my own idiosyncrasies and conditions in my environment.

Dewey (1922, p. 24) referred to such daily habits as "passive tools waiting to be called into action." Indeed, our habits are tools of a sort that we call upon to get done what we do in ordinary life. Although the habitual ways of doing almost everything we do go largely unnoticed, getting through the day without them would be unbearably cumbersome.

HABITS OF ROUTINE

The influence of habits is also found in our routine use of time. Seamon (1980) refers to such habits as time-space routines since they are ordinarily linked not only to what time it is but also to where we are or how we are moving through space. He offers the following description of such a routine:

> He would be up at seven-thirty, make his bed, perform his morning toilet, and be out of his house by eight. He would then walk to the corner cafe up the street, pick up the newspaper (which *had* to be the *New York Times*), order his usual fare (one scrambled egg, toast, and coffee), and stay there until around nine when he would walk to his nearby office. (p. 158)

Each of us will recognize similar routine use of time that characterizes our everyday patterns.

Chapin (1968) points out that our routines include not only daily habits but habits within a variety of temporal cycles:

> . . . cooking, eating and washing dishes during the twenty-four hour period of a day; the work, school, shopping, recreation or socializing routine during a seven day week; visiting out-of-town relatives and family vacation or other holiday outing routines during a year's time . . . (p. 13)

Consequently, routines may be linked to a variety of cycles. Some cycles are tied to the kind of work one does. For example, teachers have changing routines across the school term and farmers' routines depend on the seasons.

Our routine use of time serves a variety of personal needs. For example, it allows fulfillment of biological needs for nourishment, exercise, and rest and psychological needs for a rhythm of work and leisure. Our routines, even when we find them demanding, do provide a degree of structure and predictability to life. In a longitudinal study of retirement, one of the greatest challenges for older persons was to find a new routine after working (Jonsson, Josephsson, & Kielhofner, 2001). While no two days are exactly the same, most persons have and can identify a routine that is typical for a given day of the week. In industrialized societies persons generally have patterns that characterize schooldays and workdays as well as alternate patterns that characterize days off from work or school. The degree of consistency in a routine depends on one's environment. Some environments demand a fixed routine such as the grade school or factory schedule that requires persons to show up, do certain tasks, take lunch and breaks, and terminate the day at specific times. Other environments require a more flexible pattern of action.

Habits of routine help locate us effectively within the stream of time. They enable us to be where we should be and get done what we should be doing over the course of daily, weekly, and other life cycles. To a very large extent, our everyday lives are defined and shaped by these cyclical routines. They create the overall pattern by which we go about our various occupations.

HABITS OF STYLE

Dewey (1922, p. 20) noted that one's habits were reflected in a typical "style of . . . being-in-the-world." Such characteristics as being big-picture versus detail-oriented, quick versus plodding, or prompt versus procrastinating are examples of styles of performance regulated by habits. Habits of style are also found in our interpersonal behavior. Whether we tend to be quiet or talkative, direct or evasive, trusting or cautious, and formal or informal are examples of social habits of style.

Habits of style are manifest across a whole range of activities. That is, we tend to bring our personal styles to the performance of all that we do. Camic (1986) defines such habits as:

The durable and generalized disposition that suffuses a person's action throughout an entire domain of life or, in the extreme instance, throughout all of life—in which case the term comes to mean the whole manner, turn, cast, or mold of the personality. (p. 1045)

Indeed, habits of style give a unique and stable character to one's performance.

Some habits of style clearly emanate from biological dispositions such as a person's arousal and energy level. Moreover, such habits will change with biological changes, the most obvious example being the slowing down with age. Another source of influence on habits of style is culture. For example, persons from southern European cultures will tend to be more relaxed and informal than persons from northern Europe. Habits of style may also be influenced by specific contexts. Persons working in an emergency department or in a fire department must be capable of completing routines swiftly. On the other hand, work in a research laboratory may require a slow, painstaking, and careful pace of action. Not surprisingly, we seek out environments where the style of action fits our natural habits.

Habit Formation and Change

Children come into the world without internal regulators of patterned behavior save, perhaps, certain biorhythms. Soon, however, they are integrated into the rhythms, routines, and customs that make up the physical, social, and temporal world. Children first acquire routines through parental guidance and support. These are routines of day and night with the attending patterns of sleeping, waking, eating, bathing, and so on. Over the course of development, as routines, customs, and ways of doing things are reexperienced, the child incorporates complex habit patterns.

A number of these patterns remain somewhat stable throughout life, such as sleeping and eating patterns. Others change with the attainment of developmental stages such as entering the student or worker roles. Interestingly, each new environmental context has its own regular rhythms that encourage individuals to internalize a pattern of action like that of others in the social system. Eventually, a number of rhythms may interweave, such as the rhythms and patterns of home life and those of school or work life.

All habits serve to preserve patterns of action, so they are naturally resistant to change. Whenever we make alterations in our schedules or environments, we encounter the tenacity of old habits. We show up at old appointed times or we visit the wrong cabinet or office for some time after we have relocated where we keep things or where we work.

Habits resist change since they are based on our most fundamental certainties about how the world is constructed (Berger & Luckman, 1966). Habits presuppose a particular order in the physical, temporal, and social world. When habits and their background assumptions are disrupted or altered, a feeling of disorientation or unreality follows. For example, when our sleep patterns are disrupted or altered we can find ourselves waking up without the usual sense of being firmly anchored in the temporal world (i.e., thinking it is dawn when it is really dusk). A similar feeling of disorientation can occur when we are in the midst of a familiar task and lose our place (e.g., suddenly realizing we do not recognize where we are on the road when driving to a familiar destination). In such cases, we are shocked into sudden consciousness with no clear footing in what is ordinarily a familiar and taken-for-granted world.

Children remind us of how important this taken-for-granted background is when they react with extreme displeasure to disruptions of routines. Dewey (1922) referred to this aspect of habits, noting:

. . . a routine habit, when interfered with generates uneasiness, sets up a protest in favor of restoration and a sense of need of some expiatory act, or else it goes off in casual reminiscence. It is the essence of routine to insist upon its own continuation . . . (p. 76)

Habits and Disability

Habits organize our use of underlying performance capacity so that we can perform within our environment. The fit of our habits to our performance capacity and to our environment will determine how effective we are in our everyday routines. Habits play an especially important role when persons face the challenges of a disability. As the following discussions show, habits may either contribute to a disability or they may effectively compensate for underlying impairments.

DYSFUNCTIONAL HABITS

We intuitively know that the wrong habits can negatively affect us. All of us have possessed habits we would rather have been without. Sometimes, however, dysfunctional habits become more than a nuisance. They become a serious liability threatening one's welfare (Kielhofner, Barris, & Watts, 1982).

Acquired impairments can lead to an erosion of habits that further exacerbate the consequences of these functional limitations. For example, persons facing depression may be unable to pursue their routines because of limited motivation and energy (American Psychiatric Association, 2000). Over time, this can lead to an erosion of habits that contributes to inactivity (Melges, 1982). When this happens and the person loses previously effective and satisfying routines, mood and energy can be further degraded. In such cases, the disruption of habits becomes part of a downward spiral. Impairments negatively affect habits and their disruption further exacerbates the symptoms and/or consequences of the underlying condition.

Another habit problem associated with disability is that persons may learn dysfunctional habits due to their environments. For example, the inactivity imposed by hospitalization can contribute to the loss of habits. Unfortunately, opportunities for persons to practice old or new habits are often not provided during rehabilitation (Shillam, Beeman, & Loshin, 1983). Many persons with more severe emotional and cognitive impairments are placed in institutional environments. In such settings the routines can result in residents learning habits of passivity and inactivity that do not serve them well in the institution or later when they are placed in the larger community (Borell, Gustausson, Sandman, & Kielhofner, 1994; Kielhofner, 1979, 1981, 1983).

IMPACT OF IMPAIRMENTS ON HABITS

When capacities are diminished, previously established habits can be severely disrupted. One may be forced to develop new habits for many or most aspects of everyday life. Alterations in a person's functional status can totally disrupt the effectiveness of an existing habit. Zola (1982) illustrates this in his description of trying to complete his morning routine from the new viewpoint of a wheelchair:

> *When habits cannot automatically regulate what one does, additional effort and concentration are required, taking away the ease and efficiency that ordinarily accompany everyday routines.*

Washing up was a mess. Though the sink was low enough, I nevertheless managed to soak myself thoroughly. In retrospect, I should not have worn anything. Ordinarily when washing my face, chest, and arms, I would lean over the sink, and any excess water from my splashing would drip into it. My body angle in a wheelchair was different. I could not extend over the sink very far without tipping. Thus, much of the water dripped down my neck onto me. Splashing with water was out, and the use of a damp washcloth, what I once called a "sponge bath," was in. (p. 64)

When impairments are more pronounced so are the complications of everyday routines. When persons have to make extensive use of adaptive equipment or require assistance from other persons, entirely new routines must be acquired. Sometimes, new habits related to the management of the disability are required. For example, people may need to learn new habits for bowel and bladder care, for joint protection and energy conservation, or for following complicated medication regimens. Remissions and exacerbations, or progressive decreases in physical functioning, can make acquiring these necessary new habits difficult.

Disabled persons whose abilities are variable may need to develop extremely flexible habits. For example, persons with unpredictable impairments must be ready to capitalize on those times when things are better such as the following gentleman with Parkinson's disease:

I cram in to the periods when I'm flexible all the things I would have liked to have done the rest of the day . . . One day I may be nine-tenths of the day free, although that's very rare, and another much less. There's nothing I can do about it. (Pinder, 1988, p. 79)

On the other hand, steadily progressive impairments may mean that habits are to an extent replaced with conscious strategies. For example, Murphy (1987) explains how his progressive paralysis meant that everyday routines had to be calculated. As he notes, the routine of transferring from wheelchair to toilet required him to strategize how to get up, "choosing . . . supports with care, calculating the number of steps it would take to reach [the toilet]" (p. 76). When habits cannot automatically regulate what one does, additional effort and concentration are required, taking away the ease and efficiency that ordinarily accompany everyday routines.

DISRUPTION OF SPACE AND TIME

The onset of a severe impairment can radically alter the spatial and temporal dimensions of routine performance. For example, the spinal-cord–injured person must learn to organize behavior around the constraints of where one can go in a wheelchair and how long it will take (Paap, 1972). With the onset of a disability, the entire relationship of persons with their environments may change in dramatic ways, resulting in the need for new habits. In this regard Hull (1990) notes:

> On the whole, my experience has been that, if I have a bad habit, it . . . is naturally corrected . . . In other words, blindness itself imposes an iron law upon the user of the white cane. Lampposts, curbs, and stairways are the best teachers. (p. 15)

In similar fashion, wheelchairs or other devices to assist walking require their users to choose not simply the closest route to a destination, but rather the route with friendly ramps, curbs, and surfaces. The habits that accommodate a new disability must not only deal with altered performance capacity, but must also grapple with a physical world whose implications for action are radically changed. Additionally, people can become more vulnerable to external contingencies such as bad weather or crowded public places.

Time also becomes a different matter. When their impairments require additional time to conduct routine tasks, persons must develop daily routines that involve doing fewer things. Such temporal challenges can be further constrained by the necessity of adding new self-care habits to the daily routine.

Reconstructing Habits

As the previous discussions illustrated, the task of organizing daily life in the face of disability means reconstructing one's habits. Accommodations and trade-offs must take place. Some activities may need to be eliminated. New ways of doing things must be discovered and learned. Finally, one may have to delegate some tasks to family members or an attendant to have time for other more valued activities.

As Williams (1984) notes:

> If the disabled individual is to move toward "mere" impairment, eventually alternative ways of accomplishing the tasks of everyday life will be committed to memory and habit, engrained in relationships with a new world which is once again "had." (p. 110)

The path to these new habits involves leaving behind a once familiar world that has been invalidated by disability. As Merleau-Ponty (1945/1962) notes:

> It is precisely when my customary world arouses in me habitual intentions that I can no longer, if I have lost a limb, be effectively drawn into it: the utilizable objects, precisely in so far as they present themselves as utilizable, appeal to a hand I no longer have. (p. 82)

Only by reencountering the world with one's altered condition can a new relationship to the world emerge and once again become familiar and taken for granted. DeLoach and Greer describe this transformation (1981) in the following way:

> A person begins to learn new ways of doing what she did before—and ways of accomplishing, as well, some brand-new things. These new, different ways are, at first, awkward, stress-producing, and frustrating . . . little by little, a person gets accustomed to a new modus operandi. What at first was awkward, painful, or embarrassing becomes just a regular part of living, incorporated into one's routine. After such habituation, the person begins to concentrate more on participation in life now rather than on what used to be or what might have been. (p. 251)

As they indicate, the transformation of habits is a necessary pathway through which persons find their way back to the participation in everyday activities of daily living, work, and leisure.

Internalized Roles

Routine action is influenced by the fact that each of us belongs to and acts in social systems. Much of what we do is done as a spouse, parent, worker, student, and so on. Having internalized such roles, we act in ways that reflect our role status (Fein, 1990). Internalizing the role means taking on an identity, an outlook, and actions that belong to the role. Consequently, an **internalized role** is the incorporation of a socially and/or personally defined status and a related cluster of attitudes and actions.

Internalizing a role involves gaining a sense of one's relationships to others and of expected behaviors. As Sarbin and Scheibe (1983, p. 8) note, effective action depends on the "correct placements of self in the world of occurrences." Consequently, internalized roles give us the necessary social bearings to act effectively. Interaction is made less problematic when people share fundamental expectations of what it means to be in a given role relationship. When we know our role relationship to others, we recognize both how they see and should act toward us and what should be our attitudes and actions toward them.

> *When we know our role relationship to others, we recognize both how they see and should act toward us and what should be our attitudes and actions toward them.*

Role Identification

We see ourselves as students, workers, parents, and so on because we recognize ourselves as occupying certain statuses or positions and also because we experience ourselves acting as someone who holds these roles. As Sarbin and Scheibe (1983, p. 7) note, "a person's identity at any time is a function of his or her validated social positions." We identify with our roles in part because we see ourselves reflected in the

attitudes and actions of others toward us. Consequently, role identity is generated when others recognize and respond to us as occupying a particular status.

Who we are is intertwined with the roles we inhabit (Cardwell, 1971; Ruddock, 1976; Schein, 1971; Turner, 1962). This is not to say that everyone who inhabits a given role experiences the same role identity. Rather, the internalized role is highly personal. As Fein (1990, p. 13) notes, a person's "own way of understanding what she is doing defines her role. It is her intentions and understandings which make the role what it is." Identifying with any role means both internalizing elements of what society attributes to the role along with one's personal interpretation of that role. For example, one person may develop a student role identity that stresses being an intellectual. For such a person being a student may resonate with the volitional sense of having intellectual capacity, interests, and values. Another student, whose interest and values lie elsewhere, may view the student role as only instrumental to gaining a credential. Both inhabit the student role, but the ways in which they internalize it, identify with it, and enact its expectations will differ significantly.

Whatever way we come to think of and experience ourselves in a role becomes part of our self-understanding. To an extent, we see ourselves and judge our actions in terms of our own perception of the roles we inhabit. As Miller (1983) argues, personal identity reflects our awareness of all our various roles. Integrating one's various roles into a personal identity involves assigning centrality or importance to some roles over others. This process is dynamic and changes over time as different roles assume different places in our lives or demand extra effort or attention (Hall, Stevens, & Meleis, 1992; Hammel, 1999).

However, not all roles have a clearly defined social status. Some roles are more informal. Some arise out of personal circumstances (Hammel, 1999; Rosow, 1976). One example of an informal role without a clear social status is that of caregiver for a disabled spouse or parent (Schumacher, 1995). Such roles that do not correspond to a formal social status have more ambiguous meanings and expectations attached to them. Consequently, internalization of such roles requires more improvisation. Persons are often left to impart their definition on the role and to find social partners who will recognize and validate the role. This is one of the reasons that support groups are so popular. They often provide persons access to others who, like themselves, occupy a role that is not well defined. In such groups persons find validation for their role and sort out what are reasonable expectations for the role.

Role Scripts

People know how to act in a given role because of an internalized role script. Miller (1983, p. 319) notes that this script consists of "a set of schemas that organize how persons perceive, communicate, make judgments, and act toward others." These scripts allow persons to make sense of events because the script anticipates what kind of interaction or actions should occur (Mancuso & Sarbin, 1983). Similarly, Fein (1990) notes:

> Lurking behind all roles are role scripts. These are the structures that guide people during the performance of their behavior patterns. They give role players a general idea of what is expected of them and with whom they are supposed to interact. These scripts are not explicit sets of instructions, but guidelines for how to improvise a part. (p. 18)

Role scripts allow one to tacitly appreciate what social event is underway and how one should proceed in this event. For example, how we perform a greeting is guided by the role relationship we have with another. Depending on whether a pair is parent and child, worker and boss, student and teacher, or two close friends, the greeting may take on quite different forms. Consequently, we find ourselves ordinarily performing a range of role-related actions without reflection but with remarkable consistency.

Fein (1990) also notes that since roles are negotiated in interactions, the expectations and behaviors of others combine with the role script to guide the improvisation of behavior. Stryker (1968) highlights the improvisational nature of interactional role behavior, describing it as "a subtle, tentative, probing interchange among actors in given situations that continually reshapes both the form and the context of the interaction" (p. 559). Like habits, roles generate not specific actions but rather a way of acting.

Influences of Roles on Occupation

As shown in *Figure 5-3,* roles organize action in three main ways. First, they influence the manner and content of our actions. Moving from one role to another is often demarcated by such changes as how we dress, our manner of speech, and our way of relating to others. Second, each role carries with it a range of actions that makes up that role. Consequently, roles shape what kinds of things we do. For example, a student is expected to attend class, take notes, ask questions, read articles or books, complete assignments, study, and take exams. The actions expected for a role are clearly defined by some social groups. In other situations, persons must negotiate or define for themselves what actions make up the role.

Third, roles partition our daily and weekly cycles into times when we inhabit certain roles. The course of each day ordinarily involves a succession of roles and overlapping roles. Any parent who has attempted to talk on the phone with a coworker while holding a fussy baby and watching food on the stove will immediately appreciate how roles can overlap. Across our days, weeks, and lives, roles are social spaces that we enter, enact, and exit.

> *Across our days, weeks, and lives, roles are social spaces that we enter, enact, and exit.*

Socialization and Role Change

Beginning in childhood, we perceive others to fill positions that everyone takes for granted. The people who occupy such positions as mothers, teachers, and babysitters tend to behave in predictable ways. As time goes on, we discover that we too have been assigned roles. We learn that we are expected to act in certain ways because of the roles we occupy (Grossack & Gardner, 1970; Katz & Kahn, 1966; Turner, 1962).

The process of communicating role expectations is referred to as socialization (Brim & Wheeler, 1966). For example, as children develop, parents give them expectations for being a family member. These expecta-

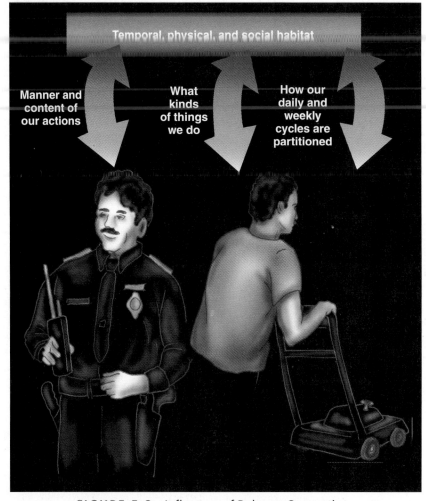

FIGURE 5-3   Influences of Roles on Occupation.

tions involve where and how to play, conformity to family routines, and the responsibilities for self-care and chores. These expectations for performance as a family member are generally more informal than the role expectations that come later in life. Thus, role socialization generally involves a developmental progression from informal to formal roles. This role progression parallels the child's growing ability to internalize role scripts and to use them as guides for action. Later in development, socialization may be much more formal, including education, practicing or apprenticing in the role, credentialing, and supervision. For many roles society goes to great lengths to socialize and regulate those who fill the role.

Persons being socialized into a new role typically negotiate their role in a give-and-take process (Heard, 1977; Schein, 1971). Each person fulfills a role uniquely but is also bound by how others are affected. An individual who enacts a role in ways that negatively affect others invites their invectives to conform to the role's expectations.

Socialization is an ongoing process because roles change throughout life. Society expects and structures role transitions at various life stages such as entering and exiting the student role, beginning work, and retiring. Persons also choose to enter and leave roles. Finally, role change is sometimes thrust on people by circumstances.

Role change is complex, involving alterations of one's identity, one's relationships to others, the tasks one is expected to perform, and how one's lifestyle is organized. An example of the complexity of role change is the experience of family members when aging parents require children to take care of them. This circumstance entails:

> A clear reversal of roles as the older generation loses power, and the authority to make the most personal kinds of decisions gravitates into the hands of their children . . . Roles need to be thoroughly redefined, often in the face of stiff resistance and understandable resentment. (Hage & Powers, 1992, p. 118)

Thus, while role change is part and parcel of human development, it is often the occasion of significant reorganization within individuals and their social systems.

Roles and Disability

Disabled persons may be barred from, have difficulty performing, or lack opportunities to learn or enter occupational roles. In addition, having a disability can assign one to unwanted, marginal roles. Consequently, living with a disability poses a number of challenges for occupying roles.

ROLE PERFORMANCE DIFFICULTIES ASSOCIATED WITH DISABILITY

Disability often presents itself as a problem with role performance. For example, a common factor that leads persons with mental illness or substance abuse problems to enter mental health care is a failure in school or work roles (Black, 1976; Mechanic, 1980). Adolescents with mental illness have more problems in academic, leisure, and work roles than their peers (Barris, Dickie, & Baron, 1988; Barris, Kielhofner, Burch, Gelinas, Klement, & Schultz,1986; Holzman & Grinker, 1974; Offer, Ostrov, & Howard, 1981).

Problems with role behavior may occur when one has not internalized appropriate role scripts and, therefore, one does not meet the expectations of the social group. By virtue of having a disability, people may have fewer experiences in which to acquire role scripts (Smith, 1972; Versluys, 1983). For example, persons with cognitive impairments are often denied access to opportunities to learn adult roles (Guskin, 1963; Kielhofner, 1983; Wolfensberger, 1975). In such cases, limitations of capacity are magnified by the lack of learning experiences.

Limitations of physical capacity may disrupt or terminate role performance. In other cases, a person can retain a role only by making major modifications in how the role is enacted. For example, a person who acquires a disability may continue as a worker but needs to engage in a new type of work. In many instances, this can mean moving to a lesser-paying job.

A disability may create problems of role performance such as being unable to discharge the role in ways consistent with one's own or others' expectations for the role. For example, persons whose impairments are not visible to others may be viewed by friends, family, or coworkers as malingering (Schiffer, Rudick, & Herndon, 1983). In other cases the conflict may be between one's own view of the role and how one is able to perform. For example, one gentleman who has multiple sclerosis, notes of his family roles: "I feel left out of discipline over the children because I am static in an armchair and cannot even phone the school. I had lost the ability to be a real father and husband" (Robinson, 1988, p. 60). Hull (1990) similarly describes how being blind has robbed him of the ability to supervise and to participate in play with his children, eroding and constricting what kind of father he can be. Such shifts in the identity and function of ongoing roles can be sources of conflict and self-devaluation.

Role strain may occur when a person cannot meet the multiple obligations or aspirations represented in several roles (Beutell & Greenhaus, 1983; Coser, 1974; Gerson, 1976; Gray; 1972). Impairments may require persons to exert more time and energy toward maintaining such major life roles as work or homemaking, requiring them to relinquish other roles (Hallet, Zasler, Maurer, & Cash, 1994; Hammel, 1999). Overall, persons with disabilities tend to occupy fewer roles than their non-disabled counterparts (Dickerson, & Oakely, 1995; Ebb, Coster, & Duncombe, 1989).

Social Barriers to Roles

Although impairments may contribute to difficulties in role performance, one of the most significant obstacles for persons with disabilities are social barriers (Hahn, 1985, 1988). For many people, the presence of a visible disability creates immediate difficulties of access to ordinary roles. Beginning in childhood, persons with disabilities may be discouraged or prevented from exploring, learning, and occupying roles. Such persons may be chronically frustrated as they are unable to attain a series of roles (Kielhofner, 1979, 1981). Social barriers to roles range from subtle attitudinal barriers that make social access difficult, to social policies whose consequence is to make roles inaccessible to persons with disabilities.

Sometimes barriers to roles are evident when people refuse to admit persons with disabilities into various social groups. One of the most dramatic examples is the area of work. Despite legislation in most industrialized countries that assures some equal access to the marketplace, persons with disabilities still have a harder time finding employment (Erikson, 1973; Trieschmann, 1989). In the United States less than one-third of severely disabled persons of working age work (Hale, Hayghe, & McNeil, 1998; Louis Harris and Associates, 1998; Trupin, Sebesta, Yelin, & LaPlante, 1997). Barriers to work include discrimination in the workplace and public policy that often penalizes persons financially or in terms of health benefits if they seek employment (Brandt & Pope, 1997; National Council on Disability, 1996).

Consequences of Role Loss and Rolelessness

Research suggests that involvement in too few roles is even more likely to be detrimental to psychosocial well-being than having too many role demands (Marks, 1977; Seiber, 1974; Spreitzer, Snyder, & Larson, 1979). Without sufficient roles one lacks identity, purpose, and structure in everyday life. For example, unemployment has been linked to suicide, depression, stress-related physical health problems, child abuse, and increased substance abuse (Borrero, 1980; Briar, 1980).

A loss of identity and self-esteem may occur as persons take on roles they believe to be less important or as they lose roles (Thomas, 1966; Werner-Beland, 1980). For example, Krefting (1989) notes:

> Most head-injured people remember parts of their old selves and recognize that the old self is gone. But they have nothing upon which to build a new self-identity. This is largely a result of lack of opportunity to fill legitimate roles in society. If an individual's personhood is not acknowledged by others, it is difficult for him or her to develop a sense of self-identity. (p. 76)

This view is echoed throughout accounts that persons with disabilities have given of themselves. There is a substantial cost to personal identity when persons no longer are recognized as the fathers, mothers, spouses, students, workers, caretakers, or friends that they used to be.

> *There is a substantial cost to personal identity when persons no longer are recognized as the fathers, mothers, spouses, students, workers, caretakers, or friends that they used to be.*

Sick and Disabled Roles

A number of writers have argued that disability may not only remove or bar one from occupational roles, but also relegate one to sick and deviant roles (Bogdan & Taylor, 1989; Parsons, 1953; Werner-Beland, 1980). When a person is ill, the normal social expectations for the worker role are typically suspended. Instead, one enters the sick role and is expected to conform to the ministrations and advice of medical personnel to get well. The sick role can be a problem for a person with a long-term illness or disability. For example, the sick role implies passivity and compliance (Parsons, 1953; McKeen, 1992), which can be counterproductive to individuals assuming responsibility for their lives and reentering occupational roles.

A case in point is Bill, diagnosed with sarcoma that required him to leave his job as a mechanic in order to undergo a regimen of surgery and chemotherapy over 3 years. Bill became accustomed to the sick role, in which others made decisions about the care that dominated his life. His identity as a cancer patient overshadowed other aspects of his identity. His interactions with others centered on his patienthood and his daily routine was dominated by the patient role. At the end of 3 years, Bill was left with an able body but found it overwhelming to consider reentry into work and other adult roles.

The reactions of others to a person with a disability can cast that person into a disabled role (Asch, 1998; Toombs, 1987; Werner-Beland, 1980). For example, others may unnecessarily lower their expectations of the person with a disability. They may become overly protective or helpful, or consider the person to be disabled beyond his or her actual limitations. Zola (1982) illustrates in the following passage how the experience of becoming a wheelchair user transformed his social interactions:

> As soon as I sat in the wheelchair I was no longer seen as a person who could fend for himself. Although Metz has known me well for nine months, and had never before done anything physical for me without asking, now he took over without permission. Suddenly, in his eyes, I was no longer able to carry things, reach for objects, or even push myself around. Though I was perfectly capable of doing all these things, I was being wheeled around, and things were being brought to me—all without my asking. Most frightening was my own compliance, my alienation from myself and from the process. (p. 52)

As he suggests, the identity of being disabled can, of itself, trigger new expectations and behaviors. This dramatic transformation validated the sensibleness of Zola's earlier attempts to avoid being cast into the role of a disabled person:

> I had separated myself early from the physically handicapped by refusing to attend a special residential school. Later, I had simply never socialized with anyone who had a chronic disease or physical handicap. I too had been seeking to gain a different identity through my associations. (Zola, 1982, p. 75)

Distancing oneself from the disabled role is understandable in light of social reactions to disability. However, by doing so people with disabilities are less likely to develop a positive identity as a disabled person or to engage in social and political action that might ameliorate social prejudice toward disability (Gill, 1997).

SELF MANAGER ROLE

Recently, Hammel (1999) has called attention to the fact that disabled persons must often take on a new self-manager role. This role involves an interrelated set of behaviors aimed at managing the medical, functional, economic, and social implications of a disability. This role includes such behaviors as engaging in necessary health maintenance behaviors, dealing with the finances of health and rehabilitative care, securing and using adaptive equipment, finding accessible housing, and hiring and supervising an attendant. Not surprisingly, this role involves substantial time and energy.

This self manager role becomes a significant part of personal identity, and the degree to which persons internalize and master this role influences the success of living in the community and assuming other life roles (Hammel, 1999). Nonetheless, this role does not carry social recognition or status. Thus, persons with disabilities must define the role for themselves and figure out on their own how to discharge it.

Habituation in Perspective

The purpose in this chapter has been to explain that which is patterned, familiar, and routine in human occupation. I have argued that these features of occupation are influenced by habituation, which consists of habits and internalized roles. We saw that habituation involves an appreciative capacity that allows us to automatically recognize and collaborate with features of the environment. Habituation plants us in the familiar territory of everyday life ready to interact with our physical, temporal, and social ecology.

All of us have encountered the disorientation and disruption that occurs when a habit or role has been altered or ended. When we have changed environments or left behind a role or habit, what was formerly familiar and comfortable becomes awkward and uneasy. We must think ahead, pay more attention, and devote more energy to what we are doing in everyday life. However, with time, most of us will have acquired new ways of doing things, new routines, new identities that make life once again predictable and familiar. When habituation is much more severely challenged by a disability, people can lose a great deal of what has given life familiarity, consistency, and relative ease. One of

the major tasks of living with disability is to reconstruct habits and roles. In the end, we all require the support of habits and roles to live effectively and comfortably in accord with our personal desires and needs.

Key Terms

Appreciation: The routine way in which we recognize the action significance of certain aspects of the environment.

Habits: Acquired tendencies to automatically respond and perform in certain, consistent ways in familiar environments or situations.

Habituation: An internalized readiness to exhibit consistent patterns of behavior guided by our habits and roles and fitted to the characteristics of routine temporal, physical, and social environments.

Internalized role: The incorporation of a socially and/or personally defined status and a related cluster of attitudes and actions.

References

American Psychiatric Association. (2000). *Diagnostic and statistical manual of mental disorders* (4th ed., text revision). Washington, DC: Author.

Asch, A. (1998). Distracted by disability. The "difference" of disability in the medical setting. *Cambridge Quarterly of Healthcare Ethics, 7,* 77–87.

Barris, R., Dickie, V., & Baron, K. (1988). A comparison of psychiatric patients and normal subjects based on the model of human occupation. *Occupational Therapy Journal of Research, 8,* 3–37.

Barris, R., Kielhofner, G., Burch, R. M., Gelinas, I., Klement, M., & Schultz, B. (1986). Occupational function and dysfunction in three groups of adolescents. *Occupational Therapy Journal of Research, 6,* 301–317.

Berger, P. L., & Luckman, T. (1966). *The social construction of reality.* New York: Doubleday/Anchor.

Beutell, N. J., & Greenhaus, J. H. (1983). Integration of home and nonhome roles: Women's conflict and coping behavior. *Journal of Applied Psychology, 68,* 43–48.

Black, M. (1976). The occupational career. *American Journal of Occupational Therapy, 30,* 225–228.

Bogdan, R., & Taylor, S. J. (1989). The social construction of humanness: Relationships with severely disabled people. *Social Problems, 36,* 135–148.

Borell, L., Gustausson, A. Sandman, P., & Kielhofner, G. (1994). Occupational programming in a day hospital for patients with dementia. *Occupational Therapy Journal of Research, 14,* 219–238.

Borrero, I. M. (1980). Psychological and emotional impact of unemployment. *Journal of Sociology and Social Welfare, 7,* 916–934.

Bourdieu, P. (1977). *Outline of a theory of practice* (R. Nice, Trans.). London: Cambridge University Press.

Brandt, E. N., & Pope, A. M. (Eds.). (1997). *Enabling America: Assessing the role of rehabilitation science and engineering.* Washington, DC: National Academy Press.

Briar, K. H. (1980). Helping the unemployed client. *Journal of Sociology and Social Welfare, 7,* 895–906.

Brim, O. J., & Wheeler, S. (1966). *Socialization after childhood: Two essays.* New York: John Wiley & Sons.

Camic, C. (1986). The matter of habit. *American Journal of Sociology, 91,* 1039–1087.

Cardwell, J. D. (1971). *Social psychology: A symbolic interaction perspective.* Philadelphia: FA Davis.

Chapin, F. S. (1968). Activity systems and urban structure: A working schema. *Journal of the American Institute of Planners, 34,* 11–18.

Clarke, A. (1997). *Being there: Putting brain, body and world together again.* Cambridge, Massachusetts: MIT Press.

Coser, L. (1974). *Greedy institutions.* New York: Free Press.

DeLoach, C. P., & Greer, B. G. (1981). *Adjustment to severe physical disability: A metamorphosis.* New York: McGraw-Hill.

Dewey, J. (1922). *Human nature and conduct.* New York: Henry Holt & Company.

Dickerson, A. E., & Oakely, F. (1995). Comparing the roles of community-living persons and patient populations. *American Journal of Occupational Therapy, 49,* 221–228.

Ebb, E. W., Coster, W., & Duncombe, L. (1989). Comparison of normal and psychosocially dysfunctional male adolescents. *Occupational Therapy in Mental Health, 9,* 53–74.

Erikson, K. T. (1973). Notes on the sociology of deviance. In H. S. Becker (Ed.), *The other side: Perspectives on deviance.* New York: Free Press.

Fein, M. L. (1990). *Role change: A resocialization perspective*. New York: Praeger.

Gerson, E. M. (1976). On "quality of life." *American Sociological Review, 41*, 793–806.

Gill, C. J. (1997). Four types of integration in disability identity development. *Journal of Vocational Rehabilitation, 9*, 39–46.

Gray, M. (1972). Effects of hospitalization on work-play behavior. *American Journal of Occupational Therapy, 26*, 180–185.

Grossack, M., & Gardner, H. (1970). *Man and men: Social psychology as social science*. Scranton, PA: International Textbook Co.

Guskin, S. L. (1963). Social psychologies of mental deficiency. In N. R. Ellis (Ed.), *Handbook of mental deficiency*. New York: McGraw-Hill.

Hage, G., & Powers, C. H. (1992). *Post-Industrial lives: Roles & relationships in the 21st Century*. Newbury Park, NJ: Sage.

Hahn, H. (1985). Disability policy and the problem of discrimination. *American Behavioral Scientist, 28,* 293–318.

Hahn, H. (1988). Toward a politics of disability: Definitions, disciplines and policies. *Social Science Journal, 22,* 87–105.

Hale, T. W., Hayghe, H. W., & McNeil, J. M. (1998). Persons with disabilities: Labor market activities, 1994. *Monthly Labor Review, 121* (9), 3–12.

Hall, J. M., Stevens, P. E., & Meleis, A. I. (1992). Developing the construct of role integration: A narrative analysis of women clerical workers' daily lives. *Research in Nursing & Health, 15,* 447–457.

Hallet, J., Zasler, N., Maurer, P. & Cash, S. (1994). Role change after traumatic brain injury in adults. *American Journal of Occupational Therapy, 48,* 241–246.

Hammel, J. (1999). The life rope: A transactional approach to exploring worker and life role development. *Work: A Journal of Prevention, Assessment and Rehabilitation, 12,* 47–60.

Heard, C. (1977). Occupational role acquisition: A perspective on the chronically disabled. *American Journal of Occupational Therapy, 41,* 243–247.

Holzman, P., & Grinker, R. (1974). Schizophrenia in adolescence. *Journal of Youth and Adolescence, 3,* 267–279.

Hull, J. M. (1990). *Touching the rock: An experience of blindness*. New York: Vintage Books.

James, W. (1950). *The principles of psychology*. New York: Dover.

Jonsson, H., Josephsson, S., & Kielhofner, G. (2001). Narratives and experience in an occupational transition: A longitudinal study of the retirement process. *American Journal of Occupational Therapy, 55,* 424–432.

Katz, D., & Kahn, R. L. (1966). *The social psychology of organizations*. New York: John Wiley & Sons.

Kielhofner, G. (1979). The temporal dimension in the lives of retarded adults. *American Journal of Occupational Therapy, 33*, 161–168.

Kielhofner, G. (1981). An ethnographic study of deinstitutionalized adults: Their community settings and daily life experiences. *Occupational Therapy Journal of Research, 1*, 125–141.

Kielhofner, G. (1983). "Teaching" retarded adults: Paradoxical effects of a pedagogical enterprise. *Urban Life, 12*, 307–326.

Kielhofner, G., Barris, R., & Watts, J. (1982). Habits and habit dysfunction: A clinical perspective for psychosocial occupational therapy. *Occupational Therapy Mental Health, 2*, 1–22.

Koestler, A. (1969). Beyond atomism and holism: The concept of the holon. In A. Koestler & J. R. Smythies (Eds.), *Beyond reductionism*. Boston, MA: Beacon Press.

Krefting, L. (1989). Reintegration into the community after head injury: The results of an ethnographic study. *Occupational Therapy Journal of Research, 9*, 67–83.

Louis Harris and Associates. (1998). *Highlights of the N.O.D/Harris 1998 Survey of Americans with Disabilities*. Washington, DC: National Organization on Disability.

Mancuso, J. C., & Sarbin, T. R. (1983). The self-narrative in the enactment of roles. In T. R. Sarbin & K. E. Scheibe (Eds.), *Studies in social identity*. New York: Praeger.

Marks, S. R. (1977). Multiple roles and role strain: Some notes on human energy, time, and commitment. *American Sociological Review, 42*, 921–936.

Mechanic, D. (1980). *Mental health and social policy* (2nd ed.). Englewood Cliffs, NJ: Prentice-Hall.

Melges, F. T. (1982). *Time and inner future: A temporal approach to psychiatric disorders*. New York: John Wiley & Sons.

Merleau-Ponty, M. (1962). *Phenomenology of perception*. (C. Smith, Trans.). London: Routledge & Kegan Paul. (Original work published 1945)

McKeen, D. G. (1992). Such a good little patient. *Disability Rag, July/August*, 43.

Miller, D. R. (1983). Self, symptom and social control. In T. R. Sarbin & K. E. Scheibe (Eds.), *Studies in social identity*. New York: Praeger.

Murphy, R. F. (1987). *The body silent*. New York: WW Norton.

National Council on Disability. (1996). *Achieving independence: The challenge for the 21st century*. Washington, DC: Author.

Offer, D., Ostrov, E., & Howard, K. (1981). *The adolescent: A psychological self-report*. New York: Basic Books.

Paap, W. R. (1972). The social reconstruction of reality: The rehabilitation of paraplegics and quadriplegics. *Disser-*

tation Abstracts International, 33, 45-A. (University Microfilms No. 72-19, 234).

Parsons, T. (1953). Illness and the role of the physician: A sociological perspective. In C. Kluckhohn, H. Murray, & D. Schneider (Eds.), *Personality in nature, society, and culture* (2nd ed.). New York: Alfred A. Knopf.

Pinder, R. (1988). Striking balances: Living with Parkinson's disease. In R. Anderson & M. Bury (Eds.), *Living with chronic illness: The experience of patients and their families*. London: Unwin Hyman.

Robinson, I. (1988). Reconstructing lives: Negotiating the meaning of multiple sclerosis. In R. Anderson & M. Bury (Eds.), *Living with chronic illness. The experience of patients and their families*. London: Unwin Hyman.

Rosow, I. (1976). Status and role change through the life span. In R.H. Binstock and E. Shanas (Eds.), *Handbook of Aging and the Social Sciences*. New York: Van Nostrand Reinhold.

Rowles, G. D. (1991). Beyond performance: Being in place as a component of occupational therapy. *American Journal of Occupational Therapy, 45*, 265–272.

Ruddock, R. (1976). *Roles and relationships*. London: Routledge & Kegan Paul.

Sarbin, T. R., & Scheibe, K. E. (1983). A model of social identity. In T. R. Sarbin & K. E. Scheibe (Eds.), *Studies in social identity*. New York: Praeger.

Schein, E. H. (1971). The individual, the organization, and the career: A conceptual scheme. *Journal of Applied Behavioral Science, 7*, 401–426.

Schiffer, R. B., Rudick, R. A., & Herndon, R. M. (1983). Psychologic aspects of multiple sclerosis. *New York State Journal of Medicine, 3*, 312–316.

Schumacher, K. L. (1995). Family Caregiver Role acquisition: Role-making through situated interaction. *Scholarly Inquiry for Nursing Practice: An International Journal, 9*, 211–226.

Seamon, D. (1980). Body-subject, time-space routines, and place-ballets. In A. Buttimer & D. Seamon (Eds.), *The human experience of space and place*. London: Croom Helm.

Seiber, S. D. (1974). Toward a theory of role accumulation. *American Sociological Review, 39*, 567–578.

Shillam, L. L., Beeman, C., & Loshin, P. (1983). Effect of occupational therapy intervention on bathing independence of disabled persons. *American Journal of Occupational Therapy, 37*, 744–748.

Smith, C. A. (1972). Body image changes after myocardial infarction. *Nursing Clinics of North America, 7*, 663–668.

Spreitzer, E., Snyder, E. E., & Larson, D. L. (1979). Multiple roles and psychological well-being. *Social Focus, 12*, 141–148.

Stryker, S. (1968). Identity salience and role performance: The reliance of symbolic interaction theory for family research. *Journal of Marriage and the Family*, November, 558–564.

Thomas, E. J. (1966). Problems of disability from the perspective of role theory. *Journal of Health and Human Behavior, 7*, 2–11.

Toombs, S. K. (1987). The meaning of illness: a phenomenological approach to the patient-physician relationship. *Journal of Medicine & Philosophy, 12*, (3), 219–240.

Trieschmann, R. B. (1989). Psychosocial adjustment to spinal cord injury. In B. W. Heller, L. M. Flohr, & L. S. Zegans (Eds.), *Psychosocial interventions with physically disabled persons*. New Brunswick, NJ: Rutgers University Press.

Trupin, L. D., Sebesta, S., Yelin, E., & LaPlante, M. P. (1997). Trends in labor force participation among persons with disabilities, 1993-94. *Disability Statistics Report, 10*, 1–39.

Turner, R. (1962). Role-taking, process versus conformity. In M. Rose (Ed.), *Human behavior and social processes*. Boston: Houghton Mifflin.

Versluys, H. P. (1983). Psychosocial adjustment to physical disability. In C. A. Trombly (Ed.), *Occupational therapy for physical dysfunction* (2nd ed.). Baltimore: Williams & Wilkins.

Werner-Beland, J. A. (Ed.) (1980). *Grief responses to long-term illness and disability*. Reston, VA: Reston Publishing.

Williams, R. S. (1984). Ability, disability and rehabilitation: A phenomenological description. *Journal of Medicine and Philosophy, 9*, 93–112.

Wolfensberger, W. (1975). *The origin and nature of our institutional models*. Syracuse, NY: Human Policy Press.

Young, M. (1988). *The metronomic society: Natural rhythms and human timetables*. Cambridge, MA: Harvard University Press.

Zola, I. K. (1982). *Missing pieces: A chronicle of living with a disability*. Philadelphia: Temple University Press.

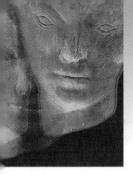

6

Performance Capacity and the Lived Body

- Gary Kielhofner
- Kerstin Tham
- Tal Baz
- Jennifer Hutson

Performance Capacity

The multitude of things we do require us to sense and interpret the world around us, move our bodies around in space, manipulate objects, plan our actions, and communicate and interact with others. Even the most ordinary activity reflects the complex and exquisite organization of our capacity to perform. As noted in Chapter 2, **performance capacity** is the ability for doing things provided by the status of underlying objective physical and mental components and corresponding subjective experience *(Fig. 6-1)*. This definition highlights that capacity involves both objective and subjective aspects.

Objective Components of Performance Capacity

Our performance depends on our being composed of musculoskeletal, neurologic, cardiopulmonary, and other body systems. The capacity to perform also depends on cognitive abilities such as memory. When we do things, we exercise these capacities.

As noted in Chapter 1, other models of practice provide detailed explanations of specific performance capacities. Collectively, these models address performance capacity by objective study of physical (e.g., muscle, bone, nerve, brain) and psychological (e.g., memory, perception, cognition) phenomena. Therefore, therapists use these models as a means to understanding and addressing specific problems of perfor-

mance capacity. Consequently, performance is explained as a function of the status of objective performance capacities. Objective description invokes a language that names, classifies, and measures systems that appraise capacity by systematically observing performance. For example, we can speak about joint range of motion measured in degrees of movement or cognition measured by test scores.

This objective approach is typically coupled with an effort to explain problems of function in terms of disturbances to underlying structures and functions. For instance, limitations of movement might be attributed to loss of muscle strength and damage to joints. Similarly, limitations in problem-solving might be attributed to disturbances of attention following brain damage. Such depictions of impairments are important and helpful because the objective understanding of their nature can provide useful cues to how they might be remediated or their negative consequences might be minimized.

Subjective Approach to Performance Capacity

Objectively describable abilities and limitations of ability are also experienced by those who have them. However, the objective approach generally views these experiences as only consequences of the real problem that must be appraised from an outsider's detached viewpoint. Even when therapists using this approach

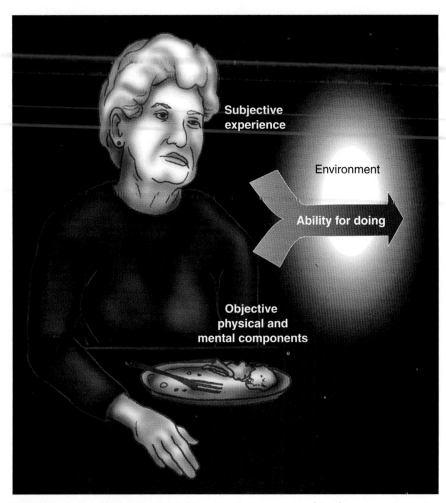

FIGURE 6-1   Objective and Subjective Components of Performance Capacity.

ask people about their subjective experience, they do so with an eye toward building an objective picture of performance capacity.

> *The observer's objective approach and the performer's subjective perspective are bound together in any instant of performance and both contribute to performance.*

Nonetheless, subjective experience also shapes how people perform (Kielhofner, 1995). Paying careful attention to subjective experience in its own right can reveal a great deal about performance capacity and limitations of performance. It can also reveal important information about how to undertake therapy.

Focusing on the subjective aspect of performance capacity is complementary to the traditional objective approach. As shown in *Figure 6-2,* the objective approach provides a view of performance capacity from the outside, while the approach offered below provides a view of performance capacity from the inside. Both the observer's objective perspective

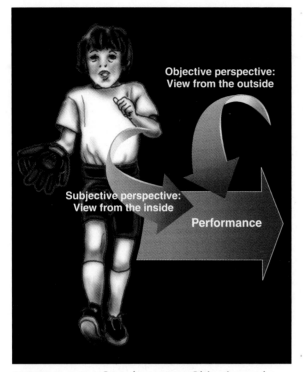

Objective perspective:
View from the outside

Subjective perspective:
View from the inside

Performance

FIGURE 6-2 Complementary Objective and Subjective Views of Performance.

and the performer's subjective experience have something to tell us about performance capacity. Neither perspective fully accounts for the other. Both the objective and the subjective are bound together in any instant of performance and both contribute to the performance. For example, in moving one arm to reach out for something, there is both how it is to perform the movement and how the arm moves in space. Both tell something about what is involved in reaching. For example, the objective approach provides a picture of how muscle contractions generate forces across joints producing degrees of extension and rotation that carry the arm through the trajectory of movement for reaching. The subjective experience will tell another story. This chapter is mainly about the nature of that story.

As is true of the objective approach, that story is told by using a particular language. This language will call our attention to the nature of subjective phenomena and their importance to performance.

The Lived Body

The basic concept used here to discuss the subjective in performance capacity is the lived body. The concept of the lived body ultimately emanates from the work of the philosopher Merleau-Ponty (1945/1962), who criticized the traditional objective approach, viewing the body as only a complex machine producing perception and action. Merleau-Ponty instead argued that the body was experienced in immediate connection with the environment. He sought and developed a view of human performance that paid careful attention to the nature of experience. He used experience as a central concept in explaining how performance was possible. Unlike the objective approach that describes performance from a detached, objective perspective, he emphasized a phenomenological approach that considered subjective experience as fundamental to understanding human perception, cognition, and action.

Using this phenomenological approach, Leder (1990, p. 1) employed the term "lived body" to emphasize how we experience, that is, live through our bodies. He describes the lived body as follows:

> Human experience is incarnated. I receive the surrounding world through my eyes, my ears, my hands . . . My legs carry me toward a desired goal seen across the distance. My hands reach out to take up tools . . . My actions are motivated by emotions, needs, desires, that well up from a corporeal self. Relations with others are based upon our mutuality of gaze and touch, our speech, our resonances of feeling and perspective. (p. 1)

Following Leder's (1990) utilization, we employ the concept of the **lived body** to refer to the experience of being and knowing the world through a particular body. The concept of the lived body applies both to human embodiment in general and to unique specific forms of embodiment associated with disability.

The body is lived or experienced in immediate connection with the environment.

> *In the course of our daily occupational life, our bodies are invisible viewpoints from which we experience and act on the world.*

The lived body concept underscores two fundamental ideas. First, mind and body are seen not as separate phenomena, but part of a single, unitary entity—namely, the lived body. Second, subjective experience of performance is not simply an artifact of performing. Rather, it is fundamental to how we perform. That is, in doing things and learning how to do things, we call on not only the objective components that make up performance capacity, but also the experience of exercising our capacities. The following sections discuss these two aspects of the lived body.

Mind-Body Unity

Understanding mind-body unity requires that we first trace the origins and meaning of mind-body duality. The tendency to view body and mind as separate has been a dominant force in Western science and culture. It began with the philosopher, Descartes, who observed that the body is an object like other objects in the physical world and, therefore, subject to the same causal laws (Leder, 1984). According to his classic and influential argument, the workings of the human body should be understood through the same objective methods with which other objects in the physical world can be investigated and understood. The other side of Descartes' philosophical argument was that the mind was immaterial and thus operated according to different, abstract principles. Hence, Cartesian dualism proclaimed that the body and mind represented completely separate realms and that understanding them required radically different approaches.

In conceptually prying apart body and mind, Cartesian dualism has left us with everyday and scientific perspectives that treat the body as unaware and that disembody the mind. The body is conceived as a physical entity without intelligence or consciousness of its own. The immaterial mind is thought to enliven and govern the otherwise inert, material body. Consequently, the mind is considered the distinct seat of reason and passion, and the body is its mere abode and tool.

To cease regarding the body and mind as two separate entities and, instead, see them as dual aspects of a single entity is not easy. Dualism is deeply ingrained in our way of thinking. Nonetheless, we can begin to understand mind-body unity by paying attention both to how the body is experienced and how the mind is embodied.

Bodily Experience

We can experience our own bodies as objects in the way Descartes identified. For example, we can look at our hands just as we gaze at other things in the world. In such looking, our experience is directed to our hands (Leder, 1990). However, this is neither the only nor the dominant way in which we experience our hands. Rather, we routinely experience from our hands to that which is outside ourselves.

When we reach into a purse for coins, grasp a door handle, pull on our socks, pat our dog, wave to our friends, or caress our loved ones, we are attending and acting to the world and from our hands. In those instances our hands are subjects not objects. Our hands are, in these instances, our point of view for reaching, grasping, pulling, patting, waving, and caressing.

Thus, the fundamental difference between experiencing our bodies as objects and as subject goes like the following. When I experience some part of my body as an object in the world, I am attending to that body part and am distinguishing between my body and myself. When I am attending to the world from my body there is no distinction between self and body. As Sartre (1970) noted, one does not just have one's body, one is one's body.

Leder (1990) describes this phenomenon in the following way. He notes that when we are doing things, our bodies disappear to us. Our experience is directed

> *We experience our body not as a "collection of adjacent organs, but a synergic system, all the functions of which are exercised and linked together in the general action of being in the world . . . "*

to that part of the world with which we are interacting and our bodies recede, vanishing from our awareness. Moreover, our bodies are that from which our attention and action is focused to what is outside us. Thus, in the course of our daily occupational lives, our bodies are invisible viewpoints from which we experience and act upon the world. We experience our bodies "as an attitude directed towards a certain existing or possible task" (Merleau-Ponty, 1945/1962, p. 100).

Because of this experience, it can seem that the body is not really part of conscious experience. For example, when we are reading a book we experience it as a mental activity, unaware that we are holding it with our hands, and seeing it with our eyes. Our bodies hold and see the book, but because the body mostly recedes from awareness when we are doing things, it can almost seem as though the body had nothing to do with reading. Of course, the body is not just part of the scene. It is the body that is doing the reading.

In everyday life, our lived bodies include both the experience of the body as object and body as subject. However, when we perform, the body is mainly experienced as subject. That is, the body is the taken-for-granted place from which we exist and from which we attend to and act on the world. We may become aware of our bodies as objects when we perceive fatigue or pain and, therefore, attend to the tired or aching limb. For the most part, however, doing things requires that we attend from the body to what we are doing.

Because our bodies are in use much of the time, our experience of our bodies is grounded in doing things. Consequently, we each experience our body as the self that is always taking in the world around us and doing things in that same world. Moreover, we experience our body not as, "a collection of adjacent organs, but as a synergic system, all the functions of which are exercised and linked together in the general action of being in the world . . . " (Merleau-Ponty, 1945/1962, p. 234). For example, when we are walking outside and viewing the scenery, we have no separate awareness of the movements of legs and arms in walking or the orientation of our head and eyes in attending to the things around us. When we raise our hands above our eyes to shade the sun it is simply part of looking, not a separate act by a separate part of the body. We experience all the parts of the body as a unified whole engaged in the action of walking and looking. Moreover, most of our experience of our bodies is the awareness we have of doing things as a body. We can imagine a walk outside, but it is only a facsimile (and a poor one at that) of feeling the sun on our brow and the ground at our feet, of apprehending the world in the midst of moving around within it. We are most aware when we are bodies in the midst of action.

When we consider the body in this way, we cannot readily separate it from what we call mind. Further, we can see that awareness is not something belonging to a separate mind and imposed on the body. Rather, the body is an intimate part of how we are aware.

EMBODIED MIND

Whatever else we might attribute to mind, it consists of knowing about things and knowing how to do things. Descartes posited knowledge as what distinguished the mind from the body. However, knowing is seated in the body. Importantly, we do not mean simply that knowledge is stored or processed biochemically in the brain. Rather, we mean that the whole of the body is the way we apprehend and thus know about how to do things. The body is the existential medium of knowing.

Knowing Things

What we know about the world around us begins with our bodies looking at, touching, and probing the world (Merleau-Ponty, 1945/1962). Abstract properties we attribute to various objects in the world echo how our bodies experience those objects. For example:

> How do I know that the ball is spherical, solid, and leathery? My moving, throwing and pressing hands reveal these properties . . . [that] do not exist solely in the ball and not at all in my hands. It is only when my hands touch the ball that these properties are revealed to me. (Engelbrecht, 1968, p.12).

Sartre (1970, p. 231) elaborates this notion in the following example of how bodily action gives us an experience of the world:

> We never have any sensation of our effort . . . We perceive the resistance of things. What I perceive when I want to lift this glass to my mouth is not my effort but the heaviness of the glass.

When we do things, we generate bodily experiences of the world that we come to interpret as properties of that world. Nevertheless, the world we know is always on the other end of something we are doing with our bodies. Perception is not simply the registration and evaluation of sense data, but rather an active taking hold of the world. When we perceive objects and their characteristics, the foundation of our knowing them always has to do with how our bodies encounter and engage them. Once again, we are speaking here not of the objective ways sensory data are taken in by sensory organs and networked through the central nervous system. Instead, we are referring to the body as a way of generating experience in response to its own questions that are posed as forms of acting toward and in the world. What the mind asks of the world and the answers that make up the mind's accumulated knowledge are asked, in large measure, through bodily action.

> **Abstract properties we attribute to various objects in the world echo how our bodies experience those objects.**

Even abstract knowledge grows out of bodily experiences. For example, only by using our bodies to do things—touching, grasping, lifting, shoving, observing, and listening to the world—do we have access to experiences that give meaning to concepts of distance, direction, temporality, clarity, resistance, resilience, and obscurity (Leder, 1990; Merleau-Ponty, 1945/1962; Sudnow, 1979). Thought itself builds on what our bodies do and experience. As Sudnow (1979) argues:

> When I sit before the piano keyboard, I am directly aligned to its center . . . I sit down and there I am, as exactly middled as before the dinner plate, the steering wheel, the bathroom faucets—before whatever action moves out from the center. Dividing in half all the body's ways, is part of the calculus, topography, trigonometry, and algebra that my body does . . . Mathematics is perhaps the purest form of human thought, not because its pictures struggle toward a perfect concept of nature, but because its pictures have their origin in the ways of the body . . . (p. 79)

The structure and content of mental operations are always based on the body's way of comprehending the world. As Leder (1990, p. 7) notes, abstract cognition "may sublimate but never fully escapes its inherence in a perceiving, active body."

Knowing How To Do Things

When we type or play piano, our fingers instinctively know where to go for the right letter or note (Sudnow, 1979). In fact, if we wish to locate a specific key on the computer or piano, our fingers can much more readily find their way than we can imagine the key's location. For example, the most efficient strategy for locating the computer key "H" is to begin to type a word beginning with that letter. Without consciously thinking about its location, the right index finger will begin to move to the right center of the keyboard where "H" is located. What is also notable in this and other instances of bodily knowing is that the body instinctively knows which part of itself should perform any action.

Our bodies readily perform all manner of things that we cannot readily describe how to do. Imagine doing any ordinary action such as a dance step, a swim stroke, whistling a tune, or tying a shoe. Imagining the action only gives us a vague trace of what it is. We must typically watch our bodies do things to notice exactly what we are doing. Compare thinking about how to tie a shoe to actually tying the shoe and one can readily see how much the knowing is in the body. Consequently, we can see how knowledge of how to do things is located in the parts of the body with which we do them. The body does not need a superimposed mind to command it through its routine performance.

Mind-Body Unity Revisited

The previous discussions noted how the body possesses characteristics of awareness we typically reserve for mind and how knowledge is bodily grounded. These discussions point to how mind and body are not sepa-

> **Perception is not simply the registration and evaluation of sense data, but rather an active taking a hold of the world with our bodies and the unique way our bodies gives us access to the world around us.**

rate phenomena but rather are "intertwined aspects of one living organism" (Leder, 1990, p. 149). The lesson of this discussion is that mind and body are not distinct things. Rather, they are different aspects of one thing.

Subjective Experience and Performance

As noted previously, every action we perform is objectively describable. It can be divided into so much flexion, extension, or rotation at joints. It can be described in terms of the trajectory, speed, and the efficiency with which movement is accomplished.

Such bodily action is known differently from within. When we reach for a cup of coffee, open a door, walk to the bus, or operate a car, we do not objectively know or do the movements involved. Instead, we are inside the movements and experience them from that vantage point. Consequently, when we use our bodies to do things, we aim for the subjective experience of doing them. Indeed, we cannot fully attend to the objective features of our performance without disrupting it in some way. For example, if we concentrate too much on how to move our hands in tying our shoes, we will interrupt our performance.

> *Learning to do something means that we must grasp the experience—to learn how it feels.*

When learning to do something, we may at first aim for the objective movements. For example, when learning to hold silverware or chopsticks, we first attend to how they are placed in the hand and how the fingers should be positioned. But learning to do something means that we must grasp the experience—to learn how it feels. Westerners who as adults have learned to use chopsticks will recall that they got the hang of it only when they could feel how to manipulate the chopsticks. Most of us will also recall when learning to ride a bicycle, roller skate, ski, or any other skilled form of doing that we began with a sense of what was objectively involved and ended up learning what the right movement felt like. Once we have grasped the feeling of how it is to do something, re-

peating the performance is altogether different. After that feeling is achieved, we no longer pay attention to the objective aspects of doing the action. Rather, we focus on the experience and use it as our guide to performing. As Sudnow (1978) describes it:

> . . . when one first gets the knack of a complex skill . . . the hang of it has been glimpsed . . . the experience is tasted. All prior ways of being seem thoroughly lacking, and the new way is encountered with a "this is it" feeling, almost as a revelation. (p. 83)

Being inside any performance allows us to assess it in a uniquely subjective way (Clarke, 1993). When we are about to reach somewhere or step somewhere, we appraise the kind of getting there that the distance entails. In moving our bodies, we do not estimate distances as so much objective distance to be traversed, but rather as so much traveling to do. We aim toward the experience of a performance, not to the objective features of performance. Consequently, learning to perform involves finding the right experience, and performance involves aiming for that experience.

The Lived Body in Perspective

Although a great deal of objective knowledge about performance capacity has been generated, the subjective experience of performance has been largely neglected. The previous section highlighted subjective experience of the lived body. The discussion covered two important themes. First, physical and mental aspects of performance do not represent separate realms. Both moving one's body to accomplish a task and planning the steps in the task are functions of a lived body that is at once both physical and mental. Second, the nature of subjective experience and its role in performance were examined. It was argued that experience is not simply an artifact or consequence of doing, but rather that experience is central to how we manage to perform. To learn any performance, we must find the experience of it—how it feels. To do any performance we

> *We aim toward the experience of a performance, not to the objective features of performance*

are guided not by the objective features of what is involved, but by how it feels to do it. Understanding both performance and limitations of performance requires attention to these features of the lived body.

Disability and the Lived Body

Although there is little systematic study of the embodied experience of disability, a number of writers who have disabilities have offered important insights to their experiences. Toombs (1992), who has multiple sclerosis, reminds us that there is a particular experience that goes with a disability. It is often radically different from experience in a nondisabled state. She notes, for example, that with a physical impairment:

> My attention is focused on my hand as hand. I must observe how it is that my fingers grasp the handle of the cup and I am conscious of my hand's unaccustomed ineffectiveness as an instrument of my action. In illness the body intrudes itself into experience. (Toombs, 1992, p. 71)

Zasetsky describes the challenges of trying to write following his traumatic brain injury:

> I didn't have enough of a vocabulary or mind left to write well . . . I'd spend ages hunting for the right words. I had to remember and turn up words that were are at least fairly similar or close enough to what I wanted to say. But after I'd put together these second choices, I still wasn't able to start writing until I figured out how to compose a sentence. (in Luria, 1972, pp. 78–79)

Others write about how the world is transformed. For example, Sechehaye (1968) describes her experience of schizophrenia as transforming the world into a place where there:

> Reigned an implacable light, blinding, leaving no place for shadow; an immense place without boundary, limitless, flat; a mineral, lunar country, cold as the wastes of the North Pole. In this stretching emptiness, all is unchangeable, immobile, congealed, crystallized. Objects are strange trappings, placed here and there, geometric cubes without meaning. (p. 44)

Similarly, Williams (1994) describes how her experiences as a child with autism placed her in a extraordinary world:

> I discovered the air was full of spots. If you looked into nothingness, there were spots. People would walk by, obstructing my magical view of nothingness. I'd move past them. (p. 3)

Others have written about the alteration of experiences that comes with medical treatments. For example, Jamison (1995) describes living with the consequences of taking lithium necessary to control her manic-depressive illness. In addition to feeling "less lively, less energetic, less high spirited" (p. 92) she also found that some of her ability to read was impaired:

> . . . I had to read the same lines repeatedly and take copious notes before I could comprehend the meaning. Even so, what I read often disappeared from my mind like snow on a hot pavement. (p. 95)

Such testimonies from persons who experience various impairments offer important windows into the experience of limitations or alterations of capacity. Systematic descriptions of the experience of impairments and the course of change over time also have the potential to offer us new ways of understanding and intervening. In what follows, we examine this potential more closely.

Understanding Transformations in the Lived Body

Collectively, we have undertaken three studies that have examined the experience of the lived body among persons with disabilities. Each focuses on:

- Nature of the experience
- Contribution of experience to disability
- Evolution of experience over time
- Role of experience in changes in performance capacity.

The following sections briefly describe the findings from the three studies. Following this are discussion of their implications for better understanding the nature of experience in disability and how experience can be used in the therapeutic process.

Recapturing Half of Self and the World

Brain damage often significantly alters experience. One of the more dramatic alterations is unilateral neglect following cerebrovascular accident. Objectively, persons with unilateral neglect are unable to orient their attention toward the left hemispace and are often unaware of the left half of their body (Bisiach & Vallar, 1988).

A study of four Swedish women with unilateral neglect (Tham, Borell, & Gustavsson, 2000) described the unfolding of lived body experiences as these women lost and then slowly began to recapture half of themselves and their worlds. Many are oblivious to their neglect (McGlynn & Schacter, 1989; Tham, Borell, & Gustavsson, 2000). The following are highlights of their discoveries.

Initially, the left half of the women's worlds did not exist for them. They lived and acted only in the remaining right half of the world, with no sense that the left half of the world had disappeared. Rather, they experienced their half-world as complete.

Only with time, as the women began to perform previously familiar tasks, did they begin to sense something vaguely unfamiliar. Their bodies, and their perceptions of space and time, felt oddly different.

As they encountered the left half of the body, it didn't feel as though it belonged to them. Each woman's arm and leg simply didn't seem like part of the self. They felt instead like objects apart from the self. One woman reported that she had to trace her left arm with her right hand to the shoulder in order to realize that it was really attached to her. Another woman, referring to her hand placed on the table in front of her, said her fingers seemed to her like five sausages just lying there. All four women spoke about the left side of the body in the third person, characterizing it as estranged and cold. One woman lamented that her left hand, "wants to reject people. It is not generous. It will just give chilliness."

In this way, as the women first became aware of their left halves, they did not experience them as an encounter with part of the self. Rather they saw the left half as something alien, not belonging to themselves.

As these women began to move about and do things, they also found that they were disoriented to space. They repeatedly found that they did not know where they were, and could not orient themselves in space. Moreover, both people and objects could suddenly disappear or appear. For example one women recalled how, "When I had dinner, I suddenly didn't know where my husband went. He just disappeared."

They also found that they could no longer rely on previously automatic ways of doing things. While they were still unaware of their neglect at this point, they could discern its consequences. They found these consequences of neglect confusing and could not fathom why they had problems in performing certain tasks. They could not link their problems of performance to their neglect since it did not yet exist for them.

Over time, they began to recognize familiar problems in performance, though they still did not comprehend that they were missing half the world. Bumping into things with their wheelchairs was a common problem. While they couldn't perceive what was happening on their left side, they could perceive certain features of the collision, such as the crashing sound and the sudden stopping of the wheelchair.

As such neglect-related experiences accumulated, they began to reflect upon them, searching for explanations for these difficulties. At first, their explanations were still not grounded in their neglect. For instance, they attributed their inability to find objects to unfamiliarity of the rehabilitation environment, expecting to find it much easier to locate objects at home. At this point, they could not consciously use any strategies to compensate for their neglect since they were unaware of their unawareness of the left half of the surrounding world.

As they regained movement in their left side, the sense of that side as belonging to the self began to return. Because improvements in mobility occurred first in the legs, the four women first felt that their left legs mostly belonged to them, although alienation of the left arm persisted.

Despite its continued estrangement, they began to feel a responsibility to the arm. One women described the experience like this:

> I have to accept it, because it is sitting here on my body. All the time when I am doing something I have to think of it, and to bring it with me. It is like I am carrying a baby all the time, a baby you can't leave on a table and then go your way. You have to bring it with you. You can't forget your hand because everything can go wrong if you do that. Instead, you bring your baby and it is the same with your hand, you can't ignore the hand, because you have it, and in the future you will need it.

While the women began to own responsibility for the left arm, they still did not own it as a part of themselves. This was highlighted by the fact that they could lose the left side of the body, as one woman noted:

> Always when I am going to bed I think that I need a pillow for my arm and if the arm is not lying there, I get scared to death. I think something is wrong because I must always have my arm with me. If I don't have that, it will become swollen. If I can't find my arm, I use the alarm to call someone and ask, 'can you find my bad arm?' And, of course, they always can.

At this point, before they could actually use it, the left hand began to reemerge as a point of view for doing things. As one woman described:

> Suddenly I forget that I can't use my left hand, especially when I am eating. For example if I find some crumbs at the table, beside my plate, I want to clean them up and to put them together. So I try to put the crumbs in my left hand, even if I know that I can't use it.

Such regaining of intentionality in the neglected side was also reflected in their beginning efforts to incorporate the left body parts in their daily life.

Next, they began to comprehend that they were missing the left half of the environment. The understanding was objective, however, and they still did not have any direct experience of this limitation. Importantly, this realization came about as others (therapists, nurses, family members, aides) told them about their neglect, explained how problems were related to neglect, or demonstrated that there were objects to the left by coaching them to search there. Thus, for these women, neglect was first understood as an objective fact, related to them by others.

Armed with this objective knowledge of their neglect and its consequences, they wanted to improve their ability to find objects and to orient to the left half of the environment. The four women gradually became more and more able to use conscious strategies to perform better by compensating for their unilateral neglect.

There appeared to emerge for each woman a kind of existential pull from the left, when objects located there were part of an occupation in which they were engaged or when circumstances on their left needed their attention. For example, one woman, while working in the kitchen, suddenly saw the toaster on her left side when she noticed that its electrical cord was hanging over the sink. She noted, "I could see the electrical cord to the left because I know it is unsafe to have it over the sink. The electricity can short, and that is dangerous."

They could also more readily locate objects that they knew should be present. For example, one woman described searching for lotion and toothpaste in her dressing case:

> I look and I look. At first I can't see the things but I know that they should be there. Then I move my eyes and I turn my head so I really can see everything because I know that the things should be there.

Increasingly, the women developed a way of reasoning that considered how things should be so that they could compare it with what they perceived. This proved effective in overcoming some problems posed by the neglect. For example, one woman noted:

> Sometimes when I am eating I think, but God, didn't I get the fish? They told us that we should be served fish today. But of course, it is placed on the left side of the plate, I think. So, I begin to search to the left, and then I can see it.

Sometimes, they were able to anticipate problems that would occur because of the neglect and use a strategy to avoid them. For example, one woman surveyed and memorized any new environment before she began to move around with the wheelchair. She could use her mental map to avoid crashing into objects that she would not see once she was moving along.

Five months after their strokes, the four women had accumulated substantial experience using such conscious compensatory strategies. Their understanding and awareness of their neglect became deeper, and their compensatory strategies became habitual.

Thus, while they still did not naturally have access to the left half of the world, they were aware that it existed outside of their immediate experience. They began to spontaneously remember to access this world. They used a number of strategies for gaining access to what was present or going on in the left half of the world. They would, for instance, use sounds that came from the left. They would search to the left by reaching and feeling for things. Finally they could actively visually search to the left. As one woman put it:

> Look to the left, look to the left, I tell myself, and then when I look to the left, I can find the thing that I am looking for.

In the end, the left half of the world existed for them, but not as before their cerebrovascular accidents. It was not an immediate presence like the rest of the world. It was a hidden place that had consequences for action, where things resided unseen. Through special efforts, objects in the left half of the world could be found and its arrangement, although unseen, could be imagined. Thus, they regained the lost half of the world in pragmatic terms, although it was forever lost to them in immediate experience.

Learning to Cycle: A Therapeutic Passage to Embodiment

Tom was a 10-year-old boy diagnosed with a regulatory disorder (i.e., difficulty in regulating his behavior and his sensory, attentional, motor, and affective processes) and somatosensory dyspraxia (i.e., difficulty formulating a plan of action necessary to sequencing and carrying out skilled motor acts). Through observation and interviews, Baz (1998) documented Tom's experience of disability and change over 8 weekly therapy sessions that are characterized in what follows.

While Tom was a bright boy with age-appropriate fine motor skills, he had extreme difficulties moving his body about in space and dealing with moving objects. His favorite occupations were reading and playing on the computer. He called these "brain things." When engaged in these activities, Tom could be static (sitting) and the focus of his attention within a specific, stable frame of acting.

According to his mother:

> [Tom] has a lot of fears . . . he's afraid of a lot of things . . . He's scared to death about learning to ride a bike because he [fears he] will fall and hurt himself . . . and he's had nightmares about it.

Similarly his occupational therapist notes:

> He's got these fears. They're really big in his head. They feel really scary to him and he doesn't seem to be able to meet those fears . . .

As his mother and therapist attest, Tom's awareness of his body and of the world was dominated by fear. This fear is not only a feeling Tom had about his body. Rather it was a way of being his body. He experienced himself as a fragile, disjointed collection of bodily parts that did not behave as a whole. Further, he could have the frightening sensation of his physical self literally coming apart.

Tom's disjointed experience of self extended to his distinction between thought and action. When he described doing ordinary things involving thinking and acting, as in the following playground vignette, he separated mind and body, objectifying his body movements:

> If you want to go down the slide but the slide's dirty . . . you gotta think what to do with the slide. Usually what I think is, "clean the slide," so I use my arm muscles to move the . . . dirt or slimy worm, or ants around with the small towel thing.

In another incident, Tom was scratching himself when someone remarked that it might be due to dry skin. He responded, "Well, I think that's why my brain is telling me to itch that." His language for describing himself and his actions is one of discontinuity—among parts of the self and between self and the world.

Not surprisingly Tom felt alienated from his body. He was not at home with it. His body was not really his through which to live. To an unusual extent, he attended to his body rather than from it. For example, his therapist noted:

> He has a tendency to keep his visual field down and low . . . looking at his hands and feet . . . as opposed to looking where he is going . . . . When attending to his body as an object, Tom loses awareness of objects in the world and loses his way in the flow of action.

Ill at ease with his body, Tom encountered things in the world with an underlying attitude of fearfulness. For Tom, fear was woven into his mode of perception. Rather than apprehending he was apprehensive. Accordingly, things in the world often appeared to him as faceless. Tom did not recognize possibilities for action in them. For instance, when Tom saw an object that he had never seen before, he found it hard to imagine what it would feel like to touch, hold, or manipulate it. He found it difficult to translate his vision to his touch. He could not envision the potential that an object held for action.

Sounds, textures, and sights faded into one amorphous, meaningless background, or they threateningly leaped out of the world. For Tom, the world could be a large abyss. Moving into it was often like stepping into thin air. Moreover, Tom's world could be downright assaulting with he, its easy victim.

Therefore, Tom often tried to avoid the world. He often did this in two ways. First he assumed a disembodied, reflective mode of perception. Not surprisingly, Tom's primary mode of relating to the world was visual. Vision is the sense considered to be closest in nature to intellect (Leder, 1990). By intellectualizing a visual image of the world, Tom was sometimes able to keep it at bay. Second, he would create a mini-world immediately in front of himself where he could engage in well-controlled fine motor actions. To do this Tom became so totally absorbed in his visual analysis and fine motor action that he was unable to respond to other events in the world. For example, Tom's mother recalls how:

> I thought he was deaf because he would concentrate so thoroughly on his play with construction toys. I mean, he would build amazing things, but a train could go through the living room and he would not react to it, and certainly not to human voices. Yeah, and it was hard to get him to establish eye contact. Whenever I was feeding him, I would work very hard to sing and be very animated and everything was always bigger and grander to engage him more.

Things were still much the same. For example, Tom describes how it was for him when his brother entered the room during his visual fixation on a toy train:

> . . . When Ray came in for a little while, I kind of ignored him, like my eyes were like glued to what I was doing . . . I was like, [I] couldn't hear him. And I couldn't understand his thoughts because I couldn't see him.

Tom approached the world analytically focusing on facts. Unfortunately, facts, by themselves, do not hold a potential for action. It is not surprising that while Tom readily acquired encyclopedic knowledge about the world, learning a new motor skill for moving about in the world was an arduous process for him.

He approached each new motor task logically and visually. However, he could not do it in his body.

Rather, he tended to overconcentrate. He would dart his attention back and forth between the world and his body, trying to direct his action from a disembodied vantage point. When the exigencies of doing a dynamic motor act called for Tom to be in his body as an actor, he faltered, as described by his therapist:

> Ask him to walk across a balance beam or to run and kick a ball or anything that has to do with propelling himself and being the agent of action where he's the doer . . . [he falls apart]. I think it's the idea of him carrying himself and being competent alone and by himself as a physical unit that he hasn't quite gotten . . .

As the therapist notes, the feeling of being fully within and in control of his body was beyond Tom's experiential grasp at the time.

Despite all this, Tom wanted to learn to ride his bicycle like others his age. When his therapist joined him at home for a first attempt, he clutched the bike, feeling it melt out of control in his hands. Throwing it to the ground, he stomped off. Afterward, just thinking about riding the bicycle triggered overwhelming fear. About subsequent attempts on the bike, his therapist notes:

> He gets on that thing and just goes limp, he's not doing anything to be active on the bike . . . he literally falls into me rather than uses his own body to catch himself . . .

Underlying Tom's surrender was a lack of knowing how to search for experience. For example, when his therapist demonstrated riding a bicycle, Tom noted that it gave him "no clue about how it would feel to me." When making his feeble attempts at riding, he was in his usual mode of apprehensiveness and intellectualizing that distanced him from being open to bodily experience. As his therapist notes:

> . . . it's hard for him to coordinate all the aspects of this [bike riding], the visual part, the postural part, the hand movements and the foot movements all together . . . He's really concentrating . . . Tom often over-concentrates until he loses the integrity and the flow of the action. He over analyzes it and then he doesn't have any flow.

Hence for Tom, the bicycle and the prospect of riding it alternately floats obscurely in shadows or looms menacingly.

Claiming His Body

An important step in Tom's transformation took place in the following therapeutic session. According to his therapist, Tom came in the room "melting to the ground." He was unresponsive and avoided eye contact. The therapist had to repeatedly call his name before Tom responded. Tom was feeling ill at ease and retreating from the world into his visual-intellectual, disembodied mode. Initially, his therapist's entreaties were a discomfort and a nuisance. Sensing his experience, the therapist invited him to engage in a sequence of gross motor activities that began with jumping on a trampoline and continued with a series of interactions between Tom and her. According to both Tom and the therapist, this activity was a turning point. Here is what happened.

Jumping up and down on the trampoline immediately engaged Tom's entire body in a rapid movement in which he could neither visually fixate nor retreat into his disembodied mode. He was, thus, shepherded into abandoning his typical objectification of his body. For the duration of his jumping, Tom had to act from his body to the routine of jumping. Moreover, the jumping prompted Tom to feel his body as a unified whole. He began to be at home with himself.

At the same time, Tom's slightest movements were immediately echoed by the trampoline. Moreover, the trampoline moved him in response to his movements. Within this dynamic, the world was taking hold of his body and moving him, but doing so in direct response to his actions. This echo of movement also served to abet and attune Tom to his moving. Moreover, because the trampoline resonated with Tom's movements, the boundary between inside and outside faded. They became part of a unitary experience. Moreover, the dynamic of the trampoline presented Tom with a specific rhythm so that he was invited go along with the natural frequency of the trampoline. Jumping on the trampoline opened for Tom a very immediate way for attuning himself to the world and reciprocating with it. For Tom, the trampoline had the exact characteristics to invite him toward something that had always remained just outside his experiential grasp. It allowed him to begin to glimpse a new way of being in his body and in his world. Tom began to live his body in a new way.

Next, the therapist introduced tossing a basketball that Tom was to catch and toss into a basket while still jumping on the trampoline. As if by magic, Tom saw the oncoming ball not as a threat but as an invitation to act. In his state of attending to the world from his body he was able to apprehend the ball's trajectory and catch it. Later he had the same experience with juggling beanbags. Notably the therapist was able to sense Tom's readiness to catch and toss and found the rhythm that enabled him to do so.

In the midst of these experiences Tom's action evolved as follows. Initially Tom's movements were very rigid and constricted. His knees were unbent and locked. His hands hung stiffly alongside his body. His mouth was near motionless when he talked and his intonation was flat. He held his breath in anxiety. He looked away from the therapist.

Gradually, while jumping on the trampoline, his movements became more fluid. His breathing became more rhythmic. His face began to show expression. His intonations grew richer. His language was more and more interactive. He made eye-contact with the therapist. Tom's fearful stance turned into one of involvement. He did not wince or fall apart when the ball was thrown to him and even tolerated being occasionally bombarded with beanbags. His eye-hand coordination and timing in catching and throwing steadily improved. He began to take risks in how he moved. He became more humorous and playful.

After the session Tom noted his own surprise at being able to try something new:

> [The therapist got me] from something that I did know about [basketball] to something that I didn't know about [juggling] . . . I was surprised because before I was afraid to juggle and I was like no, I couldn't do it, but she got me to juggle and now I know that practice makes perfect . . .

In a later session, when Tom again attempted riding the bicycle, his therapist noted the following changes:

> I was having to do less work. He was doing more. And although he was leaning, it was not as much . . . last week I felt like a training wheel. He was just leaning on me like he would lean on a training wheel and I was correcting him out of that, but today . . . I could feel him balancing and then leaning more at the end of the motion.

Within a couple of weeks, Tom mastered riding his bicycle. More importantly, a deeper transformation took place. Tom was beginning to inhabit his body and his world in a new way.

The "Hand and Me," Then "We"

Curtis, a 42-year-old African American, worked for a catering company and routinely clocked more than 40 hours a week. Curtis threw himself into his work, believing that "you should be able to go as far and do as much in anything that you think you want to do." His work was mostly "hands on." Of himself, he says:

> Um, I'm pretty good with figuring things out . . . if you just sit back and think about it for a minute. . .it only takes common sense. So, add a little common sense with a little intelligence, What you got? A person that can figure out problems (Curtis, 7/13/98, first audiotaped interview).

When problems developed at work, Curtis would jump in and solve the problem. He particularly enjoyed accomplishing tasks and solving problems that required using his hands.

One weekend, while replacing the floorboards on his work truck, Curtis lacerated his left hand with a power saw. The cut was so severe that the third, fourth, and fifth digits were almost completely severed. Alone at the time of injury, he explains that:

> [I] grabbed a towel, wrapped my hand up, then got some duct tape and taped it up around the towel. Then I went in the house, got my wallet with my insurance card, got my I.D., got my keys, locked the door . . . moved the stuff out from under the garage door opener because the door wouldn't come down . . . let the garage door down, got in the truck and drove myself to [the hospital].

Seventeen hours of surgery successfully reattached his fingers. Based on interviews over a 2-month period, Hutson (1998) chronicled changes in Curtis' embodiment that occurred as a result of his hand amputation and reattachment.

In the days after surgery, Curtis could not move his hand. He felt suddenly plucked out of his usual mode of being, as his hand was no longer available as an immediate and reliable resource for doing things. Just as importantly as the inability to move his fingers was that he could no longer do many things that used to be automatic:

> I couldn't do things, and I'm not that type. These [hands] are . . . these here's my life, right. Without these (hands) I was . . . so mad and crazy.

In addition to its no longer being available as a potential for action, Curtis noted that the reattached hand:

> Don't feel like a hand. It's hard to describe how it feel. You know how when you crush your fingertip and it gets black at the nail, you know how it throbs. It feels like that. Or, it don't feel like nothin at all. Nothin. Or sometimes it's all tingly.

Not only did he find the sensation of the hand different, but Curtis also felt that his hand was no longer part of himself:

> I don't know. I don't consider, for some . . . for some strange reason I, it, two thing. I think of it as two things now. It's me and the hand. It's not just me. It's me and the hand. Uh, why I don't know. Well I don't even know how I came up with that but I guess ever since I been, ever since the accident it's been me and the hand.

Later, as Curtis began to be able to move the hand, his relationship to it changed, but it was still not the same as before. He shifted from using the phrase "me and the hand" to using the term "we." Curtis explains his new use of the term "we":

> I guess because I'm gonna have to do it, but the hand gonna have to perform it, I would assume. And if the hand don't perform it then it's just me. But, when the hand start movin, I said we did it. I didn't say I did it. We did it, because the hand still had to move. So ever since then it's been we. . . . It's always gonna be we.

His language clearly illustrates that while Curtis' hand was reattached and partly functional, it was not part of the self as it had been before. His distinction between the self that would do and the hand that would perform underscores the separation of the hand that moves from the self that intends the motion. Nonetheless, unlike the prior, nonfunctional hand that was simply not part of himself, he had formed an unusual partnership with the new performing hand.

What kept the hand from being part of the self, despite his growing ability to move his hand in a functional way, was that he still attended to the hand instead of from it. This also created practical problems in how he completed tasks. Because Curtis could not use the hand as an automatic point of view for doing things, he had to monitor the hand's action and any objects it held. For example:

> So, I have to squeeze [something I hold] tight enough where I can feel it in my hand because if I don't, it'll just [slip out], and it takes a lot of concentration . . . I pick something up with this hand. I have to keep my eye on what I have in this hand. If I take my mind and go someplace else with it, it'll just slip because I won't feel it. It's kind of hard actually. I try to do a lot with it but it's awful hard because you, you have to concentrate too much on this one thing. And you know, like it should be, it's not automatic like what I'm doing right now [with the right hand]. I can still talk to you and hold this cup at the same time. With this left hand I can't do that.

Because Curtis was not able to act from his left hand, many two-handed tasks took too much attention for ease in everyday performance. So, while his left hand had objectively regained functional movement, he initially preferred not to use it in routine activities. Instead he learned to do things with his right hand alone. For example:

> I had to learn how to button up my shirt with one hand. But it have to be short sleeve shirt, 'cause I can't button this up right here (referring to the right cuff) I can't do that. I can do this one with this hand (pointing to left cuff) and these right here (front buttons) but I can't do this one (right cuff). It wasn't difficult, but in a way it was because of the way that, well you know that men are used to buttoning up the sleeve with one hand anyway. So, it, the point of it was I couldn't grab it and get it over. I just had to keep practicing to get it. But now, it's easy.

As Curtis describes it, after an initial period of clumsiness, he mastered and thus achieved ease in putting on his shirt with one hand. This ease was something he could not achieve when the left hand was incorporated into anything he did.

The left hand was uneasy when doing things, and it also needed tending. He had to consciously monitor its involvement in any activity and to make sure it was not exposed to danger. Consequently, it was easier to leave it out of doing things. For a while this is how things were.

After several weeks Curtis approached his occupational therapist about returning to work because he was tired of sitting at home. The therapist, in consultation with the surgeon, determined that Curtis could return to work on light duty. He was instructed to avoid hot and cold and not to lift anything over 15 pounds using the left hand.

Because of his excellent work history, the employer invited Curtis to return to work full-time as the supervisor with responsibility of organizing and managing other workers. Although the new role was actually a promotion, Curtis did not see it positively. For him, doing things with his hands was essential to his satisfaction. Indicating his hands, he notes, "I like to do things with this." Consequently, Curtis experienced much of his new job as still "doin nothin." He explains:

> Because I really don't do nothin. I don't do much. Just driving. I do a lot of deliveries, box lunches, 'cause I do deliver a lot of lunches and a lot of dinners. Mostly driving, but I don't do.

Because he was not much of a paper pusher, Curtis, by his own admission, began to engage in two-handed tasks he "had no business doin." Despite his recognition of possible danger to his hand and the cumbersome process of having to concentrate on his left hand whenever he used it, he nonetheless began to feel an irresistible urge to use his injured hand at work:

> I have to do things. Okay, uh it's just like telling a new born baby when he gets up and starts to walking and you tell him no, he can't walk. Uh, you holding him down instead of letting him go and explore the world that is what I'm gonna have to do anyway with this [left] hand, is explore and find. And I'm gonna have to learn how to compensate for things I can't do to come up with a way of doing it anyhow.

Curtis had the growing feeling that if he did not make use of the hand he might as well "just sit around and let the hand die," in which case it would have been better to "just cut the hand on off." Thus, while his injured hand still offered Curtis no experience of operating from it to the world, he nevertheless began to feel a call to involve the hand in doing.

While Curtis still could not experience the hand as part of his intentional self, he decided to breathe a kind of life into the hand by making it part of his doing things.

His final assessment was that, "it's always gonna be we." Clearly, he does not expect the hand to become fully part of himself as before. Nonetheless, his references to the hand as a baby worthy of life, needing soothing and the opportunity to explore and grow, suggests that he has found in the metaphor of parent and child a way to exist with this hand. The hand is not fully part of himself, but adopted as part of a new "we."

Discussion

The three studies just presented systematically examined the lived body experience. These studies illuminated both the nature of disability experience and the role of experience in how persons managed to overcome or adapt to their impairments.

Disability Experience

Disability always represents a particular way of being embodied. This is an altered way of existing that thrusts itself on the person with a disability. Hence, persons with disabilities must live the reality of their embodiment. Moreover, they are challenged to adapt to their experiences. Any change in capacity must often be in terms of those experiences. As Csordas (1994) reminds us, people with disabilities must take up an existential position in the world that reflects their particular embodiment.

> *Altered experience alters performance.*

There appear to be some phenomena that are more general to the disability experience and others that are particular to a type of impairment. Still others are unique to the individual. For example, all the subjects in the studies we examined experienced some form of alienation from their bodies or parts of their bodies. Both Murphy (1987) and Sachs (1993) have also described the experience of disability as including alienation from one's own body.

While alienation involves the common feature of not experiencing the body or some part of the body as belonging to the self, the particular experience of alienation varied. For the women with neglect, there was at one stage disbelief that their left side was attached to the rest of them. For Curtis, his hand was clearly attached to his body, but it no longer felt like part of his intentional self. For Tom there was an element of never having fully owned his body or experienced it as a whole.

Despite these differences, all the subjects had to find ways of coming to terms with this alienation. Tom was able to achieve ownership and integration of his body; the women regained the sense of acting from their left side. Curtis continued to experience his hand as separate from self, but decided in the end to bring it into his routine way of doing things. These findings suggest that coming to terms with bodily alienation may be an important task in regaining capacity for a range of persons with disabilities.

Understanding disability in terms of subjective experience is important because it often explains aspects of a person's functional capacity not accounted for in objective approaches. Curtis exemplifies how an objective description of his performance capacity could not fully account for his performance. Whereas part of his performance capacity is reflected in his objectively describable ability to move his hand, how he experienced his hand was equally important to his functional capacity. Curtis' ability to use his hand cannot be described fully from an objective viewpoint alone.

Consequently, we see that how people perform does not only reflect the objective status of performance components. It also emanates from how they experience themselves and their worlds. Altered experience alters performance.

Importance of Experience for Transforming Capacity

Each of the three cases presented could be described from an objective view of the body and mind. For example, Tom's integration of sensory information can be seen as due to changes in the brain structure, the women's acquisition of ways to deal with world-neglect can be described in terms of new learning compensatory strategies, and Curtis' hand function could be described as return of strength, range, and sensation. These objective descriptions are certainly valid and important for understanding what happens to such persons as their impairments change over time. However, as the studies clearly illustrate, these descriptions would only partly explain how change took place.

In all three studies, it was through the realm of experience that effective strategies of change were discovered. The actual events and human actions that resulted in change were a function of experience. Each of these persons had to use their experience as a way of solving their own problems and challenges. For example, only when Tom is able to locate the experience of being in relationship to the world in another way, only when he can feel the new experience, does he begin to change. Similarly, the women with neglect had to come to know a new reality in which their practical world consisted not just of what they could perceive, but also of something outside perception. Learning to exist effectively in such a world meant that they had to come to a way of understanding their new experiences. Both these examples indicate how transformation in performance capacity depends on a transformation in experience.

Conclusion

This chapter offered a subjective approach to understanding performance capacity that is complementary to the usual objective approach. The concept of the lived body derived from phenomenology offers a unique way of conceptualizing subjective experience and its role in performance. Through careful attention to this subjective experience we have a way to better understand performance capacity.

Key Terms

Lived body: The experience of being and knowing the world through a particular body.

Performance capacity: Ability for doing things provided by the status of underlying objective physical and mental components and corresponding subjective experience.

References

Baz, T. (1998). *The experience of change in therapy.* Masters Thesis, Department of Occupational Therapy, University of Illinois at Chicago.

Bisiach, E., & Vallar, G. (1988). Hemi neglect in humans. In F. Boller & J. Grafman (Eds.), *Handbook of neuropsychology.* Amsterdam: Elsevier Science Publishers.

Clark, F. (1993). Occupation embedded in a real life: Interweaving occupational science and occupational therapy. *American Journal of Occupational Therapy, 47,* 1067–1078.

Csordas, T. (Ed.). (1994). *Embodiment and experience: The existential ground of culture and self.* New York: Cambridge University Press.

Engelbrecht, F. (1968). *The phenomenology of the human body.* South Africa: Sovenga.

Hutson, J. (1998). *Qualitative study of the experience of an injured worker.* Masters Thesis, Department of Occupational Therapy, University of Illinois at Chicago.

Jamison, K. R. (1995). *An unquiet mind: A memoir of moods and madness.* New York: Vintage Books.

Kielhofner, G. (1995). A meditation on the use of hands. *Scandinavian Journal of Occupational Therapy, 2,* 153–166.

Leder, D. (1984). Medicine's paradigm of embodiment. *Journal of Medical Philosophy, 9,* 29–43.

Leder, D. (1990). *The absent body.* Chicago: University of Chicago Press.

Luria, A. R. (1972). *The man with a shattered world: The history of a brain wound.* New York: Basic Books.

McGlynn, S. M., & Schacter, D. L. (1989). Unawareness of deficits in neuropsychological syndromes. *Journal of Clinical Experimental Neuropsychology, 11,* 143–205.

Merleau-Ponty, M. (1962). *Phenomenology of perception.* (C. Smith, Trans.). London: Routledge & Kegan Paul. (Original work published 1945)

Murphy, R. (1987). *The body silent.* New York: Henry Holt & Company.

Sachs, O. (1993). *A leg to stand on.* New York: Harper Collins Publishers.

Sartre, J. P. (1970). The body. In S. F. Spricher (Ed.), *The phi-*

losophy of the body: Reflections on Cartesian dualism. Chicago: Quadrangle Books.

Sechehaye, M. (1968). *Autobiography of a schizophrenic girl: The true story of Renee.* (G. Rubin Rabson, Trans.). New York: Grune & Stratton.

Sudnow, D. (1978). *Ways of the hand: The organization of improvised conduct.* Cambridge: Harvard University Press.

Sudnow, D. (1979). *Talk's body: A meditation between two keyboards.* New York: Knopf.

Tham, K., Borell, L., & Gustavsson, A. (2000).The discovery of disability: A phenomenological study of unilateral neglect. *American Journal of Occupational Therapy, 54,* 398–406.

Toombs, K. (1992). *The meaning of illness. A phenomenological account of the different perspectives of physician and patient.* Boston: Kluwer Academic Publishers.

Williams, D. (1994). *Nobody nowhere: The extraordinary autobiography of an autistic.* New York: Avon Books.

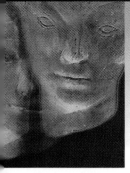

7

The Environment and Occupation

● Gary Kielhofner

Previous chapters acknowledged the role of the environment in choices for doing, routine patterns of behavior, and performance. This chapter further examines the influence of the environment on occupation. Two important questions are addressed: 1) How does the environment influence what we choose to do and the way we do it? and 2) What factors in the environment influence occupation? In answering these questions, this chapter provides a way of conceptualizing environmental influences and contributions to what we do in the course of daily life.

In addition, this chapter considers the role of the environment in disability. It emphasizes that disability always involves a relationship between the person and the environment. Accordingly, the environment may contribute to disabling or enabling a person who has an impairment.

Nature of Environment

We exist in multiple contexts. We are located in a particular geographic area and are part of a society. We are members of and are influenced by particular cultures. We live in some kind of abode and routinely move about in a neighborhood, the countryside, or our town and/or city. We have belongings and tools that surround us and that we use. We live among people with whom we routinely interact. These are all our environments.

The primary concern of this chapter is with those aspects of the environment that most impact upon doing things. Consequently, for our purposes, the **environment** can be defined as the particular physical and social features of the specific context in which one does something that impacts upon what one does, and how it is done.

Given this definition, we recognize that most people operate in a variety of environments in the course of a day. As we move about in these different contexts, we encounter different physical spaces, objects, groups of people, and kinds of things that are done in those contexts. The configuration of these elements in any setting influences what we chose to do and how we go about doing it.

Role of Culture

Since the physical and social environments are interpreted and shaped by culture, (Altman & Chemers, 1980) it is important to recognize culture as a pervasive feature of the environment. **Culture** is defined as the beliefs and perceptions, values and norms, customs and behaviors that are shared by a group or society and are passed from one generation to the next through both formal and informal education (Altman & Chemers, 1980; Brake, 1980; Ogbu, 1981; Rapoport, 1980).

Within most cultures there are also a variety of subcultures. For example, in American society, there are urban, rural, ethnic, and other subcultures. Each shows important differences from the dominant culture and, in particular, influences the organization of various groups.

The impact of culture is not homogeneous. We may experience several different sources of cultural influence, depending on the range of environments in

> *Culture influences not only what is within the environment, but also how a person is predisposed to interact with the environment.*

which we do things. For example, I live in a farming community in rural southern Wisconsin, commute to urban Chicago to work, and am responsible for educational and clinical programs that have a mission of serving minority populations that bring me into contact with Hispanic and African-American subcultures. In addition, I travel abroad regularly and count among my friends persons living in Europe, Canada, South America, and Asia. All these experiences expose me to a significant range of cultural influences. Although my experience is more diverse than that of many people, it is increasingly probable that persons will experience an array of cultural influences in a world with increasing resources for communication and mobility. The insulated and homogeneous cultural experiences of persons who lived a century ago are less and less likely in today's world (Gergen, 1991).

We can readily see how the social world, the world of human relationships and activities, is shaped by culture. Nevertheless, there is an equally important influence of culture on the physical environment. Culture determines how our physical context is organized and what artifacts we are likely to encounter within it. Culture also gives us a way of seeing and encountering the physical environment, including the world of nature.

When we consider any aspect of the physical or social environment, it is important to remember that culture is in the background shaping and defining it. Because culture is a pervasive force in the environment, I will repeatedly refer to its role in discussing the physical and social environment. Moreover, it is important to recognize that culture is also internalized by people. A person's values, sense of competence, interests, and internalized roles and habits are all reflections of that person's belonging to a particular culture. Culture influences not only what is within the environment but also how a person is predisposed to interact with the environment.

Opportunities and Resources for Choosing and Doing

Elements of the physical and social environment provide opportunities and resources that evoke and enable choosing and doing things (Dunn, Brown, & McGuigan, 1994; Gibson, 1979; Law, 1991; Law, Cooper, Strong, Stewart, Rigby, & Letts, 1996; Nelson, 1988; Reed, 1982). These opportunities and resources emanate from the places we inhabit, the objects we use, the others we encounter, and what is available to do.

Most environments offer a range of opportunities to choose what to do. For example, a natural resource such as a lake or forest affords one the opportunity to enjoy the view, to photograph the scene, or to go hiking or swimming. Even objects designed for specific purposes such as an automobile may provide the choices of driving to work, tuning the engine, washing and waxing, or cruising downtown.

The environment may also provide resources to sustain our motivation. Family members and friends may offer us emotional support and reassurance to sustain effort toward a goal. Others' confidence in us may encourage us to try harder, and their feedback may help us make better choices for what to undertake.

The environment provides resources that facilitate our performance. Tools, instructions, and guidance from others are examples of environmental resources that enable performance. Moreover, those aspects of the environment that we do not readily recognize as enabling behavior contribute to our performance. Consider, for example, piecing together a jigsaw puzzle. As we fit the pieces together, we store information about the solutions we have already achieved and we progressively eliminate pieces that would otherwise be inappropriate candidates for being included in future solutions. The pieces that make up the puzzle are not just objects we use, but also resources that help us solve the problem of how to put it together. In this way, all elements of the environment contribute to how we go about doing things. They are intimately part of our performance.

Familiar aspects of the physical and social environment are necessary to our routine behaviors. We rely on stable and recurring features of the environment to acquire and enact our habits and roles. To perform our daily routines competently, the familiar arrangement of spaces and objects and the recurrent events and predictable behavior patterns of others are all essential. Consequently, those elements of the environment that are consistent and reliable are crucial resources for our habits and roles.

chapter 7

Demands and Constraints on Choosing and Doing

Each environment poses a variety of conditions that place limits on or strongly direct our action (Dunn, Brown, & Mcguigan, 1994; Law, 1991; Law et al., 1996; Lawton, 1980). Fences, walls, steps, and other features of the physical environment constrain where we go or how much effort it takes. Time limitations and task complexity determine how much we can do. Others' desires, laws and regulations, job requirements, and social norms require or forbid certain behaviors.

In each environment we encounter expectations that demand particular behaviors and discourage or disallow others. For example, in an airport the counters and agents, roped areas, security checkpoints and guards, posted rules and announcements, gates, and lines of passengers influence and, in part, dictate the sequence of things we do. Standing in line, obtaining a boarding pass, checking luggage, going to the gate, and boarding the plane are all done according to environmental demands and constraints.

The various expectations and requirements of our environments can obviously constrain choices. They also appear to sustain motivation. For example, some retirees who no longer have the demands of the work routine find it more difficult to maintain their motivation for doing things (Jonsson, Josephsson, & Kielhofner, 2000).

Barriers and challenges in the physical environment, informal and formal rules governing how various occupations must be done, and expectations for productivity are examples of environmental features that shape how we perform. Environmental demands and constraints also influence the development of habits and roles. Thus, for example, when we enter school, specific courses must be taken, we must go to designated rooms to attend those courses, and certain public and private behaviors are expected (e.g., joining class discussions, dressing a certain way by virtue of school code or peer pressure, studying, using the library, taking exams, and completing papers). A school's physical arrangement and rules and requirements, combined with teachers, peers, and others' perceptions of the student role, all funnel and shape the attitudes and actions that come to make up each student's role.

Many of the demands and constraints in an environment are present to maintain order in social processes. Therefore, they help shape individuals toward competent participation in the environment. However, demands and constraints of an environment can also negatively constrain motives and action. For example, some features of a school environment may interfere with learning (Kielhofner, 1983). Many service environments have also been noted to have adverse effects on their occupants. For example, Borell, Gustavsson, Sandman, and Kielhofner (1994) studied how the rules, organized events, and concerns of staff in a day hospital for persons with dementia actually stifled clients' attempts to engage in spontaneous behaviors and encouraged passivity and inactivity.

Environmental Impact

Each environment offers a number of opportunities and resources, demands and constraints. Whether these are noticed or felt, and whether they influence behavior, depends on each person's current values, interests, personal causation, roles, habits, and performance capacities. Let us take as an example the relationship between environmental demands and performance capacities. Environments that challenge a person's capacities tend to evoke involvement, attentiveness, and maximal performance (Csikszentmihalyi, 1990; Kiernat, 1983; Lawton & Nahemow, 1973). On the other hand, when environments demand performance well below capacity, they can evoke boredom and disinterest and even result in, "the type of negative affect and behavior seen in sensory deprivation" (Kiernat, 1983, p. 6). When demands are too far beyond capacity, they can make a person feel anxious, overwhelmed, or hopeless. Since persons have different capacities and beliefs in their own abilities, the

Each environment offers a number of opportunities and resources, demands and constraints. Whether these are noticed or felt, and whether they influence behavior, depends on each person's current values, interests, personal causation, roles, habits, and performance capacities.

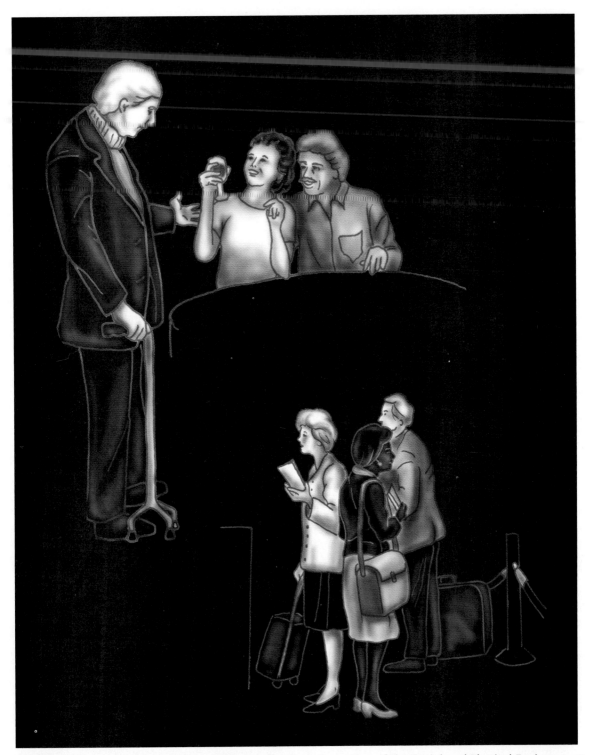

FIGURE 7-1   Environmental Impact Depends on the Intersection of the Social and Physical Environment with the Values, Interests, Personal Causation, Habits, Roles, and Performance Capacities of those within the Environment.

same environment may engage and excite one person, bore another, and overwhelm a third.

It is important to note the difference between features of an environment and its actual influence on specific persons within that environment. The opportunity, support, demand, and constraint that the physical and social aspects of the environment have on a particular individual will be referred to as **environmental impact**. Environmental impact is not a feature of the environment alone. Rather, as shown in *Figure 7-1*, it results from the interaction between features of the environment and characteristics of the person.

Physical Environment

All that we experience and can do is, in some measure, a function of our placement in a physical world. The spaces in which we act (Lawton, 1983) and the objects we encounter within them impact our doing things (Csikszentmihalyi & Rochberg-Halton, 1981). Notably, access to objects and spaces is profoundly affected by the economic resources that persons have at their disposal.

Spaces

Occupation takes place in both natural and built spaces. As shown in *Figure 7-2*, these spaces have unique features that shape what we do within them. The physical properties of natural spaces along with the weather offer opportunities, supports, and demands for behavior. Consider, for example, the different possibilities for doing things on a beach during a hot summer day and in a forest during a winter snowstorm.

Occupations often take place in specific built spaces, such as a school, stadium, shopping mall, or salon. Built spaces reflect and are instrumental to culture. They are readily recognized by members of the culture as having a designated purpose and as intended for certain persons' use (Rubinstein, 1989). Consequently, they offer specific opportunities and constraints for doing. For example, a library invites browsing and reading and discourages speaking aloud, whereas a football stadium encourages spectators to watch and cheer for their team.

Objects

Within the physical environment we encounter a variety of objects. **Objects** are defined as naturally occurring or fabricated things with which we interact and whose properties influence what we do with them (*Fig. 7-3*). While objects in natural environments occur according to the scheme of nature, those in built environments are placed there by human design. Which objects are present and how they are organized generally depends on the purpose of the space and cultural convention (Rubinstein, 1989).

Objects also strongly influence occupation. For instance, whether children engage in solitary or social play depends on what types of toys and equipment are present (Quilitch & Risley, 1973). Raw materials (boxes, sand, tires) lend themselves to active exploration (Csikszentmihalyi & Rochberg-Halton, 1981), whereas fixed equipment in playgrounds can constrain what play occurs (Haywood, Rothenberg, & Beasley, 1974). Objects also influence behavior simply by virtue of their intrinsic properties (Hocking, 1994). The weight, size, pliability, texture, and other physical attributes of objects may influence whether we toss, carry, bend, or otherwise handle them. Simple and familiar objects may give comfort and invite relaxing behavior, whereas complex objects tend to demand specialized and skilled behavior.

We tend to surround ourselves with objects that reflect our established patterns of interest and activity and that reflect who we are. Adolescents, for example, frequently mention musical instruments and stereo equipment as being their most prized possessions (Csikszentmihalyi & Rochberg-Halton, 1981). Objects often take on the most value when they signify something very personal about one's experiences or accomplishments, or one's connections to others (Csikszentmihalyi & Rochberg-Halton, 1981). For example, objects handed down in families may also convey the "sense of having roots or of belonging in a particular setting" (Ljungström, 1989). On the other hand, Rubinstein (1989) notes how an elderly woman's collection of figurines, "marked and filled her space, gave her sensory pleasure, had a story and gave her stories to tell, and added texture to her rooms" (p. 49).

The symbolic meaning of objects may influence how they support or demand ways of using them. For example: when a car is a symbol of independence and

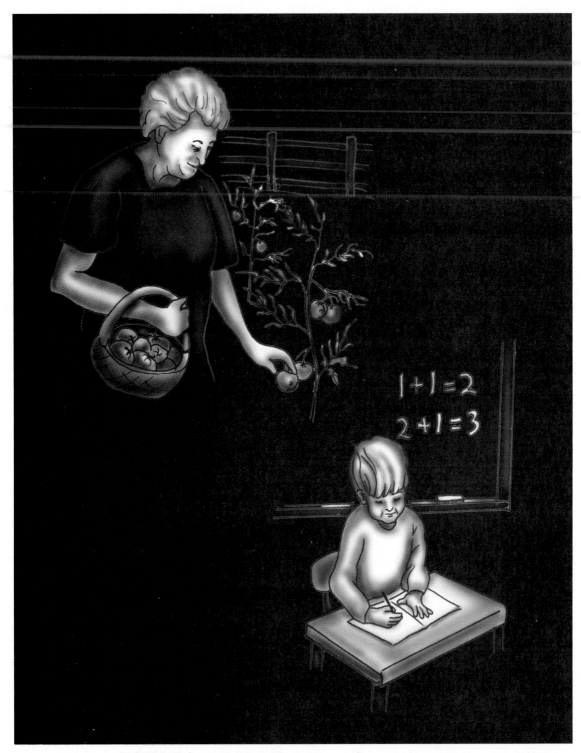

FIGURE 7-2   Natural and Built Spaces Influence What We Do.

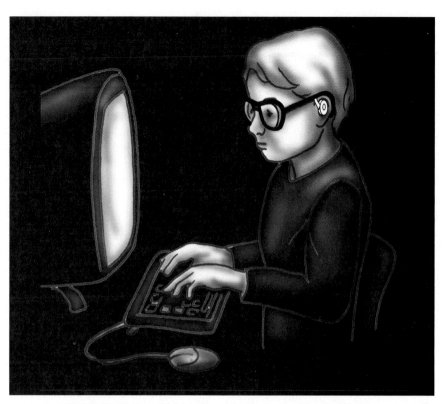

FIGURE 7-3 Objects Provide Opportunities for Doing.

responsibility, the young adult owner may feel increased demands for competence in understanding its maintenance. A practical object with strong sentimental value may be restricted from use to avoid its becoming damaged or destroyed.

Impact of the Physical Environment on Persons with Disabilities

Physical spaces can pose multiple problems for persons with disabilities. The most obvious are natural and architectural barriers that interfere with the performance of work, play, and daily living tasks. The onset of a physical disability can transform a house into a virtual prison (Rockwell-Dylla, 1992). Ordinary features of a house may become significant barriers, as Murphy (1987) observed:

In common with all old houses, our floors sag in places, creating little hills and valleys so small that they are undetectable to the normal person. But

when you are using weakened arms to push a wheel chair across them, you get to know every one of them. (p. 190)

As laws and social consciousness change, many architectural barriers are being eliminated. Nevertheless, much of the built environment is designed without consideration of inhabitants' possible impairments, thereby limiting opportunities and posing constraints on those with disabilities.

Familiar spaces can provide a variety of supports that make it possible to function despite impairments. For example, Rowles (1991) describes an elderly couple, Walter and Beatrice, who have lived in the same house for more than half a century:

Intimate familiarity with the layout of [Walter's] home had served him well as he had grown increasingly constrained by failing vision. Beatrice's use of this environment was also facilitated by her bodily awareness of the placement of furniture.

The configuration of furniture had gradually evolved over the years in a manner that provided places for her to hold on should she experience one of the dizzy spells to which she had become prone. (p. 268)

Natural spaces similarly can provide a variety of problems for the person with a disability. For example, Hull (1990), who is blind, notes that snow is a particular problem because snow blunts the sounds he relies on and makes use of the cane difficult. As this example illustrates, the kind of problems the physical environment poses will differ depending on whether one's impairment is emotional, sensory, motor, or cognitive.

Most fabricated objects in the environment are naturally geared via their size, shape, weight, complexity, and functions for able-bodied, sighted, hearing, and cognitively intact individuals. Impairments often make it impossible or dangerous to handle or interact with the objects of everyday life. Zola (1982) offers the following litany of problems posed by objects for persons like himself with motor impairments:

Chairs without arms to push myself up from; unpadded seats which all too quickly produce sores; showers and toilets without handrails to maintain my balance; surfaces too slippery to walk on; staircases without banisters to help me hoist myself; buildings without ramps, making ascent exhausting if not dangerous; every curbstone a precipice; car, plane, and theater seats too cramped for my braced leg; and trousers too narrow for my leg brace to pass through. With such trivia is my life plagued. (p. 208)

Of course, while some objects can pose constraints, others are important resources. A very large number of objects have been designed and are available to compensate for impairments. Such adaptive aids range from simple tools with build-up handles to compensate for limited grip to complex computer-based systems that control environments and allow communication.

Although these objects have tremendous potential to support a higher level of function, they also pose demands. Persons with disabilities often must live with a plethora of objects that extend or substitute for motor function, replace lost senses, provide protection, or manage disease processes. Wheelchairs, braces, adaptive equipment, bottles of medication, the disability

check, ramps into one's home, catheterization supplies, and grab bars may be welcome resources or necessary nuisances.

They also carry deep symbolic messages. Simply being in a wheelchair can change one's social identity and interactions. Since objects can symbolize dependency or disability, some persons will not use otherwise functionally helpful objects. For example, I recall vividly young men in a spinal cord unit who adamantly refused to wear splints during their Friday night poker games. For all their functional virtues, the splints simply spoiled the ambiance of the poker game and stifled the bravado of the players. Another poignant example provided by a colleague was that older adults in the inner city often did not use mobility aids such as canes and walkers because they felt it increased their visibility as easy targets of crime.

Bates, Spencer, Young, and Hopkins-Rintala (1993) chronicle how one spinal-cord–injured man, Russell, struggled over the meaning of a wheelchair in his life. When first learning sitting tolerance in a wheelchair he could not yet propel, he notes:

I hate that time then because I can't do nothing. They might as well stick me in a damn closet. Can't move, can't do nothing . . . all you can do is sit there and think how helpless you are. (p. 1016)

Later the chair became a constant reminder that his goal of walking again might not be viable. Over time, he vacillated between wanting to take a blowtorch to the chair and finding it necessary as a means of mobility. Even after discharge from rehabilitation his feelings about the chair were ambivalent. The kinds of extraordinary objects that disabled persons use can invoke intense emotional responses. These feelings influence not only what the object means to the individual, but also how that individual will learn about and use the object, and whether it will be integrated into an acceptable life (Bates et al., 1993).

Specialized settings such as residential facilities are frequently devoid of many ordinary objects. Several years ago, in a study of persons with mental retardation living in board and care homes, I was struck by how barren were the rooms and apartments. Personal belongings, decorations, comfortable furniture, minor appliances, and the many other things that most members of our society take for granted as part of our living spaces were absent. A lack of objects in one's living space can contribute to apathy and feelings of helplessness (Gray, 1972; Magill & Vargo, 1977). Everyday objects that provide opportunities for activity choices can be more important than specialized or adapted objects in stimulating functional behavior (Simmons & Barris, 1984).

The arrangement of objects in a space can also support or constrain behavior. For example, how furniture is placed in a room or how food is served in an institution can encourage or discourage social interaction (Holahan, 1979; Melin & Gotestam, 1981). Too often, objects in institutional settings serve organizational efficiency but negatively affect what inhabitants do. A final, important consideration is that disability and poverty often go hand in hand. As a result, many persons lack access to the physical resources that might otherwise enable them (Helfrich, Fisher, & Kielhofner, 2000).

Social Environment

The social environment includes groups of persons that one joins and the occupational forms that one performs. Both provide resources and opportunities for doing while demanding and constraining action.

Social Groups

Much of what we do involves interacting with others in social groups. **Social groups** are defined as collections of people who come together for various formal and informal purposes, and influence what we do within them. Groups give us opportunities and demand that we take on roles. As shown in *Figure 7-4*, they also constitute a social space (Knowles, 1982) in which our habits are shaped according to group ambiance, norms, and climate.

Most social groups endure over time and have an internal organization. The nature and organization of groups can range from an informal gathering of acquaintances at a local bar, to formalized organizations developed for the explicit purpose of achieving some goal (Etzioni, 1964; Katz & Kahn, 1966). Since an enduring climate of values and interests is characteristic of most groups (Moos, 1974), people will tend to acquire those same values and interests (Newcomb, 1943; Pervin, 1968).

Social groups have a major impact on the development of role behavior. Because roles are learned in the context of groups (Versluys, 1980), the groups that are available to a person will influence the roles available to

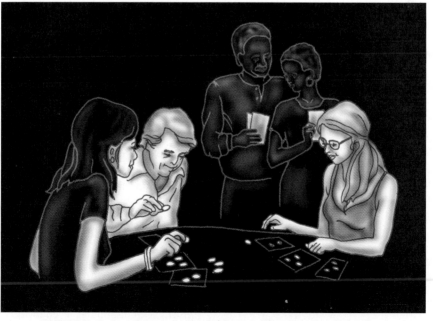

FIGURE 7-4 Groups as Social Spaces Shaping Our Behavior.

that person. An infant's role repertoire is limited primarily to family-derived roles in dyadic or small group relationships—daughter, son, niece, nephew, sister, brother. When children enter school, they have opportunities to participate in more groups such as clubs, choruses, bands, and sports teams. By adulthood, individuals are generally involved in a complex of work, religious, political, fraternal, and other types of groups (Allen, Wilder, & Atkinson, 1983). Throughout life the range of groups open to a person may expand or narrow.

Occupational Forms

Each culture is made up of a range of things that its members do to undertake everyday life. For example, each culture develops means for acquiring and preparing food. Generations of trial and error, creative refinement, and invention of new techniques and tools result in organized and sometimes ritualized ways of getting and preparing food. Cultures have generated such conventionalized ways of doing things for most aspects of life.

These conventionalized ways of doing things are referred to as occupational forms (Nelson, 1988). The notion of form refers to the specific manner, actions, meanings, and so on that characterize doing something. When we perform, we go through or enact the form. Each culture includes a wide range of occupational forms that constitute the opportunities and demands that the culture will put on its members for doing things.

Each of these forms has its own internal coherence. That is, the actions and manners that make up the form are connected to its meaning and purpose. For example, when people are playing a game of cards, their behaviors will reflect the purpose or objectives of the game and their attitude will be relaxed and playful. Woodworking, jogging, and shopping are all names for occupational forms. Because occupational forms are routinely done by members of a group and can be

named, they are readily recognized by members of the culture. Consequently, most of the time when we observe others we are able to say what they are doing. In so doing, we name the occupational form they are performing.

Given these considerations, **occupational forms** can be defined as conventionalized sequences of action that are at once coherent, oriented to a purpose, sustained in collective knowledge, culturally recognizable, and named. Occupational forms are conventionalized in that there is a typical or correct way of doing them. Cultures specify procedures, outcomes, and standards for doing an occupational form that are passed on to those who wish to learn the form. The conventions for doing some occupational forms are quite fixed. Taking an exam, for instance, requires someone to be in a particular place at a particular time and to answer a previously prepared set of questions. Success is contingent on answering correctly a preestablished percentage of these questions. Some occupational forms, such as driving, are governed by laws that specify how they are to be done and what is not allowed. In other cases, conventions for doing the form are open, such as going for a walk or dressing oneself. However, even those occupational forms that are more open-ended will conform to recognizable cultural parameters.

Occupational forms are always directed at some recognizable end even if the end is simply to experience the behavior, as in dancing or going for a walk. Indeed, it is the purposiveness of occupational forms that guarantees their maintenance as culturally recognizable acts.

By creating and sustaining occupational forms and their meanings, cultures provide opportunities to do things. The things we do have a form that existed long before we learned to do them. Moreover, the occupational form itself exerts a specific influence on us each time we undertake to perform it. The conventions that make up the occupational form constrain and demand certain actions. As shown in *Figure 7-5*, occupational forms are available in our social environment for us to do.

> *By creating and sustaining occupational forms and their meanings, cultures provide opportunities to do things.*

Social Environment and Disability

Most social groups have a deep ambivalence toward persons with disabilities. Even in societies whose laws, health care, and welfare systems are organized so as to

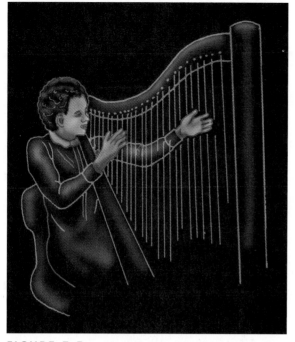

FIGURE 7-5   Occupational Forms as Things We Do.

support persons with disabilities, the attitudes of individuals and the practices of groups often betray discomfort with disabled persons (Gill, 1997; Hahn, 1993; Longmore, 1995). Personal accounts of individuals with disabilities are replete with stories of others' negative reactions and attitudes and of outright discrimination and rejection.

Onset of a physical disability can transform one's social environment. As Murphy observes, "The onset of quadriplegia, I discovered, had placed me in a new social dimension" (1987, p. 195).

Emotional or intellectual disabilities can equally set persons apart from the rest of society. Western cultures place a high value on intelligence, so that an implied deficit in this area is tantamount to the most serious kind of personal flaw—something that strikes at the very worth of the individual (Dexter, 1956, 1960; Edgerton, 1967).

Persons who acquire a disability may find themselves temporarily or permanently removed from the groups in which they previously enacted their roles (Sarbin, 1954). Further, those social groups in which the individual does things may be fundamentally changed. For example, coworkers may attribute an injured worker's accident to carelessness and thereby fear working alongside him or her. Coworkers may resent accommodations made for an emotionally disabled colleague. Disabled persons may also experience a shrinking social world as old friends and acquaintances are uneasy or unwilling to continue relationships or when the activities that were the basis of association are no longer possible (Hull, 1990; Murphy, Scheer, Murphy, & Mack, 1988; Oliver, Zarb, Silver, Moore, & Salisbury, 1988; Vash, 1981).

The family is both greatly affected by and influential on a member with a disability. For example, parents share in the suffering and grief that may be a part of a child's disability (Kornblum & Anderson, 1982). Household routines, family member responsibilities, organization of the physical home, and restraints on family spontaneity, travel, and other factors may all be part and parcel of having a disabled member in the family. Families may be extremely taxed by the work of caring for a disabled family member. Activities such as social contact and leisure may suffer (Breslau, 1983). A great deal of stress may be placed on family members who must accommodate the limitations of the person with a disability (Trombly, 1983).

Because persons with disabilities frequently have access to fewer non-kindred relationships they may depend significantly on the family for emotional, financial, and other forms of support. Consequently, the family can be a vital influence on the disabled person. Families that positively influence their disabled members include them in their routines and rituals and give them meaningful roles in the family (Bogdan & Taylor, 1989).

Disabled persons often end up spending significant portions of their lives in specialized social groups. These groups may include substitutes for home such as halfway houses, residential facilities, or nursing homes. They may be short-term treatment settings such as hospitals, community mental health centers, rehabilitation facilities, or long-term social and work settings such as senior centers and sheltered workshops. Such settings aim to provide services that support or enhance the performance and quality of life of persons with disabilities. However, a variety of factors, from constrained resources to organizational incentives and demands, can result in less than optimal conditions for achieving their ends. Consequently, many of these social groups may contribute to the very problems they seek to alleviate (Edgerton, 1967; Emerson, Rochford, & Shaw, 1983; Kielhofner, 1983; Scull, 1977; Test & Stein, 1978). For example, Suto and Frank (1994) observed that persons with schizophrenia in a residential setting faced, " . . . predominantly passive free time activities, a lack of involvement in traditional social roles, and many hours of free time" (p. 14). The combination of being severed from ordinary social groups and being placed in groups where the normal opportunities for roles and activities are severely restricted can have a profound effect on everyday occupational life.

The vast majority of occupational forms in any culture have been developed without consideration of how persons with impairments might do them. Consequently, the availability of occupational forms can be dramatically altered by disability. Performance limitations can make some occupational forms impossible. Disabled persons may forego or relinquish to others occupational forms that have become impossible to do. The temporal and social nature of occupational forms may be radically altered. For example, more time may be required for performance. Previously private occupational forms may require assistance from others. Incorporating necessary adaptive equipment into occupational forms may change their character.

Access to occupational forms is often unnecessarily restricted for disabled persons. For example, an elderly person who is, "asked to make his or her own bed but is capable of much more . . . feels self-incompetence and helplessness" (Miller & Oertel, 1983, p. 110).

For a variety of reasons disabled persons are given access to underchallenging occupational forms. Zola offers the following reflection on this issue:

> The jobs here were too simple, too fragmented, too mindless, too meaningless. Granted that my fellow residents might have limited physical capacity but why such busy work, why industrial products that were marketable only with a subsidy? Could the workers possibly feel they were doing something worthwhile? Of course, many jobs in the outside world were as repetitive and meaningless but at least those workers may have had a rationalization of the job's being a means to

an end. To what end were these tasks oriented? Why was work created from the point of view of the limitations of the workers rather than their potentialities? (1982, p. 71)

Such questions have been raised repeatedly by both observers and disabled persons. Yet access to occupational forms that are meaningful and that convey respect remains, all too frequently, a problem.

Occupational Settings

The physical and social are intertwined in the environments we encounter. Together they constitute occupational settings. An **occupational setting** is a composite of spaces, objects, occupational forms, and/or social groups that cohere and constitute a meaningful context for performance. Occupational settings are not merely collections of people, objects, and forms in places where we perform. They are life worlds that resonate with meaning and action that make up coherent wholes (Rockwell-Dyla, 1992; Rowles, 1991). Consider, for example, the hot, vibrant, light-sound-people atmosphere of a night spot; the peaceful shade of autumn woods; the monotonous machinery in a factory where workers perform in synchrony; the quiet low-light, soft music, furniture-and-rug atmosphere of a family room; or the bright, orderly, rows of packaged food in a supermarket occupied by people pushing metal carts. Each of these has an organization and rhythm all of its own. These life world features present opportunities, resources, demands, and constraints for doing. Occupational settings are places of being and acting.

Occupational settings that ordinarily make up the course of daily life are the home, the neighborhood, the workplace, and gathering/recreation/resource sites (e.g., theaters, churches, temples, beaches, clubs, libraries, galleries, ski lodges, restaurants, health clubs, and stores). A given environment may serve as a different type of occupational setting for different individuals, depending on

> *Occupation is, after all, action that occupies a particular social and physical space.*

what they do in it. For example, a restaurant is a workplace for the waiters, cook, and others who labor in it, but a gathering and recreation site for those who frequent it for a meal with family or friends.

For most people, everyday life involves rounds of doing things in a number of occupational settings. As we move from setting to setting the different spaces, objects, social groups, and occupational forms we find there provide us with opportunities, resources, demands, and constraints. Much of what we choose to do and how we go about doing it is owing to the features of these settings.

Inseparability of Environment and Occupation

The relationship between humans and their environments is intimate and reciprocal. As has been discussed, the environment impacts what people do and how they do it. Humans constantly seek out certain types of environments and seek to change their environments toward their ends. For example, Rubinstein (1989) tells the story of an elderly woman who lives in a studio apartment and conducts most of her occupational life there. As her day progresses she meticulously rearranges the apartment to accommodate sleeping, receiving guests, and leisure.

Such modification of the environment to make it suitable for different occupations illustrates how much we depend on context for our experience and action.

The environment also figures centrally in the experience of disability. In fact, a person's degree of access and integration into the physical and social environment can be used as an index of disability (Brandt & Pope, 1997). Disability can be prevented or reduced when the environment is free of barriers and offers adequate support. Consequently, the extent of an individual's disability results in large measure from the surrounding environment (Brandt & Pope, 1997).

In the end, we owe our very humanness and our most essential selves to our environments. As Eisenberg (1977) argues:

> What determines the similarity between my behavior last year and what it is likely to be during the next is not nearly so much a matter of that which is "I" as it is of the social fields of force in which that "I" moves. That is, having acquired a repertoire of behaviors, I maximize their adaptive utility by seeking out the familiar and avoiding the strange in the social world around me. The apparent consistency in the self is the result, not merely of what has gone before, but of the continuation into the future of the same social forces that have given rise to it. (p. 233)

In fact, the environment is so intimately linked with the person that it can be considered "part of the organism" (Sameroff, 1983, p. 242). The central lesson of this chapter is that if we want to understand human occupation, we must also understand the environments in which it takes place. Occupation is, after all, action that occupies a particular social and physical space.

Key Terms

Culture: Beliefs and perceptions, values and norms, customs and behaviors that are shared by a group or society and are passed from one generation to the next through both formal and informal education.

Environment: Particular physical and social features of the specific context in which one does something that impacts upon what one does, and how it is done.

Environmental impact: Actual influence (in the form of opportunity, support, demand, or constraint) that the physical and social aspects of the environment have on a particular individual.

Objects: Naturally occurring or fabricated things with which we interact and whose properties influence what we do with them.

Occupational forms: Conventionalized sequences of action that are at once coherent, oriented to a purpose, sustained in collective knowledge, culturally recognizable, and named.

Occupational settings: Composite of spaces, objects, occupational forms, and/or social groups that cohere and constitute a meaningful context for performance.

Social groups: Collections of people who come together for various formal and informal purposes, and influence what we do within them.

References

Allen, V. L., Wilder, D. A., & Atkinson, M. L. (1983). Multiple group membership and social identity. In T. R. Sarbin & K. E. Scheibe (Eds.), *Studies in social identity.* New York: Praeger.

Altman, I., & Chemers, M. (1980). *Culture and environment.* Monterey, CA: Brooks/Cole.

Bates, P. S., Spencer, J. C., Young, M. E., & Hopkins Rintala, D. H. (1993). Assistive technology and the newly disabled adult: Adaptation to wheelchair use. *American Journal of Occupational Therapy, 47,* 1014–1021.

Bogdan, R., & Taylor, S. J. (1989). The social construction of humanness: Relationships with severely disabled people. *Social Problems, 36,* 135–148.

Borell, L., Gustavsson, A., Sandman, P., & Kielhofner, G. (1994). Occupational programming in a day hospital for patients with dementia. *Occupational Therapy Journal of Research, 14,* 219–238.

Brake, M. (1980). *The sociology of youth culture and youth cultures.* London: Routledge & Kegan Paul.

Brandt, E. N., & Pope, A. M. (1997). *Enabling America: Assessing the role of rehabilitation science and engineering.* Washington, DC: National Academy Press.

Breslau, N. (1983). Family care: Effects on siblings and mothers. In G. H. Thompson, I. L. Rubin, & R. M. Belenker (Eds.), *Comprehensive management of cerebral palsy.* New York: Grune & Stratton.

Csikszentmihalyi, M. (1990). *Flow: The psychology of optimal experience.* New York: Harper & Row.

Csikszentmihalyi, M., & Rochberg-Halton, E. (1981). *The meaning of things.* Cambridge, MA: Cambridge University Press.

Dexter, L. A. (1956). Towards a sociology of mentally defective. *American Journal of Mental Deficiency, 61,* 10–16.

Dexter, L. A. (1960). Research on problems of mental subnormality. *American Journal of Mental Deficiency, 64,* 835–838.

Dunn, W., Brown, C., & McGuigan, A. (1994). The ecology of human performance: A framework for considering the effect of context. *American Journal of Occupational Therapy, 48,* 595–607.

Edgerton, R. B. (1967). *The cloak of competence: Stigma in the lives of the mentally retarded.* Berkeley, CA: University of California Press.

Eisenberg, L. (1977). Development as a unifying concept in psychiatry. *British Journal of Psychiatry, 131,* 225–237.

Emerson, R. M., Rochford, E. B., & Shaw, L. L. (1983). The micropolitics of trouble in a psychiatric board and care facility. *Urban Life, 12,* 349–366.

Etzioni, A. (1964). *Modern organizations.* Englewood Cliffs, NJ: Prentice-Hall.

Gergen, K. J. (1991). *The saturated self: Dilemmas of identity in contemporary life.* Philadelphia: Basic Books.

Gibson, J. J. (1979). *The ecological approach to visual perception.* Boston: Houghton Mifflin.

Gill, C. J. (1997). Four types of integration in disability identity development. *Journal of Vocational Rehabilitation, 9,* 39–46.

Gray, M. (1972). Effects of hospitalization on work-play behavior. *American Journal of Occupational Therapy, 26,* 180–185.

Hahn, H. (1993). The political implications of disability definitions and data. *Journal of Disability Policy Studies, 4 (2),* 41–52.

Haywood, D. G., Rothenberg, M., & Beasley, R. R. (1974). Children's play and urban playground environments. *Environmental Behavior, 6,* 131–168.

Helfrich, C. A., Fisher, G., & Kielhofner, G. (2000). Definitions of allied health services in urban community contexts: Consumer perspectives. *Journal of Allied Health, 29,* 93–100.

Hocking, C. (1994). *Objects in the environment: A critique of the model of human occupation dimensions.* Paper presented at World Federation of Occupational Therapy, Symposium, International Perspectives on the Model of Human Occupation, London, England.

Holahan, C. J. (1979). Environmental psychology in psychiatric hospital settings. In D. Canter & S. Canter (Eds.), *Designing for therapeutic environments: A review of research.* New York: John Wiley & Sons.

Hull, J. M. (1990). *Touching the rock: An experience of blindness.* New York: Vintage Books.

Jonsson, H., Josephsson, S., & Kielhofner, G. (2000). Evolving narratives in the course of retirement: A longitudinal study. *American Journal of Occupational Therapy, 54,* 263–270.

Katz, D., & Kahn, R. L. (1966). *The social psychology of organizations.* New York: John Wiley & Sons.

Kielhofner, G. (1983). "Teaching" retarded adults: Paradoxical effects of a pedagogical enterprise. *Urban Life, 12,* 307–326.

Kiernat, J. M. (1983). Environment: The hidden modality. *Physical & Occupational Therapy in Geriatrics, 2 (1),* 3–12.

Knowles, E. S. (1982). From individuals to group members: A dialectic for the social sciences. In W. Ickes & E. S. Knowles (Eds.), *Personality, roles and social behavior.* New York: Springer-Verlag.

Kornblum, H., & Anderson, B. (1982). Acceptance: Reassessed—a point of view. *Child Psychiatry and Human Development, 12,* 171–178.

Law, M. (1991). The environment: A focus for occupational

therapy. *Canadian Journal of Occupational Therapy, 58,* 171–179.

Law, M., Cooper, B., Strong, S., Stewart, D., Rigby, P., & Letts, L. (1996). Person-environment occupational model: A transactive approach to occupational performance. *Canadian Journal of Occupational Therapy, 63,* 9–23.

Lawton, M. P. (1980). *Environment and aging.* Monterey, CA: Brooks/Cole.

Lawton, M. P. (1983). Environment and other detriments of well-being in older people. *Gerontologist, 23,* 349–357.

Lawton, M. P., & Nahemow, L. (1973). Ecology and the aging process. In C. Eisdorfer & M. P. Lawton (Eds.), *Psychology of adult development and aging.* Washington, DC: American Psychological Association.

Ljungström, Å. (1989). Craft artifacts: Keys to the past. Narratives from a craft documentation project in Sweden. *Journal of Ethnological Studies, 28,* 75–87.

Longmore, P. K. (1995). The second phase: From disability rights to disability culture. *The Disability Rag and Resource, 16,* 4–11.

Magill, J., & Vargo, J. (1977). Helplessness, hope, and the occupational therapist. *Canadian Journal of Occupational Therapy, 44,* 65–69.

Melin, L., & Gotestam, G. (1981). The effects of rearranging ward routines on communication and eating behaviors of psychogeriatric patients. *Journal of Applied Behavioral Analysis, 14,* 47–51.

Miller, J. F., & Oertel, C. B. (1983). Powerlessness in the elderly: Preventing hopelessness. In J. F. Miller (Ed.), *Coping with chronic illness: Overcoming powerlessness.* Philadelphia: FA Davis.

Moos, R. H. (1974). *Evaluating treatment environments: A social ecological approach.* New York: John Wiley & Sons.

Murphy, R. F. (1987). *The body silent.* New York: WW Norton.

Murphy, R. F., Scheer, J., Murphy, Y., & Mack, R. (1988). Physical disability and social liminality: A study in the rituals of adversity. *Social Science and Medicine, 26,* 235–242.

Nelson, D. (1988). Occupation: Form and performance. *American Journal of Occupational Therapy, 42,* 633–641.

Newcomb, T. M. (1943). *Personality and social change.* New York: Dryden Press.

Ogbu, J. U. (1981). Origins of human competence: A cultural-ecological perspective. *Child Development, 52,* 413–429.

Oliver, M., Zarb, G., Silver, J., Moore, M., & Salisbury, V. (1988). *Walking into darkness: The experience of spinal cord injury.* London: Macmillan Press.

Pervin, L. A. (1968). Performance and satisfaction as a function of individual-environment fit. *Pyschological Bulletin, 69,* 56–68.

Quilitch, H. R., & Risley, T. R. (1973). The effects of play materials on social play. *Journal of Applied Behavioral Analysis, 6,* 573–578.

Rapoport, A. (1980). Cross-cultural aspects of environmental design. In I. Altman, A. Rapoport, & J. F. Wohlwill (Eds.), *Human behavior and environment* (Vol. 4). New York: Plenum.

Reed, E. S. (1982). An outline of a theory of action systems. *Journal of Motor Behavior, 14,* 98–134.

Rockwell-Dylla, L. (1992). *Older adults' meaning of environment: Hospital and home.* Unpublished master's thesis, University of Illinois at Chicago.

Rowles, G. (1991). Beyond performance: Being in place as a component of occupational therapy. *American Journal of Occupational Therapy, 45,* 265–271.

Rubinstein, R. L. (1989). The home environments of older people: A description of the psychosocial processes linking person to place. *Journal of Gerontology, 44,* 45–53.

Sameroff, A. J. (1983). Developmental systems: Contexts and evolution. In P. H. Mussen (Ed.), *Handbook of child psychology.* New York: John Wiley & Sons.

Sarbin, T. R. (1954). Role theory. In G. Lindzey & E. Aronson (Eds.), *The Hand-book of social psychology* (Vol. 1). Reading, MA: Addison-Wesley.

Scull, A. T. (1977). *Decarceration: Community treatment and the deviant—A radical view.* Englewood Cliffs, NJ: Prentice-Hall.

Simmons, J. E., & Barris, R. (1984). *The relationship between the home environment and the occupational behavior in the post-CVA patient.* Unpublished manuscript.

Suto, M., & Frank, G. (1994). Future time perspective and daily occupations of persons with chronic schizophrenia in a board and care home. *American Journal of Occupational Therapy, 48,* 7–18.

Test, M. A., & Stein, L. I. (1978). Community treatment of the chronic patient: A research overview. *Schizophrenia Bulletin, 4,* 350–364.

Trombly, C. A. (1983). *Occupational therapy for physical dysfunction* (2nd ed.). Baltimore: Williams & Wilkins.

Vash, C. L. (1981). *The psychology of disability.* New York: Springer-Verlag.

Versluys, H. P. (1980). The remediation of role disorders through focused groupwork. *American Journal of Occupational Therapy, 34,* 609–614.

Zola, I. K. (1982). *Missing pieces: A chronicle of living with a disability.* Philadelphia: Temple University Press.

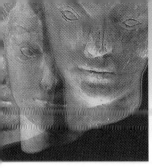

8

Dimensions of Doing

- Gary Kielhofner

Previous chapters examined personal and environmental influences on doing. They discussed:

- How personal causation, values, and interests motivate doing
- The influence of habits and roles in shaping routine patterns
- How underlying capacities and subjective experience make possible the details of what people do
- How the environment provides opportunities, resources, demands, and constraints on doing.

This chapter examines the nature of doing occupation and the consequence of doing over time in an individual's life. This chapter thus presents a cross-sectional and longitudinal perspective on occupation.

Levels of Doing

When considering what people do in the course of their occupations, different levels of doing can be identified (Haglund & Henriksson, 1995). For example, consider a mechanic who attended to an engine problem. The question, "What has the mechanic done?" can be answered in the following ways:

- The mechanic engaged in a type of work
- The mechanic tuned an engine
- The mechanic made a series of calculated judgments and motor actions.

All these responses are accurate. However, each describes what the mechanic did at different levels of analysis. Three levels of doing that correspond to this example can be identified, as shown in *Figure 8-1*. These levels are:

- Occupational participation
- Occupational performance
- Occupational skill.

Participation refers to doing in the broadest sense. It attends to engaging in occupation at the level of work, play, and activities of daily living that make up a person's life. Performance denotes the larger chunks of action that make up a coherent undertaking. The concept of skill provides the most detailed or fine-grained look at what a person does, attending to purposeful units of action.

Occupational Participation

The World Health Organization and the Occupational Therapy Practice Framework use the term participation to refer to a person's involvement in life situations (American Occupational Therapy Association, 2001; World Health Organization, 1999). Participation connotes persons' taking part in society along with their experiences within their life contexts (World Health Organization, 1999, p. 19).

Consistent with this usage, the term **occupational**

When considering what people do in the course of their occupations, different levels of doing can be identified.

A disability may alter, but need not prevent, occupational participation if adequate environmental supports are in place.

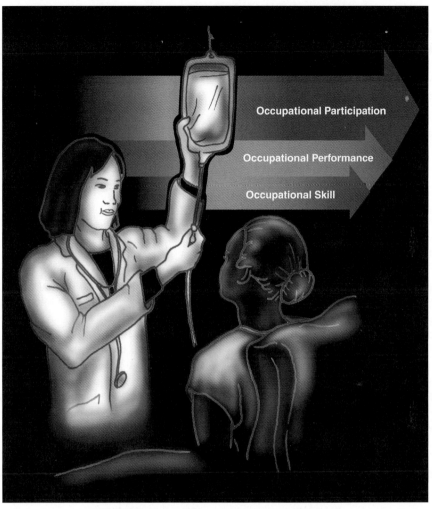

FIGURE 8-1   Three Dimensions of Doing.

participation is used here to refer to engagement in work, play, or activities of daily living that are part of one's sociocultural context and that are desired and/or necessary to one's well-being. Engagement involves not only performance but also subjective experience (Yerxa, 1980). Thus, occupational participation connotes doing things with personal and social significance. Examples of occupational participation are volunteering for an organization, working in a full- or part-time job, recre- ating regularly with friends, doing self-care, maintain- ing one's living space, and attending school.[a]

---

[a]No single categorization of the areas of occupational participation is proposed here. Readers may wish to examine the WHO classification and the AOTA Practice framework classification (AOTA, 2001; WHO, 1999) as examples of how areas of participation can be identified. Be- cause each person organizes his or her occupational participation into a unique overall life pattern, a useful approach in practice is to pay attention to how the client defines and enacts participation.

Each area of occupational participation involves a cluster of related things that one does. For example, maintaining one's living space may include paying the rent, doing repairs, dusting furniture, decorating, and attending monthly meetings of a resident's association.

Occupational participation is collectively influenced by:

- Performance capacities
- Habituation
- Volition
- Environmental conditions.

Thus, occupational participation is both personal and contextual. It is personal in that the types of participation in which a person will engage is influenced by the individual's unique motives, roles, habits, and abilities and limitations. It is contextual in that the environment can either enable or restrict occupational participation.

A 10-year-old's areas of occupational participation may include doing personal hygiene and dressing, routine chores at home, school attendance and homework, participation in sports, family activities, and free play. The child's school attendance and family activities are primarily shaped by societal expectation and social roles assigned to the child. What kind of sports the child plays may depend on capacities, interests, and available opportunities in the environment. Free play activities are a result of activity choices that reflect the child's personal causation, values, and interests as well as the opportunities provided in the physical and social environment. Thus, we can see that a complex interaction of personal and environmental factors ultimately shapes the full spectrum of occupational participation in a person's life.

A disability may alter, but need not prevent, occupational participation if adequate environmental supports are in place. For example, consider a young woman with spinal cord injury. Her occupational participation may include doing personal hygiene and grooming with a personal assistant. Use of the personal assistant may reflect both her performance limitations and her volitional choice to dispatch self-care with minimum personal effort and time in order to focus personal resources on work. For the same reason, she may rely on someone else to acquire and prepare food. She may be highly invested in her professional career and

in managing a range of health maintenance tasks necessary to spinal cord injury (e.g., assuring proper diet and exercise, dealing with health providers, accessing and getting adaptive equipment and other resources paid for, hiring and supervising an attendant, or engaging in social activism related to disability rights). Finally, she may pursue discretionary social and solitary leisure activities that are possible within her performance limitations, motivated by her volition, and facilitated by her physical and social environment. As this example indicates, performance limitations may influence, but need not prevent, occupational participation, if a person can make volitional choices and has adequate environmental supports.

Occupational Performance

As noted above, participation in an occupation may involve doing a variety of things. For example, a carpenter's work may include such things as framing a wall, shingling a roof, and installing a door or window. The carpenter's play may include a weekly game of poker, going fishing, bicycling, and attending sports events with friends. This person's activities of daily living can include such things as taking a shower, dressing, balancing a checkbook, or preparing a meal. As we saw in Chapter 7, these discrete things we do are occupational forms. As such, they have a unique purpose, structure, and appearance so that we are able to recognize and name them.

Each time a person does one of these discrete acts, he or she is performing (i.e., completing or—literally—going through the form). Thus, **occupational performance** refers to doing an occupational form (Nelson, 1988). For example, when persons do such tasks as shining shoes, baking a cake, mowing the lawn, and painting a room, they are performing those occupational forms.

Since most of our performance of occupational forms includes things that are part of our everyday routines, habituation has an important influence on performance. Roles influence the type and range of occupational forms in which we will engage. Habits also influence what things we include in our routines and they influence how we go about doing the occupational forms that make up our daily lives.

Performance is also greatly affected by the environment. The occupational forms we perform in the course of daily life require the use of objects and spaces and many occur within social groups. Environmental factors are also critical to whether and how impairments affect performance. For example, environmental supports ranging from adapted equipment to memory aids may make it possible for a person to complete an occupational form despite limitations of performance capacity.

Skills

Within any occupational performance we can discern a number of discrete purposeful actions. For example, making a sandwich is a culturally recognizable occupational form in many Western cultures. To make a sandwich one engages in such purposeful actions as gathering together sandwich ingredients, handling these materials, and sequencing the steps necessary to assemble the sandwich.

Such actions that make up occupational performance are referred to as skills. **Skills** are defined as observable, goal-directed actions that a person uses while performing (Fisher, 1999; Fisher & Kielhofner, 1995; Forsyth, Salamy, Simon, & Kielhofner, 1997). In contrast to performance capacity that refers to underlying ability, skill refers to the concrete actions that are done in the midst of undertaking an occupational form. As shown in *Figure 8-2*, a person's characteristics (including volition, habituation, and performance capacity) interact with the environment, resulting in skill.

Three types of skills are recognized: motor skills, process skills, and communication and interaction skills *(Fig. 8-3)*. Detailed taxonomies of the skills have been developed as part of creating assessments of motor, process, and communication/interaction skills (see Chapter 12 for further information on these assessments). Fisher and colleagues have developed the taxonomies of motor and process skills, which make up an Assessment of Motor and Process Skills (Berspang & Fisher, 1995; Doble, 1991; Fisher, 1993, 1997). Forsyth and colleagues have developed a taxonomy of communication/interaction skills, which make up the Assessment of Communication/Interaction Skills (Forsyth et al., 1997; Forsyth & Kielhofner, 1999).

Motor skills refer to moving self or task objects (Fisher, 1999). They include such actions as stabilizing and bending one's body and manipulating, lifting, and

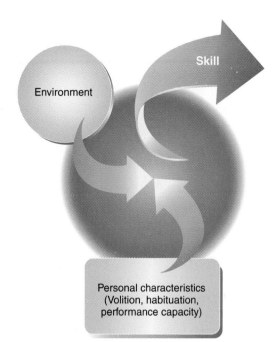

FIGURE 8-2   Skill as a Function of the Interaction Between Personal Characteristics and the Environment.

transporting objects. **Process skills** refer to logically sequencing actions over time, selecting and using appropriate tools and materials, and adapting performance when encountering problems (Fisher, 1999). They include such actions as choosing and organizing objects in space as well as initiating and terminating steps in performance. **Communication and interaction skills** refer to conveying intentions and needs and coordinating social action to act together with people (Forsyth et al., 1997; Forsyth & Kielhofner, 1999). They include such things as gesturing, physically contacting others, speaking, engaging and collaborating with others, and asserting oneself.

Embedded Levels of Doing

As the previous discussions illustrated, skill is embedded within performance, and the latter within participation. So, whenever persons are participating in occupations, they complete a number of occupational forms and use a wide range of skills. Let us consider

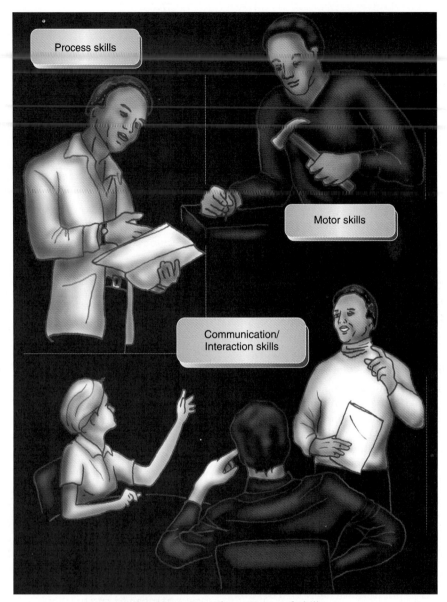

Process skills

Motor skills

Communication/
Interaction skills

FIGURE 8-3   Three Types of Skills.

some examples, which are illustrated in *Table 8-1*. Occupational participation may include working as a nurse, maintaining one's house, and socializing with

> **Skill is embedded within performance, and the latter within participation.**

friends. As we have noted, within each of these occupations, one will complete a number of occupational forms. For example, while working as a nurse one might give an injection. While maintaining the house, one might vacuum the floor. While socializing with friends, one might play a game of scrabble. While doing self-care, one may take a bath. In the course of performing these things, one would employ a number of skills required to complete that particular occupational

TABLE 8-1 Three Levels of Doing

Level of Doing	Examples			
Occupational Participation	Self-grooming	Working as a nurse	Maintaining one's apartment	Socializing routinely with friends
Occupational performance	Brushing teeth	Giving an injection	Vacuuming the floor	Playing Scrabble
Occupational skill	Calibrating Reaching Sequencing Manipulating	Speaking Reaching Sequencing Manipulating	Reaching Sequencing Manipulating Walking	Reaching Sequencing Manipulating Speaking

form. Thus, several skills make up an occupational performance just as several occupational performances make up an area of occupational participation.

The extent of our success in completing occupational forms will depend on proficiency of the skills we employ to do them. The fullness of a person's participation in work, play, or activities of daily living will similarly depend on the degree to which he or she is able to successfully complete the occupational forms that make up an area of occupational performance. For example, professors' success at lecturing depends primarily on their communication/interaction skills, and their participation in professorial work depends on their success at lecturing and at other occupational forms such as planning courses, creating and giving exams, and advising students.

Consequences of Doing: Occupational Identity, Competence, and Adaptation

As the previous discussion demonstrated, most persons' lives consist of several types of occupational participation. In this section we see how, over time, this participation results in occupational adaptation and its components, occupational identity and competence.

The term adaptation has been used in occupational therapy literature to refer to the extent to which persons are able to develop, change in response to challenges, or otherwise achieve a state of well-being through what they do (Fidler & Fidler, 1978; King, 1978; Nelson, 1988; Reilly, 1962). In earlier versions of MOHO, adaptation was defined as meeting personal needs and desires while meeting reasonable environmental ex-

pectations through one's occupation (Kielhofner, 1985, 1995).

Schkade and Schultz (1992, p. 831) first used the term occupational adaptation to refer to "a state of competency in occupational functioning toward which human beings aspire." Their definition suggested that adaptation involved dual aspects of competency and aspiration. Spencer, Davidson, and White (1996) added that occupational adaptation was a cumulative process emanating from one's life history.

Mallinson, Mahaffey, and Kielhofner (1998) reported evidence from a study of life history interviews that a person's adaptation consists of two distinct elements, identity and competence. A subsequent study of persons' life histories generated further evidence of occupational identity and occupational competence as distinct components of occupational adaptation (Kielhofner, Mallinson, Forsyth, & Lai, 2001). Building on this theoretical and empirical work, the following presents a definition of occupational adaptation and its two components, identity and competence.

Occupational Identity

Christiansen (1999) notes that identity refers to a composite definition of the self, including roles and relationships, values, self-concept, and personal desires and goals. He further argues that our participation in occupations help to create our identities. Building on his argument, as well as the empirical work referred to earlier, **occupational identity** is defined here as a composite sense of who one is and wishes to become as an occupational being generated from one's history of occupational participation. One's volition, habituation, and experience as a lived body are all integrated into occupational identity.

Consequently, occupational identity includes a composite of:

- One's sense of capacity and effectiveness for doing
- What things one finds interesting and satisfying to do
- Who one is, as defined by one's roles and relationships
- What one feels obligated to do and holds as important
- A sense of the familiar routines of life
- Perceptions of one's environment and what it supports and expects.

These elements are garnered over time and become part of one's identity. Their implications for the future are also part of occupational identity.

Thus, occupational identity reflects accumulated life experiences that are organized into an understanding of who one has been and a sense of desired and possible direction for one's future. Occupational identity serves both as a means of self-definition and as a blueprint for upcoming action.

Preliminary evidence suggests that occupational identity is represented in a continuum that begins with self-appraisal and extends toward the more challenging elements of accepting responsibility for and knowing what one wants from life (Kielhofner et al., 2001). Thus, it would appear that building an occupational identity starts with self-knowledge of our capacities and interests from past experience and extends to constructing a value-based vision of the future we desire.

Occupational Competence

Occupational competence is the degree to which one sustains a pattern of occupational participation that reflects one's occupational identity. Thus, while identity has to do with the subjective meaning of one's occupational life, competence has to do with putting that identity into action in an ongoing way. Occupational competence includes:

- Fulfilling the expectations of one's roles and one's own values and standards for performance
- Maintaining a routine that allows one to discharge responsibilities
- Participating in a range of occupations that provide a sense of ability, control, satisfaction, and fulfillment
- Pursuing one's values and taking action to achieve desired life outcomes.

Competence appears to begin with organizing one's life to meet basic responsibilities and personal standards and extends to meeting role obligations and then achieving a satisfying and interesting life (Kielhofner & Forsyth, 2001).

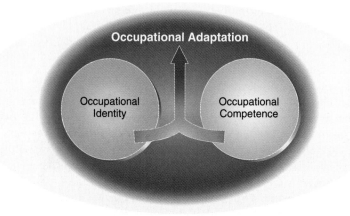

FIGURE 8-4   Occupational Adaptation and Its Two Components.

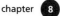

Occupational Adaptation

Occupational adaptation is defined here as the construction of a positive occupational identity and achieving occupational competence over time in the context of one's environment. This definition acknowledges that occupational adaptation has two distinct and interrelated elements *(Fig. 8-4)*. It also specifies that adaptation takes place in a specific context with its opportunities, supports, constraints, and demands.

While occupational identity and competence co-develop over time, one cannot operationalize a view of self and life that one has not developed. Evidence also suggests that while disability can affect both identity and competence, its effects are more pronounced in competence (Kielhofner et al., 2001; Mallinson et al., 1998).

Development and Threats to Occupational Adaptation

As noted earlier, occupational adaptation is the consequence of one's history of participation in life occupations *(Fig. 8-5)*. From the time we learn our first occu-

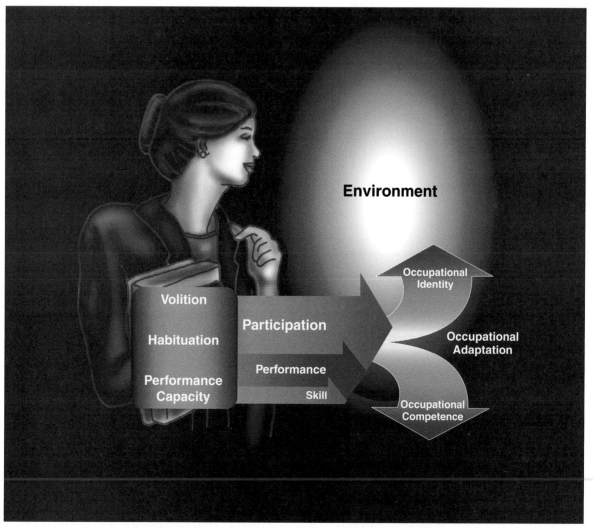

FIGURE 8-5 The Process of Occupational Adaptation.

> *Most people will, at one time or another, experience a threat to or problems in occupational adaptation requiring the rebuilding of occupational identity and competence.*

pational forms and begin to participate in the world around us by doing things, we shape our own volition, habituation, and performance capacity. Throughout this process, we are in constant interaction with the physical and social environment that shapes the development of our volition, habituation, and performance capacity as well. These personal characteristics, in interaction with the environment, influence our occupational participation.

Over time, we construct our occupational identity and competence through ongoing occupational participation. Occupational identity and competence are realized as we develop and respond to life changes (including illness and impairment). Identity and competence describe, then, the unfolding state in which we find ourselves at any point in our lives.

Our degree of success in occupational adaptation, as reflected in the identities we construct and our extent of competently enacting them, varies over time. Most people will, at one time or another, experience a threat to or problems in occupational adaptation requiring the rebuilding of occupational identity and competence. The next chapter examines this process in more depth by considering the occupational adaptation of persons challenged by disability.

Key Terms

Communication and interaction skills: Conveying intentions and needs and coordinating social action in order to act together with people.

Motor skills: Moving self or task objects.

Occupational adaptation: Constructing a positive occupational identity and achieving occupational competence over time in the context of one's environment.

Occupational competence: Degree to which one is able to sustain a pattern of occupational participation that reflects one's occupational identity.

Occupational identity: Composite sense of who one is and wishes to become as an occupational being generated from one's history of occupational participation.

Occupational participation: Engagement in work, play, or activities of daily living that are part of one's sociocultural context and that are desired and/or necessary to one's well-being.

Occupational performance: Doing an occupational form.

Process skills: Logically sequencing actions over time, selecting and using appropriate tools and materials, and adapting performance when encountering problems.

Skills: Observable, goal-directed actions that a person uses while performing.

References

Berspang, B., & Fisher, A. G. (1995). Validation of the Assessment of Motor and Process Skills for use in Sweden. *Scandinavian Journal of Occupational therapy, 2,* 3–9.

Christiansen, C. H. (1999). Defining lives: Occupation as identity: An essay on competence, coherence, and the creation of meaning. *American Journal of Occupational Therapy, 53,* 547–558.

Commission on Practice, American Occupational Therapy Association. (2001). *Occupational Therapy Practice Framework.* Unpublished Working Paper.

Doble, S. (1991). Test-retest and inter-rater reliability of a process skills assessment. *Occupational Therapy Journal of Research, 11,* 8–23.

Fidler, G. S., & Fidler, J. W. (1978). Doing and becoming: Purposeful action and self-actualization. *American Journal of Occupational Therapy, 32,* 305–310.

Fisher, A. G. (1993). The assessment of IADL motor skills: An application of many-faceted Rasch analysis. *American Journal of Occupational Therapy, 47,* 319–338.

Fisher, A. G. (1997). Multifaceted measurement of daily life task performance: Conceptualizing a test of instrumental ADL and validating the addition of personal ADL tasks. *Archives of Physical Medicine and Rehabilitation: State of the Art Reviews, 11,* 289–303.

Fisher A. G. (1999). *Assessment of Motor and Process Skills* (3rd ed.). Ft. Collins, CO: Three Star Press.

Fisher, A. G., & Kielhofner, G. (1995). Skills in occupational performance. *A model of human occupation: Theory and application* (second edition). Baltimore: Williams & Wilkins.

Forsyth, K., & Kielhofner, G. (1999). Validity of the assessment of communication and interaction skills. *British Journal of Occupational Therapy, 62,* 69–74.

Forsyth, K., Salamy, M., Simon, S., & Kielhofner, G. (1997). *Assessment of Communication and Interaction Skills.* Chicago: University of Illinois, Model of Human Occupation Clearinghouse.

Haglund, L., & Henriksson, C. (1995). Activity—From action to activity. *Scandinavian Journal of Caring Sciences, 9,* 227–234.

Kielhofner, G. (1985). *A model of human occupation: Theory and application.* Baltimore: Williams & Wilkins.

Kielhofner, G. (1995). *A model of human occupation: Theory and application* (2nd ed.). Baltimore: Williams & Wilkins.

Kielhofner, G., & Forsyth, K. Development of a client self-report for treatment planning and documenting therapy outcomes. *Scandinavian Journal of Occupational Therapy, 8,* 131–139.

Kielhofner, G., Mallinson, T., Forsyth, K., & Lai, J. S. (2001). Psychometric properties of the second version of the Occupational Performance History Interview (OPHI-II). *American Journal of Occupational Therapy, 55,* 260–267.

King, L. J. (1978). Toward a science of adaptive responses. *American Journal of Occupational Therapy, 32,* 429–437.

Mallinson, T., Mahaffey, L., & Kielhofner, G. (1998). The occupational performance history interview: Evidence for three underlying constructs of occupational adaptation. *Canadian Journal of Occupational Therapy, 65,* 219–228.

Nelson, D. (1988). Occupation: Form and performance. *American Journal of Occupational Therapy, 42,* 633.

Reilly, M. (1962). Occupational therapy can be one of the great ideas of 20th century medicine. *American Journal of Occupational Therapy, 16,* 1–9.

Schkade, J. K., & Schultz, S. (1992). Occupational adaptation: Toward a holistic approach for contemporary practice. Part 1. *American Journal of Occupational Therapy, 46,* 829–837.

Spencer, J. C., Davidson, H. A., & White, V. K. (1996). Continuity and change: Past experience as adaptive repertoire in occupational adaptation. *American Journal of Occupational Therapy, 50,* 526–534.

World Health Organization. (1999). *ICIDH-2: International classification of functioning and disability.* Beta-2 draft, full version. Geneva: Author.

Yerxa, E. J. (1980). Occupational therapy's role in creating a future climate of caring. *American Journal of Occupational Therapy, 34,* 529–534.

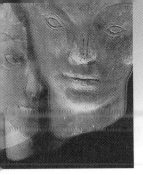

9

Crafting Occupational Life

- Gary Kielhofner
- Lena Borell
- Ladonna Freidheim
- Karen Goldstein
- Christine Helfrich
- Hans Jonsson
- Staffan Josephsson
- Trudy Mallinson
- Louise Nygård

Introduction

Chapter 8 noted that occupational identity represents a composite sense of oneself and one's future generated from ongoing occupational participation. It further noted that occupational competence involves sustaining a pattern of participation that reflects one's identity. The purpose of this chapter is to consider further how persons generate and maintain occupational identity and competence—in short, how they craft their occupational lives.

Both occupational identity and competence encompass how volition, habituation, and performance capacity collectively orient each of us to our own unique lives. Consider that this includes:

- What we hold as important
- Our unique sense of pleasure and satisfaction in doing things
- Our knowledge of our own capacities, limitations, and relative effectiveness
- Our awareness of who we are in reference to the social world
- Our familiarity with the rhythms and routines of life
- Our lived experience as embodied beings
- Our unique apprehension of the world around us.

These elements are always in the background, shaping how we craft our ongoing occupational lives in the stream of time.

How do we manage to synthesize all the many elements of the self and the world, which are also spread over time, into some kind of comprehensible whole? How do we navigate our sometimes conflicting urges, desires, hopes, and fears? How do we manage to choose from among the many messages, expectations, and opportunities of our environments? How do we select what to do next and have a sense of where it fits? How do we get a handle on our lives and go about living them?

When considering the previous questions, we might add two more. Why are we not perennially confused, unable to synthesize the vast array of life experiences? How do we select among potential choices and respond to others' perceptions and expectations of us? While life sometimes reflects exactly this kind of confusion and dilemma, most people manage to navigate life and see the journey as having some kind of coherence and meaning. What, then, makes this possible?

Narrative Organization of Occupational Life

Answers to the above questions are at least partly answered by the argument that we conduct and draw meaning from life by locating ourselves in unfolding narratives that integrate our past, present, and future selves (Geertz, 1986; Gergen & Gergen, 1988; Helfrich, Kielhofner, & Mattingly, 1994; Mattingly, 1991; Schafer, 1981; Spence, 1982; Taylor, 1989). How narratives manage this synthesis and impart meaning on many elements and episodes of life has been the topic of ongoing discourse. At least two important features of narratives—plot and metaphor—account for this. The following sections examine these two features of narrative.

Plot

Gergen and Gergen (1988) refer to plot as the fore-structure of narrative that determines how we think and talk when we use stories. The plot of a story represents the intersection between the progression of time and the direction (for better or worse) that life takes. Consequently, the plot is the shape of events over time as they get better or worse (Gergen & Gergen, 1988; Jonsson, Kielhofner, & Borell, 1997).

The plot of a narrative reveals the overall meaning because it sums up where life has been and is going. For example, the tragic plot is found in a life when some event results in a steep downward turn in a previously good or improving life *(Fig. 9-1)*. The melodramatic plot involves a series of upward and downward turns. The tragic plot illuminates a life ruined. In con-

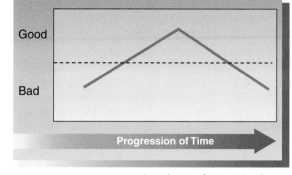

FIGURE 9-1 Narrative Slope of a Tragic Plot.

trast, the melodramatic plot reveals a life of struggle. Emplotting life events links them together in a way that makes sense of the life as a whole. Consequently, the various life episodes derive their meaning from the overall shape of the plot.

When we succeed or fail in something substantial and when events (good or bad) happen to us, we are always drawn to understand what they mean. We seek to evaluate these events in terms of their significance for our lives. Evaluating what we have done, and what happens to us, is always in terms of its impact on the unfolding life story. Most often, events represent a continuation of the basic direction of our lives. Others encourage or threaten our sense of where life is headed. In evaluating ongoing events of life, the underlying plot (the direction for better or worse that life will take) is always at stake.

Plot is not only implied in how we anticipate the significance of events for the future, but also in how we draw on our past experiences to understand what present circumstances might mean. We evaluate each new unfolding circumstance of life in terms of how such things have gone before and in terms of where it might lead. For example, Jonsson, Kielhofner, & Borell (1997) studied how older persons anticipated their retirement. What each person expected in retirement was always intimately tied to how past and present occupational life, especially work, had been experienced. If work was negative, then retirement could be seen as an escape. In this case, life after retirement could be expected to get better. If work was positive, then re-

> *. . . we conduct and draw meaning from life by locating ourselves in unfolding narratives that integrate our past, present, and future selves*

tirement could continue a good life by providing opportunities to do other valued things or it could be a loss that would make life worse.

How past and future are linked depends on and reveals the plot. If, for example, one is living a tragic narrative, past successes do not portend that things will go well in the future. On the other hand, if one is in a story where things are getting better, past failures will be lessons that provided the person with new strengths or obstacles that were overcome. The significance of the past for the present and the future depends on and reflects the plot of one's narrative. In a similar fashion, inevitable or likely events in the future take on their significance with reference to the past and present. How they are seen to relate to past or present also depends on and reflects the underlying plot.

Metaphor

Stories are also given meaning by metaphors (Ganzer, 1993). Metaphor is the use of a familiar object or phenomenon to stand in the place of the less-understood event or situation (Ortony, 1979). The value of metaphor is that it imparts a succinct characterization on a complex or emotionally difficult circumstance. The metaphor does this by evoking something familiar or readily understood to stand in the place of that which is difficult to grasp and/or face.

Metaphors thus provide a way of dealing with that which is otherwise unmanageable. For example, when faced with serious, life-threatening illness, people often evoke the metaphor of battle. This metaphor casts the disease as a threatening enemy that must be fought and expelled or destroyed. We all understand that there are important literal differences between having a disease and going into a battle. Nonetheless, the power of the metaphor is that the whole overwhelming and alien situation of life-threatening illness is recast into a succinct way of viewing and responding to it: the disease is an invading enemy that must be fought.

Persons also evoke metaphors to make sense of their disabilities. For example, Mallinson, Kielhofner, and Mattingly (1996) identified metaphors of momentum and entrapment in the narratives of persons with mental illness. People hospitalized because of their mental illness often referred to their lives in terms of speed, inertia, impetus, acceleration, and deceleration. They related images such as getting one's life going again, life slowing down, life passing one by, life grinding to a halt, or life going nowhere when they were summing up or evaluating the events of their lives. They used the metaphor of momentum to characterize their struggles, motives, life junctures, and life events by evaluating them in terms of the progression and direction of their lives. Importantly, the way in which they lived their lives also embodied such slowing down, coming to a halt, heading off in wrong directions, and so on.

Other persons with mental illness described their lives as being severely restricted or confined by life circumstances. Their stories were imbued with the wish for escape or for finding a way out of the maze. They saw their situations as both intolerable and inexorable. Importantly, they also acted as individuals who were trapped. They could not make decisions. They sometimes exhibited symptoms of agoraphobia and were literally confined in their rooms or homes. They stayed in dissatisfying relationships, jobs, and life situations.

How Metaphors Shape Narrative Meaning

Schön (1979) noted that metaphors are a primary vehicle through which persons comprehend things that have gone wrong in life. Consequently, when lives are troubled and when people are struggling to comprehend difficult, painful, and incomprehensible things that have happened, metaphors are effective ways of assigning meaning to them. Moreover, metaphors sum up "what needs fixing" (Schön, 1979, p. 255). In pinpointing the essential nature of life's problems, struggles, and dilemmas, they also imply how they can be solved or overcome. For example, the metaphors of momentum imply solutions of going in a new direction, getting things going, or slowing down. Metaphors of entrapment suggest that one must escape or be freed.

Narrative, Meaning, and Doing

Narratives, with their plots and metaphors, shape how we perceive ongoing life. They are a way of making

> *Occupation both emanates from and influences where one's story is going.*

meaning as life unfolds and as new circumstances present themselves. Consequently, there is always openness in narrative that can take and make meaning of whatever emerges in an unpredictable life (Bruner, 1990a, 1990b; Ricoeur, 1984). Moreover, what we do continues our stories, sometimes aiming toward a particular turn of events or outcome, sometimes moving things along, and sometimes acquiescing to what seems inevitable (Jonsson, Josephsson, & Kielhofner, 2000; Jonsson et al., 1997). Occupation both emanates from and influences where one's story is going (Clark, 1993; Helfrich et al., 1994).

For this reason, narratives can either impede or focus action. For example, if someone already sees his or her life as a tragedy, there is little reason to work toward goals because the tragic plot pronounces that things are ruined. On the other hand, if someone sees his or her life as getting better, he or she will likely be motivated to work hard toward that outcome.

Summary

Thus far we have argued that the coherence and meaning we achieve in our lives is facilitated through narratives. We noted the following features of narratives that give them this integrating and meaning-making potential:

- Narratives tie together past, present, and future as well as integrate multiple themes of self and the world
- Narratives integrate and impart meaning through the use of plot and metaphor

> *Both our identity and our competence are reflected and enacted in the stories with which we makes sense of and go about doing our occupational lives.*

- Narratives are open-ended and thus allow us to comprehend emergent events and circumstances of life, tying them to what has gone before and what might come next
- Narratives are not only told but are also done
- What one does continues the unfolding of one's narrative

Given these considerations, we can define **occupational narratives**[a] as stories (both told and enacted) that integrate across time our unfolding volition, habituation, performance capacity, and environments through plots and metaphors that sum up and assign meaning to these elements. Both our identity and our competence are reflected and enacted in the stories with which we make sense of and go about doing our occupational lives. In the end, our adaptation, or lack thereof, is reflected in how we tell and enact our occupational narratives.

Five Occupational Narratives

How occupational narratives figure in ongoing life can best be appreciated by detailed examination of such stories. The following sections present five occupational narratives. Each narrative tells about living with an impairment. Three are rendered in the third person, because the text was shaped by someone other than the story's character. Two are in the first person because they are primarily authored by the persons described in the narrative.

Tom

Twelve years ago, Tom graduated from high school with honors. As a student he was the school newspaper editor, National Honor Society President, Quill & Scroll President, and a debate club member. He spent summers writing for a city-wide student

---

[a] Previous discussions of narrative in relationship to MOHO have referred to the concept of volitional narrative. This concept argued that narratives incorporate the essential themes of volition (one's ability and control in life, one's interest and satisfaction, and one's values). We have linked the concept of narrative to the broader constructs of occupational identity and competence in this chapter. Consequently, narratives are now seen as embracing a larger scope of occupational life and experience than previously thought.

newspaper and taking advanced journalism training. He graduated as class valedictorian of a prestigious private university with a degree in journalism, having completed successful internships in two major city daily newspapers. After 16 months of work as a city reporter on a daily paper, he landed a job on a big city paper as a bureau reporter covering several beats.

Six years later, Tom has been out of work for the better part of a year. He worries constantly about getting a new job. He is palpably embarrassed about his departure from what promised to be a brilliant career. He wonders what would happen if an old professor would spy him back at his university placement office. He agonizes over how he will explain several glaring gaps of unemployment in his resume. Despite these torturous anxieties, Tom drags himself to an interview for an editing position in a monthly political newsletter. This job is admittedly several rungs below investigative journalism.

Afterward, Tom characteristically jokes about the interview experience. All went well. He simply explained his career gaps as being due to leprosy and imprisonment. He sobers. Truth be told, he lied. He sat there and said his resume gaps were due to a recurrent eye problem. Of course, this explanation was not completely fictitious; he had an eye problem once in the past. Anyhow, Tom got the job! He muses:

> What I am doing is about a million light years from what I originally ever thought I would be doing. I never thought I'd ever be going into the trade, the trade publications. That's what these are called. When I was in the beginning of, well, when I was towards the end of high school, I probably would have envisioned myself eventually working for the *Chicago Tribune*. Towards the middle of college I probably had changed that to working for a medium-sized daily paper. I really realized that with my illness you can't plan much of anything, any real long-term plans. You can't say this is the first step on the rest of my career, and in five years I plan to be in such and such a city, and in ten years I plan to be an editor of this paper. And people who don't get sick make those kinds of plans. Every plan that I've made has eventually been defeated and I've had to shift to another sub-plan. I

used to have—my motto in life after my first episode was—and I'd gotten this out of the newspaper was, "What counts in life is what you do with plan B," okay? Well, I've, I've got to about plan F now. You just have to keep changing your goal. You just have to be practical, and try to be realistic, and settle for less than what you had envisioned before. You really learn to take things at, sort of, at the most, a year at a time. I was never planning more than a year ahead. Now, you know, I'm not making any plans at all. The future is, is just, a very, foggy, unclear place.

Tom has a bipolar disorder. His employment gaps and unfulfilled career hopes are due to recurring periods of depression and mania that usually result in hospitalization. It all began after his stellar high school experience, when he had started the serious study of journalism at college:

> I started panicking and really worrying a lot about my classes, thinking I was failing them. But there was no evidence for this, because I was doing really well in my classes—if you looked at test scores. Nothing could convince me that I wasn't going to fail. I couldn't figure out why this was happening to me. I tried to figure out all kind of reasons why, but I couldn't come up with anything. I was crying a lot and eventually stopped going to classes completely. It was a really, sad, sad day at the end of the quarter when my Mom and I went and we took all my stuff from the dorm room home. I went into the hospital January 2, 1982, because I had become delusional and the depression was getting worse. I was there for three months and it really messed up my academic career for a while.

Scathed but not destroyed, Tom returned to college. He graduated with highest honors. He even made it to a major city newspaper. Nevertheless, this and other journalism jobs have ended with exacerbations of bipolar disorder. Yet Tom struggles on:

> It's awful! Its like, you know, a little ant crawling up a hill, and you just kick him down every so often, and he'll . . . he'll climb back up and continue, but its gonna take him a long time. I'm just trying to get back on any track that I can. Because once you get another job, you could just as easily lose it—like you lost the last one. Every time you lose a

job it becomes harder to get another one. You have to explain the last one. You try to keep a positive attitude and think that you will find a job and that somehow, if you do go through another episode, that it won't be bad, or that you'll be able to catch it early enough that you'll cut it short, somehow. You can't predict these things. You know, you stop predicting.

Each time illness interrupts Tom's life, he revises his life story to accommodate it. Hopeful, he half-expects further setbacks. Tom bridges the distance between his adolescent dreams, his present job in the trade publications, and the future as follows:

One of the keys is that you realize that you don't have to move ahead—that you can stay in the same place, that it's not such a terrible thing to give up ambition to some extent. You don't have to share the same amount of ambition as your friends. I'm realizing that I have to sort of stop thinking of myself in the same peer group that I used to. My peer group was once all my college friends who are now climbing their ladders in their respective newspapers, whatever, publishing companies. I really think that if I keep comparing myself to them it's only gonna' make me angry and envious and hostile. So, really, now what's emerging as my new peer group is all the other people with chronic illnesses who, like me, are just having to do the best that we can. I think you learn to scale down what you expect, but that doesn't mean that you stop enjoying life. It just means that you have to find enjoyment in other things.

Lisa

A visitor has just come to talk with Lisa, who is 54, divorced, and lives by herself in her own house near her parents' home in a suburb of Stockholm. After greeting her guest, she sits down but rises immediately, asking, "Do you want a sandwich?"

"No thanks," the guest says.

Then she fetches some cookies and puts them on the table. She goes to the refrigerator, opens it,

and looks inside, saying something to herself about buns. Then she seems to catch herself, embarrassed. Her guest wonders aloud what she said and Lisa responds, "I was looking for the buns, but I suppose I already ate them." Lisa takes some dark bread from the refrigerator and says, matter-of-factly, "Do you want a sandwich?"

The guest repeats, "No, thanks."

Lisa returns to the table. She looks around. She goes to the sink, saying, "What was I looking for?"

Later, after her lunch, she wipes the wash bowl and then says, "I wonder where I took this from? Where do I keep it? I have no idea!" She looks under the sink. She turns. She looks around more. "No, I think I keep it in the laundry," she says.

In her typically Swedish, practical view of the world it is important to Lisa to remain active and be useful. She announces, "If there is laundry to do, I just start doing it." One of her favorite activities is ironing. When an observer notes that she looks so peaceful ironing, Lisa explains that when she irons, "It gets nice . . . and then I like having clean and ironed shirts in the closet . . . and then you feel useful doing it . . ." Lisa goes on to tell about how, on good days, she becomes adventuresome and goes into the city to shop for food on sale. Being practical and useful sums up much of how life should be in Lisa's common sense view; however, she has a secret that makes this difficult.

In autumn 1990, Lisa's dementia first showed at work when she experienced depression, memory loss, and difficulty concentrating. Her symptoms were interpreted as depression and she began taking antidepressive medication without any benefit. Her difficulties increased and she was assigned to less demanding tasks. By the deep winter, she could not handle work at all and had to leave her job with disability benefits. By spring she was hospitalized.

At this time Lisa had severe memory deficits. She could not, for example, recall her own age. As Lisa describes it, she feels "somewhat of a chaos inside." Today, her cognition continues to deteriorate. Lisa is considered to suffer from a degeneration of the frontal cortex.

Lisa makes it clear that she must not show her

disease to the world, but it is hard work to conceal her difficulties. She wonders, "Perhaps everybody can see I'm this dizzy and crazy," and then she repeats how hard she works to conceal what she is like. Even Lisa's mother, who is the person closest to her, is not entirely aware of her problems. Lisa considers aloud what might happen if her mother knew the facts of her dementia, "Maybe they would take my house away from me, or something like that, and believe I can't manage at all . . . " Then there is the worry about what will happen when her mother is no longer nearby as a source of support. "I worry about the day she dies. Then I will be all by myself with this sticky mess in my head. Then I won't manage and everything will fall apart."

The impending chaos when Lisa's life will come apart hovers relentlessly around her little house. It causes Lisa anxiety over all the many things that might go wrong and overwhelm her. Thus, "All small things become huge houses. I get a lot of Christmas cards, and I worry about having to first find cards to send in return, and then I have to write them out. And find addresses. And then they need stamps and I have to get out to buy stamps. And then I have to mail them and all . . . " So go Lisa's worries about how she is going to manage.

Lisa reminisces to her guest about the frequent bus trips into Stockholm that were a part of her routine. She is very hesitant to take these trips now. She tells how, a few weeks ago, she was going to meet her daughter in a large shopping center in the city. When the time came, she could not imagine how to get into the city or return home, so she did not go. Today, she starts to look for her telephone books so she can call the bus company with a question about the schedule. She finds the books in the cleaning cupboard but just stares at them, apparently wondering which one she should consult. Finally, she sighs, "No, today I feel bad. I don't want to do it." Then, as if to explain, Lisa tells her guest, slowly and solemnly, "I'm not that strong anymore. I'm weak and I can't make it. It feels like I just could break down. Before this I was strong, but I'm not anymore."

Jon

I was born in 1951 on the southwest side of Chicago. My sister is older and she was married when I was nine. My father died when I was 16. I was an unremarkable student, graduating high school by the skin of my teeth. I enrolled in the local community college, but this was during the Vietnam era. During my first year of college I joined the Air Force Reserves. I spent most of 1970 on active duty in Texas, returning to school the following spring semester. At that time I met a girl and within weeks became engaged.

I was very involved in school activities. I became editor of the college newspaper and was elected to the Student Congress. My junior year I transferred to the University of Illinois at Chicago with a major in accounting. I got married at the end of my first quarter. I took a very heavy course load, trying to make up for lost time, but I was still not a good student. What got me through college was remembering that growing up, my parents were insistent about college, telling me, "You will go to college! You will go to college!" If I hadn't graduated from college, the sense of personal failure would have been unbearable. Nothing else, just nothing else, was more important.

It wasn't easy, but I graduated and went to work for a small accounting firm. Within a year I moved on to one of the largest CPA firms in the country. I worked there for four years. In the meantime, I bought a house and my first son was born. I left the firm in 1979 just as my second son was born and started a small accounting and tax service working with small businesses. I also began getting involved in local government, and was appointed as a town planning commissioner and a district trustee of schools.

Within a year I purchased a small tax business to operate in addition to my primary practice. I was maintaining things, but the economy was getting worse. When an opportunity came to join a larger firm again, I took it.

Throughout my twenties I focused on my career. Most of my time went toward practice development. I loved being a dad, but my wife and I were fighting all the time. Much of the fighting had to do with my constant working. Eventually we separated. I took an apartment and tried to sort things out. I was working and seeing my boys on weekends, while evaluating both my marriage and career choices. I was feeling the pressures from the practice, the new firm, and my marriage. It was not a good time.

I was trying to work through these things when I was in a car accident on my way home from work. It was February 1983. I was sitting at a red light when a drunken driver rear-ended my car. The car seat collapsed on impact and I was thrown head first into the back seat. I sustained a compression fracture on the C5–6 level. My only recollection of the accident spans about 30 seconds. It was about eight in the evening, a clear and cold night. I was lying on my back inside the car, and I could see the sky because the roof had been cut away. I felt light snowflakes on my face and it was very cold, yet everything else felt warm. I heard police radios and saw the reflections of flashing red lights. I heard voices, one of them was mine, but I have no idea what was being said.

I'm told that in the hospital I kept asking the same questions over and over, "What's going on?" and "Am I going to die?" The next morning the shock was wearing off and I began to understand about the accident and the nature of my injury. No one used the word quadriplegia. I think that would have bothered me more. They told me about loss of movement and function. I remember hoping that it was temporary, but I understood that it might be permanent.

I asked, early on, if my hand function would return. I thought, if so, I could get my guitar and play all day. I had purchased a new guitar just prior to the accident. The enjoyment of playing was in developing the technique—the coordination of both hands toward a sound and a rhythm. The doctor said maybe in time, but it was a long shot. While I was in rehabilitation, one of the therapists brought me brochures for adaptable guitar equipment. The device enabled the user to construct chords on the guitar, one at a time, and then strum the strings. The technique and style of playing the guitar was lost in the process. I told the

therapist I was not interested in playing the guitar in that fashion.

I knew that the Jon Smith who existed before the accident was gone. This Jon Smith was very different, at least physically. I took stock of what assets I had left, namely my mind and a certain amount of tenacity, and decided to take it from there. I concluded that I needed to have my own agenda for the rehabilitation process. In addition to the therapy sessions, which were intended to develop my abilities, I knew that the rehabilitation setting was the best place for me to test and discover my limits as well. I tried to come to grips with how things would or could be when I was out living on my own. Obvious questions, such as whether I would need 24-hour attendant care would actually be determined by less obvious questions, which unfortunately the staff was all too ready to answer for me by assumption rather than logic or deduction.

As an example, I was told I would need to turn in bed every four hours to avoid skin breakdown; however, at the time I could not turn myself. The staff response was that I would need an attendant at night to assist in turning me. I asked, "What happens if I don't get turned?" They responded that I had to be turned every four hours—they had a schedule. I suggested trying every six hours to see what would happen. "Nobody goes six hours," I was told. I argued with the doctor, the nurses, and the therapists that if I could get by without being turned then I wouldn't need an attendant at night. They finally agreed to the logic and we tried no turns as an experiment, carefully checking for any signs of skin breakdown. We found none and after a few days the doctor approved a schedule with no turns at night; the prospect of a nighttime attendant was avoided.

After eight months in rehabilitation I was discharged and went to live in my mother's home. We had a large family room put on the house after my father died. I finished all of the interior carpentry and now, 16 years later, I was living in this room. There was an irony to it, but it did give me an opportunity to really get a feel for what it would take for me to live on my own. I was able to identify those skills that I needed to develop. I returned to rehabilitation three months later with very definite goals. I began to feel more sure of myself as I accomplished the goals. Within days of my final discharge I bought a van with a lift and hand controls. I just drove all summer. It was therapeutic. I started taking the kids with me at least one day a week and they helped me a lot. They made me experiment and asked me to try new things. Because of them I stared venturing out more into public. I think nothing of it now, but it was their idea to go to a movie theater the first time. I went to a mall by myself because my son asked me to pick something up for him. I worked very hard at having our relationship work. My priorities always started with my sons. We may have a better relationship now than we would have had without the accident.

I was realizing that I was not helpless and I was getting bored. About that time someone I knew at a Center for Independent Living suggested I apply to the center as Finance Director. Working at the Center I was able to experiment with different files and desk layouts to best accommodate my limited hand function. Most important though was my introduction to computers. Over time I found myself far more productive with computers than I had ever been before the accident.

I was still living at my mother's, but looking for my own place. I found a local apartment complex and met with the construction people who were rehabbing six apartment buildings. We talked about making as many apartments as they could accessible. They specifically selected one building with no steps and made some minor modifications. I was getting ready to move into one of the apartments, but the day before I was supposed to sign the lease the owner called, suggesting that I not come. He was vague, but said he didn't think the apartment was appropriate for me and that I would be happier living elsewhere. I began to realize that I was being discriminated against because of my disability.

I called the ACLU who referred me to the State Department of Human Rights. I obtained help from Northwestern University's law school legal aid clinic and filed a complaint. The whole pro-

cess took over two years to complete. I found a different apartment in the meantime but I stayed with the case as a matter of principle. We were preparing for trial when the owner offered to settle. The owner agreed to an order of nondiscrimination, and advertised the building as available to others with physical disabilities. I won the right to the apartment and a monetary settlement for damages.

Living on my own was an experience. I needed some help setting up the apartment; however, once I was organized I found it to be very accommodating. I felt like I was getting on with my life.

Later that year I applied to Northwestern University's graduate management program. Graduate school was an excellent opportunity to develop skills and become more competitive in spite of my disability. I was working at the Center, attending school part-time, and feeling pretty productive.

During my second year of graduate school I learned of additional state funding available for the creation of new Centers for Independent Living. I organized a group to start a new Center providing services to people with disabilities in Suburban Chicagoland. I served as Chairman of the organizing committee. We lobbied the state legislature, played politics, and fought the government bureaucracy to establish the new Center. We were frustrated at times, but overall it was a very interesting and rewarding experience. After nearly 2 years of effort, we were successful in securing the state funding to open the second largest Center in the Midwest.

As the Center was becoming a reality, I considered taking the position of Executive Director; however, I decided it was important for me to make my career choices in spite of my disability, not because of it. I continued with the Center, but only as a volunteer, serving as Chairman of the Board of Directors. Over the six years since the Center opened, we've seen it grow to a staff of 13 with a budget approaching $700,000.

I moved on to my current job, finance officer of a rapidly growing child welfare agency. In addition, I continued to focus on career development, obtaining another graduate degree and passing the

CPA exam. Looking back, I may have been trying to overcompensate professionally. I wanted to keep open as many career opportunities as possible.

The accident obviously changed my life. Whatever plans I had for my life were gone. The pressures I was feeling at the time of the accident were taken out of my hands, and I was forced to start over with a clean slate. I had always been a planner, but whatever I had planned for my life was gone. Whatever road I had been on, I wasn't on that road anymore.

What I was going to do with my life, my time, what my relationship with my kids would be like, who I might spend my life with . . . all of those things were unknown to me. Some still are, but I realized that I needed to start asking those questions of myself. I was making choices because life goes on. Even though I had lost so much of how I had been, I was still in a position to ask myself, "What should I do with the rest of my life?"

I think I'm stronger and more determined than before becoming disabled. I do feel a certain sense of accomplishment, although I feel I still have a lot to do. I've worked hard to maintain a strong relationship with my sons. I hope I'm more sensitive to the circumstances of other people. Before the accident, I would never have envisioned the events of my life so far.

Ladonna

"I can't make my leg bend."

The doctor responds, "It's bending now."

"I mean when I want it to bend, like when I land from a *grande jete*. I tell the knee to bend and it won't. It's been bending when I land for almost my whole life and now it won't."

"Let me see you walk."

The doctor observes, "You walk fine."

I say, "I know that, but I can't land right from a *grande jete*."

"Then don't do that."

"Then don't do that." How frustratingly simple. The countless doctors, specialists, surgeons, and physical therapists enlisted to aid me in my struggle each in their turn uttered those hopeless words, "Then don't do that."

The career of a ballerina starts young. I began taking ballet lessons at the age of 5. I was forced to relinquish life as a ballerina at the age of 20. During this early part of my life, I performed as a member of the corps de ballet of the Beverly Dance Ensemble and was featured as a guest artist in numerous recitals, dance concerts, and musical theater productions. Most recently, I held the position of Managing Director of the dance company in residence at the Chicago Cultural Center, Hedwig Dances. I moved into arts administration after multiple injuries ended my budding career as a dancer.

The end began with recurring dislocations of my left patella, which would later be attributed to a joint malformation responsible for patella subluxations. My recovery was complicated by a series of chronic ailments resulting in pain and loss of function. Today, my condition is further complicated by localized degenerative joint disease and fibromyalgia.

My first tutu was blue, not pink like the other 5 year olds. I was a quiet, shy child, but you wouldn't have known it to see me on stage—blowing kisses and bowing long after the other little girls had already left the stage. Nine years later, at my first professional performance, my parents gave me a gold rose pendant—a flower that would never die. Six years later the chain broke and I lost it. That same year I lost the ability to dance.

The doctors were confounded by my symptoms, and it took years for them to sort it all out. During those years I fought for the ability to dance, and in the years of recovery that followed, I had 4 operations, made 9 trips to the emergency room, was subjected to countless tests and consultations with specialists, took thousands of pills, and endured almost 10 years of physical therapy. I guess all this helped. Some.

The first joint to go was the left knee. For years I viewed this knee as the enemy. Despite our adversarial relationship, I coddled it, trying to cajole it into behaving for me. Then in frustration I would curse "the damn leg that wouldn't do what I told it."

When I began to experience significant difficulties with other joints, as well as some neurologic and internal medical problems, it was as though my entire body had turned on me. My will and my body were engaged in a battle. The body was winning.

The only word to describe what I felt then is betrayal. I had been betrayed by my own body. That body once could whip out 32 *fouete* turns like the black swan in Swan Lake. That body once felt the movement in the music without needing to count it out. Now, that body refused to comply.

I began to detach myself from that body. It became increasingly separate, as it was increasingly not under my control. I estranged myself from the noncompliant body the way anyone would seek to withdraw from a betrayer.

My condition worsened. My dreams of ballet were being steadily, slowly ripped to shreds. As this happened, I began to be ostracized by the dance community. Instructors said I was bad for morale. Seeing an injured dancer was just too depressing. Worst of all were the hushed voices of the other dancers, "I would kill myself if that happened to me. That's what a real dancer would do." Cruel? How could I blame them? I wasn't sure myself that I wanted to live a life without ballet. I was losing my source of pride, of joy, of beauty, and of grace.

Life without ballet. What would I do? Who would I be? Would anyone love me if I couldn't dance? Would I be desirable, if I had no gift to offer, no special talent? It may seem silly now, but I had known nothing else for my entire lifetime.

In dance, the body is "besouled, bespirited, and beminded." One's entire self shapes, and is shaped by, the dance (Fraleigh, 1987). When I was dancing I did not "think" about what to do next. My mind did not consciously instruct my feet to point, my neck to elongate, my arms to float, my fingers to curve, my hips to turn out, one leg to kick while the opposite knee pulled up, my head to tilt, my torso to align, my lips to smile—all simultaneously. My body required only the simple command—battement—and it knew exactly what to do. This movement, like hundreds of others, had become, through experience, part of my

body's repertoire. The development of such a repertoire was accomplished through devoted practice. However, movement of the body alone is not enough. It is the expression of the soul through movement that transforms moving body parts into art. The difference between someone who dances (a person who is merely capable of executing the steps) and a dancer (a person whose movement inspires the use of such words as magical, ethereal, magnificent) is the expression of the soul. The body, mind, and soul must fuse to succeed in dance.

Injury disrupts that union. Without that fusion the dancer fails. The body long separated from the mind soon loses its meaning. The meaningless body cannot realize expression. A soul without means of expression soon ceases to be the soul (Fraleigh, 1987). This was the fear, the terror, the loss. I believed that my soul was dying and I didn't know how to save it.

As I learn more about this body-mind-soul relationship, I realize that to some extent it was true. My soul, as it had been experienced and expressed, did die. Perhaps it is better to say that it was transformed by new life experiences. But before that transformation could take place, I had to grieve for the loss. The loss of what had been my life, my way of thinking, my way of being, my essence.

My family also needed to grieve. It would be 5 years after I lost the ability to dance before my parents stopped telling people that their daughter *is* a ballerina. It was even longer before they could come to terms with my need for help getting up and down stairs. I am capable of limping up and down the stairs without assistance. However, when people help me it is less painful. The more often I am helped throughout the day, the less pain I am in that day. The less painful life is, the more productive I can be. So, if I am to live well and accomplish much, I do need such help.

As ballerinas, we were motivated by the phrase, "no pain, no gain." My motivation has changed. I have come to realize that the more I can do to keep my pain under control, the more I can accomplish. Minimize pain. Maximize productivity.

The greatest struggle I had to overcome, after dealing with the reactions and attitudes of others, was coping with the loss of my gift. I was not simply losing an ability, a career, a meaningful occupation—I was losing my defining gift. My great gift, that intrinsic thing that gave my life meaning and purpose. My greatest fear was that we only get one great gift, and that I had lost mine.

The other dancers understood that. Only non-dancers recommended that I embark on a related career. Become a choreographer, or an actress. Or my personal favorite, "Don't worry, you're a pretty girl. You'll marry well."

I didn't need a new job or someone to support me. I needed meaning and purpose. I needed to know that our worth does not lie in what we are capable of doing, but in the doing—in experiencing life and interacting with others.

My identity as a ballerina had provided me with a sense of belonging and understanding of my place in the world. Without that identity, I felt lost. It took me years to realize that in losing my identity I had not lost who I am. Perhaps I would have, had I not found a new way to manifest the essential qualities of my original gift. The gift was not simply the physical ability to execute the steps. Rather it was the ability to bring to life an expression of great emotion. That gift remains mine. I realized this while in college at the University of Illinois, Champaign-Urbana.

When all avenues for recovery had been exhausted, and I had wound up on the operating table for a fourth time, even I had to acknowledge defeat. I had to relinquish dance. But what now? My parents made that decision. They said, "No way are you going to sit around our house and cry. You're going back to school." Their response to my fear, my complete lack of direction: "You won't figure it out here. Take some classes, you'll find something else." And off I went.

The University of Illinois has an excellent wheelchair athletics program housed in their Rehabilitation Center. These athletes took me in and helped me to discover what it is be a person first and an ability second. I played wheelchair football and trained for wheelchair basketball. I was terrible. But it gave me something I desperately needed—a place to belong.

I also learned new ways to use my body, new habits to promote function with as little pain as possible. The embodiment of these new abilities and habits gradually allowed me to adapt to my new way of being in the world. My experiences at the center also inspired my passion for working to improve the lives of people with disabilities. I have taught dance classes for people with developmental and physical disabilities, volunteered for the Wirtz Sports program at the Rehabilitation Institute of Chicago, cared for patients at Children's Memorial and Thorek Hospitals, consulted with the Chicago theater community and St. Clement's church on accessibility issues, served on the Board of Directors of the Ministry to the Disadvantaged, and assisted a gentleman with cerebral palsy in starting his own business. As of this writing, I am enrolled in the Professional Master's Program in Occupational Therapy at the University of Illinois, Chicago.

I still have chronic pain. My joints still collapse periodically. My other chronic ailments persist. But I have learned to live with these circumstances. I have come to treasure those precious moments when I am pain-free. Then my heart is light and my head is giddy—the way I felt when I danced.

When the pain returns, a heaviness comes with it. Severe acute pain is like a blackness that engulfs you. Chronic pain is that same blackness hovering just inches away, at times engulfing part or all of you, at other times merely threatening to do so. You learn to ignore it as much as possible until a fluctuation of intensity or impact on function forces you to acknowledge its presence.

Sometimes I wish that I could just curl up and cry, and go to sleep until the pain goes away. But I choose more than that for my life, for myself. I am in pain more often than not. So I believe that it is important for me to see pain as part of my life, not as an intrusion or disruption. Otherwise, I would spend more time being disrupted than living life.

So I sit here writing. What I want to do is scream because I hurt so much! Today is a particularly bad pain day. But I go through the motions, getting as much done as I can while trying not to let on to others just how much pain I am in. It's hard, but the rewards are worth it. Joy can pierce through the pain.

Life after ballet is better than I thought it would be. My life has meaning. This is not because of any particular thing that I am capable of doing. It is because of the way that I relate with my uniqueness to the world and to the people in it.

I didn't replace ballet. Nothing can replace ballet. I learned to live without it. I learned to focus on what I value most: passion, kindness, and compassion. I've learned not to be defined by a particular ability, or a particular job, or the opinions of others (although admittedly I still struggle with that last one).

The hardest thing about living with chronic conditions remains the negative and often hurtful reactions of others. But I have been blessed with amazing people in my life who lighten my load. My family has come around, my faith brings me peace, and my volunteer work gives me joy. I still have my great gift; I just have a new way of expressing it.

David

David holds Fine Arts Bachelor's and Master's degrees from a prominent private university. Classical music is singularly important to David, and his identity is as an artistic person. He has been playing the violin since he was 7 years old. Because of his passion for music, he feels obligated to make practicing a part of his daily routine. However, David cannot find the time, energy, or support with which to practice and become skilled once again. Lately his playing has been "horrendous."

After graduate school, David taught music in four different public and private schools. His longest job was 6 months. He was fired from three of the positions. In David's view, he was repeatedly fired because his educational philosophy conflicted with each school's mission. There were also the "difficult" teachers and staff.

Feeling defeated, David stopped teaching and was unemployed for several years—a "victim of society." The word "victim" surfaces often when David talks about his life. He feels he is powerless to enact his own desires and that he is constrained by external forces.

David eventually found employment at a museum exhibit that focused on the history of classical music. In this job, he thoroughly enjoyed the teaching and interactions with children and their parents. He found a way to use an education that had seemed a waste. He felt useful and appreciated. He enjoyed the sense of accomplishment. Moreover, because the job was part time, he had time to practice the violin and improve his skills and technique. Things were looking up.

Then David learned he had AIDS. His doctor prescribed AZT and told David that he had 6 months to live. He was devastated but continued to work because it gave him structure. After a few months, feeling that he was the target of both subtle and blatant discrimination related to his AIDS status, he quit his job. Now a "broken victim," he began receiving Social Security Disability Income but did not feel it was enough to maintain his lifestyle. With his financial resources diminishing, he decided to move back home with his aging and ailing mother. Now David is his mother's primary caregiver.

With the move back home, David began a long, downward spiral of depression that continues to this day. He feels acutely the "shame of not being an independent adult who is able to take care of himself." He now relies on the financial support of his mother to cover the costs of health care, rent, bills, food, and other needs.

David is deeply conflicted about being his mother's primary caregiver. This role of caregiver is his primary identity. The responsibilities that come along with it define his daily routine and constitute most of his activities. He resents his mother's needs and the way they dictate his daily routine and rob time from his music. He finds the combination of household chores and taking care of both his own and his mother's self-care and health needs to be overwhelming. Nonetheless, he has refused numerous offers of caregiving assistance from outside sources.

David feels ensnared between two extremes. He longs to be the best possible caregiver. In contrast, he feels that "nothing in the house" gets accomplished. He simply does not have the "strength, will, expertise, or emotional wherewithal" to get things done. His high expectations of himself and the reality of what he can accomplish pull him in opposite directions.

David refers to himself as the "adult child acting as parent, but who is still treated as a child by that parent." He enjoyed his relationship to his mother in the past. Becoming a caregiver has changed that. It leaves him feeling incompetent.

Extremely frustrated, David feels trapped by the fear of making changes that would disrupt his mother's routine. His life is shaped by conditions beyond his control. He is a "victim of circumstances." According to David, he wishes to but cannot make his life otherwise. Although he experiences life as stressful and unsatisfying, he sees his only alternative as "suffering through it."

David's convictions about his situation are always reinforced when he makes an attempt to break out of his situation. For example, he tried to spend some time away from his mother by volunteering at an AIDS service organization one day a week. However, he ended up feeling overwhelmed by his "job as a person with AIDS." Being associated with the AIDS organization underscored his lack of control over the virus. He stopped volunteering.

Next David attempted to take piano composition class. After a couple of weeks, the class was not going as well as he hoped. He felt a strong sense of failure at bringing musical interest back into his life. His caregiving role was "all-consuming" and, as he had done before, David continued to feel that he had no control of his life's events.

David recently came to the top of a long waiting list for an independent housing program. Once again, he declined. He will continue to live with his mother.

The Narratives in Perspective

Each person's story reflects a unique and personal journey with its own challenges, failures, and accomplishments. Yet, woven into each of these stories are all the components of occupational identity. That is, each person seeks to make sense of his or her own capacity. Each seeks to find enjoyment and satisfaction in the activities that fill their lives. Each tries to sort out what is important. Each aims to find and enact roles. Each must deal with the routines of everyday life. Each seeks to comprehend changed physical or mental abilities and experiences.

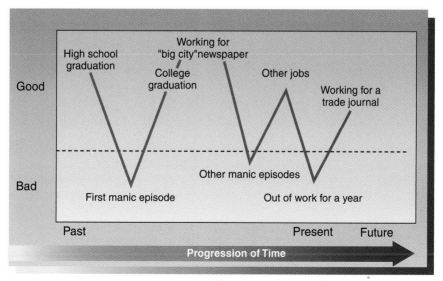

FIGURE 9-2 Tom's Narrative Slope.

These narratives also make comprehensible the things each person does (or does not) do. For example, they reveal why Tom chose to leave reporting for a trade journal, why Lisa gave up her habit of taking the bus into the city, why Jon decided to earn graduate degrees, why Ladonna did not turn from dancing to choreography, and why David does not practice piano. These decisions and actions all take meaning from and enact the fundamental plot of the narrative to which they belong.

As shown in *Figure 9-2*, Tom's is a melodramatic plot, with its repeated struggles and accomplishments. Tom also makes sense out of his occupational life in the face of bipolar disorder by evoking the metaphor of struggling against a large and formidable foe. His struggle and the nature of his powerful adversary make his ongoing adjustment of career aims reasonable and admirable. Importantly, the central meaning in his occupational life is greatly summed up in his narrative with its complementary plot and metaphor.

The downward slope of Lisa's narrative takes her to the edge of a precipice *(Fig. 9-3)*. In any moment she may be found out as incompetent, losing her house and her freedom as she had lost her job. One mistake, she believes, could bring her world crashing down on her. Lisa's story is largely lived and articulated only in sporadic bits. She does not employ a deep overriding metaphor but evokes the household images of a "sticky mess" in her head and the small tasks that become like managing big houses. Nonetheless, her story illustrates that even persons with cognitive limitations manage to emplot their occupational lives. As Bruner (1990a) notes, narrative is basic to how we think about our lives.

The upward slopes of Jon's and Ladonna's narratives *(Figs. 9-4 and 9-5)* follow devastating events. Ladonna's metaphor of treasure (her gift), lost and found again, permeates her story. Implied in Jon's story is a metaphor of salvation, of losing the old self and finding a new inner strength that results in his becoming a better person as a result of his injury and disability. David's story has both the shape of a tragedy and the metaphor of entrapment *(Fig. 9-6)*.

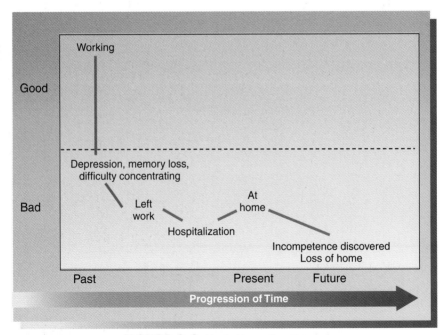

FIGURE 9-3 Lisa's Narrative Slope.

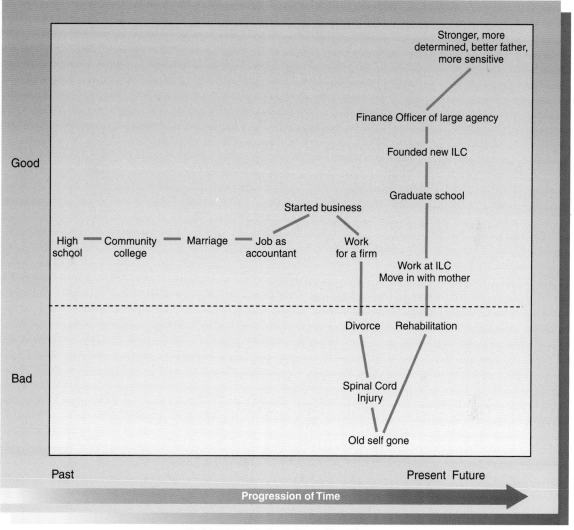

FIGURE 9-4 Jon's Narrative Slope.

Ultimately, how these persons go about life—their occupational competence—is tied to the underlying plots and metaphors of their stories. The stories of Jon, Ladonna, and Tom empower them to keep going despite substantial losses and challenges. David lives out his story of entrapment by avoiding choices that could extract him from circumstances he finds dissatisfying. Lisa lives cautiously to avoid a dreaded outcome in her story. These persons all clearly conduct their lives in terms of their narratives.

Influences on the Occupational Narrative

The disparity of the narratives presented in this chapter also raises important questions about why some persons end up with a positive occupational narrative and others with life stories that constrain and rob them of quality of life. It is tempting to conclude in cases such as Lisa's that it is the circumstances of life (i.e., a progressive disease) that shape the direction of

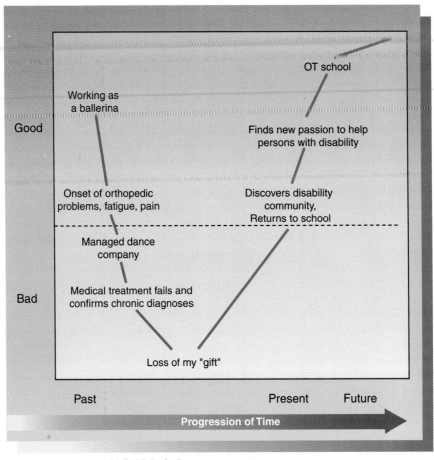

FIGURE 9-5 Ladonna's Narrative Slope.

the narrative. However, in the original study (Nygård, 1996), of which Lisa's narrative was a part, there was another woman with dementia who was able to construct for herself a positive narrative emphasizing her remaining abilities. Consequently, something more must account for the nature of narratives people craft for themselves.

Whereas the question of how narratives are ultimately shaped will no doubt require several answers, there are three factors that appear to have an important impact. These are the unfolding events of life, social forces, and the presence or absence of an engaging occupation. The following sections examine each of these factors.

Unfolding Events and Circumstances of Life

Each of the five narratives in this chapter indicates that ongoing events and circumstances of life insert themselves into narratives, having a significant influence on how they unfold. In a longitudinal study, Jonsson et al. (2000) examined how narratives shape and are shaped by what happens as lives unfold. The study began when a group of older persons were anticipating retirement and continued as they continued into their retirement. Over time, the actual direction that retirees' lives took was reflective of an interaction between their original narrative and unfolding events and circumstances. Subjects' narratives readied them to re-

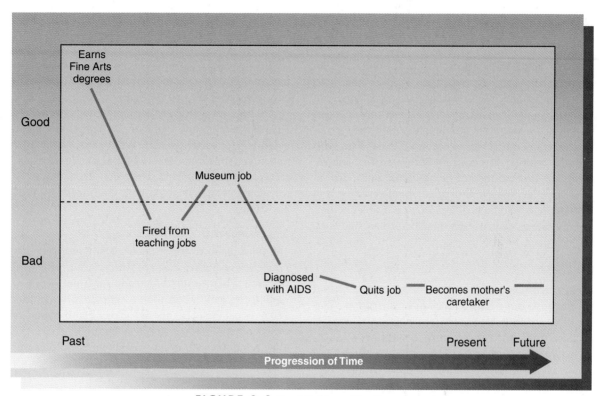

FIGURE 9-6 David's Narrative Slope.

A dynamic tension always exists between how we narrate our lives and what is around the next corner.

spond in particular ways to ongoing life events and circumstances. Nonetheless, differences in those external circumstances and events could also nudge the narrative in one direction or another. Thus, stories tended to be resilient, that is, to maintain their own plot. However, whereas life events and circumstances were usually integrated into the existing plot, they sometimes changed. In either case, the narrative had to come to terms with new events and circumstances.

Sociocultural Influences on Narrative

A dynamic tension always exists between how we narrate our lives and what is around the next corner.

While each person constructs his or her occupational narrative, there are also important and pervasive influences by the sociocultural context. First, each person derives a sense of narrative plot and various metaphors from surrounding cultures. The themes and images that populate our narratives are those derived from the kinds of discourse we encounter in our everyday worlds. Prevailing plots and metaphors that are part of the language and behavior of any culture serve as templates for how persons can make sense of and enact their lives. Moreover, in the course of socialization and

. . . in the course of socialization and throughout life, societies show to members what kinds of stories can be brought to bear on certain situations or problems.

throughout life, societies show to members what kinds of stories can be brought to bear on certain situations or problems.

We can see this influence in how the narratives we presented are couched in the themes, ideas, and viewpoints provided by everyday culture. Tom, Jon, Ladonna, and David all reflect the American values of career accomplishment and ambition and they struggle, as many others do, to reconcile themselves with cultural notions of success and achievement. Lisa reflects the Swedish idea of being useful and practical. All five reflect the Western ideal of individualism and autonomy as guiding and organizing principles in their commonsense views of how they should live their lives.

> *Because our occupational lives unfold in interaction with others, our narratives are also invariably tied to how others act toward us and how we act toward them. Those who enter and find a place in our lives, and their characteristics and actions, affect our occupational narratives.*

Each person has borrowed heavily from the dominant social themes in constructing his or her occupational narrative. To the extent that societies provide prevailing narrative themes, they may have an impact on the kinds of narratives persons within them construct for themselves. For example, Kielhofner and Barrett (1997) document how a woman living in poverty is located in a narrative of seeking escape and refuge from the ongoing circumstances of her life in the inner city. Such a narrative arises out of social conditions and appears common among those who share such conditions.

Because our occupational lives unfold in interaction with others, our narratives are also invariably tied to how others act toward us and how we act toward them. Those who enter and find a place in our lives, and their characteristics and actions, affect our occupational narratives. This feature of narratives was illustrated in the study of retirees when family members

were mobilized to do things that avoided the negative turn of events anticipated by their relatives (Jonsson et al., 2000). It is an important feature of social life that we note and seek to influence the occupational narratives of those whose lives intersect with our own. In the end, our stories are tied to theirs.

In sum, social influences on narrative are twofold. First, the content and shape of our narratives are provided by the social context. We invariably construct narratives that draw on socially available plots and metaphors. Second, since we live our occupational narratives in interaction with others, they inevitably affect our stories.

ENGAGING OCCUPATIONS

The third phase of the study of elderly retirees noted previously suggests that constructing a positive life story requires a person to find and participate in an engaging occupation (Jonsson, Josephsson, & Kielhofner, 2001). Engaging occupations evoke a depth of passion or feeling and become a central feature in a narrative. They are done with great commitment and perseverance and stand out from the other things a person does. They are infused with positive meaning connected to interest (i.e., pleasure, challenge, enjoyment), personal causation (i.e., challenge, indication of one's competence), and value (i.e., something worth doing, important, contribution to family or society). Thus, the engaging occupation resonates with all aspects of volition. It is typically done with regularity over a long period of involvement and includes several occupational forms that cohere or constitute an interrelated whole. Involvement in an engaging occupation also represents a commitment or sense of duty to the occupation and a connection to a community of people who share a common interest in that occupation. In summary, an **engaging occupation** is a coherent and meaningful set of occupational forms that cohere and evoke deep feeling, a sense of duty, commitment, and

> *Engaging occupations evoke a depth of passion or feeling and become a central feature in a narrative.*

perseverance leading to regular involvement over time in relation to a community of people who share the engaging occupation.

The narratives shared in this chapter appear to support the concept of engaging occupations and their potential centrality to achieving a positive occupational narrative. Each person was struggling with the loss of, the challenge of maintaining, or the need to replace an engaging occupation.

Conclusion

We began this chapter by asserting that people conduct and make meaning out of their occupational lives by locating themselves in an unfolding occupational narrative. We further argued that this story integrates past, present, and future selves, imparting meaning on the events and circumstances of life through the use of plot and metaphor. We presented the occupational narratives of five persons to illustrate how these stories made sense of and provided a framework for undertaking occupational life.

In this chapter we have spoken of occupational narratives. Implied in this term is that other types of narratives exist. That is, people may have more than a single narrative that defines the self. Narratives outside the occupational domain may be, for example, those associated with sexuality/intimacy or spirituality. Different narratives may certainly intersect and influence each other, but they represent distinct aspects of life. For example, it is not uncommon for the occupational narrative to be moving in an upward direction at the same time one's most intimate personal relationship is dissolving. Conversely, when occupational life is disrupted (e.g., job loss, school failure) persons may turn to and depend on intimate relationships or spiritual beliefs for consolation.

We further linked occupational narratives to the concepts of identity and competence discussed in the previous chapter. Our argument in this chapter has been that as each person lives life, he or she develops an occupational identity and occupational competence that represents ongoing patterns of thinking, feeling, and doing. Occupational identity is reflected in the relative success the person has in formulating a vision of life that carries him or her forward. Occupational competence is reflected in each person's relative success in putting that vision into effect.

Inasmuch as narratives are both told and done, they interweave identity and competence. This is not to suggest that identity and competence are always integrated. Indeed, there are situations in which one is unable to enact the life story one envisions and desires. There is evidence that following onset of disability, many persons may initially experience a gap between the identity reflected in their narratives and what they are able to enact (Kielhofner, Mallinson, Forsyth, & Lai, 2001; Mallinson, Mahaffey, & Kielhofner, 1998). These same studies also suggest that one cannot have competence without an intact identity. Crafting life appears to begin with what we imagine when we begin to fashion our occupational narratives. This reflects the fact that narrative is the great mediator between self and life. We always apprehend ourselves and the world around us in terms of our stories. Narrative is both the meaning we assign to occupational life and the medium within which we enact it.

Key Terms

Engaging occupation: A coherent and meaningful set of occupational forms that cohere and evoke deep feeling, a sense of duty, commitment, and perseverance leading to regular involvement over time in relation to a community of people who share the engaging occupation.

Occupational narratives: Stories (both told and enacted) that integrate across time our unfolding volition, habituation, performance capacity, and environments through plots and metaphors that sum up and assign meaning to all these various elements.

References

Bruner, J. (1990a). *Acts of meaning.* Cambridge, MA: Harvard University Press.

Bruner, J. (1990b). Culture and human development: A new look. *Human Development, 33,* 344–355.

Clark, F. (1993). Occupation embedded in a real life: Interweaving occupational science and occupational therapy: 1993 Eleanor Clarke Slagle lecture. *American Journal of Occupational Therapy, 47,* 1067–1078.

Fraleigh, S. (1987). *Dance and the lived body: A descriptive aesthetics*. Pittsburgh, PA: University of Pittsburgh Press.

Ganzer, C. (1993). Metaphor in narrative inquiry: Using literature as an aid to practice. Paper presented at the 15th Allied Health Research Forum, Chicago, IL.

Geertz, C. (1986). Making experiences, authoring selves. In V. Turner & E. Bruner (Eds.), *The anthropology of experience*. Urbana, IL: University of Illinois Press.

Gergen, K. J., & Gergen, M. M. (1988). Narrative and the self as relationship. In L. Berkowitz (Ed.), *Advances in experimental social psychology*. San Diego: Academic Press.

Helfrich, C., Kielhofner, G., & Mattingly, C. (1994). Volition as narrative: Understanding motivation in chronic illness. *American Journal of Occupational Therapy, 48*, 311–317.

Jonsson, H., Josephsson, S., & Kielhofner, G. (2000). Evolving narratives in the course of retirement: A longitudinal study. *American Journal of Occupational Therapy, 54*, 463–470.

Jonsson, H., Josephsson, S., & Kielhofner, G. (2001). Narratives and experience in an occupational transition: A longitudinal study of the retirement process. *American Journal of Occupational Therapy, 55*, 424–432.

Jonsson, H., Kielhofner, G., & Borell, L. (1997). Anticipating retirement: The formation of narratives concerning an occupational transition. *American Journal of Occupational Therapy, 51*, 49–56.

Kielhofner G., & Barrett L. (1997). Meaning and misunderstanding in occupational forms: A study of therapeutic goal setting. *American Journal of Occupational Therapy, 52*, 345–353.

Kielhofner, G., Mallinson, T., Forsyth, K., & Lai, J-S. (2001). Psychometric properties of the second version of the Occupational Performance History Interview. *American Journal of Occupational Therapy, 55,* 260–267.

Mallinson, T., Kielhofner, G., & Mattingly, C. (1996). Metaphor and meaning in a clinical interview. *American Journal of Occupational Therapy, 50,* 338–346.

Mallinson, T., Mahaffey, L., & Kielhofner, G. (1998). The occupational performance history interview: Evidence for three underlying constructs of occupational adaptation. *Canadian Journal of Occupational Therapy, 65,* 219–228.

Mattingly, C. (1991). The narrative nature of clinical reasoning. *American Journal of Occupational Therapy, 45,* 998–1005.

Nygård, L. (1996). *Everyday life with dementia: Aspects of assessing and understanding the consequences and experiences of living with dementia*. Stockholm: Norstedts Tryckeri AB.

Ortony, A. (1979). *Metaphor and thought*. Cambridge, MA: Cambridge University Press.

Ricoeur, P. (1984). *Time and narrative: Vol. 1*. Chicago: University of Chicago Press.

Schafer, R. (1981). *Narration in the psychoanalytic dialogue*. In W. J. T. Mitchell (Ed.), *On narrative* (pp. 25–49). Chicago: University of Chicago Press.

Schön, D. (1979). Generative metaphor: A perspective on problem-setting in social policy. In A. Ortony (Ed.), *Metaphor and thought*. Cambridge, MA: Cambridge University Press.

Spence, D. P. (1982). *Narrative truth and historical truth: Meaning and interpretation in psychoanalysis*. New York: WW Norton.

Taylor, C. (1989). *Sources of the self: The making of the modern identity*. Cambridge, MA: Harvard University Press.

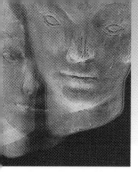

10

Doing and Becoming: Occupational Change and Development

● Gary Kielhofner

In combination with innate, biologically based potentials, what we do propels each of us through a trajectory of lifelong change. Fidler and Fidler (1983) referred to this process as "doing and becoming," underscoring how the course of life is shaped by what we do day by day.

Each successive occasion of doing something increases our capacity and propensity for what was done. When we work, play, and perform activities of daily living we shape our capacities, our patterns of living and interacting with others, and our comprehension of our world and ourselves. To a large extent, we each author our own development through what we do.

Change Processes Underlying Development

Occupational development involves complex processes of change in volition, habituation, and performance capacity. These changes result from the convergence of internal and external factors carried along by doing. We saw in Chapter 3 that there are three elements involved in any permanent change (Fig. 10-1). First, an al-

teration of some internal or external component contributes something new to the total dynamic, out of which new thoughts, feelings, and actions emerge. Second, if these conditions are repeated sufficiently, volition, habituation, and/or performance capacity coalesce toward a new internal organization. Third, ongoing interaction of the new internal organization with consistent environmental conditions maintains a new stable pattern of thinking, feeling, and acting.

Ordinarily, volition, habituation, and performance capacity change in concert. During this process of change, these elements will resonate with and sometimes amplify each other. For example, increases in capacity tend to be accompanied by stronger personal causation. The latter leads to choices to do things that further develop that capacity. The process can also go in the other direction as illustrated in the following example. Older persons whose diminished capacities increase the risk of falling may develop, as part of personal causation, a fear of falling that leads to choices to curtail action. However, by curtailing action, elders may further reduce their capacity and increase the actual risk of falling (Peterson et al., 1999).

Changes in environmental impact are also an important part of any change trajectory. The environment may be the factor that initiates change. Even when this is not the case, change usually means that persons will begin to interact with different aspects of the environment, modify the environment, seek out new environments, or avoid certain past environments. The influence of these altered person-environment interactions is essential to the change process and, eventually, to the maintenance of new patterns of thinking, feeling, and doing that are the result of change.

> *When we work, play, and perform activities of daily living we shape our capacities, our patterns of living and interacting with others, and our comprehension of our world and ourselves. To a large extent, we each author our own development through what we do.*

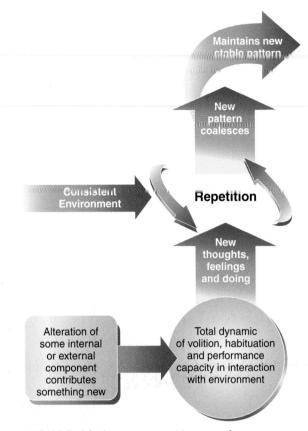

FIGURE 10-1   Necessary Elements for Permanent Change.

In any process of change multiple factors will intersect, contributing both synergistic and divergent forces. For example, adolescents discover new capacities and begin to see themselves as more autonomous. Such volitional changes lead adolescents to interpret what they do differently (refusals and defiance, previously viewed as transgressions, now become assertions of autonomy) and to select new action that tests limits and explores risk. Parents and others in the environment may not consistently agree with the adolescent's desires for autonomy and risk-taking. Moreover, the adolescent's own habituation may assert old patterns such as childhood habits of reliance on parents. Accordingly, the process of change can sometimes be characterized by disorganization, alterations in the pace of change, and backsliding. Change is seldom neat and orderly.

Types of Change

Not all change is the same. The following sections consider three different patterns of change. These are referred to as incremental, transformational, and catastrophic change.

Incremental change refers to a gradual alteration such as change in amount, intensity, or degree. The following are examples of incremental change:

- Increases in learning and sense of capacity that take place as a child masters a new occupational form
- The growing sense of familiarity that occurs over time as one enacts a new role
- The slow waning of physical and mental abilities that accompanies aging and requires gradual accommodations.

Incremental change occurs within the context of one's existing occupational identity and competence. Incremental change often occurs almost imperceptibly because it is ordinary, follows normative pathways, and occurs at a relatively unremarkable pace. Nonetheless, incremental change pervades the course of development.

Incremental change can precipitate more dramatic change when it results in alteration of some component of the self beyond a critical threshold, changing the dynamics of one's situation and leading to new, emergent thoughts, feelings, and actions. Examples of this are the growing familiarity of a job that leads one to seek a new, more exciting one or the steady decline of functioning in old age that leads to the necessity of changing one's living situation. When such significant alterations in life occur, another form of change takes over. It is discussed next.

Transformational change occurs when one fundamentally or qualitatively alters an established pattern of thinking, feeling, and doing. Thus, unlike incremental change, transformational change involves a fundamental modification of one's occupational identity and competence. The following are examples. Children enter the terrible twos, during which their increasing sense of efficacy leads them to insist that they do things by themselves. A 7th grader, who has always been perceived as a studious nerd, decides he wants to be seen as cool, embarking on a whole new attitude, dress, and behaviors. A college freshman lives away from home for the first time and develops a whole new sense of independence and autonomy in managing everyday life. A middle-aged man leaves a high achievement career to spend more time with family and friends. A woman who has been a homemaker for many years decides to return to school to enter a career. As the examples illustrate, transformational change involves a fundamentally new way of seeing and doing things.

Transformational change is much less frequent than incremental change, but generally has a much larger impact on development because it results in a substantial difference in how a person goes about some aspect of occupational life. Some types of transformational change are typical for the course of development. Others are unique to the person.

Transformational change tends to be chaotic. It may involve some undoing of old patterns before new ones are established. It often results in a temporary mismatch between the person and the environment. For example, parents confronted with a newly autonomous toddler or defiant teenager are often caught off guard and must, themselves, adjust to the new situation. The toddler and the teenager, who want new autonomy, often do not have a commensurate sense of what their abilities and limitations are. Thus, mistakes, struggles, failures, and disappointments are often part of the process.

Catastrophic change occurs when internal or external circumstances dramatically alter one's occupational life situation, requiring a fundamental reorganization. The circumstances precipitating catastrophic change are imposed without choice. They are dramatic and unwelcome. Examples of events leading to catastrophic change are the onset of a chronic illness or disability, death of a spouse, suddenly losing a long-term job, becoming a victim of violence or war, or becoming homeless.

Catastrophic change can present a severe challenge to occupational adaptation. It often requires persons to reconstruct both occupational identity and competence. The event precipitating catastrophic change often makes it impossible to go forward within the existing occupational narrative and may, for a while, leave the person without a coherent narrative. Hence, the person must both cope with the breakdown of a previous identity and embark on crafting a new one.

Interplay of Types of Change

The course of development is marked by all three kinds of change. Incremental and transformational changes often intersect in the course of development. Although we tend to think of development as a progressive linear process (at least until the decline of old age), the course of life actually tends to be much more complex. Transformational and catastrophic change can take life in new directions. The latter, in particular, can result in difficulty and struggle as well as periods of poor adaptation.

Following transformational and catastrophic change, a period of incremental change is typical. During the latter a new pattern of thinking, feeling, and doing is gradually established and increasingly becomes routine and familiar. Just as surely as these new patterns become the way of things, some internal or external alterations will come along and precipitate a new round of change. Consequently, life tends to alternate between periods of relative stability and periods of reorganization.

Stages of Change

Occupational change ordinarily occurs across a continuum from exploration to competence to achievement (Reilly, 1974). This continuum is usually involved in transformational and catastrophic change. That is, people typically progress through these levels of function when they move into new roles, encounter new environments, make lifestyle changes, or when they reorganize their lives in response to a major disruptive circumstance or event.

This continuum of development may involve all areas of one's occupational life, as when persons who have acquired a major disability must reorganize how they view themselves and their abilities, how they achieve satisfaction and meaning in life, and how they go about their work, leisure, and activities of daily living. The continuum may also apply to only one aspect of a person's occupational life. The person who is retiring, the mother who decides to return to work after her children have left home, and the person who takes up a new serious hobby are examples of persons who may develop new occupational participation through the stages discussed below.

Exploration is the first stage of change in which persons try out new things and, consequently, learn about their own capacities, preferences, and values. Persons explore when they are learning to do new occupational forms, making role changes, or searching for new sources of meaning. Exploration provides the opportunity for learning, discovering new modes of doing, and discovering new ways of expressing ability and apprehending life. It yields a sense of how well one performs, how enjoyable the task is, and what meaning it can have for one's life. Exploration requires a relatively safe and undemanding environment. Since a person who is exploring is still unsure about capacity or desire, the resources and opportunities in the environment are critical.

Competency is the stage of change when persons begin to solidify new ways of doing that were discovered through exploration. During this stage of change persons strive to be adequate to the demands of a situation by improving themselves or adjusting to environmental demands and expectations. Individuals at a competence level of change focus on consistent, adequate performance. The process of striving for competence leads to the development of new skills, the refinement of old skills, and the organization of these skills into habits that support occupational performance. Competency affords an individual a growing sense of personal control. As persons strive to organize their performances into routines of competent behavior that are relevant to their environment, they immerse themselves in a process of becoming, growing, and arriving at a greater sense of efficacy.

Achievement is the stage of change when persons have sufficient skills and habits that allow them to participate fully in some new work, leisure activity, or activity of daily living. During the achievement stage of change, the person integrates a new area of occupational participation into his or her total life. Occupational identity is reshaped to incorporate the new area of occupational participation. Other roles and routines must be altered to accommodate the new overall pattern to sustain occupational competence.

In the case in which all areas of a person's occupational participation are changing, some areas may attain achievement before others. For example, following a traumatic spinal cord injury, a person may first concentrate on redeveloping ways to manage activities of daily living that include moving to an independent living setting after a period of rehabilitation or living in an institutional setting. Developing patterns of leisure in the new context and returning to work may come later.

Progression Through the Stages of Change

It should also be recognized that persons might move back and forth between stages. For example, having explored various career options and made a choice to enter an educational program, students sometimes find that the choice was not right and return to exploration. As another example, Hammel (1999) observed that persons with spinal cord injury often moved back and forth between these stages.

The three stages of change broadly describe the trajectory that occupational change is likely to take. The actual pattern of events, actions, thoughts, and feelings that transpires when someone goes through change will be unique for each person and for each episode of change.

Readiness for Change

The three stages of change describe a typical pathway once a person has embarked on the process of change. This presumes that a person is ready to begin making change. For a variety of reasons this may not be the case. Even persons whose occupational participation is not adaptive are sometimes reluctant to make a change or do not believe a change is possible in their lives. Another factor limiting readiness to change may be proximity to a catastrophic event. Hammel (1999) found that following spinal cord injury, people went through a process of adjustment that preceded concrete steps toward change. At first, people were dominated by the sense of loss and a disruption of previous life. Following this, she observed, persons enter a period of reaction marked by strong feelings of anger, frustration, fear, and/or depression. Next, they began to acknowledge going on with life and begin to formulate intentions to make change. Following this, they began the exploratory stage of change. Such research suggests that catastrophic change may be marked by a period between the initial event and circumstance that precipitates or necessitates change and the beginning of making the change.

Centrality of the Environment in Change

As already noted, the environment has a pervasive influence in any process of change. The environment can be the source of alterations that precipitate change. Many of the changes that occur in the course of development occur according to socially defined timetables and expectations for change.

The environment can also be a barrier to change. Social definitions of a person's identity or expected behaviors can conflict with personal desires and attempts to change. Realizing change is difficult when the environment fails to support or reward the alterations a person is trying to make. The stages of change presented above also suggest that appropriate environments exist for persons to advance through the stages. For example, to engage in the process of exploration or competency, the environment must allow for persons to try out and/or strengthen new action.

Contributions of Change to the Course of Development

As noted previously, the course of development is characterized by an ongoing process of change. The course of any life involves ongoing incremental and transformational change. Most lives will be affected by one or more periods of catastrophic change.

A cross-sectional view of development will show that, at any point in the life cycle, aspects of one's occupational life will be at different stages. For example, the older child who has mastered self-care and has integrated it into daily routines (achievement) will be at the beginning of exploring the vocational interests in play and school. Achievement in work will follow years later. Underlying development, then, is a complex collection of change processes that follow one another, overlap, and interweave.

Transformation of Work, Play, and Activities of Daily Living

Discussions of development often emphasize that particular courses or processes of development are normal. For example, most discussions of childhood development describe various attainments that, on average, have occurred by a particular age. However, great variation in the course of development occurs across persons. Too much emphasis on norms can distract us from the more important change processes that underlie development. Development is first and foremost a change process through which the individual is transformed throughout life.

The most obvious outward manifestation of occupational development is that persons engage in different occupations over the course of their lives. For example, younger children play, older children and adolescents attend school, and adults work. The transformation of occupation across the life span reflects an underlying order realized in the individual but sustained by the sociocultural environment. Socially established and culturally defined patterns of work, play, and self-care over the life span influence the sequence of occupational participation reflected in development.

The following sections provide an overview of the course of occupational development using the typical divisions of childhood, adolescence, adulthood, and later adulthood. The discussions are not meant to be exhaustive or detailed accounts of occupational development. Rather, they offer a perspective from which to consider how volition, habituation, performance capacity, and environment contribute to and undergo change throughout the life course.

Ongoing Tasks of Occupational Adaptation: Identity and Competence

During each stage of development, as internal changes occur and as the environments in which we do things change, we face two fundamental tasks. These are:

- Constructing an occupational identity by which we know ourselves and our lives
- Establishing occupational competence in our patterns of doing.

In each culture the pattern of development is narratively structured. That is, the culture carries a dominant narrative describing the life course (Luborsky, 1993). For example, the typical narrative of a white middle class male in most Western societies goes something like the following: "At first you are a child, during which time you play and learn to take care of your-

> *How each person constructs an occupational identity and realizes it in everyday patterns of doing will vary from person to person.*

self and participate in family life. Then you go to school to prepare for adult responsibilities. After school, you get a job, get married, have children, buy a house, and undertake a work career. When your children are reared, your house is paid for, and you have worked sufficient years to earn a retirement pension, you retire and live a life of leisure." Of course, such dominant narratives may differ according to one's gender, race, and social class. For example, until the latter part of the 20th century, the dominant female narrative involved marrying someone who would earn the family income and maintaining a household while raising children.

Although the cultural narratives about life's course do reflect what is normative or considered socially desirable, they are, to varying degrees, ill suited to define the individual life course (Luborsky, 1993). For example, dropping out of school, changing career choices, getting divorced, becoming widowed, or being fired or laid off from a job all present variations in the life course story that people grapple with in forming their identity. More dramatically, being homosexual, having or acquiring a disability, or wanting to live life outside the culturally defined narrative present major challenges for achieving an occupational identity. Consequently, dominant cultural narratives can be sources of constraint that hinder adaptation.

How each person constructs an occupational identity and realizes it in everyday patterns of doing will vary from person to person. Some will more or less readily accept the dominant narratives shared by the group to which they belong. Others will choose a more individualistic course. Still others will be thrust by life circumstances into charting a different path for themselves. Nonetheless, the challenge of adaptation remains the same: to identify and enact a self and a way of living that is experienced as worthy or correct, yields a sense of accomplishment, provides grounding in familiar routines, and allows one to realize one's unique

potentials, limitations, and desires. This is sometimes within and sometimes beyond our grasp. Hence, both the challenge and precariousness of development.

Childhood

Through the course of childhood, extensive transformation of volition, habituation, and performance capacity takes place. These changes allow the child to emerge as an occupational being with personal ways of doing, thinking, and feeling. Childhood occupation is both unique in its own character and serves as a foundation for later competence (Case-Smith & Shortridge, 1996; Hurt, 1980).

Volition

As children experience themselves doing things, their personal causation, interests, and values emerge. The volitional choices of early childhood are mainly activity choices. Later, children begin to make occupational choices to take on personal projects (e.g., learning to play a musical instrument) or discretionary roles (e.g., joining scouts, a club in school, or a sports team). Occupational choices may be, at first, assisted or coached by parents who supply for children the rationale for projects, habits, and roles.

Play is a major vehicle through which the child first develops a sense of personal causation (Bundy, 1997). As noted in Chapter 4, personal causation begins with children's awareness that they can cause things to happen. The desire to have effects in the environment becomes a strong motive and manifests itself in the child's play (Bundy, 1997; Ferland, 1997). Children's awareness of their capacities is gained through engaging with the environment in play, in social interaction, and eventually in other occupational spheres (Lindquist, Mack, & Parham, 1982). At first, children's sense of their abilities is very general (e.g., effort and capacity are not distinguished and not always accurate) (Nicholls, 1984). Through the child's experiences of failure and success, the child's knowledge of capacity and feelings of efficacy become more complex and accurate.

Cultural messages about values influence the child early in life. Adult approval and disapproval of actions guide the child's understanding of the social value of doing certain things. Growing awareness of what parents, siblings, and others value increasingly influences activity and occupational choices. For example, as children learn the value of being productive in occupations (e.g., chores and schoolwork), they increasingly assume responsibility for such behaviors and, in turn, experience the approval of others that solidifies the commitment to behave accordingly.

Childhood interests reflect expanding capacities. Children are attracted to activities that allow exercise of capacity and yield new experiences. Much of childhood pleasure comes from the mastery of new actions (Mailloux & Burke, 1997). As new capacities emerge, interest turns toward their utilization and expansion. For example, increased hand dexterity invites, and results from, the child engaging in play requiring fine motor control, such as constructing simple projects. Linguistic competence leads to interest in verbal humor and rhymes. Children find particular interest in those activities that provide optimal arousal by challenging capacity (Burke, 1977, 1993; Ferland, 1997).

Habituation

The young child's major occupational roles are player and family member (Florey, 1998; Hinojosa & Kramer, 1993). Parents and others see play as the normal business of the child. The player role has its own expectations, as when parents specify where and with what objects children may play. In addition, play is a means of trying out roles in sociodramatic play and games.

The family member role emerges as parents expect and value productive contributions of the child to the routines of family life by engaging in such occupational forms as picking up toys, doing small chores, and carrying out self-care. As childhood progresses, the range of roles increases to include the student role and the role of friend and membership in various childhood groups.

Biological rhythms provide the child's first consistent patterns. Environmental rhythms allow the child to internalize routines such as sleeping, waking, bathing, eating, playing, and self-care. In time, the child becomes more and more able to organize behaviors to accomplish chores and routines of self-care. Moreover, children find repetition a source of security, predictability, and comfort. Many habits that will be resources throughout life are acquired in childhood. Whereas the major influence on habits is the family

routine, the child is affected by each new occupational setting, such as day care and school.

Performance Capacity

Performance capacity undergoes dramatic transformation as the child gains experience, especially from play (Pierce, 1997; Robinson, 1977). Throughout childhood, increasing competence for interacting with the environment leads to the desire and capacity to seek out novel experiences. As children's capacities increase, their world expands (e.g., entering formal education). This process results in exposure to new environments that further impact on the development of capacity.

Occupational Identity and Competence

Occupational identity emerges in childhood. As children acquire the ability to integrate past, present, and future and to imagine themselves in an unfolding story, they begin to narrate parts of their lives and to sort out meanings through stories (Burke & Schaaf, 1997). By late childhood, children have a fairly developed sense of who they are. The occupational competence developed during childhood similarly tends to follow social norms and expectations. Nonetheless, each child begins to discover and pursue unique interests and aptitudes that individualize identity and competence.

Adolescence

Adolescence is typically a period of stress and turmoil due to both intrapersonal and sociocultural factors (Hendry, 1983). In addition to being a time of accelerated and dramatic biological change, adolescence can also be an uncertain social transition from childhood to adulthood. The beginning of adolescence is associated with both biological (puberty) and institutional (junior high school) changes. The end of adolescence was traditionally associated with entry into the worker role, but the timing of work entry can differ radically depending on whether one works directly after high school, attends college, or obtains postgraduate education. Consequently, adolescence has no firm boundaries.

Volition

Adolescence is characterized by an increasing drive for autonomy (Mitchell, 1975; Santrock, 1981). Adolescents must successfully learn to make activity and occupational choices that bring personal satisfaction and meaning while meeting expanding environmental expectations. The most pressing occupational choice of adolescence is selecting a type of work (Allport, 1961).

Adolescents are challenged to maintain a sense of efficacy while facing new social expectations for responsibility and having to acquire an expanding repertoire of occupational forms. Adolescents also begin to assess their capacity in terms of expected performance in future roles. During adolescence, belief in one's ability to control life outcomes ordinarily increases (Hendry, 1983). Increased freedom of choice challenges adolescents to clarify and establish their values. Rejection of some previous or parental values leads to a more personalized worldview and confirms for adolescents that their values are their own. Establishing values is challenging since the sources of values in society are many and sometimes contradictory. Not surprisingly, many adolescents experiment and struggle in the process of value formation, often moving between ideal values and the realities of life (Florey, 1998).

Interests also undergo substantial transformation during adolescence. What interests emerge depend very much on the social context. One of the primary influences on interest change is movement out of the family setting, where interests are often family-centered, into a peer group where new interests are espoused. Interests also change because the adolescent can do new things such as dating and driving a car. Adolescents' interests also become more of an expression of identity (Csikszentmihalyi & Rochberg-Halton, 1981). What one enjoys becomes a kind of statement about what kind of person one is.

Habituation

Adolescence is a period of transformation in the roles and habits that regulate everyday behavior. Adolescents try out many of the roles they will hold as adults. Such role experimentation fills several needs for adolescents. It helps them to consolidate their identity, to satisfy the desire for status and independence, and to recognize their abilities for particular roles.

Although some roles continue from childhood into adolescence, the nature of those roles and the expectations associated with them begin to change. For example, in the family context adolescents become more responsible for taking care of themselves (e.g., buying their own clothes, cooking meals for themselves) and contributing to household (e.g., through part-time work). While there are increasing opportunities to try on a variety of roles, adolescents may be frustrated that certain adult roles are not yet available to them (Hendry, 1983).

For the adolescent, the peer group is a source of information about the world outside the family and is a testing ground for new ideas and behaviors. The role of friend is increasingly important and may undergo several changes during adolescence. Part-time jobs and volunteer work expose many adolescents to the work world and afford opportunity to develop skill in getting and keeping jobs, budgeting time and money, and taking pride in accomplishments. Volunteer work can also serve as a means for exploring future vocations.

New habits are required for the changing circumstances of adolescence and for the world of work. Adolescent habits take over much routine behavior that was previously externally regulated in the family and by the other social contexts. A major impact on the habits of the adolescent is the movement from grammar school to junior high and high school. No longer in a single classroom with a series of daily activities for the entire class, students have individual schedules and must be responsible for being in the right place at the right time. More of adolescents' time is at their personal discretion. They must use time to establish a routine for the student and other roles.

Performance Capacity

Physical growth and change is central to the transformation of performance capacity in adolescence. Adolescents reach or approximate their adult size and begin bodily processes that characterize adulthood. Intellectual, cognitive, and emotional capacities expand in adolescence, allowing greater depths of awareness and comprehension of the world (Mitchell, 1975; Santrock, 1981). The adolescent also expands capacities for communication and interaction.

Occupational Identity and Competence

Adolescents begin to seriously see themselves as the authors of their own lives and to connect present actions with future outcomes and possibilities (Case-Smith & Shortridge, 1996). Adolescents' need to craft their own occupational identity and competence culminates in several important occupational choices, such as selecting a career and finding a partner.

The early adolescent's identity is more concerned with issues of enjoyment. Later, the adolescent gives increasing consideration to sense of capacity and feelings of efficacy and chooses occupations according to internalized values. By late adolescence occupational identity is much more sophisticated and centers on the occupational choices necessary to enter adult life. Nonetheless, this process is highly variable and proceeds at different paces for different persons (Ginzberg, 1971). In fact, because identity and competence are continually evolving and changing with growth and experience, the process of occupational choice is continuous and dynamic.

Adulthood

The boundaries of adulthood are closely tied to one's working life. Adulthood typically begins with the assumption of a more or less permanent full-time job or other productive occupation and ends with retirement (Hasselkus, 1998). Adulthood is the longest period of life. Contrary to popular views of adulthood as a period of stability or a state of maturity that is achieved and sustained, adults undergo considerable change. Some of these changes are externally recognizable, as the person passes through a series of steps, crises, or transitions: marriage or divorce, starting a family, changing jobs, and bidding farewell to grown children. Other changes are internal, as the individual sorts out the various meanings, goals, and purposes that guide choice and self-evaluation in adult life.

Volition

Diverse factors such as economic constraints and obligations of parenthood affect adult decisions, but for most people adulthood is the time when one truly begins to live one's own life. Adulthood ordinarily is ac-complished by an increasing desire to achieve and to work autonomously. For most people, this is accompanied by an increased sense of efficacy.

Early adulthood is generally a period of acquiring and refining abilities for one's line of work. Young workers see themselves as learning and increasing their efficacy. By middle adulthood, individuals have generally realized their peak performance. While the sense of efficacy is often dominated by work, other adult experiences such as rearing a family and maintaining a household are also areas that evoke strong feelings about one's effectiveness. Parents often find themselves facing great responsibilities with minimal preparation, such as the challenge of a newborn or confronting an adolescent's rebelliousness. Similarly, such adult responsibilities as maintaining a household and managing personal finances can be sources of stress, accomplishment, and failure.

During adulthood, values usually become increasingly important as a motivating force and a source of self-evaluation. Although personal values related to occupation tend to remain relatively stable throughout adulthood, a generalized shift does often occur. The goals of early adulthood are focused on instrumental and material values, such as getting ahead at work and earning a satisfactory living. Middle-aged workers may begin to focus more on humanitarian concerns and on themes of legacy (e.g., what one will leave to the future or how one will be remembered by children). Although this particular pattern of value change will not characterize all adults, some shift in values is likely in the course of adult life.

Leisure and work interests are relatively stable. Many adults entered their work because it embodied the opportunity to channel and develop personal interests. However, it is not a universal phenomenon that adults find their work interesting. Many adults pursue their interests avidly and seriously during their leisure time. Other adults use interests as a means of relaxing and regenerating themselves for work.

Habituation

Adulthood is characterized by a variety of socially prescribed and individually chosen roles that structure the adult's daily life and provide identity. Apart from family roles, most of these roles are enacted in community settings (Hasselkus, 1998). Typical adult role transitions include the initiation or end of partnerships, parenthood, changes in work roles, and joining civic and social organizations.

The one pervasive feature of adult life is work. Working requires learning new behaviors, forming new interpersonal relationships, reapportioning one's use of time and, frequently, developing a new identity. The work role also influences other adult roles, especially friendship and leisure roles. Workers often share confidences and decision-making with coworkers and may develop strong friendship ties with colleagues.

Most adults have to divide their time among work, family, community, and leisure roles. Participation in organizational and social roles, volunteering, and participating in religious organizations are other roles that many adults pursue. Because each of these roles can involve substantial investments of energy and time, a large number of people find inevitable conflicts in their use of time. Despite the potential for conflicts in time use, having a combination of roles appears to enhance well-being (Baruch, Barnett, & Rivers, 1980).

Habits of adulthood are necessarily concerned with the efficient allocation of time to various roles and the occupational forms they require. The division of the weekly routine into time for work, play, rest, self-care, and family is to some extent contingent on the norms of society (e.g., the typical 9-to-5, Monday-through-Friday work week). Adult habits are influenced by their context in other ways as well. For example, factory and hospital work requires a rather rigid adherence to schedules, whereas farmers and university professors must develop their own routines around seasonal variations in work. Marriage, purchasing a home, and the arrival of children also place demands on persons to develop habits for home maintenance and caretaking. Previously accustomed to a routine organized around personal needs and desires, adults typically find themselves having to orient their routines to a broader set of concerns.

Performance Capacity

Adulthood represents both the peaking and declining of abilities. Young adults are still acquiring new abilities, whereas middle and later adulthood is characterized by some waning in capacity (Bonder, 1994). Physical changes affect the occupational performance of adults. Over time, adults experience a decrease in energy and strength along with some decrement in sensory perception. For example, it is in adulthood that many people first require glasses or bifocals. Others find that they must cut back on some rigorous activities.

Identity and Competence

Adults assess and reassess their unfolding life stories (Handel, 1987; Kimmel, 1980). Narrative reassessment typically reflects a transformation from an early concern with competence and achievement to a later concern with value and personal satisfaction. This transformation, sometimes referred to as a mid-life crisis, may lead persons to recraft their stories, change work careers, or enact similarly drastic alterations in their occupational lifestyles. Whatever life course they choose or life events they must grapple with, adults continue the narrative process of knowing themselves, exploring the worth and meaning of their lives, and seeking to control the circumstances and direction of their lives. For some adults this struggle results in a high level of well-being. Others fail to find a satisfactory and meaningful life course and, instead, live lives characterized by compromise, conflict, or catastrophe.

Later Adulthood

Later adulthood is defined both by biological changes and social convention. Retirement and eligibility for social benefits demarcates entry into this period of later adulthood (Bonder, 1994). It is difficult to define later adulthood by chronologic age alone. Rather, it is useful to think of later adulthood as demarked by changes in lifestyle as determined by waning capacity, personal choice, and social convention.

Volition

Older adults' volition is important to help direct the many choices that drive or are in response to necessary changes in lifestyle. Old age is generally accompanied by losses of capacity, and lack of opportunities to use abilities can lead elderly persons to experience diminution of personal causation. Since the loss of capacity may have important implications for independence and lifestyle, some older adults may be especially inventive in sustaining a sense of efficacy while others may hold unrealistic views of their abilities.

Values typically undergo some transformation and have a pervasive influence on occupational choices in old age. One view holds that older adults shift from instrumental values such as being ambitious, intellectual, capable, and responsible toward terminal values such as a sense of accomplishment, freedom, equality, and comfort. Whereas this pattern may be true of many older adults, it is most accurate to say that the nature and direction of any value change depend on past and current life circumstances. Nonetheless, for most older adults the importance of work and achievement wanes while other values concerning family, community, and leisure become more significant (Antonovsky & Sagy, 1990). As abilities decline, elderly persons must redefine their standards and revise the way in which values are satisfied. Nonetheless, value commitments are important to maintaining morale in later life.

For many older adults, the relative freedom from obligations in old age provides opportunity to pursue a variety of interests more seriously or fully than before. However, constrained capacity and resources in later life can prevent some persons from pursuing interests. For example, some older adults are involved in solitary and passive occupations although they prefer to be involved in social and more active occupations (McGuire, 1980). Older adults can be constrained in their activity choices by a lack of transportation, facilities, money, and companions; by fears of injury, learning new things, or disapproval; and by no longer feeling a sense of satisfaction (McAvoy, 1979; McGuire, 1983).

Habituation

Role changes in later life can sometimes be involuntary and unpleasant. For example, elderly persons may lose the spouse and friend roles through death. Many lost roles are not easily replaced. Older adults who cannot replace lost or diminished roles may experience boredom, loneliness, and depression. Many older adults rely on family, community, or other institutions to provide roles. For example, Elliot & Barris (1987) found that older adults' role identification was greater in nursing homes that provided more opportunities for activity.

Some persons continue to work beyond ordinary

retirement age for income; to feel satisfied, useful, and respected; and/or to have a major role in organizing their lives (Sterns, Laier, & Dorsett, 1994). When it does occur, retirement can be a far-reaching event, because so much of life is geared toward preparation for, entry into, and advancement in work and because work structures a great deal of time and activity. Consequently, the transition from work to retirement is full of both possibilities and pitfalls. Retirement is an entirely individual process (Jonsson, Kielhofner, & Borell, 1997). For one individual it may mean escape from arduous labor and an opportunity to devote time to occupations of a higher priority, such as family involvement, a second career, or hobbies. For another, it may mean loss of social contact and severance from a primary source of self-worth and meaning. Whatever the implications, retirement is a major life event that reshapes an individual's occupational life.

Family roles and relationships are important and often change dramatically in the lives of older adults (Cutler-Louis, 1989). Older adults often spend significant time with adult children and grandchildren. Relationships with adult children can be an important source of gratification sustained by a reciprocal exchange in the form of affection, gifts, and services. For example, older adults often act as babysitters, confidantes and advisors, house sitters, and providers of income. As older adults become frail, disabled, or chronically ill, adult children may assume responsibility for the care of their aging parents. This role reversal is often complicated and challenging for all involved.

Friendship is another important role of older adults. Although having extensive friendships is not necessary, the person who has a number of friendships is less vulnerable to loss of friends through death. Loss of one's partner in old age may severely disrupt life. One may lose a friend, homemaker, financial supporter, and caretaker depending on the nature of the relationship. Other role changes may accompany the loss of a partner. The surviving partner may have to take over many things previously done by the spouse.

Elderly persons often possess habits developed over a long period in a stable environment. Changes in underlying capacity and changes in environment can challenge these habits. At the same time, changing circumstances, such as widowhood or retirement, often impose demands for acquiring new habits. Moreover, as capacities decline, habits become increasingly important to sustain functional performance and quality of life.

Performance Capacity

Aging involves a natural decline in performance capacity and is associated with a high frequency of health conditions that affect capacity (Kauffman, 1994; Riley, 1994). However, substantial losses of ability are not inevitable and may be forestalled if the elderly person remains active. Consequently, age-related changes are unique to each person. Moreover, the impact of such decrements may be mitigated by adapting one's habits and environment.

Occupational Identity and Competence

With aging, the composition and telling of one's life story seems to gain importance. As older adults approach the end of life, both the need to make the most of the time one has and to make sense of the life one has lived become important (Ebersole & Hess, 1981; Hasselkus, 1998). The sense of whether one's life story has fulfilled the cultural ideal can be a source of comfort and fulfillment or of distress (Luborsky, 1993).

For most older adults the central fixture in the life narrative is the transition to retirement, which can mean vastly different things to retirees (Jonsson et al., 1997; Jonsson, Josephsson, & Kielhofner, 2000, 2001). As discussed in the previous chapter, a major factor affecting the extent to which occupational identity and

> *Indeed, the most remarkable characteristics of any individual journey through life are the singular incidents, the crises, the personal transformations, the setbacks, and other features that deviate from any neat or normative portrayal of development.*

competence are positive for the elderly person appears to be whether the person has an engaging occupation (Jonsson et al., 2001).

Conclusion

This chapter identified some of the major transformations and patterns that characterize the course of occupational development. In attempting to portray what may be typical or ordinary in the developmental course, individual differences were necessarily ignored. However, these differences are critical to development. Indeed, the most remarkable characteristics of any individual journey through life are the singular incidents, the crises, the personal transformations, the setbacks, and other features that deviate from any neat or normative portrayal of development. Moreover, these unique events, struggles, and transformations give each life its special direction, pace, and meaning and hold the key to understanding that particular life.

Key Terms

Achievement: The stage of change when persons have sufficient skills and habits that allow them to participate fully in some new work, leisure activity, or activity of daily living.

Catastrophic change: Stage of change that occurs when internal or external circumstances dramatically alter one's occupational life situation, requiring a fundamental reorganization.

Competency: Stage of change when persons begin to solidify new ways of doing that were discovered through exploration.

Exploration: First stage of change in which persons try out new things and, consequently, learn about their own capacities, preferences, and values.

Incremental change: A gradual alteration such as change in amount, intensity, or degree.

Transformational change: Change that occurs when one fundamentally or qualitatively alters an established pattern of thinking, feeling, and doing.

References

Allport, G. (1961). *Pattern and growth in personality*. New York: Holt, Rinehart & Winston.

Antonovsky, A., & Sagy, S. (1990). Confronting develop-

mental tasks in the retirement transition. *Gerontologist, 30,* 362–368.

Baruch, G., Barnett, R., & Rivers, C. (1980, December 7). A

new start for women at midlife. *New York Times Sunday Magazine*, pp. 196–200.

Bonder, B. R. (1994). Growing old in the United States. In B. R. Bonder & M. B. Wagner (Eds.), *Functional performance in older adults* (pp. 4–14). Philadelphia: FA Davis.

Bundy, A. C. (1997). Play and playfulness: What to look for. In L. D. Parham & L. S. Fazio (Eds.), *Play in occupational therapy for children* (pp. 52–66). St. Louis, MO: Mosby.

Burke, J. P. (1977). A clinical perspective on motivation: Pawn versus origin. *American Journal of Occupational Therapy, 31,* 254–258.

Burke, J. P. (1993). Play: The life role of the infant and young child. In J. Case-Smith (Ed.), *Pediatric occupational therapy and early intervention* (pp. 198–224). Stoneham, MA: Andover Medical Publishers.

Burke, J. P., & Schaaf, R. C. (1997). Family narratives and play assessment. In L. D. Parham & L. S. Fazio (Eds.), *Play in occupational therapy for children* (pp. 67–84). St. Louis, MO: Mosby.

Case-Smith, J., & Shortridge, S. D. (1996). The developmental process: Prenatal to adolescence. In J. Case-Smith, A. S. Allen, & P. N. Pratt (Eds.), *Occupational therapy for children* (pp. 46–66). St. Louis, MO: Mosby.

Csikszentmihalyi, M., & Rochberg-Halton, E. (1981). *The meaning of things.* Cambridge, MA: Cambridge University Press.

Cutler-Lewis, S. (1989). *Elder care.* New York: McGraw-Hill, Inc.

Ebersole, P., & Hess, P. (1981). *Toward healthy aging: Human needs and nursing response.* St. Louis, MO: CV Mosby.

Elliot, M. S., & Barris, R. (1987). Occupational role performance and life satisfaction in elderly persons. *Occupational Therapy Journal of Research, 7,* 215–224.

Ferland, F. (1997). *Play, children with physical disabilities and occupational therapy: The ludic model.* Ottawa, Canada: University of Ottawa Press.

Fidler, G., & Fidler, J. (1983). Doing and becoming: The occupational therapy experience. In G. Kielhofner (Ed.), *Health through occupation: Theory and practice in occupational therapy.* Philadelphia: FA Davis.

Florey, L. (1998). Psychosocial dysfunction in childhood and adolescence. In M. E. Neistadt & E. B. Crepeau (Eds.), *Occupational therapy* (pp. 622–635). Philadelphia: Lippincott.

Ginzberg, E. (1971). Toward a theory of occupational choice. In H. J. Peters & J. C. Hansen (Eds.), *Vocational guidance and career development* (2nd ed.). New York: Macmillan.

Hammel, J. (1999). The life rope: A transactional approach to exploring worker and life role development. *Work: A Journal of Prevention, Assessment and Rehabilitation, 12,* 47–60.

Handel, A. (1987). Personal theories about the life-span development of one's self in autobiographical self-presentations of adults. *Human Development, 30,* 83–98.

Hasselkus, B. R. (1998). Introduction to adult and older adult populations. In M. E. Neistadt & E. B. Crepeau (Eds.), *Occupational therapy* (pp. 651–659). Philadelphia: Lippincott.

Hendry, L. B. (1983). *Growing up and going out: Adolescents and leisure.* Aberdeen: Aberdeen University Press.

Hinojosa, J., & Kramer, P. (1993). Developmental perspective: Fundamentals of developmental theory. In P. Kramer & J. Hinojosa (Eds.), *Pediatric occupational therapy* (pp. 3–8). Philadelphia: Lippincott Williams & Wilkins.

Hurt, J. M. (1980). A play skills inventory: A competency monitoring tool for the 10-year-old. *American Journal of Occupational Therapy, 34,* 651–656.

Jonsson, H., Josephsson, S., & Kielhofner, G. (2000). Evolving narratives in the course of retirement: A longitudinal study. *American Journal of Occupational Therapy, 54,* 463–470.

Jonsson, H., Josephsson, S., & Kielhofner, G. (2001). Narratives and experience in an occupational transition: A longitudinal study of the retirement process. *American Journal of Occupational Therapy, 55,* 424–432.

Jonsson, H., Kielhofner, G., & Borell, L. (1997). Anticipating retirement: The formation of narratives concerning an occupational transition. *American Journal of Occupational Therapy, 51,* 49–56.

Kauffman, T. (1994). Mobility. In B. R. Bonder & M. B. Wagner (Eds.), *Functional performance in older adults* (pp. 42–61). Philadelphia: FA Davis.

Kimmel, D. C. (1980). *Adulthood and aging* (2nd ed.). New York: John Wiley & Sons.

Lindquist, J. E., Mack, W., & Parham, L. D. (1982). A synthesis of occupational behavior and sensory integration concepts in theory and practice, part 1. Theoretical foundations. *American Journal of Occupational Therapy, 36,* 365–374.

Luborsky, M. (1993). The romance with personal meaning: Gerontology, cultural aspects of life themes. *The Gerontologist, 33,* 445–452.

Mailloux, Z., & Burke, J. P. (1997). Play and the sensory integrative approach. In L. D. Parham & L. S. Fazio (Eds.), *Play in occupational therapy for children* (pp. 112–125). St. Louis, MO: Mosby.

McAvoy, L. L. (1979). The leisure preferences, problems, and needs of the elderly. *Journal of Leisure Resources, 11,* 40–47.

McGuire, F. (1980). The incongruence between actual and desired leisure involvement in advanced adulthood. *Active Adaptive Aging, 1,* 77–89.

McGuire, F. (1985). Constraints on leisure involvement in the later years. *Active Adaptive Aging, 3,* 17–24.

Mitchell, J. J. (1975). *The adolescent predicament.* Toronto: Holt, Rinehart & Winston.

Nicholls, J. G. (1984). Achievement motivation: Conceptions of ability, subjective experience, task choice, and performance. *Psychological Review, 3,* 328–346.

Peterson, E., Howland, J., Kielhofner, G., Lachman, M. E., Assmann, S., Cote, J., & Jette, A. (1999). Falls self-efficacy and occupational adaptation among elders. *Physical & Occupational Therapy in Geriatrics, 16,* 1–16.

Pierce, D. (1997) The power of object play for infants and toddlers at risk for developmental delays. In L. D. Parham & L. S. Fazio (Eds.), *Play in occupational therapy for children* (pp. 86–111). St. Louis, MO: Mosby.

Reilly, M. (1974). *Play as exploratory learning.* Beverly Hills, CA: Sage Publications.

Riley, K. P. (1994). Cognitive development. In B. R. Bonder & M. B. Wagner (Eds.), *Functional performance in older adults* (pp. 4–14). Philadelphia: FA Davis.

Robinson, A. L. (1977). Play, the arena for acquisition of rules for competent behavior. *American Journal of Occupational Therapy, 31,* 248–253.

Santrock, J. W. (1981). *Adolescence: An introduction.* Dubuque, IA: Brown.

Sterns, H. L., Laier, M. P., & Dorsett, J. G. (1994). Work and retirement. In B. R. Bonder & M. B. Wagner (Eds.), *Functional performance in older adults* (pp. 148–164). Philadelphia: FA Davis.

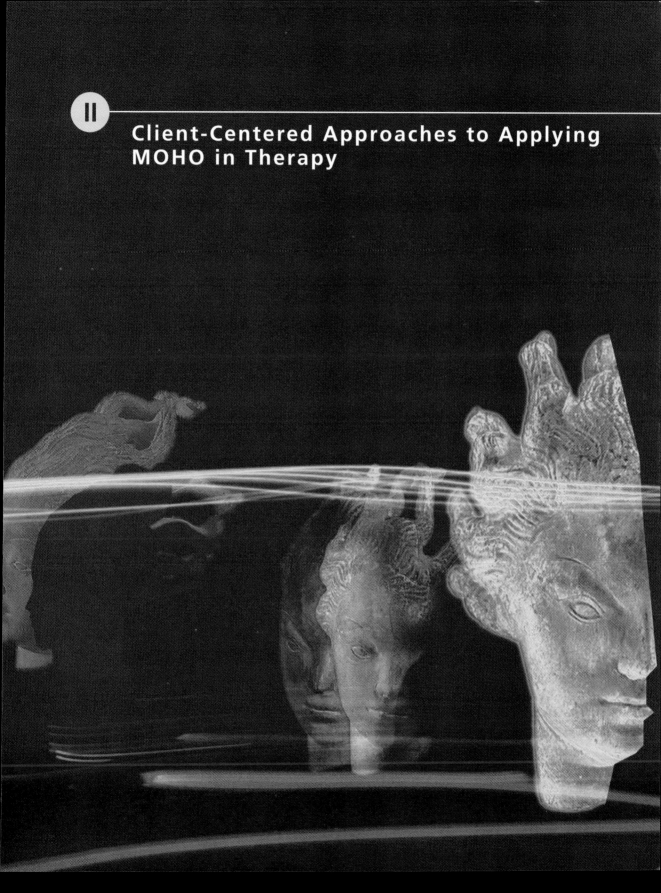

II

Client-Centered Approaches to Applying MOHO in Therapy

Introduction to Section II

This section includes 10 chapters (11 through 20) that discuss application of MOHO in therapy. Chapter 11 begins the process of linking the theoretical concepts offered in Section I to practice by offering a framework for therapeutic reasoning. This chapter discusses how to combine information about the client with MOHO theory to arrive at a conceptualization of the client's situation that provides the rationale for therapy. This chapter also offers a set of questions that use MOHO concepts and propositions to ask about the client. Finally, it offers examples of the kinds of client problems and strengths that might be found in response to these questions.

Chapters 12 through 17 discuss means of achieving answers to the kinds of questions posed in Chapter 11. Chapter 12 provides an overview of the information gathering process that makes up client assessment. It discusses the role of both formal and informal means of information gathering. Chapters 13 through 16 present and illustrate the use of formal assessments developed for use with MOHO. These chapters respectively present assessments that collect information through:

- Observing clients
- Client self-report on checklists and questionnaires
- Client interviews
- Some combination of the above methods.

Together the chapters present all the MOHO-based assessments available at the time of this writing. Each of these assessments have different purposes, formats, and relevance to populations and contexts of practice. Therefore, therapists must judiciously select which assessments to use in their practices. Chapter 17 addresses this process, discussing how to select the most appropriate assessment(s) for a given client and context.

Chapters 18 and 19 cover what takes place in MOHO-based therapy. Chapter 18 discusses client change, noting the kinds of changes that MOHO conceptualizes and that MOHO-based therapy seeks to achieve. It also discusses the centrality of the client's occupational engagement (i.e., actions, thoughts, and feelings) for achieving change. The chapter presents a taxonomy of client occupational engagement that results in change. Chapter 19 continues the discussion of change, focusing on what therapists do to support

client change. This chapter begins with an overview of the therapeutic use of self and then proposes a taxonomy of therapist strategies that will support client engagement and changes and that make up therapeutic use of self as conceptualized by MOHO. Chapter 20 aims to bring together the discussions of this section by presenting a scheme for formulating, communicating, and documenting therapy.

All the chapters emphasize the importance of client-centeredness in therapy. MOHO concepts require therapists to have knowledge of their client's values, sense of capacity and efficacy, interests, roles, habits, performance experience, and personal environment. MOHO-based assessments are designed to gather information on and provide clients opportunities to provide their perspectives on these factors. The client's unique characteristics, in combination with the theory, guide the development of an understanding of the client's unique situation. The understanding of the client, in turn, provides the rationale for therapy. Moreover, since MOHO conceptualizes the client's own doing, thinking, and feeling as the central dynamic in achieving change, therapy must support the client's choice, action, and experience.

The chapters in this section illustrate how to enact a particular form of client-centered practice guided by a theory-based understanding of the client. Together they emphasize:

- Respect for the client's unique circumstances and perspectives, including the complexity of client challenges and problems
- The importance of client-centered assessments that provide insight into client strengths and weaknesses by both soliciting client views and gathering objective data using validated means
- The responsibility of the therapist to have and exercise expertise in generating a theory-based understanding of the client's situation that reflects the client's unique perspectives and characteristics
- The importance of collaboration with the client and the necessity of empowering clients to author their own lives by selecting and working toward change in therapy
- The centrality of the client's occupational engagement (i.e., actions, thought, and feelings) to change
- The therapist's role in supporting clients to engage in occupations that will result in desired change.

The chapters in this section illustrate that the application of MOHO in practice is neither simple nor formulaic. Rather, such application requires:

- Mastery of and ability to think with MOHO concepts
- A working knowledge of MOHO assessments relevant to a client population
- Active and reflective reasoning that moves between client information and theory to achieve conceptual understanding of the client and of the therapy process
- Ability to grapple with the complexity of client problems, the uncertainty and dynamic course of change, and the ongoing need to monitor and think about what is happening in therapy as well as negotiating ongoing goals and strategies with the client.

Any approach to therapy that seeks to be more simple or formula-driven is not adequately client-centered because it neither fully appreciates the client's unique situation nor brings a sufficiently sophisticated understanding to bear on client problems. Occupational therapy clients deserve to be heard and understood. MOHO provides an avenue for achieving both these goals with thoroughness and depth.

Because applying MOHO is challenging, this section is designed to provide a number of concrete tools to support therapists in its application. These, of course, make up the technology for practice discussed in Chapter 1. They include concrete strategies for therapeutic reasoning, structured assessments, detailed discussions of what should take place in therapy, and ample case illustrations. Finally, at the end of this section (pages 346–355) a master Section II Table synthesizes information presented across several chapters in this section. The table presents:

- MOHO concepts
- Corresponding questions proposed in Chapter 11
- Client problems and strengths, which may be found in response to the questions (also from Chapter 11)
- The kinds of client change that could overcome/compensate for problems (from Chapter 18)
- The kinds of client doing that generates such changes (from Chapter 18)
- Therapist strategies that support such changes (from Chapter 19).

This table combines information from several chapters to provide a comprehensive and coherent resource for thinking about the application of MOHO. It represents a logical continuum from theory to therapeutic action. In effect, the table answers the following questions:

- What does this theory lead one to ask about the client?
- How does this theory help one understand the client?
- What kinds of change does this theory propose as part of therapy?
- How does therapy based on this theory enable the client to achieve this change?
- What is the role of the therapist in supporting change?

Chapters 11, 18, 19, and 20 will make reference to this master table, which is readily located by noting the pages marked by purple borders.

The materials in this section represent the most detailed guidelines for application of MOHO available to date. They should provide the reader with a wealth of information and strategies for putting MOHO theory into practice.

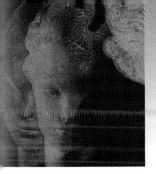

11

Thinking With Theory: A Framework for Therapeutic Reasoning

- **Gary Kielhofner**

- **Kirsty Forsyth**

The chapters in Section I offered a range of concepts aimed at explaining the motivation, patterning, and performance of occupation. At this point, one can ask the following question. How does a therapist use all these concepts to understand a client and proceed with therapy? This chapter begins to answer the question by offering a framework for relating MOHO concepts to reasoning about clients and their life circumstances.

The Framework

The framework introduced in this chapter identifies a therapeutic reasoning[a] process, whereby a therapist uses theory to understand a client and to develop a plan of therapy with a client. This framework emphasizes the thinking process involved in using theory. Later chapters build on this framework to describe further the process of applying theory in planning, implementing, evaluating, communicating, and documenting therapy.

As illustrated in Figure 11-1, therapeutic reasoning can be described as a four-phased process. First, therapists use the theory to derive questions that identify

what they want to learn about the client. The questions should reflect both what is initially known about the client and what MOHO theory calls attention to about the client. Second, therapists use these questions as guides for collecting information about and from the client. Third, the therapist uses the information gathered to create an explanation of the client's situation. This phase combines the specific information about a particular client with generic concepts and propositions offered by the theory to create a client-centered and theory-based conceptualization of the client's situation. In the fourth phase, the therapist generates goals and strategies for therapy that emanate from the conceptualization of the client's situation and from the client's desires.

Importantly, the phases of therapeutic reasoning are not strictly sequential. That is, a therapist will move back and forth between phases over the course of therapy. Ordinarily, the therapist will generate at least some questions from the theory at the beginning of the therapeutic reasoning process. Moreover, some information about and from the client must be collected before deciding on and beginning therapy. Once therapy begins additional questions are likely to arise, leading the therapist to collect new information, deepen understanding of the client, and generate new ideas and strategies for therapy. Moreover, as *Figure 11-1* shows, each phase is informed by:

- The client's characteristics and viewpoints
- The therapist's knowledge of the theory.

Consequently, therapeutic reasoning using MOHO is both client-centered and theoretically driven.

---

[a]The term clinical reasoning is used by authors to refer to the process by which therapists generate an understanding of clients and make decisions in therapy (e.g., Mattingly, 1991; Mattingly & Fleming, 1993). The term therapeutic reasoning is used here, instead, to avoid medical model connotations of the term "clinical" and to highlight the client-focused collaborative nature of the proposed reasoning process.

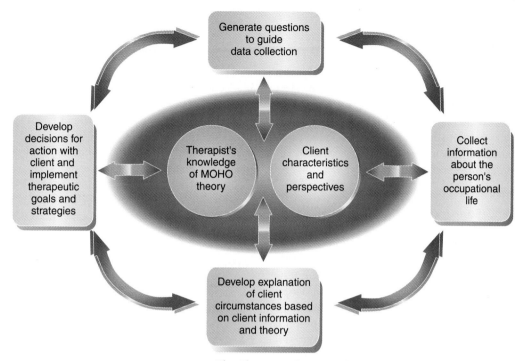

FIGURE 11-1   The Therapeutic Reasoning Process.

Client-Centeredness in Therapeutic Reasoning with MOHO

An important aspect of MOHO-based therapeutic reasoning is its client-centered nature. Canadian occupational therapists have led the profession in articulating the importance of client-centered practice (Law, 1998). Client-centered principles define therapy as a process that respects, informs, and enables clients to become active partners in determining the goals and strategies of therapy. However, client-centered principles do not provide concepts and postulates for conceptualizing the client's situation or determining the intervention approach. Therefore, a model of practice must be selected and used within client-centered practice.

MOHO is recognized as a model consistent with client-centered practice (Law, 1998). In fact, MOHO is inherently a client-centered model in two important ways:

- It views each client as a unique individual whose characteristics determine the rationale for and nature of the therapy goals and strategies

- It views what the client does, thinks, and feels as the central mechanism of change.

FOCUS ON CLIENT UNIQUENESS

Therapeutic reasoning with MOHO focuses on understanding clients in terms of their own values, interests, sense of capacity and efficacy, roles, habits, and performance-related experiences within the relevant environments. Therefore, the concepts of the theory call attention to the importance of knowing the details of a client's beliefs, perspectives, lifestyle, experience, and context. MOHO theory both focuses the therapist on the client's uniqueness and provides concepts that al-

> *MOHO theory both focuses the therapist on the client's uniqueness and provides concepts that allow the therapist to more deeply appreciate the client's perspective and situation.*

low the therapist to more deeply appreciate the client's perspective and situation.

Moreover, since the logic of therapy emanates from a conceptual understanding informed by client characteristics in combination with the theory, the client's uniqueness always defines where therapy aims and of what it consists. For this reason, the model does not offer a single approach for all clients. Rather, it provides concepts and propositions for making sense of individual client information and for generating related therapy goals and plans.

CENTRALITY OF CLIENT ENGAGEMENT TO THERAPY

As elaborated in Chapter 18, MOHO concepts also propose that the client's occupational engagement (i.e., what the client does, thinks, and feels) is the central dynamic of therapy. MOHO-based intervention supports the client's doing, thinking, and feeling in order to achieve change desired by the client and/or indicated by the client's situation. As discussed in Chapter 19, MOHO-based practice requires a client-therapist relationship in which the therapist must understand, respect, and support client choices, actions, and experiences.

Theory-Driven Therapeutic Reasoning

Effectiveness in using MOHO as a practice model depends on the therapist's understanding of the theory. MOHO concepts are relatively complex, since they seek (as noted in Chapter 2) to address a wide range of phenomena and to approach them in depth. On the other hand, when a therapist has mastered the concepts, thinking with theory becomes natural and enhances decision-making with and on behalf of the client.

Learning the theory evolves over time as the therapist uses it in practice. Importantly, engaging in therapeutic reasoning will enrich the therapist's under-

> *Since reasoning involves moving between theory and the circumstances of clients, knowledge of theory grows as the therapist sees it represented in the client's circumstances.*

standing of the theory. Since reasoning involves moving between theory and the circumstances of clients, knowledge of theory grows as the therapist sees it represented in clients' circumstances. Each time the therapist applies a concept to a client, the client's situation reveals another instance of that concept. For example, each client reveals a unique instance of personal causation. By seeing how numerous clients conceive of, understand, and feel about their capacity and efficacy, a therapist's understanding of what personal causation means will deepen.

Therapists' growth in knowledge of the theory will also include a deepened appreciation of its implications in practice. For example, experience will reveal what therapeutic processes and strategies are generally most helpful for particular kinds of client problems. Notably, having a consistent set of theoretical concepts allows the therapist to think more systematically about clients and the therapy process, thereby enhancing what the therapist learns from experience.

Illustration of Therapeutic Reasoning

The following case example illustrates the therapeutic reasoning process. In discussing the case, we will focus on volitional concepts and propositions.

Dan

Dan was a client in a long-term treatment facility for adolescents with psychiatric disabilities. Dan had experienced school performance problems and family difficulties related to depression. He also had a history of substance abuse. Dan appeared nervous and uneasy most of the time. The concept of volition naturally led the therapist to wonder about several things about Dan:

- What are Dan's thoughts and feelings about his capacity and efficacy, and do they account for his anxious demeanor?
- Does Dan have interests and act on them, and does he enjoy the things he does?
- What are Dan's values, and is he able to realize them in what he does?
- What kinds of decisions does Dan make about do-

ing things, and how do his personal causation, values, and interests influence these decisions?

These and related questions arose as the therapist came to know Dan. Moreover, they guided the collection of information about him.

The therapist observed Dan in several situations. The therapist also interviewed Dan about the things he did in his life, his experiences at home, in school, and with friends. Finally, Dan filled out some paper-and-pencil assessments that allowed him to tell the therapist about his interests and values. Guided by the MOHO theory of volition, the therapist was able to use the information to construct the following understanding of Dan *(Fig. 11-2)*.

At this point in Dan's life, his personal causation was dominated by a sense of incapacity and in-

efficacy. He felt very little control over most aspects of his life. He showed little interest in most of the things other adolescents enjoyed, and even when doing something that he felt some attraction to, Dan's experience was dominated by anxiety over his performance. His anxiety was fueled at home by an extremely critical parent who constantly anticipated and pointed out Dan's failures. Moreover, because Dan had gained a reputation in school as a difficult student, he faced a similar judgmental attitude from several teachers. Dan felt very pressured by these attitudes because he disliked very much feeling that others perceived him as "bad." Finally, Dan's peers tended to view him as different and did not readily include him in the things they did.

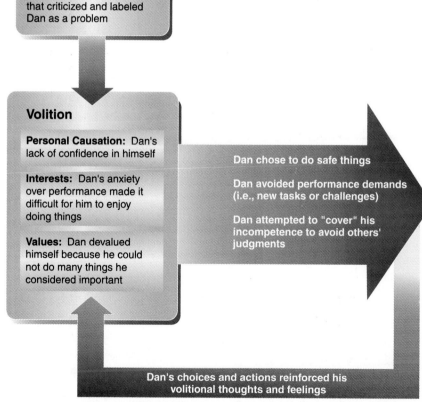

Environment

Attitudes at home and school that criticized and labeled Dan as a problem

Volition

Personal Causation: Dan's lack of confidence in himself

Interests: Dan's anxiety over performance made it difficult for him to enjoy doing things

Values: Dan devalued himself because he could not do many things he considered important

Dan chose to do safe things

Dan avoided performance demands (i.e., new tasks or challenges)

Dan attempted to "cover" his incompetence to avoid others' judgments

Dan's choices and actions reinforced his volitional thoughts and feelings

FIGURE 11-2   A Theory-Based Understanding of a Client's Volition.

Because of his anxiety over performance, Dan was unable to feel a sense of enjoyment or satisfaction in doing most things. His few interests were solitary, since he was fearful of performing around peers. He very much valued and wanted to be able to do the same things as other adolescents and to be included by them. Because he viewed himself as lacking capacity for these things, he devalued himself, often making disparaging comments about his own performance. This, briefly, was the therapist's conceptualization of Dan's volition and the environmental factors that impacted upon it.

According to MOHO theory, volition—in combination with environmental conditions—influences activity choices. The therapist observed the following characteristics of Dan's choices that emanated from his volition and environment. He consistently avoided doing anything new or facing any kinds of performance demands. When allowed to make his own choices he always chose to do things that were familiar, safe, and solitary. He was extremely uncomfortable around peers and put forth a great deal of effort to avoid situations in which peers could judge his performance. For example, he would sometimes privately admit his lack of confidence about performance to the therapist, but in a group therapy session with peers present, he insisted that all the things available to do were "stupid," thereby avoiding having to perform in front of his peers.

With this additional information, the therapist could recognize how Dan's volition, along with corresponding environmental conditions, was sustaining him in a maladaptive pattern. That is, his choices to do things were designed to avoid failure and judgment of others, but these choices also assured he would neither learn new skills nor develop a stronger sense of capacity and efficacy.

Using lay terms that he could understand, the therapist shared his understanding of Dan's situation with him to determine whether he agreed. This served not only to make sure that the therapist had accurately comprehended Dan, but also to inform Dan, in terms he could understand, of the theoretical ideas the therapist was using. Dan reluctantly agreed with what the therapist proposed and added some of his own concerns and interpretations. This discussion gave the therapist further insights to Dan and helped Dan learn more about himself. As they came to a mutual understanding of Dan's situation, they discussed some ideas for goals in therapy. This discussion informed Dan of how the therapist was conceptualizing his therapy and what it was designed to achieve for him.

Using the theory to make sense of Dan's situation and sharing the therapist's formulation with him helped them arrive at mutually agreeable goals for his therapy. Dan's long-term volition-related goals included:

- Increasing Dan's belief in skill and sense of efficacy so that he could make choices to do things he valued and that would lead to improving his performance
- Increasing his range of interests and ability to enjoy doing things, both alone and with peers
- Enabling him to gain competence, and thereby a feeling of efficacy, in doing what he most valued.

These long-term goals were translated into short-term measurable goals in language Dan understood. For example, one short-term goal was that at the end of every session Dan would be able to report at least one thing he enjoyed about the activity he did.

Next, the therapist and Dan had to decide how to go about achieving these goals. MOHO theory indicates that these volitional changes require the following process. First, environmental conditions outside Dan needed to change to allow a new dynamic out of which new volitional thoughts, feelings, and actions could emerge for Dan. Second, the therapist needed to repeat this situation sufficiently so that Dan's volition could begin to reorganize around a sense of capacity, a desire and enjoyment of doing things, and a positive valuation of himself.

Consequently, the therapist began with the therapeutic strategy of advising and supporting Dan to choose projects in which he could readily succeed and that he saw as valuable. Dan decided to engage in leatherwork and woodwork. Both occupational forms involved the use of tools—something important to Dan. Handling the tools symbolized competence to him. Moreover, they allowed

Dan to create products that would tangibly affirm his competence. During therapy the therapist gave him constant feedback on his successes and invited Dan to review each session, identifying what he had enjoyed, accomplished, and learned. They dealt with problems and challenges that arose by working together to see how he could achieve good outcomes by problem solving and/or asking for help. This meant redefining help-seeking from being a sign of failure to being yet another method Dan could choose and use to accomplish what he wanted. Dan's therapy began with individual sessions in which he could be free of the worry about what his peers would think about his performance. He progressed to doing things in parallel groups when he had developed sufficient capacity and belief in his own abilities to demonstrate his new-found competence in front of peers.

The therapist's understanding of Dan's volition also guided the therapist in the details of his intervention. The therapist knew that when he was reluctant to engage in activities it was because they were too threatening. The therapist observed Dan carefully for signs of anxiety in performance and consistently reoriented him to simply enjoy the activity and use the opportunity to develop some skills (exploration stage of change).

Later when he had gained some sense of capacity and efficacy, Dan was able to choose and succeed at greater (competence level) challenges, requiring a role within cooperative groups and a routine of performance. For instance, he became part of an adolescent woodworking team that met daily in the woodshop to work on fabricating a game table for their common recreation room.

As they began to plan for Dan's discharge from therapy, the therapist also knew that maintaining the volitional changes he had gained in therapy would require consistent, supportive environmental conditions to allow him to continue his new pattern of thinking, feeling, and acting. Consequently, the therapist made recommendations for Dan's parents and teachers, which were shared with them by the psychologist who managed Dan's case and conducted family therapy with Dan and his parents.

This case example illustrated how:

- MOHO theory can be used to construct a particular conceptualization of a client situation
- How the unique characteristics of the client are combined with MOHO theory to arrive at this conceptualization
- The conceptualization guides selection of therapy goals and the therapy process.

Additionally, the case illustrated that the therapeutic reasoning process can be shared actively with the client, who becomes a partner in each phase. To the extent they are capable and willing, clients should always be given an opportunity to participate in the process of thinking with theory. When this happens, the theory not only enriches the therapist's view, but enhances the client's self-understanding.

Questions to Guide Information Gathering

The first phase of using theory to generate questions about clients is often the most challenging step in applying theory in practice, since it initiates the process of moving between theory and the client. Therefore, the next section presents an initial set of questions that therapists can use in going back and forth between the theory and clients.

There is no single or best set of questions for applying MOHO. Many factors, including the type of clients to whom one provides services, the context, the amount of time for therapy, and therapists' styles of reasoning will influence what questions are most appropriate to guide information gathering. Therefore, the questions suggested here should be seen as a beginning framework from which therapists can go on to construct their own questions and adapt questions to the unique situation of each client.

This framework offers broad questions designed to be potentially relevant to a range of clients. Therefore, it should always be kept in mind that the questions in the framework may need to be reframed in light of factors emanating from the client and the therapeutic situation. These factors may include:

- Age of the client
- Nature and timing of onset of the client's disability

- Educational, rehabilitative, or preventive mission of therapy
- Anticipated duration of therapy, and the hospital, home, school, work or other setting in which therapy will be implemented.

Moreover, not all the questions listed as part of this framework will be pertinent to every client. For example, the client's age or level of functioning may make some questions irrelevant or impossible to answer. Moreover, constraints of time may necessitate selecting from among questions those that are most important to ask about a given client.

It is also important to recognize that the questions offered here are not exhaustive. Therapists should use these questions as a starting point for developing more specific questions tailored to each client's unique characteristics. Moreover, the best questions emerge over time as the therapist interacts with and comes to know the client. As therapists learn more about each of their clients, they should think of newer and more refined questions that emerge from their theoretical perspective.

General Questions

We begin with very broad questions and proceed to more detailed ones. The seven general questions (shown in *Figure 11-3*) represent a comprehensive approach in which major factors in any person's occupational life are considered. They include a concern for the person's characteristics, life history, environment, and actual doing. Taken together they present a broad framework for creating an occupational profile (Youngstrom et. al., 2001) of the client. Proceeding clockwise on Figure 11-3, the first two questions aim at understanding a person's occupational adaptation, that is, the person's construction of a positive occupational identity and maintenance of occupational competence over time. These two questions orient the therapists to consider the person's pattern of adaptation over time and also call attention to the occupational narrative the person is living. These broad questions are aimed at determining the extent to which a person's occupational life may be in difficulty or threatened. They serve also to orient the therapist to understand the client's overall perspective on his or her life.

The depth with which a therapist will seek to answer these questions depends on the client. In some case, it may be sufficient to gather a brief overview of the client's perspectives. In other situations, it may be necessary to gather a detailed history of a person's occupational life.

The next three questions explore what the person does at the levels of participation, performance, and skill. The first question examines doing at the most global level, asking about the person's work, play, and activities of daily living. The second question asks about the person's ability to complete the occupational forms that are a part of these occupations. The third question asks whether the person exhibits the skills necessary for carrying out those occupational forms.

What a person does is a function of both personal characteristics and the environment. Thus, the next two questions orient the therapist to ask about how personal (volition, habituation, and performance capacity) and environmental (physical and social) characteristics contribute to what the person does.

These seven general questions lead to a more detailed level of examination. For example, if a client does not appear to have a positive occupational identity and competence, more detailed questions will be useful in examining this aspect of the client's circumstances. Consequently, the seven general questions are primarily designed as screening questions aimed at determining whether the area bears further exploration. When it does, the kinds of detailed questions that are examined next will be necessary.

Occupational Identity and Competence

As shown in *Figure 11-4*, the questions of identity and competence are concerned with characterizing the person's life in terms of critical events that have occurred and changes in the direction of life, for better or worse. They also consider how persons impart meaning on their lives through the plots and metaphors of their occupational narratives. Finally, they consider how the person has enacted the narrative through choices and patterns of behavior over time, along with considering the impact these have had for the person's welfare.

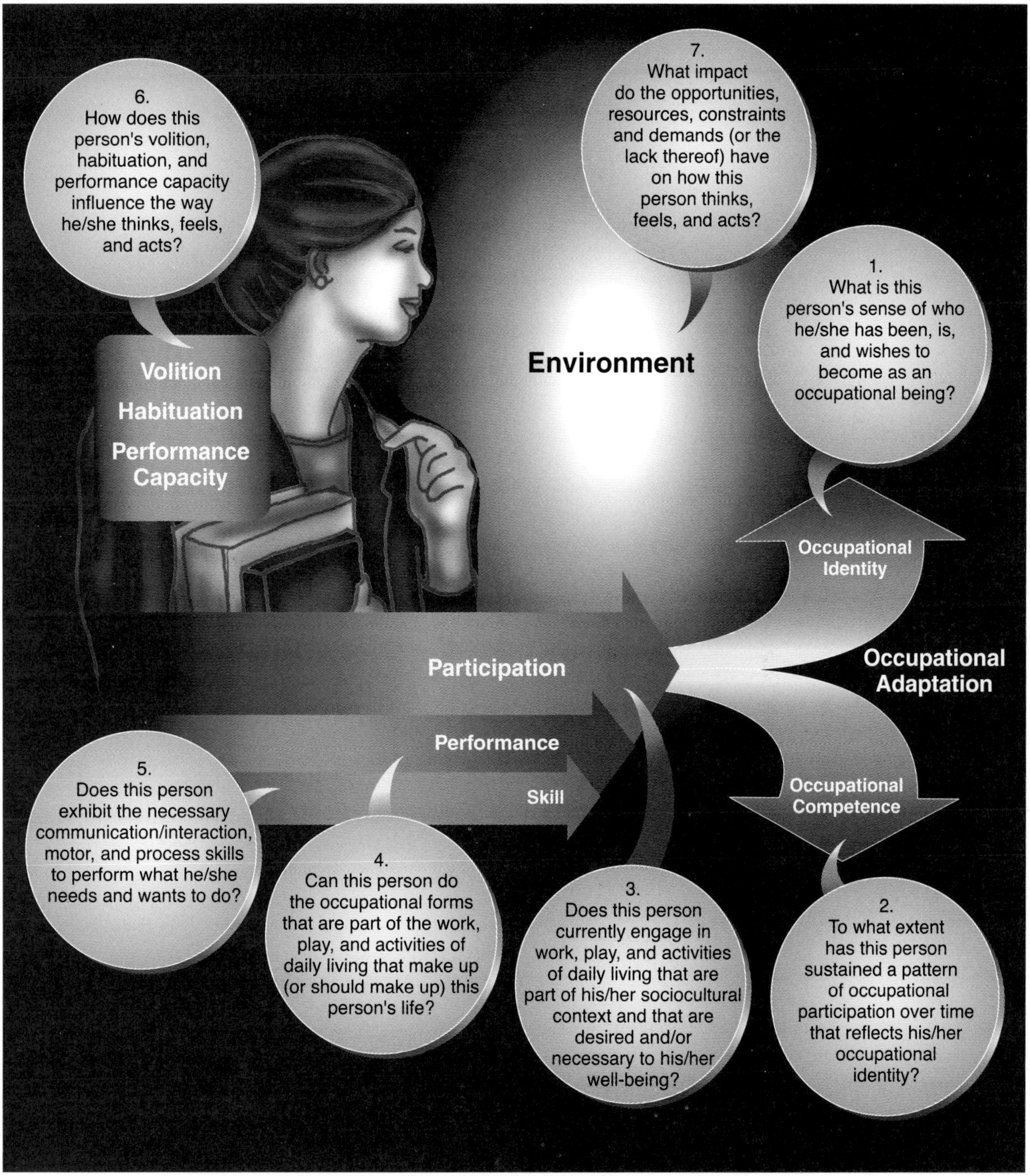

FIGURE 11-3 Seven General Questions Generated From the Theory.

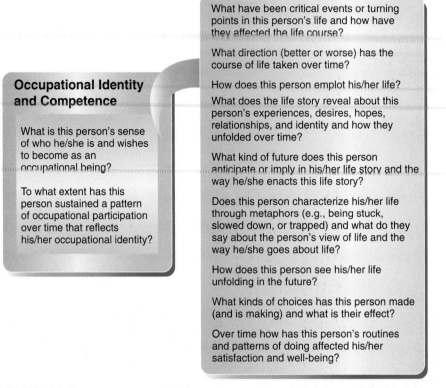

Occupational Identity and Competence

What is this person's sense of who he/she is and wishes to become as an occupational being?

To what extent has this person sustained a pattern of occupational participation over time that reflects his/her occupational identity?

What have been critical events or turning points in this person's life and how have they affected the life course?

What direction (better or worse) has the course of life taken over time?

How does this person emplot his/her life?

What does the life story reveal about this person's experiences, desires, hopes, relationships, and identity and how they unfolded over time?

What kind of future does this person anticipate or imply in his/her life story and the way he/she enacts this life story?

Does this person characterize his/her life through metaphors (e.g., being stuck, slowed down, or trapped) and what do they say about the person's view of life and the way he/she goes about life?

How does this person see his/her life unfolding in the future?

What kinds of choices has this person made (and is making) and what is their effect?

Over time how has this person's routines and patterns of doing affected his/her satisfaction and well-being?

FIGURE 11-4   Questions Pertaining to Occupational Identity and Competence.

Levels of Doing

The three questions reflecting levels of doing (Questions 3–5 in Figure 11-3) progress from broad to specific. Thus, they represent a sequence in which the therapist would ordinarily proceed. The first question asks about the person's current engagement in work, play, and activities of daily living. If a person has problems or cannot participate in one of these areas of occupational participation, the next question aims at identifying any difficulty he or she has in doing the occupational forms that make up an area of participation. For example, if a person is unable to do self-care to the extent that he or she wishes (participation), then the therapist could proceed to ask which occupational forms (e.g., bathing, dressing, toileting) present difficulty. If the person is having difficulty with one or more occupational forms, then one can ask what skills are giving the person difficulty in performance.

It may not be necessary to address all three questions. For example, if a client is able to perform all the occupational forms necessary to his or her work, leisure, and activities of daily living, then it will be unnecessary to ask about skills unless some other reason exists for examining skills, such as the possibility that the client wants to undertake new occupational forms for which his or her skills are questionable.

Personal Characteristics

Examination of personal characteristics requires the therapist to ask about volition, habituation, and performance capacity. *Figure 11-5* shows a next level of six more detailed questions that examine these components. Each of these six questions can be broken down into even more detailed questions, which are discussed below.

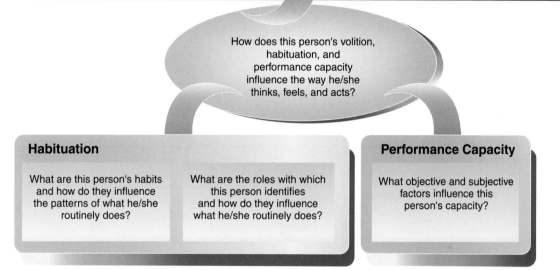

Volition

What is this person's view of personal capacity and effectiveness and how does it affect the choice, experience, interpretation, and anticipation of doing things?

What convictions and sense of obligation does this person have and how do they affect his/her choice, experience, interpretation, and anticipation of doing things?

What are this person's interests, and how do they affect his/her choice, experience, interpretation, and anticipation of doing things?

How does this person's volition, habituation, and performance capacity influence the way he/she thinks, feels, and acts?

Habituation

What are this person's habits and how do they influence the patterns of what he/she routinely does?

What are the roles with which this person identifies and how do they influence what he/she routinely does?

Performance Capacity

What objective and subjective factors influence this person's capacity?

FIGURE 11-5 Questions Pertaining to Personal Characteristics (Volition, Habituation, and Performance Capacity).

VOLITION

Figure 11-6 shows the more detailed questions pertaining to volition. Questions in the area of personal causation guide therapists to inquire about how persons organize their commonsense understanding of abilities, their accuracy, and the feelings and thoughts associated with belief in capacity and sense of efficacy. Questions related to values are concerned with what persons hold as significant and important in their lives and the extent to which these views are the person's own, consistent with personal abilities and differentiated. Questions related to interests ask whether a person has and pursues interests and can experience enjoyment in doing things.

HABITUATION

Figure 11-7 provides the more detailed questions pertaining to habituation. Questions related to roles ask

about the person's pattern of role involvement and its impact on identity, action, and social involvement as well as the person's ability to meet role obligations. Habit questions focus on the extent to which habits are established, effective, and provide quality of life.

PERFORMANCE CAPACITY

Questions related to performance capacity are shown in *Figure 11-8*. As noted in Chapter 6, performance capacity consists of both objective and subjective components, and other models of practice address objective components. Therefore, the question which asks about underlying impairments, if affirmatively answered, directs the therapist to identify and select other models of practice relevant to the impairment. For example, if the impairment is related to the musculoskeletal system, the biomechanical model (Kielhofner, 1997; Trombly, 1995) would be appropriate to consult. The

Personal Causation

What is this person's view of personal capacity and effectiveness and how does it affect the choice, experience, interpretation, and anticipation of doing things?

What abilities or limitations stand out in a person's view of self?

Is the sense of capacity accurate?

Is this person aware of abilities and limitations?

Does this person feel in control of his or her own thoughts, feelings, and actions and their consequences?

Does this person expect to achieve desired outcomes?

Does this person have confidence, anxiety, or other feelings in the face of performance?

Values

What convictions and sense of obligation does this person have and how do they affect the choice, experience, interpretation, and anticipation of doing things?

What is the organizing theme in this person's sense of values?

What things are most important to this person to do?

What standards or other criteria does this person use to judge his/her own performance?

Are the values to which this person ascribes really his or her own?

Can this person prioritize among what is important?

Is this person clear as to what his or her values are?

How do this person's values match or conflict with his or her abilities?

Does this person hold values that lead to adaptive choices?

Interests

What are this person's interests and how do they affect the choice, experience, interpretation, and anticipation of doing things?

Can this person identify personal interests?

What occupations does this person enjoy doing?

What are the aspects of doing that this person enjoys most (e.g., physical challenge, intellectual stimulation, social contact, aesthetic experience)?

Does this person do the things he/she enjoys?

Is anything interfering with this person's feeling of pleasure and satisfaction in performance?

FIGURE 11-6   Questions Pertaining to Volition.

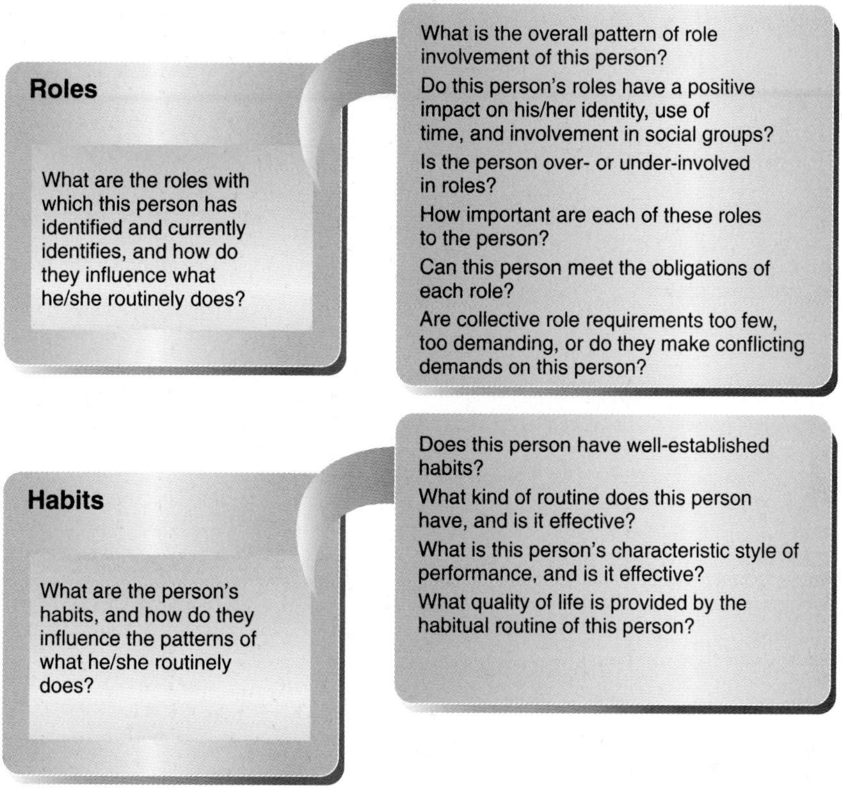

Roles

What are the roles with which this person has identified and currently identifies, and how do they influence what he/she routinely does?

What is the overall pattern of role involvement of this person?

Do this person's roles have a positive impact on his/her identity, use of time, and involvement in social groups?

Is the person over- or under-involved in roles?

How important are each of these roles to the person?

Can this person meet the obligations of each role?

Are collective role requirements too few, too demanding, or do they make conflicting demands on this person?

Habits

What are the person's habits, and how do they influence the patterns of what he/she routinely does?

Does this person have well-established habits?

What kind of routine does this person have, and is it effective?

What is this person's characteristic style of performance, and is it effective?

What quality of life is provided by the habitual routine of this person?

FIGURE 11-7   Questions Pertaining to Habituation.

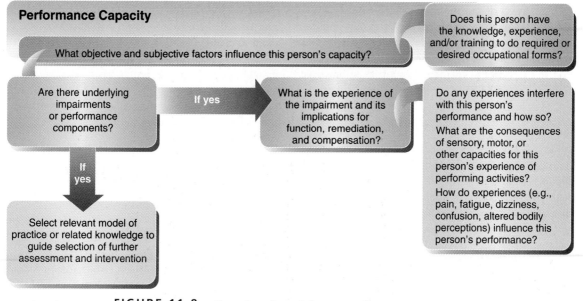

Performance Capacity

What objective and subjective factors influence this person's capacity?

Does this person have the knowledge, experience, and/or training to do required or desired occupational forms?

Are there underlying impairments or performance components?

If yes → What is the experience of the impairment and its implications for function, remediation, and compensation?

Do any experiences interfere with this person's performance and how so?

What are the consequences of sensory, motor, or other capacities for this person's experience of performing activities?

How do experiences (e.g., pain, fatigue, dizziness, confusion, altered bodily perceptions) influence this person's performance?

If yes ↓

Select relevant model of practice or related knowledge to guide selection of further assessment and intervention

FIGURE 11-8   Questions Pertaining to Performance Capacity.

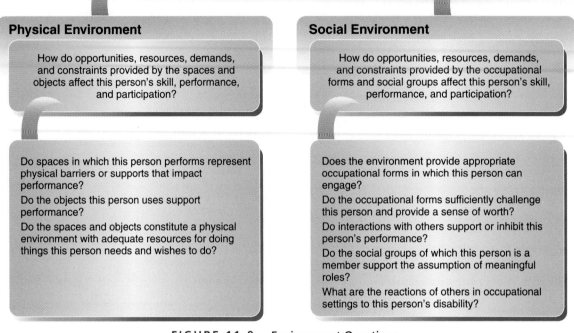

What impact do the opportunities, resources, constraints, and demands (or the lack thereof) have on how this person thinks, feels, and acts?

Physical Environment

How do opportunities, resources, demands, and constraints provided by the spaces and objects affect this person's skill, performance, and participation?

Do spaces in which this person performs represent physical barriers or supports that impact performance?

Do the objects this person uses support performance?

Do the spaces and objects constitute a physical environment with adequate resources for doing things this person needs and wishes to do?

Social Environment

How do opportunities, resources, demands, and constraints provided by the occupational forms and social groups affect this person's skill, performance, and participation?

Does the environment provide appropriate occupational forms in which this person can engage?

Do the occupational forms sufficiently challenge this person and provide a sense of worth?

Do interactions with others support or inhibit this person's performance?

Do the social groups of which this person is a member support the assumption of meaningful roles?

What are the reactions of others in occupational settings to this person's disability?

FIGURE 11-9   Environment Questions.

other pathway of questioning focuses on subjective components of performance capacity and asks implications of the experience of the impairment. Finally, because the capacity to do something may be related to what the person has learned through experience or training, a question about these factors is included.

Environment

Within the environmental arena, questions are raised about how a person's social and physical environments influence what a persons thinks, feels, and does *(Fig. 11-9)*. The questions ask about the impact of spaces, objects, occupational forms, and social groups.

Using the Questions

We have just examined a series of questions for guiding the process of gathering information about a client

based on the MOHO. *Figure 11-10* illustrates all the questions (in abbreviated form) and illustrates how the more detailed questions branch from the seven central questions. Taken together, these questions provide a map of how to gather information about a client. Therapists who are first learning to use MOHO may find it helpful to refer to this map as a guide or checklist of things to consider about a client.

Tailoring Questions

As already noted, a therapist will generally need to tailor these questions and to generate additional questions to fit the emerging circumstances of gathering information on each particular patient. When translating concepts into theoretical questions the therapist is seeking the relevance of the theory for a particular person's life. Questions will always need to be tailored for each particular client if the therapeutic reasoning process is to remain client-centered. The process of tailoring occurs when initial questions lead to information that influences what subsequent questions are generated.

For example, in response to the first of several detailed questions in the framework about interests (i.e., can this person identify personal interests?), a therapist may find one of the following:

- The client cannot identify any interest
- The client identifies several interests
- The client is unable to respond verbally to any questions about interests.

Each of these three different situations suggests different questions that should follow. In the first case, the therapist may wish to ask why the client cannot identify interests. For example:

- Has the client lacked opportunity to develop interests?
- Has the client lost interests because of the interference of an impairment?

In the second case, when the client identifies several interests, the therapist may wish to go on to ask whether the client participates in these interests and what common themes, if any, exist in the interests. In the third case the therapist might ask whether the client's behavior indicates that he or she enjoys certain occupations. How one proceeds with a line of questioning is always informed by the answers to previous questions.

Reasoning in Partnership with Clients

At the beginning of this chapter it was emphasized that therapeutic reasoning with MOHO is client-centered. This means that the therapist should pursue answers to the questions with guidance from the client's unique characteristics, perspectives, and, whenever possible, direct input. Indeed, the ideal way for the therapist to apply the framework is in collaboration with a client (or the client's caretaker if the client is not able).

Getting answers to the questions requires a give and take between therapists and clients. The client will be essential to answering questions since they pertain to the thoughts and feelings that are the client's intimate possessions. The therapist generates the questions and guides interpretation of the information about and provided by the client. Both client and therapist bring complementary expertise to the therapeutic reasoning process.

Identifying Strengths and Challenges

The questions outlined in this chapter will lead occupational therapists to have an understanding of their clients' occupational strengths and challenges. The Section II Master Table on pages 346–355 lists the questions proposed earlier and also notes client strengths and weaknesses that might be revealed by gathering information to answer the questions. This information is located in the table along with further information that will be covered in later chapters. By referring to the table, the reader will find organized together:

- MOHO concepts
- Related questions
- Problems and challenges that might be identified
- Types of client changes that therapy may produce
- Forms of client occupational engagement that engender such changes
- Therapist strategies that support the client's engagement and change.

The Section II Master Table lists a range of strengths and weaknesses that might characterize any given client. Of course, each client will have a unique profile of strengths and challenges revealed by answers to the questions. For example, a person may have:

- A poor sense of his or her own abilities leading to a difficulty making choices to engage in occupational forms
- Difficulty structuring the day due to the lack of role responsibilities
- Limited motor skills
- A physical environment that is not supportive of performance capacity.

However, the same person may:

- Be able to identify and prioritize among occupational goals
- Have strong interests
- Possess good process skills
- Experience a supportive social environment.

As this example illustrates, the questions offered in this chapter should enable the therapist to generate a more detailed understanding of the client's occupational life including a unique profile of strengths and challenges. The composite of these strengths and challenges provides a comprehensive understanding of a client's functioning. Such a view of functioning considers not only a client's underlying capacity or skill. It also

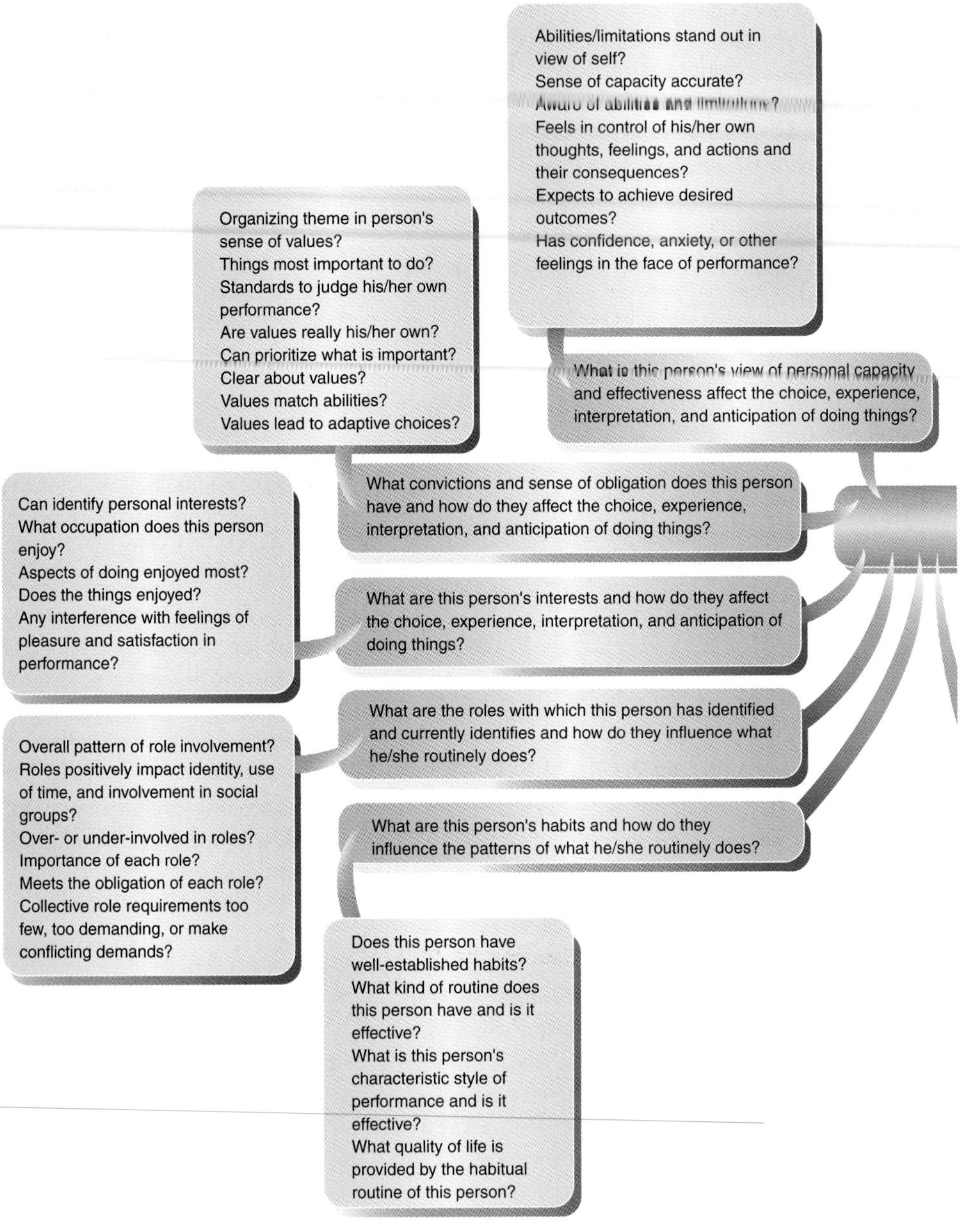

Abilities/limitations stand out in view of self?
Sense of capacity accurate?
Aware of abilities and limitations?
Feels in control of his/her own thoughts, feelings, and actions and their consequences?
Expects to achieve desired outcomes?
Has confidence, anxiety, or other feelings in the face of performance?

Organizing theme in person's sense of values?
Things most important to do?
Standards to judge his/her own performance?
Are values really his/her own?
Can prioritize what is important?
Clear about values?
Values match abilities?
Values lead to adaptive choices?

What is this person's view of personal capacity and effectiveness affect the choice, experience, interpretation, and anticipation of doing things?

Can identify personal interests?
What occupation does this person enjoy?
Aspects of doing enjoyed most?
Does the things enjoyed?
Any interference with feelings of pleasure and satisfaction in performance?

What convictions and sense of obligation does this person have and how do they affect the choice, experience, interpretation, and anticipation of doing things?

What are this person's interests and how do they affect the choice, experience, interpretation, and anticipation of doing things?

Overall pattern of role involvement?
Roles positively impact identity, use of time, and involvement in social groups?
Over- or under-involved in roles?
Importance of each role?
Meets the obligation of each role?
Collective role requirements too few, too demanding, or make conflicting demands?

What are the roles with which this person has identified and currently identifies and how do they influence what he/she routinely does?

What are this person's habits and how do they influence the patterns of what he/she routinely does?

Does this person have well-established habits?
What kind of routine does this person have and is it effective?
What is this person's characteristic style of performance and is it effective?
What quality of life is provided by the habitual routine of this person?

FIGURE 11-10   Summary Figure for Chapter 11.

Spaces represent physical barriers or supports? Objects this person uses support performance? Spaces and objects constitute a physical environment with adequate resources for doing things?

Does the environment provide appropriate occupational forms in which this person can engage?
Do the occupational forms sufficiently challenge this person and provide a sense of worth?
Do interactions with others support or inhibit this person's performance?
Do the social groups of which this person is a member support the assumption of meaningful roles?
What are the reactions of others in occupational settings to this person's disability?

How do opportunities, resources, demands, and constraints provided by the spaces and objects affect this person's skill, performance, and participation?

How do opportunities, resources, demands, and constraints provided by the occupational forms and social groups affect this person's skill, performance, and participation?

What impact do the opportunities, resources, constraints, and demands (or the lack thereof) have on how this person thinks, feels, and acts.

What is this person's sense of who he/she has been, is, and wishes to become as an occupational being?

What have been critical events or turning points and how have they affected the life course?
What direction (better or worse) has the course of life taken over time?
How does this person emplot his/her life?
What does the life story reveal about the person's experiences, desires, hopes, relationships, and identity, and how they have unfolded over time?
What kind of future does this person anticipate or imply in his/her life story and the way he/she enacts this life story?
Does this person characterize his or her life through metaphors (e.g., being stuck, slowed down, or trapped) and what do they say about the person's view of life and the way he/she goes about life?
How does this person see his/her life unfolding in the future?
What kinds of choices has this person made and is making and what is their effect?
Over time, how has this person's routines and patterns of doing affected his/her satisfaction and well-being?

How does this person's volition, habituation, and performance capacity influence the way he/she thinks, feels, and acts?

To what extent has this person sustained a pattern of occupational participation over time that reflects his/her occupational identity?

Does this person exhibit the necessary communication/interaction, motor, and process skills to perform what he/she needs and wants to do?

Can this person do the occupational forms that are part of the work, play, and activities of daily living that make up (or should make up) this person's life?

Does this person currently engage in work, play, and activities of daily living that are part of his/her sociocultural context and that are desired and/or necessary to his/her well-being?

Performance Capacity
What objective and subjective factors influence this person's capacity?

Does this person have the knowledge, experience and/or training to do required or desired occupational forms?

Are there underlying impairments of performance components?

If yes

What is the experience of the impairment and its implications for function, remediation, compensation?

If yes

How does this person describe the experience of his/her body and mind?
Do any experiences interfere with this person's performance and how so?
What are the consequences of sensory, motor, or the other capacities for this person's experience of performing activities?
How do experiences such as pain, fatigue, dizziness, or confusion influence this person's performance?

Select relevant model of practice or related knowledge to guide selection of further assessment and interaction includes the volitional, habituation, and environmental factors that impact on the client's success in participating in occupations over time and crafting a unique and satisfying occupational identity and competence.

A Look Ahead: Other Phases of Therapeutic Reasoning

Generating questions is only one phase of the therapeutic reasoning process introduced at the beginning of this chapter. The phase of gathering information requires that the therapist have a comprehensive knowledge of strategies and tools for gathering information. Chapters 12 through 16 overview and introduce the information gathering strategies that therapists can use to obtain the answers to these questions with reference to a particular client. Chapters 17 through 20 discuss change in therapy, how therapy supports the change process, and how to translate understanding of a client into therapy goals and strategies.

References

Kielhofner, G. (1997). *Conceptual foundations of occupational therapy* (2nd ed.). Philadelphia: FA Davis.

Law, M. (Ed.). (1998). *Client-centered occupational therapy.* Thorofare: Slack.

Mattingly, C. (1991). The narrative nature of clinical reasoning. *American Journal of Occupational Therapy, 45,* 998–1005.

Mattingly, C., & Fleming, M. (1993). *Clinical reasoning: Forms of inquiry in a therapeutic practice.* Philadelphia: FA Davis.

Trombly, C. (1995). *Occupational therapy for physical dysfunction* (4th ed.). Philadelphia: FA Davis.

Youngstrom, M. J., Anthony, P., Brinson, M., Browning, S., Clark, G. F., Oldham, J., Roley, S. S., Sellers, J., Van Slyke, N. L., Radomski, M. V., Hertfeldr, S. D., & Peterson, M. F. (2001, April). *Occupational therapy practice framework.* Paper presented at the American Occupational Therapy Association Conference, Philadelphia, PA.

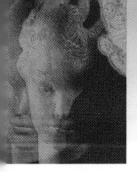

12

Gathering Client Information

● Gary Kielhofner

Chapter 11 identified a therapeutic reasoning process in which collecting information about clients is the second step. How does a therapist using MOHO go about collecting information on clients? This chapter discusses methods that can be used to gather information relevant to MOHO concepts. It also discusses some guidelines for going about the information-gathering process that are important to therapeutic reasoning.

Two Approaches to Collecting Client Information

Therapists can gather information about their clients using:

● Structured assessments
● Unstructured approaches.

A therapist using structured assessments follows a set protocol. A therapist using an unstructured approach takes advantage of naturally occurring opportunities to gather information.

Both structured assessments and unstructured approaches for information gathering have their place. Structured assessments use means for information gathering that have been refined and tested. They guard against bias and provide information that is readily interpretable. Unstructured approaches capitalize on unique opportunities that arise for obtaining useful information in informal, spontaneous, and creative ways.

Gathering information on and from clients ordinarily requires therapists to use both structured assessments and unstructured approaches. Therapists should approach data gathering systematically and thoughtfully with concern for:

● The kinds of information that are needed
● The best method to gather that information given the client and the circumstances.

The following sections discuss both structured assessments and unstructured approaches, exploring how each can best be used.

Structured Assessments

Structured assessments are fixed procedures for collecting client information that have been systematically developed and studied. Ordinarily, they will have the following characteristics:

● A specified protocol or guidelines for use, including forms for recording, scoring, and reporting the information gathered
● Evidence that the assessment is dependable
● A formal basis for interpreting the information they gather.

Each of these characteristics is examined below.

PROTOCOL FOR USE

Through experience, field-testing, and research, developers of structured approaches seek to determine optimal methods for gathering, recording, and interpreting particular information. Once these methods have been determined, they become part of the formal protocol of the assessment. Protocols may consist of:

● Guidelines to follow in administering the assessment
● Specific forms to use in recording, scoring, and reporting the information gathered.

Guidelines for administration explain what the therapist and/or client should do to gather or report the information that the assessment is designed to gather. These guidelines reflect what has been learned about optimal ways to gather and make sense of the information. They help guard against bias in the information gathered. They also help assure that the procedure generates information that is relevant, detailed, and focused on the purpose of the assessment. Guidelines may include such things as:

- A standard context in which observation may be performed
- A set of questions to ask in an interview
- Instructions for what a therapist may or may not say or do while information is being gathered.

Forms used as part of structured assessments assure that the information is recorded in a way that makes it most useful for the purposes of the assessment. Forms may include such things as:

- A questionnaire with items to be rated or questions to be answered
- Categories for recording reports, observation, or comments
- Outlines or layouts for visually illustrating information or writing descriptive narratives.

Depending on the nature of the assessment, protocols may be very specific or they may allow flexible adaptation to circumstances. Ordinarily the protocol of a structured assessment is explained in a manual. Sometimes this may also involve or require training. Using a structured assessment requires that one first carefully learn its purpose and procedures.

EVIDENCE OF DEPENDABILITY

When an information-gathering method is considered dependable, two things are meant (Benson & Schell, 1997). First, a dependable information-gathering method is reliable. That is, it will give the same information within reasonable variations of administration such as:

- In different circumstances
- At different times
- With different clients
- When different therapists administer it.

Reliability assures that a structured assessment is capable of gathering information in a consistent way that is not unduly affected by variations of administration that occur in ordinary use of the assessment. The reliability of an assessment is ordinarily studied by comparing information obtained under different conditions such as those noted above. When the assessment yields information across conditions that are found to be stable, then the instrument is considered reliable. Reliability is always a matter of the degree of consistency found. Generally, there are accepted guidelines for how much consistency is expected, depending on the statistical method that is used to assess it.

Second, a dependable information-gathering method is valid. Being valid means that it provides the information it is intended to provide. This may seem a rather straightforward thing, but it can be quite complex. Minimally, it requires careful attention to the details of the kind of information every part of an assessment is designed to capture. For example, when we developed an observational assessment designed to provide information on volition, we had to make sure that a client's skill was not confused with volition when making the rating. There is an item on the assessment that asks whether a client *tries to solve problems.* Careful instructions had to be developed for the therapist to rate the item based on whether the client showed the motivation (i.e., confidence and interest) to try to solve a problem, and not on whether the client was successful in solving the problem. The latter was an indication of skill, not to be confused with volition.

Validity is a particularly important feature of structured assessments, since it gives therapists some assurance about exactly what kind of information is being gathered when an assessment is administered. This is important to the therapeutic reasoning process because it enables therapists to create an accurate understanding of the client. Theoretical concepts point toward certain phenomena. Structured assessments provide proven means to capture information on these specific phenomena. If an assessment lacks validity, it may provide ambiguous information that leads a therapist to construct an erroneous conceptualization of a client's situation.

The science of developing assessments employs a variety of statistical approaches to examine their properties. Ordinarily, a series of studies are conducted to appraise whether a particular information-gathering procedure provides the kind of information intended. Such studies are likely to examine:

- Whether the content of the assessment is coherent and representative of what is intended to be gathered (content or internal validity). Thus, items on an assessment may be examined for the extent to which they cohere to reflect the underlying concept. For example, we examined whether the items on an assessment of communication/interaction skills worked well together to capture this area of skill (Forsyth, Lai, & Kielhofner, 1999)

- Whether information gathered with the assessment is associated with other information with which it should bear a relationship (concurrent validity). For example, information gathered on volition should be associated with the kinds of activity choices a person makes
- Whether information gathered with the assessment differs from information that has no relationship to it (convergent validity). For example, a person's values should have little or a limited relationship to their skills
- Whether information gathered with the assessment can tell the difference between disparate groups of people. For example, children who are succeeding in school would be expected to have better personal causation than children who are failing. An assessment designed to gather information on children's personal causation should be able to discriminate between those children who are and are not having school performance difficulties
- Whether information gathered with an assessment can predict relevant future action or circumstances (predictive validity). For example, an assessment that gathers information on a person's communication/interaction skills should be able to predict how well that person will be able to perform in a situation requiring those skills.

The development of any assessment ordinarily involves a series of studies that examine whether there is evidence of one or more of the types of validity noted above. The more consistent evidence that exists, the more confidence one can have in the validity of an assessment. Validity is never simply present or absent. It is always a matter of degree as represented in the number and scope of studies providing evidence of an assessment's validity.

EVALUATING DEPENDABILITY

In the course of research to determine reliability and validity, refinements in the assessment are made that improve dependability. Ordinarily, assessments that

have been more thoroughly researched will be more dependable. Structured assessments, including those presented in the following chapters, vary widely in how thoroughly they have been studied. Moreover, all assessments—no matter how thoroughly researched—have some limitations. Therapists should have an awareness of the evidence of dependability for any structured assessment they use. This knowledge allows one to know how much confidence should be placed in the information collected with a particular assessment.

MEANS OF INTERPRETATION

Structured approaches generate information through observing a client, listening to a client, and/or asking a client to respond to a written form. To determine what the information means, therapists must have some way of synthesizing or ordering it. One of the most common ways of doing this is the use of rating scales.

Rating Scales

Rating scales may be completed by either the therapist or the client. The assessments discussed in the following chapters all use rating scales for the therapist to record information gathered from observation. An example of this is The Occupational Self Assessment (OSA) (Baron, Kielhofner, Iyenger, Goldhammer, & Wolenski, 2002). This assessment allows clients to rate how competently they do a number of things related to occupational life. For instance, on the OSA a client encounters the item, *working toward my goals,* and then rates the item using one of the following four categories:

- I do this extremely well
- I do this well
- I have some difficulty doing this
- I have a lot of problem doing this.

All the items on the OSA are designed to capture information about occupational competence. Therefore, each time clients rate an item on the scale, they are providing some information about their occupational competence.

One of the most common and useful ways of interpreting data from such rating scales is to treat them as a profile of strengths and weaknesses. For example, how clients rate themselves across all the OSA items indicates areas in which they have more or less competence. Another more precise way to make sense of the information given on rating scales is to derive measures from them.

Measurements

Rating scales yield ordinal information. That is, they provide some kind of ordering or ranking, such as the OSA's determination of how well one does each of the things listed on the instrument. It is possible to take such ordinal information and create measures. That is, statistical methods can translate the ordinal information obtained on rating scales into interval measures (Wright & Linacre, 1989).

A measure determines the specific amount of a characteristic someone has. Everyday examples of measurement are height and weight. Such measures allow us to say not only that one person is taller than another (an ordinal judgment), but also how much taller (e.g., 3 inches). This kind of precision in characterizing a person is possible because measures are interval. That is, the numbers that are used to quantify the characteristic (and thus answer the question, "How much?") are composed of evenly spaced intervals, allowing mathematical calculations (e.g., subtracting the height of one person from that of another to calculate the difference in their heights). One can readily see how such mathematical manipulability is useful in practice. One can, for example, ask, "How much has a person's occupational performance improved in the course of therapy?" By deriving a measure from a client's self-ratings on the OSA, it is possible to generate a measure that allows such a question to be answered.

Most of the assessments using rating scales that are discussed in the following chapters use a statistical approach (Wright & Linacre, 1989) that converts the ordinal information they gather into interval measures. The most sophisticated example is the Assessment of Motor and Process Skills (AMPS) that provides precise measures of a client's level of skill (Fisher, 1999). The AMPS requires computer scoring of the therapist's ordinal ratings. Therapists can obtain a program for use on a personal computer to score the assessment.

Other model-based assessments can be similarly scored by computer. However, there are no publicly available programs for doing this on one's own personal computer. The plan for these assessments is to make available an alternative, paper-and-pencil key for converting the ordinal ratings into interval measures. The first of these scoring keys are now becoming available, as discussed in the following chapters.

Other Means of Interpreting Information

Many structured approaches yield qualitative information. Interpreting qualitative information gathered by structured assessments is often helped by the structure of the assessment itself (that categorizes information) as well as by guidelines for interpretation provided along with the assessment. In some cases, a particular approach to interpreting the qualitative information will be provided. For example, the Occupational Performance History Interview (OPHI-II) (Kielhofner et al., 1998) provides a specific means of analyzing and interpreting the life story that emerges in that interview.

BENEFITS OF STRUCTURED INFORMATION COLLECTION METHODS

Writers have correctly encouraged occupational therapists to make use of structured assessments (Bonder, 1993; Fisher & Short-DeGraff, 1993; Watts, Brollier, Bauer, & Schmidt, 1989). Some of the benefits of structured methods are:

- Use of structured assessments benefits from the systematic effort that has gone into making them dependable
- Consumers and other professionals have some assurance that the assessment is worth the therapist's time and effort because it yields useful and dependable information.
- Such methods are less likely to yield information that is misleading or biased.

Consequently, when appropriate structured information-collection methods are available and feasible, therapists are well advised to use them.

Structured Information Collection Methods Used With MOHO

Structured assessments developed for or used with MOHO employ observation, client self-report questionnaires and checklists, and interviews as the means of gathering information. Some assessments combine more than one of these approaches and are, therefore,

FIGURE 12-1   Model of Human Occupation Assessments, Concepts They Cover, and Populations for Which They Are Intended.

INSTRUMENT NAME	CONCEPTS TARGETED	POPULATION
Observational Tools (Chapter 13)		
Assessment of Communication and Interaction Skills (ACIS)	Communication/interaction skills	Adolescents, adults, elderly (potentially relevant to children)
Assessment of Motor and Process Skills (AMPS)	Motor and process skills	Children (3–4 years and older), adolescents, adults, elderly
Pediatric Volitional Questionnaire (PVQ)	Volition (personal causation, values, and interests), influence of environment on volition	Children (2–6 years)
Volitional Questionnaire (VQ)	Volition (personal causation, values, and interests), influence of environment on volition	Children over 6 years, adolescents, adults, elderly (especially appropriate for persons who cannot readily self report)
Self Report Checklists and Questionnaires (Chapter 14)		
Modified Interest Checklist	Interests (past, present, and desired participation, degree of attraction)	Adolescents, adults, elderly
NIH Activity Record	Habits, roles, values, interests, and personal causation reflected in routine, degree of performance difficulty, and lived body experience of pain and fatigue	Adolescents, adults, elderly
Occupational Self Assessment (OSA) and Child occupational Self Assessment (COSA)	Occupational competence, values, and environmental impact	OSA: children over 11 years, adolescents, adults, and elderly COSA: children ages 8–11
Role Checklist	Roles and values	Adolescents and adults
Occupational Questionnaire	Habits, roles, values, interests, and personal causation reflected in routine	Adolescents, adults, elderly
Pediatric Interest Profile	Interests (strength of attraction, feeling of competence and participation)	Children (6–12 years), adolescents (12–21 years)

(continued)

FIGURE 12-1   *(continued)*

INSTRUMENT NAME	CONCEPTS TARGETED	POPULATION
Interviews (Chapter 15)		
Occupational Circumstances Assessment: Interview and Rating Scale (OCAIRS-Version 2.0)	Values, interests, personal causation, roles, habits, performance, environment	Adolescents, adults, elderly
Occupational Perforamnce History Interview-2nd Version (OPHI-II)	Occupational competence, occupational identity, environment, values, interests, personal causation, roles, habits	Adolescents, adults, elderly
School Setting Interview (SSI)	Needs for accommodation to deal with objects, spaces, occupational forms, and social groups in school setting	Children of school age
Worker Role Interview (WRI)	Personal causation, values, interests, roles, habits, perception of work and environment	Adults
Work Environment Impact Scale (WEIS)	Physical (objects and spaces) and social (occupational forms and social groups) environment	Adults
Mixed Method Assessments (Chapter 16)		
Assessment of Occupational Functioning (AOF-CV)	Values, interests, personal causation, roles, habits, performance	Adolescents, adults, elderly
Model of Human Occupation Screening Tool (MOHOST)	Personal causation, values, interests, roles, and habits	Adolescents, adults, elderly
Occupational Therapy Psychosocial Assessment of Learning (OT PAL)	Volition (ability to make choices), habituation (roles and routines), and environmental impact	Children of school age

referred to as mixed method assessments. *Figure 12-1* shows tools that have been developed or modified for use with MOHO and are covered in subsequent chapters. The figure also notes the concepts on which the assessments gather data and the age groups for which they are appropriate.

Selecting and Using Other Structured Assessments

Therapists using MOHO also use structured assessments other than or along with assessments developed to specifically reflect MOHO concepts. They do so for a variety of reasons. First, therapists often use MOHO in association with other conceptual practice models that

have their own assessments. Second, therapists may choose other assessments that specifically target occupational performance in ways that MOHO-based assessments do not. Such assessments include activities of daily living assessments, standardized development assessments, and formal work evaluations. These kinds of assessments are used when the therapist needs information on the client's capacity to do specific occupational forms such as dressing, bathing, or driving. Although such assessments were not developed specifically for use with MOHO, they are certainly compatible with it. Third, a therapist may choose assessments that gather information directly or partly related to constructs in MOHO. An example is the use of structured interest inventories. Since the existing MOHO-based interest assessments focus mainly on leisure interests, therapists wishing to gather information on work-related interests will ordinarily use one of a number of available standardized vocational interest assessments.

Unstructured Approaches to Gathering Information

As noted previously, unstructured approaches to gathering information take advantage of natural circumstances that arise for learning about a client. They serve a complementary role to the structured approaches already discussed. Unstructured information collection simply involves observing and/or talking with the client.

The following are some common circumstances in which therapists will make use of unstructured methods:

- There is no appropriate structured assessment available
- The client is uncomfortable with or unable to complete a structured assessment
- The therapist wishes to augment information collected by structured assessments
- Structured assessments take more time than is available
- An unexpected opportunity to obtain useful information arises.

Unstructured methods are also an important means of continuing the information-gathering process throughout the course of therapy. Every opportunity the therapist has to observe and/or talk with a client will potentially yield useful information. If therapists use such opportunities wisely, they can gather a wealth of information efficiently and effectively.

Therapists will often find it helpful to use the kinds of questions identified in the previous chapter to guide their use of unstructured approaches. As unstructured methods do not follow an established protocol, such questions enable therapists to know what to pay attention to or to ask about.

One of the advantages of unstructured approaches is that they can be adapted to unfolding situations in therapy. The therapist can periodically obtain information relevant to conceptual questions that are still unanswered or that emerge in the course of intervention. Unstructured information collection can occur in a wide range of circumstances such as:

- Having a conversation with a client while beginning a therapy session
- Observing a student's performance when visiting the classroom
- Listening to a client's comments about the workplace where he was injured
- Noting the affect of a client during a group session
- Listening to a client's occasional stories about what happened since the last therapy session.

Because unstructured methods often occur serendipitously and are informal, they can appear to be less important than structured methods. However, all unstructured information collection is potentially very valuable if it is carefully gathered and interpreted.

GATHERING INFORMATION ON THE LIVED BODY

Since no structured assessments exist for gathering information on the lived body experience, therapists must always use unstructured methods for this purpose. As discussed and illustrated in Chapter 6, understanding a person's performance experience can be extremely important. However, because disability can radically alter experience from what is ordinary, therapists must take special care in gathering such information. Grasping what the client is experiencing is complicated by the fact that it might differ radically from the therapist's own experience. The suggestions offered below are based on methods developed in a study of unilateral neglect (Tham, Borell, & Gustavsson, 2000).

A combination of observation and informal interviewing appears to be the most effective approach. Because it is often very difficult for clients to describe their lived body experiences, therapists should begin by explaining that such information will help the therapist and client better plan therapy and by reminding clients that they are experts on their own experience.

It is also helpful to talk to clients while they are performing tasks or immediately thereafter. This strategy both calls clients' attention to their experience and allows them to tell about it while the memory of the experience is fresh. Another useful strategy is to ask clients to describe how performing in the present differs from how it used to feel before the onset of the disability. Sometimes it is helpful to share what other clients have previously described to see if clients recognize it as similar to their own experiences. The kind of description given in Chapter 6 can also be a good starting point for asking clients about their own experiences. Finally, the therapist should refine what is asked as clients are able to begin talking about their experiences. Using phrases that the client used and asking for their meaning can help focus discussion.

PROPER USE OF UNSTRUCTURED METHODS TO ASSURE DEPENDABILITY

When using unstructured methods to gather information, therapists use much of the same kind of logic and safeguards that qualitative researchers use when they gather information from field observation and interviews (Denzin & Lincoln, 1994; Hagner & Helm, 1994; Hammersly, 1992; Krefting, 1989; Miles & Huberman, 1994; Wolcott, 1990). Although it is not possible to review here all the kinds of concerns and practices that qualitative researchers have in mind when collecting and interpreting information, three important strategies for assuring dependability of information gathered by unstructured methods will be discussed:

- Evaluating context
- Triangulation
- Validity checks.

Evaluating Context

Circumstances have an important influence on the information one receives. For example, a client struggling with some problem suddenly confides in a therapist about all his fears for the future. From such an encounter, the therapist may have much more honest and useful information than the information previously gathered in a formal interview. On the other hand, circumstance may make the information suspect. For example, if a client is reporting on her performance in a group where it is clear she is trying to impress another group member, the therapist may have reasons to suspect that the report is exaggerated. Circumstances often tell the therapist how much confidence to place in the information and how to interpret it.

Triangulation

Triangulation is a method of helping to assure that information is accurate by comparing it with information from another source (Denzin & Lincoln, 1994). Thus, for example, one may compare what clients say they can do with observation of their performance or with what a spouse or caretaker says the person can do. Another method of triangulation is to compare the same type of information collected over time. Observing performance or asking about a client's view of the future more than once is a way of checking whether one observation or response was truly representative of how the person performs or feels.

Validity Checks

When using unstructured methods therapists should be vigilant to assure that their interpretation of the meaning of the information is valid. First, a therapist should ask whether an interpretation corresponds logically and structurally with the general picture obtained from earlier information. If it does, then one has a stronger basis to consider the interpretation. The therapist may also ask whether the interpretation corresponds with case examples and other discussions offered by the theory that guided the information gathering.

Another important method of checking the validity of one's interpretations is to continue to collect information that will either support or refute the interpretation of the previous information's meaning. Finally and importantly, one can and should check interpretations of information by asking the client if the interpretations are valid. For example, observation of a client's behavior in a task situation suggests that the client was anxious and the therapist interprets this information as meaning the client's sense of efficacy in a particular task is poor. The therapist can check the validity of this interpretation by sharing it with the client to ask whether he or she agrees. In sum, a therapist using unstructured methods can assure validity by employing a careful and reflective attitude and by checking up on information and its interpretation.

AN ILLUSTRATION OF UNSTRUCTURED INFORMATION COLLECTION

The following example is used to illustrate how unstructured information gathering can be used in therapeutic reasoning. This example shows how unstructured observation and interviewing were used with a very young, severely impaired child to assess volition.

Mary

Mary was a 3 year old whose case was being followed in a developmental clinic. She had a rare genetic disorder that resulted in extreme delays in growth and development of cognitive, motor, and social functions. Mary's therapist used unstructured observation and conversations with Mary's mother throughout the course of therapy to understand Mary's volition and how it influenced her activity choices.

The occupational therapist made the following observations of Mary. While she had no formal language, Mary was effective in communicating desires and displeasures. She strategically cried or made sounds of disapproval when things were not going as she wanted. For example, the therapist presented a toy that made music, and when the music stopped, Mary began crying. The therapist started the music again and Mary immediately stopped crying, demonstrating her communicative intent. In contrast to her obvious sense that she could have control and achieve desires by influencing those around her, Mary appeared to have very little awareness of how to make things happen through movement. She kept her flexed arms tight against her chest. She made no attempts to reach for objects, grasp, or otherwise motorically act on her environment. It appears that Mary did not have the intention or desire to physically do things to the environment.

These observations led the therapist to conclude that Mary's belief in capacity and sense of efficacy were organized around her basic awareness of being able to influence others. This was corroborated by her mother. At home, Mary was surrounded by many family members who readily understood much of her primitive communication and did things for her that she wanted. In contrast, she rarely attempted to move her body.

The therapist also observed that Mary valued and responded intensely to human contact. She also displayed a number of interests through orienting and maintaining attention toward things such as a toy that played music and a vibrating pillow. Additionally, she vocalized pleasure at vestibular stimulation through a pleasant grunting sound while being bounced on a ball. Thus, the therapist concluded that while Mary had a highly developed volition, it was focused on getting others to do things and passively enjoying things that others initiated.

The therapist used this conceptualization of Mary's volition to construct a treatment plan in which the occupational therapist challenged Mary to reach, touch, grasp, and so on to generate the social, vestibular, auditory, and tactile experiences that she valued and enjoyed. Careful observation of her volitional responses during therapy sessions to determine, for example, when she was too challenged by the demands presented or when she was attending to an interest, was important for the occupational therapist to guide therapy. The occupational therapist also instructed the family in how to encourage Mary to generate these experiences with their help instead of doing everything for her. During the course of 1 month, Mary improved significantly. She began to actively reach for and pick up objects. She was able to operate a switch to turn on a mechanical toy that played music. Finally, she showed more interest in her environment and in what she could do herself to make things happen.

As the example illustrates, the occupational therapist was able to gather information from unstructured observation and discussion with Mary's mother. This information allowed the therapist to generate an understanding of Mary's volition and used it to guide therapy. Finally, it should be noted that at the time Mary was in therapy, the Pediatric Volitional Questionnaire (PVQ) (Geist, Kielhofner, Basu, & Kafkes, 2002) had not yet been developed. Such an instrument would be quite appropriate to incorporate along with unstructured methods in the evaluation of such a child.

Comprehensive Information Gathering

Both structured assessments and unstructured methods of information gathering have their special strengths and contributions to therapeutic reasoning. Structured assessments provide essential information in a format that is highly organized. Unstructured methods typically provide qualitative details that complement the information gathered in structured assessments. Therapists should begin by asking themselves the kinds of conceptual questions that were discussed in the previous chapter. Then, they should select and use the most appropriate structured assessments and unstructured methods to get answers to those questions.

Social Nature of Information Gathering

Asking people to give out personal information is not a neutral process (Luborsky, 1997). Clients often have strong feelings about the kinds of information therapists ask of them. After all, therapists use this information to form an opinion about clients. Further, therapists may, based on what they learn, take action or make recommendations that have profound influences on their clients' lives. What is determined from gathering information may affect such things as where a client is allowed or helped to live, whether a client returns to work, or if a client is eligible for further therapy or training.

Clients may be ambivalent about, distrust, or fear the therapist's assessment process. After all, what if it reveals something the client does not want to face or want others to know? When clients fear or distrust the assessment process, they will be less likely to share information openly. Sometimes, clients may actively mislead the therapist or selectively share information to manage what the therapist learns.

Clients may also feel that the assessment process is an invasion of privacy. In addition, when persons reveal things about themselves to someone who retains his or her own private identity, there is an uneven distribution of information. Giving someone else highly personal information potentially gives that person power over oneself. One person with a chronic disability recently told me that she did not feel like telling her life story to professionals because they would impart their own significance to it. She wanted her story to be her own and to control its meaning for herself. In her experience, professionals had not helped her manage her own life story, but rather questioned and interfered with her occupational identity.

Clients completing information-gathering procedures (e.g., interviews and written self reports) may see their answers as a reflection of their "social skills, competence, and self-image" (Luborsky, 1993, p. 11). Therefore, their responses can be influenced by how they perceive a therapist and believe the therapist is viewing them.

As a consequence, therapists should always pay careful attention to their demeanor in asking clients for information. Establishing a sense of trust and rapport with the client is essential to gaining dependable information. This is best achieved when the therapist:

- Is honest and direct with the client
- Informs the client about the nature and purpose of any data gathering
- Assures the client through word and action that the therapist has the client's best interests in mind
- Shows empathy for the client's experiences
- Demonstrates a genuine interest in knowing the client as a person.

A therapist who is mindful of how the client is feeling during any information gathering and consciously attempts to meets the needs of clients will gather much more dependable and in-depth information.

Getting Adequate Information

A therapist who does not take time to gather adequate information risks doing harm to the client in therapy. For example, an occupational therapist recently shared the following story. When the therapist asked her father, who recently had a stroke, about his experience in occupational therapy, he replied, "I hope I don't have to go back there, but I sure would like to find someone who could help me to shave myself." Unfortunately, while the occupational therapist had identified this man's perceptual and motor deficits, she had missed the most important point: to find out what he wanted to be able to do. Instead, he was putting pegs in an overhead board, a task that he found demeaning and depressing. Although the harm done to this gentleman may have been limited, it nevertheless contributed negatively to the quality of his remaining life. He died shortly thereafter.

Therapists are generally working under time constraints that do not allow endless information gathering. Thus, we must ask, "How much information is enough?" The answer to this question is not simple and will involve many considerations. Among them are the complexity of the client's problems and the amount of time allocated for intervention as well as assessment. The basic principle should always be that whatever action is taken in therapy, the therapist should have adequate information about the client to be sure that the therapy is in the best interest of the client and, whenever possible, that the client agrees with both the aim and method of the therapy.

Because there are always limitations on time and resources for gathering information, therapists should be careful to maximize the efficiency of their information gathering. One way of doing this is to proceed with information gathering at the broadest level, progressing to more detailed levels as the need is indicated by any problems (Trombly, 1993). For example, before therapists commence examining the underlying capacity of clients, they should first determine whether a client is able to fully participate in occupations and perform necessary occupational forms.

The questions offered in Chapter 11 can be a resource for guiding such an approach since they begin with broad issues and become more fine-tuned. If one follows such an approach in information gathering, it is unlikely that the therapist will miss something critical about the client. In the end, however, the approach to assessment should always be client centered—that is, based on the client's characteristics, needs, and wishes. After all, the purpose of information gathering is to come to know another human being to provide services useful to that person.

References

Baron, K., Kielhofner, G., Iyenger, A., Goldhammer, V., & Wolenski, J. (2002). *The Occupational Self Assessment (OSA) (Version 2.0)*. Chicago: Model of Human Occupation Clearinghouse, Department of Occupational Therapy, College of Applied Health Sciences, University of Illinois at Chicago.

Benson, J., & Schell, B. A. (1997). Measurement theory: Application to occupational and physical therapy. In J. Van Deusen & D. Brunt (Eds.), *Assessment in occupational therapy and physical therapy* (pp. 3–24). Philadelphia: WB Saunders.

Bonder, B. (1993). Issues in assessment of psychosocial components of function. *American Journal of Occupational Therapy, 47*, 211–216.

Denzin, N. K., & Lincoln, Y. S. (Eds.). (1994). *Handbook of qualitative research.* Thousand Oaks, CA: Sage Publications.

Fisher, A. G. (1999). *Assessment of motor and process skills* (3rd ed.). Ft. Collins, CO: Three Star Press.

Fisher, A. G., & Short-DeGraff, M. (1993). Improving functional assessment in occupational therapy: Recommendations and philosophy for change. *American Journal of Occupational Therapy, 47*, 199–201.

Forsyth, K., Lai, J., & Kielhofner, G. (1999). The assessment of communication and interaction skills (ACIS): Measurement properties. *British Journal of Occupational Therapy, 62*, 69–74.

Geist, R., Kielhofner, G., Basu, S., & Kafkes, A. (2002). *The Pediatric Volitional Questionnaire. (PVQ) (Version 2.0)*. Chicago: Model of Human Occupation Clearinghouse, Department of Occupational Therapy, College of Applied Health Sciences, University of Illinois at Chicago.

Hagner, D. C., & Helm, D. T. (1994).Qualitative methods in rehabilitation research. *Rehabilitation Counseling Bulletin, 37*, 290–303.

Hammersly, M. (1992). Some reflections on ethnography and validity. *Internal Journal of Qualitative Studies in Education, 5*, 195–203.

Kielhofner, G., Mallinson, T., Crawford, C., Nowak, M., Rigby, M., Henry, A., & Walens, D. (1998). *The Occupational Performance History Interview, (OPHI-II) (Version 2.0)*. Chicago: Model of Human Occupation Clearinghouse, Department of Occupational Therapy, College of Applied Health Sciences, University of Illinois at Chicago.

Krefting, L. (1989). Disability ethnography: A methodological approach for occupational therapy research. *Canadian Journal of Occupational Therapy, 56*, 61–66.

Luborsky, M. (1993). The romance with personal meaning in gerontology: Cultural aspects of life themes. *Gerontologist, 33*, 445–452.

Luborsky, M. (1997). Attuning assessment to the client: Recent advances in theory and methodology. *Generations, 21*, 10–15.

Miles, M. B., & Huberman, A. M. (Eds.). (1994). *Qualitative data analysis*. Thousand Oaks, CA: Sage Publications.

Tham K., Borell L., & Gustavsson A. (2000). The discovery of disability: A phenomenological study of unilateral neglect. *American Journal of Occupational Therapy, 54,* 398–406.

Trombly, C. (1993). Anticipating the future: Assessment of occupational function. *American Journal of Occupational Therapy, 47,* 253–257.

Watts, J. H., Brollier, C., Bauer, D., & Schmidt, W. (1989). The assessment of occupational functioning: The second revision. *Occupational Therapy in Mental Health, 8(4),* 61–87.

Wolcott, H. F. (1990). On seeking and rejecting validity in qualitative research. In E. W. Eisner & A. Peshkin (Eds.) *Qualitative inquiry in education: The continuing debate* (pp. 121–152). New York: Teachers College Press.

Wright B. D., & Linacre J. M. (1989). Observations are always ordinal: Measurements, however, must be interval. *Archives of Physical Medicine and Rehabilitation, 70,* 857–860.

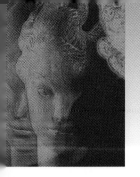

13

Observational Assessments

- **Gary Kielhofner**
- **Kirsty Forsyth**
- **Carmen Gloria de las Heras**
- **Junko Hayashi**
- **Jane Melton**
- **Laurie Raymond**

The four assessments discussed in this chapter gather information from observation of a client's behavior. Two of these assessments provide information on a client's skills:

- The Assessment of Motor and Process Skills
- The Assessment of Communication/Interaction Skills.

The other two provide information on a client's volition:

- The Volitional Questionnaire
- The Pediatric Volitional Questionnaire.

All four assessments are designed to capture qualitative information about the client that is entered as comments on the rating scale forms. The ratings provide profiles of strengths and weaknesses of the client and can be scored to provide measures of skill or volition.

Assessments of Skills

The Assessment of Motor and Process Skills (AMPS) (Fisher, 1999) and the Assessment of Communication and Interaction Skills (ACIS) (Forsyth, Salamy, Simon, & Kielhofner, 1998) have been developed to gather information on skills. Both the AMPS and the ACIS employ observation of clients performing occupational forms. The AMPS and ACIS represent a unique approach to assessing a client's ability to perform in every day occupational forms. These assessments provide detailed information about actual performance. They identify both strengths and difficulties a person demonstrates in doing a given occupational form.

Assessment of Motor and Process Skills

The Assessment of Motor and Process Skills (AMPS) (Fisher, 1999) gathers information on skills by observing the person doing selected activities of daily living, including personal activities of daily living as well as domestic or instrumental activities of daily living. A wide range of internationally and cross-culturally standardized tasks can be drawn on when administering the AMPS. The AMPS can be used with children (3-4 years of age and older), adolescents, and adults.

The AMPS consists of two scales that separately measure process and motor skills. The two scales are administered simultaneously, and this allows for direct evaluation of the interactive nature of motor and process skills such as the use of process skills to compensate for limitations in motor skills.

Each item on the two scales is scored with a four-point rating that considers the effectiveness, efficiency, and safety of a client's performance. The motor skills scale gathers information on the actions done to move oneself or objects. The process skills scale gathers information on the logical sequencing of actions, selec-

Assessment of Motor and Process Skills (AMPS)	*Gathers information about the motor and process skills that a person displays while engaging in occupation*	*Information on training at:* *AMPS Project* *Occupational Therapy Building* *Colorado State University* *Fort Collins, CO 80523* *or* *Visit http://www.colostate.edu/Programs/ AMPS*

tion and appropriate use of tools and materials, and adaptation to problems.

The AMPS yields a measure of both process and motor skills that takes into consideration the level of difficulty of the occupational forms the client was observed doing and that also adjusts for the tendency of the particular rater to be more severe or lenient in assigning ratings. To make these adjustments, the AMPS is scored by a computer. Moreover, raters must first be trained and calibrated as to their severity/leniency. After training, therapists are provided with software for computer scoring of the AMPS.

The AMPS provides detailed and useful information about how a person performs. For persons who have difficulty performing, the AMPS identifies what aspects of performance (i.e., skills) are problematic and how complex an occupational form the person can perform. The ratings of the items on both scales indicate areas of skill that are intact and areas in which the person is having difficulty. The AMPS also determines whether a person has the necessary motor and process skills needed for community living. Research has determined cut-off scores for both motor and process skills, below which persons have difficulty with community living.

ADMINISTRATION

Administration and scoring of the AMPS takes 30–60 minutes. The therapist first interviews the client and/or the client's caregiver to ensure that the client will be observed doing things he or she has experience performing and that are relevant. The therapist then selects four or five of the standardized occupational forms that are of an appropriate level of difficulty and relevant to the client. Next, the client chooses two or three that he or she will perform.

After observing the client's performance, the therapist scores the 16 motor and 20 process skill items and enters these scores into the computer. The AMPS computer program is used to generate AMPS instrumental activities of daily living (IADL) motor and process ability measures and a variety of reports that can be used for documentation, treatment planning, and research.

DEPENDABILITY

Numerous studies support the validity and reliability of the AMPS (Atchison, Fisher, & Bryze, 1998; Baron, 1994; Bernspång & Fisher, 1995, 1999; Darragh, Sample, & Fisher, 1998; Dickerson & Fisher, 1993; Doble, Fisk, Fisher, Ritvo, & Murray, 1994; Doble, Fisk, Lewis, & Rockwood, 1999; Duran & Fisher, 1996; Fisher, 1993, 1997; Fisher & Fisher, 1993; Nygård, Bernspång, Fisher, & Winblad, 1994; Pan & Fisher, 1994; Park, Fisher, & Velozo, 1994; Puderbaugh & Fisher, 1992; Robinson & Fisher, 1996). These studies support the internal consistency of the motor and process skills scales, the stability of the AMPS measures over time, and the ability of the measures to remain stable when the AMPS is scored by different raters. The AMPS scales are sensitive in detecting subtle but clinically meaningful differences in motor and process skills within and between individuals. The precision of the AMPS is based on its standardization on more than 12,000 subjects. The AMPS also has been shown to be valid in cross-cultural applications (Fisher, Liu, Velozo, & Pan, 1992; Goto, Fisher, Mayberry, 1996).

Andrew

Using the AMPS to Generate Environmental Supports for Independence

Andrew is a 50-year-old man with moderate intellectual impairment and chronic back pain that he has experienced since being in a car accident some years ago. Andrew is very tall and obese. He was referred to the occupational therapist and other members of a multidisciplinary team by his family physician due to concern that he was increasingly becoming unable to manage living independently.

Andrew had been living in a rented house in the English countryside outside London for 10 years, since his immediate family members had died. During this time, he managed to live in the house but his living conditions were often marginal. He had not attempted to organize or maintain his home environment. He had survived on preprepared convenience foods purchased from a local supermarket—a diet that contributed to his obesity. He had no awareness of the value of the money that he had accumulated from his state benefit. He had become increasingly isolated, and his only access to support was via a neighbor who assisted him with financial matters such as paying his rent and other household bills. Andrew was increasingly facing situations he could not manage without help. His hygiene had deteriorated. Moreover, he was growing more and more anxious about his situation.

Andrew identified that he had difficulty in carrying out many household chores. Among these were building the coal fire that heated his house and getting into the bath. The latter problem he perceived as due mainly to his back pain. Andrew was unemployed but had formerly worked as a farm and forestry laborer. He expressed a strong desire to learn to better control his environment and to have more social interaction. However, he was unsure as to whether or how this could be possible.

Choice and Use of the AMPS

Because Andrew was having difficulty performing his activities of daily living, the occupational therapist chose to use the AMPS to gather information on Andrew's motor and process skills. This assessment would also highlight his strengths and weaknesses in performing daily living tasks necessary for community living that he desired to improve.

The therapist identified five tasks of appropriate challenge for Andrew from the standardized tasks available in the AMPS. From these, Andrew chose to perform three tasks: preparing a cheese sandwich, preparing a fresh fruit salad, and hand washing dishes. He considered these occupational forms to be meaningful in his life.

The evaluation was carried out in the occupational therapy kitchen, as Andrew did not have all tools and equipment required for these tasks at home. Andrew engaged in a few practice sessions before the formal AMPS administration to allow him to become familiar and practiced in the activities and the environment.

Results of the Evaluation

Andrew scored 2.0 on the motor skill scale and 1.1 on the process scale. Both scores indicate that he is on the borderline where skill deficits begin to negatively impact on performance of daily living tasks and where the majority of people experience difficulty with independent living.

AMPS also identified Andrew's adequate motor and process skills along with specific areas of difficulty during performance, as indicated in *Figure 13-1.*

Andrew demonstrated ineffective motor skills across all his performance in the following areas:

- Positioning and bending the body appropriately to the task
- Coordinating two body parts to securely stabilize task objects
- Maintaining a secure grasp on task objects.

In the area of process skills, Andrew experienced difficulty in:

- Choosing appropriate tools and materials
- Using objects according to their intended purpose
- Heeding (attending to the purpose of) the specific occupational form he was doing
- Inquiring about necessary information
- Initiating actions or steps without hesitation
- Organizing tools and materials in an orderly, logical, and spatially appropriate fashion

FIGURE 13-1   Andrew's Strengths and Problems Observed During the Administration of the AMPS.

Motor Skills	A	D	MD
Posture			
STABILIZING the body for balance	X		
ALIGNING the body in vertical position	X		
POSITIONING the body or arms appropriate to task		X	
Mobility			
WALKING: moving about the task environment (level surface)	X		
REACHING for task objects	X		
BENDING or rotating the body appropriate to the task		X	
Coordination			
COORDINATING two body parts to securely stabilize task objects		X	
MANIPULATING task objects	X		
FLOWS: executing smooth and fluid arm and hand movements	X		
Strength and Effort			
MOVES: pushing and pulling task objects or level surfaces or opening and closing doors or drawers	X		
TRANSPORTING task objects from one place to another	X		
LIFTING objects used during the task	X		
CALIBRATES: regulating the force and extent of movements	X		
GRIPS: maintaining a secure grasp on task objects		X	
Energy			
ENDURING for the duration of the task performance	X		
Maintaining an even and appropriate PACE during task performance	X		
Process Skills			
Energy			
Maintaining an even and appropriate PACE during task performance	X		
Maintaining focused ATTENTION throughout task performance	X		
Using Knowledge			
CHOOSING appropriate tools and materials needed for task performance		X	
USING task objects according to their intended purposes		X	
Knowing when and how to stabilize and support or HANDLE task objects	X		
HEEDING the goal of the specified task		X	
INQUIRES: asking for needed information		X	
Temporal Organization			
INITIATING actions or steps of task without hesitation		X	
CONTINUING actions through to completion	X		
Logically SEQUENCING the steps of the tasks	X		
TERMINATING actions or steps at the appropriate time	X		

Rating Key: **A** = Adequate, **D** = Difficulty, **MD** = Markedly Deficient

continued

FIGURE 13-1 (*Continued*)

Process Skills (continued)	A	D	MD
Space and Objects			
SEARCHING for AND LOCATING tools nd materials	X		
GATHERING tools and materials into the task workforce	X		
ORGANIZING tools and materials in an orderly, logical, and spatially appropriate fashion		X	
RESTORES: putting away tools and materials or straightening the workplace			X
NAVIGATES: maneuvering the hand and body around obstacles	X		
Adaptation			
NOTICING AND RESPONDING appropriately to nonverbal task-related environmental cues		X	
ACCOMMODATES: modifying one's actions to overcome problems		X	
ADJUSTS: changing the workspace to overcome problems	X		
BENEFITS: preventing problems from recurring or persisting		X	

Rating Key: **A** = Adequate, **D** = Difficulty, **MD** = Markedly Deficient

- Navigating (appropriately moving) his hands and body around objects
- Noticing and responding to nonverbal task-related environmental cues
- Accommodating his actions to overcome problems
- Benefiting from experience to prevent reoccurrence of problems.

Finally, his skill in restoring (i.e., putting away tools and materials or clearing work surfaces) was markedly deficient.

Interpretation of the Results

In the area of motor skills, the following qualitative observations also were made during the AMPS assessment. Andrew used inappropriate biomechanical lifting techniques that, combined with his old back injury impairment, limited his ability to effectively bend or lift from a low height. These problems were exacerbated by the fact that standard work surfaces were not ergonomically suitable for Andrew. Because of his physique, his body and arm positioning in relation to work surfaces and objects made performance more difficult for him.

Andrew's problem with gripping objects appears related to his experience. The therapist determined through interviewing Andrew that he had mainly used gross motor skills in most of his lifetime occupations. Thus, his fine motor finger and hand function was not well developed and limited his performance in occupational forms that required fine motor skill.

In the area of process skills, it was clear Andrew had problems in performing the newly learned tasks. For example, when preparing the sandwich he did not incorporate some ingredients he had previously decided to include. When asked about this following the evaluation, Andrew said that he had "forgotten." This exemplifies Andrews's general difficulty with completing all the steps or components of an occupational form. This same problem is echoed within other skill areas, such as restoration of objects to their original condition and location after finishing. Andrew also appeared to misinterpret or misunderstand some information that he received. This is made more problematic since Andrew did not seek clarification.

Andrew hesitated when beginning and during familiar tasks. He organized his workspace so that it was crammed. He used some tools in such a way that he could have injured himself. He generally had difficulty adapting to his environment and responding to environmental changes.

Despite Andrew's problems in both motor and process skills, he did have many adequate skills. These strengths indicated that he did not require assistance at all times during performance. Identification of Andrew's problem areas pointed to the specific kinds of supports that would allow him the opportunity and confidence to engage safely in routine occupational performance. By examining each area of weakness, the therapist was able to identify and implement corresponding strategies of environmental support.

Usefulness of the Information for Therapeutic Reasoning

With the information provided by the motor scale, the occupational therapist was able to make specific recommendations that Andrew's environment be suitably adapted to accommodate his motor needs. His motor skills problems were linked to two factors:

- His use of poor body mechanics related to his back
- The lack of fit between household objects and his unusually large stature.

Consequently, the following strategies were undertaken to assist him. His kitchen was modified with consideration to his height. Household equipment was purchased and installed to limit difficult bending or lifting. For example, he purchased a front-loading washing machine and his small refrigerator was elevated to waist height. His bathroom was altered to incorporate a walk-in shower and a raised toilet. His bed was modified to be suitably supportive and of the correct height. A chair to suit his stature was purchased. Finally, a referral was made to physiotherapy to teach him proper techniques and exercises for his back.

By identifying his weaknesses, the process scale highlighted Andrew's need for regular assistance with some tasks and prompting with others, as well as the need for support for problem-solving when faced with difficult or novel situations. The following resources were developed to address these ongoing needs. The occupational therapist and community support worker developed protocols for empowering Andrew to carry out tasks as independently as possible but within his skill capacity. For example, they created pictorial shopping lists, recipe cards, and telephone number lists for Andrew. Methods of carrying out the routine things that Andrew did were developed to consider his process skills. The information generated about process skills identified strengths and weaknesses An-

drew would bring to performance and, thereby, pointed to environmental supports he would need. For example, tending to the fire that heated his home was split into component parts; Andrew does what he can safely complete, and his care worker completes the other parts.

Andrew also attended a community group run by the occupational therapist and community nurse to address issues of safety at home. Furthermore, with support Andrew enrolled in a basic literacy college course. As Andrew gained awareness of his own capacities, his sense of efficacy improved significantly. With the regular support he received at home, he was able to function safely and with a reasonable degree of independence.

As this case illustrates, the AMPS provides critical, objective information concerning occupational performance that guides therapists in making decisions about therapy. It is also useful for documenting the need for resources that enable persons to perform in the community. The comprehensiveness and precision of the AMPS in providing detailed and research-based information makes it an important asset in understanding and meeting a client's performance needs.

Assessment of Communication and Interaction Skills

The Assessment of Communication and Interaction Skills (ACIS) is a formal observational tool designed to measure an individual's performance in an occupational form within a social group (Forsyth et al., 1998). The instrument allows occupational therapists to determine a client's strengths and weaknesses in interacting and communicating with others in the course of daily occupations. The ACIS has been developed for use in a wide range of settings.

ACIS observations are carried out in contexts that are meaningful and relevant to the clients' lives. Because social situations cannot be standardized with the same precision as solitary occupational forms (such as those used in the AMPS), the ACIS does not adjust scores for the type of social group or task in which the person is observed. Rather, a format exists for classifying the context of observation and its degree of ap-

Assessment of Communication and Interaction Skills (ACIS)	*Gathers information about the communication skills that a person displays while engaged in occupation*	*Information on ordering can be found on the Model of Human Occupation Clearinghouse web site at:* *http://www.uic.edu/hsc/acad/cahp/OT/MOHOC* *Or go to: http://www.uic.edu* *Link to:* *1) Academic Departments* *2) Applied Health Sciences* *3) Occupational Therapy* *4) MOHO*

proximation to the kind of everyday social situations in which the client does or wants to perform. The therapist seeks to make observations in the client's actual environment or in contexts that resemble the client's environment as much as possible. The group context can range from a dyadic interaction to participation in a large group. A wide range of group contexts can be used for observation. These include task-oriented groups, meetings, work teams, games, and other leisure events.

The ACIS contains a single scale that consists of 20 skill items divided into 3 communication and interaction domains: physicality, information exchange, and relations. The items are rated on a four-point scale similar to that of the AMPS but with a focus on the impact of the skills on both the progression of the social interaction and occupational form, as well as the impact on other persons with whom the client interacts. For example, the scale considers whether others are made comfortable, appropriately informed, and helped by the actions of the client. Because the rating of communication and interaction requires judgment about appropriateness to the social context, the therapist using the scale must have social competence to understand the norms and expectations of the context.

Although formal development of the instrument has centered on clients with psychiatric impairments, the instrument has been successfully used with clients who have a wide range of impairments. The ACIS is used when a client appears to have difficulty in communication and interaction or when the client reports such difficulty. Research to date has focused on adolescents and adults, but the scale appears to be appropriate for children who are at the age when the full range

of basic communication and interaction skills are ordinarily developed (i.e., older than 3–4 years).

ADMINISTRATION

The ACIS is supported by a detailed manual designed to instruct and guide the therapist in its use (Forsyth et al., 1998). The manual provides criteria for applying the rating to each item, supported by examples. The therapist begins by interviewing the client (or a significant other) to ascertain what types of contexts would be appropriate and meaningful for observing the client. To administer the ACIS, the occupational therapist observes clients' communication and social interaction while they engage with others as part of completing an occupational form. The observing therapist can be the group leader or participant. Therefore, the ACIS can be administered during a therapeutic group.

The total administration time for the ACIS varies from 20–60 minutes. Observation time ranges from 15–45 minutes. The rating is completed after conclusion of the session. Rating time ranges from 5–20 minutes depending on the amount of qualitative comments the therapist wishes to enter into the form. It may be possible to observe more than one person during an observation session; however, the dependability of doing so has not yet been examined in research.

In its current state of development, the ACIS is most effectively used to generate a profile of strengths and weaknesses and qualitative details about any client's problems. This profile is the most important source of information for deciding what skills to target for change. In addition, the qualitative information gained in the course of administering the ACIS is often helpful for understanding why a particular client is having difficulty with some communication/interaction skills. A final use of the ACIS is to identify social environments that have the most positive impact on the client's communication and interaction. Since ACIS scores may vary with the environmental context, the more supportive contexts will produce higher scores. Such information can be useful in deciding what kinds of group assignment or living placement is best for a client.

DEPENDABILITY

Simon (1989) found modest interrater reliability with the first version of the ACIS. Salamy (1993) revised the ACIS and found evidence that the items worked well together to constitute a single scale of communication/interaction. Her findings also indicated the need for further revision. Subsequently, Forsyth (1996) made extensive revisions in the ACIS scale. In a study of persons who had a wide range of psychosocial impairments, findings suggested the revised scale items work together to form a single valid measure of communication/interaction skills (Forsyth, Lai, & Kielhofner, 1999). Moreover, consistency was found between and within a large sample of raters. Further research examining the dependability of the ACIS is currently underway. Future plans include developing a paper-and-pencil method of obtaining an interval measure from the ratings. Measures for research purposes can be generated via computer analysis, but because the plans are to provide a method of manual scoring, no computer program for clinical scoring has been developed.

Doug

Using the ACIS to Understand and Address Problematic Social Behavior

Doug was a 17-year-old student in a special education classroom for students with intellectual deficits. He had a diagnosis of Down's syndrome and was considered to have moderate intellectual impairment. Doug sometimes exhibited aggressive behavior and was deemed a troublemaker in and outside the classroom by the teacher and an aide. They had attempted for some time to use punishments and rewards to change Doug's interactional problems.

However, their efforts had little effect on Doug. Consequently, the occupational therapist was asked to evaluate Doug's social skills and make recommendations concerning managing his disruptiveness and aggression.

The occupational therapist observed Doug in the classroom, during recess, and during lunchtime (all natural contexts in which Doug was expected to perform in the school). Ratings and comments based on these three observations are shown in *Figure 13-2*. The comments reflect the composite of these observations. Doug demonstrated mostly adequate skills in the area of information exchange. In contrast, he had problems with physicality and relations.

In the area of physicality Doug had the following skill problems. When he was excited or angry he tended to use physical forms of contact (e.g., hugging, kissing, shoving, and grabbing) that made others uncomfortable or upset. He often failed to make eye contact, except when he was angry. In the latter situation he would "stare down" the person with whom he was angry. Doug had a tendency to stand too close to people, making them uncomfortable. He appeared to have little awareness of others' reactions to his behaviors. In fact, when others withdrew in reaction to some of his inappropriate physical interaction, he would continue or intensify the offending behavior. For example, he would try to move closer and closer to someone who was uncomfortable with his proximity, or shove someone harder when they tried to ignore him after a first push.

Doug also had problems with engaging others. He often initiated interactions in ways that made others uncomfortable. He often failed to respect social norms such as picking up and using others' possessions and going ahead of others in line. He also had difficulties asserting himself. Doug seemed to be unaware of how to make requests and tended to "bully" others when he wanted something. He often did this with a playful attitude. Nevertheless, this playful aggressiveness tended to make others uncomfortable.

As with his difficulties in the physical domain, Doug seemed to engage in these behaviors with

FIGURE 13-2   Doug's Scores and Comments on the ACIS.

	Observational Situation			Comments
	Classsroom	Recess	Lunchtime	
PHYSICALITY				
Contacts	1	1	1	Hits others to get attention. Hits others when angry
Gazes	1	2	1	Avoids eye contact in many interactions. When angry, he stares
Gestures	3	2	2	Sometimes exaggerates gestures
Maneuvers	3	2	2	Accidentally bumps into others
Orients	2	2	1	Sometimes turns away from social action
Postures	2	1	1	Sometimes looms threateningly over others
INFORMATION EXCHANGE				
Articulates	3	3	3	No major problems; often talks very fast
Asserts	2	2	2	Is aggresive instead of assertive
Asks	3	3	3	Generally okay, sometimes gets a bit demanding
Engages				Is effective at initiating conversation, often uses poor strategies to engage others (e.g., hitting, hugging)
Expresses	3	3	2	Can share information and feelings effectively, except when he is upset
Modulates	2	3	2	Tends to speak too loudly
Shares	3	3	3	Can respond when others ask
Speaks	3	3	3	Generally can make himself understood
Sustains	3	3	3	Is able to keep up interaction if he is interested
RELATIONS				
Collaborates	2	1	1	Can work for a while with others in a structured game or task with clear supervision, but tends to break rules or goof off in an apparent attempt to gain attention
Conforms	2	1	1	Often transgresses social rules. For example, he takes other people's food; forces his way in line
Focuses	2	2	2	Can maintain focus for a while, but is easily distracted or bored
Relates	2	3	2	Can be genuinely nice to be with, but has problems when upset. Can become overly aggressive in seeking attention, or trying to get his way
Respects	2	1	1	Has trouble reading others' cues and seems unaware of their discomfort with his behavior

Rating Key : **4** = Competent, **3** = Questionable, **2** = Ineffective, **1** = Deficit

limited understanding of how his behavior was received by others. Doug was clearly motivated to interact with others and liked their attention to him when he received it. His difficulty in being able to get his social needs met in ways that fit the needs or expectations of others meant that he was often engaged in tense interactions with others who were either fleeing or avoiding him or reacting angrily to his transgressions. Therefore, much of Doug's social interaction was marked by strain, conflict, and negative affect. The assessment revealed that while Doug was motivated for positive interactions, he lacked the skill to be able to accomplish his desires. He did not so much disregard others as he had difficulty in being able to "see" his own behavior and "read" its impact on others.

Using the ACIS Information in Deciding Intervention

Based on the assessment, the therapist undertook social skills training, using two major strategies. The first was to enable Doug to be more aware of his own social actions and their impact on others. The therapist first reviewed videotapes of Doug in the classroom with him, guiding him to watch himself and to watch others' reactions to him. To assist Doug in being better able to read others, reactions to his behavior, the therapist practiced with Doug identifying and labeling various facial expressions and gestures of others. These exercises were aimed at helping Doug identify how people felt inside based on how they appeared to him. As the practice sessions took place, it was clear that Doug had limited awareness of what others were feeling and trying to communicate to him. With practice he was able to identify basic emotions of others from various cues they gave.

The second strategy was to provide Doug with specific training related to the skills in which he had shown the most difficulty. For example, he practiced how to initiate interactions with others, how to assert himself without becoming aggressive, and how to make socially acceptable physical contact. The therapist devised simple role-playing situations in which Doug could practice appropriate skills such as greeting others, asking for things, and waiting in line. These role-play situations were based on everyday occurrences in the classroom and playground, so that Doug would not be expected to generalize his social behaviors to situations he had not practiced. It was clear that his understanding of social contexts was limited, so he did best when he learned a behavior in the actual context in which he was expected to display it. Once again, videotape was used to allow Doug to see his own behavior and to illustrate differences between acceptable and unacceptable behavior.

As this case illustrates, the ACIS is useful for providing a detailed profile of strengths and weaknesses in communication and interaction skills. The structured observation also allows the therapist to identify a profile of strengths and weaknesses and to collect qualitative information that helps pinpoint the nature of a person's problem in communication and interaction. Such information enables the therapist to target specific skills for intervention and to devise strategies that are most likely to help the client improve skills.

Volitional Questionnaire and Pediatric Volitional Questionnaire

The Volitional Questionnaire (VQ) (de las Heras, Geist, Kielhofner, & Li, 2002), and the Pediatric Volitional Questionnaire (PVQ) (Geist, Kielhofner, Basu, & Kafkes, 2002) are assessments designed to gather information on volition from observation. These two assessments were developed for use with persons who could not effectively report their own volition because they had more severe functional impairments and/or severely restricted volition. Before the development of the VQ and PVQ, there was no structured volitional assessment available for use with persons who were unable to complete the checklists or respond to the interviews otherwise used to gather data on volition. The PVQ is designed for toddlers (ages 2–6), and the VQ is used with older children, adolescents, and adults.

Both assessments are used as part of direct interventions. However, because persons with severe functional problems and/or volitional difficulties often receive services from a variety of caregivers including family members, the assessments are also used as a basis for consultation. They have proven particularly useful in this regard because they generate information about both the client's volitional traits and how environmental factors affect volition. Such information can readily translate into recommendations for multidisciplinary intervention strategies and for family members to enhance clients' motivation and involvement in doing things. The instruments can also be useful in revealing motivational factors that contribute to problematic behaviors and, therefore, in identifying effective strategies for reducing or eliminating such behaviors.

Volitional Questionnaire (VQ) Pediatric Volitional Questionnaire (PVQ)	*Gather information about volition (motivation) and about impact of environment on volition*	*Information on ordering can be found on the Model of Human Occupation Clearinghouse web site at:* http://www.uic.edu/hsc/acad/cahp/OT/MOHOC *Or go to:* http://www.uic.edu *Link to:* **1) Academic Departments** **2) Applied Health Sciences** **3) Occupational Therapy** **4) MOHO**

Volitional Questionnaire

The Volitional Questionnaire (VQ) is appropriate for any individual for whom self-report assessment of volition is not readily feasible (e.g., individuals with dementia or brain damage or persons with extreme volitional problems due to environmental stresses or social traumas). The VQ is based on the recognition that clients, who have difficulty formulating goals or expressing their interests and values verbally, routinely communicate them through actions. For example, persons indicate interest by how much energy they direct to doing something or the affect they display while doing it. Thus, the VQ scale is composed of 14 items that describe behaviors reflecting values, interests, and personal causation. The items are scored using a four-point rating (passive, hesitant, involved, and spontaneous). The rating indicates the extent to which the client readily exhibits volitional behaviors versus the amount of support, encouragement, and structure that is necessary to elicit volitionally relevant action. The scale reflects the fact that persons with higher volition choose action and demonstrate positive affect more readily, whereas persons with more limited volition need additional environmental resources and supports.

The VQ recognizes that a client's motivation will vary in different environments according to how much the features of each environment match the client's interests, values, and personal causation. Consequently, the client is observed in a number of contexts (ordinarily three to five) in which the physical and social environmental conditions are varied. An environmental form can be used to record information about relevant features of the environment that affect volition. Con-

sequently, the therapists using the VQ gather information on how various environmental features affect the client's volition as well as information about the client's volitional strengths and weaknesses.

Research on the VQ (Chern, Kielhofner, de las Heras, & Magalhaes, 1996) shows that the items on the scale are ordered in a particular sequence from less to more volition. This sequence indicates a volitional continuum that begins with basic behaviors such as being able to indicate preferences and initiate action. Higher levels of volition are indicated by the client's willingness to try to solve problems or correct mistakes and in the display of pride. The highest level of volition is indicated by such behaviors as seeking challenges and new responsibilities. Practical experience with the VQ indicates that a client's improvement in volition ordinarily reflects the sequence of lower to higher volition noted above. A specific intervention protocol, the re-motivation process, has been developed for persons with volitional problems (de las Heras, Llerena, & Kielhofner, 2002). This protocol involves constant use of the VQ to guide intervention and monitor client progress.

ADMINISTRATION

The VQ is supported by a detailed manual that discusses the purpose and uses of the VQ and describes the administration protocol in detail (de las Heras et al., 2002). Each of the items on the VQ scale is explained in terms of what it is intended to capture. Guidelines for rating each item are supported by multiple examples. The manual is designed for therapists who wish to learn administration of the VQ through self-study.

Occupational therapists administer this scale by observing and rating patients while they engage in work, leisure, or daily living tasks. As noted above, the four-point rating indicates the amount of volitional spontaneity (versus passivity or need for support and encouragement) the individual demonstrates. Because of the nature of the rating scale, the observing therapist can provide support and structure if it is necessary to elicit volition. This feature of the VQ means that it can be administered as part of a therapy session and that it can be used to explore what kind of environmental supports enhance a given client's volition.

As noted above, the therapist selects three to five contexts in which to observe a client. The strategies for selecting the contexts of observation vary with each client, but the underlying goals are to identify:

- Those factors in the social and physical environment that most affect volition both positively and negatively
- How stable or variable volition is across environments
- The level of motivation a client typically displays
- The kinds of environmental supports that enhance the individual's volition
- The client's interests and values.

This kind of information allows the therapist to determine the environmental contexts and strategies that will facilitate positive development of the individual's volition.

Following each observation, the therapist completes the environmental form and the rating scale. When therapists have completed the planned observations, they conclude by writing a brief narrative that describes:

- The client's interests and values
- The amount and kind of support required for the client to accomplish a behavior
- The influence of values, interests, and personal causation on the client's motivation to engage in activities
- The influence of different environments on the client's volition.

Observation periods ordinarily last approximately 15–30 minutes. The scale and the environmental form can be completed in less than 10 minutes. Because the assessment can be administered as part of a therapy session in which the environment is systematically var-

ied, it can be used efficiently to explore how different environmental factors influence volition. The VQ is also useful for monitoring volitional change over time.

DEPENDABILITY

The first study to examine the reliability and validity of the VQ was completed by de las Heras (1993a, 1993b). Content validity was verified by a panel of experts. The instrument also showed adequate interrater reliability. Differences in client volition across environments supported the conclusion that volition is influenced by the environment and highlighted the importance of evaluating volition in different settings.

In two studies Chern, Kielhofner, de las Heras, & Magalhaes (1996) examined the validity of this instrument. The first of these studies indicated that the items of the VQ reflect a single construct of volition. However, this study also found that the instrument was not as sensitive as desired in discriminating between persons with different levels of volition. Following revision of the scale, the second study found that the revised scale was more discriminating. Additional revision of the scale has been undertaken to improve its dependability further, and empirical examination of the revised scale's properties is planned. There are also plans to develop a paper-and-pencil method of determining a measure of volition. In the meantime, noting the person's profile of strengths and weaknesses and the degree to which the person demonstrates higher-level volitional behaviors provide a qualitative index of the person's level of volition.

Reiko

Using the VQ to Enhance Intervention Effectiveness

Reiko is a 75-year old woman who until recently lived in an apartment in Hiroshima. For 15 years Reiko had lived alone after her only daughter and husband both died. She had been very active and self-sufficient. Nine months ago she moved into a nursing home because of mild dementia. Most recently, she had a stroke that left her with incomplete left hemiplegia and some unilateral neglect. She has just begun a 3-month term of rehabilitation that is standard in Japan. The rehabilitation goal is to maximize Rieko's independence in the nursing home.

Since her stroke, Reiko has taken no initiative or responsibility. She passively follows the schedule decided by the medical staff. She attends and complies with therapies daily but lacks energy and autonomy. Moreover, her degree of dependence in self-care is greater than would be expected given the nature of her impairments. She does not initiate any activity on her own, needing to be encouraged and led by someone throughout the day. All these factors are indicative of low volition. Therefore, the VQ was used to better understand Reiko's volition and how the environment impacted on it.

The therapist used the VQ to observe Reiko four times over a 5-day period. Three of the four observations were done as part of a regularly scheduled therapy session. A fourth took place during lunchtime. In this way, the therapist's actual time for administration was minimal.

Reiko's VQ scores differed significantly across these observations, as shown in *Figure 13-3*. This indicates that her volition was very dependent on context. During the first observation, Reiko was painting a simple picture (a flower) as part of a craft group. The painting had been chosen by the therapist who led the group to increase attention to the left side of her visual space. Reiko passively followed all the therapist's instructions and continued painting until the therapist told her the session was over. Her volition scores were mainly passive in this context. When asked, she indicated she was unaware of the therapeutic goal of the painting and did not like doing it.

Reiko was observed the second time while having lunch in the ward dining area. She had to use a spoon instead of chopsticks and had to be prompted to find some of her food because of her neglect. Although there were others in the area, she chose to sit and eat alone and not interact. In this context her VQ scores were mostly in the hesitant range.

In session 3, Reiko was changing into pajamas as part of activities of daily living training. The therapist was very supportive, gave cues, and pointed out mistakes. Reiko was cooperative but seemed overwhelmed by the dressing task. She only did what the therapist prompted her to do and did not seem to take an active interest in the dressing task.

FIGURE 13.3   Reiko's Scores on the VQ.

Environmental Context	Painting				Eating				Dressing				Making Rice Cake Balls			
1. Shows curiosity	P	H	I	S	P	H	I	S	P	H	I	S	P	H	I	S
2. Initiates actions/tasks	P	H	I	S	P	H	I	S	P	H	I	S	P	H	I	S
3. Tries new things	P	H	I	S	P	H	I	S	P	H	I	S	P	H	I	S
4. Shows pride	P	H	I	S	P	H	I	S	P	H	I	S	P	H	I	S
5. Attempts challenges	P	H	I	S	P	H	I	S	P	H	I	S	P	H	I	S
6. Seeks additional responsibilities	P	H	I	S	P	H	I	S	P	H	I	S	P	H	I	S
7. Tries to correct mistakes	P	H	I	S	P	H	I	S	P	H	I	S	P	H	I	S
8. Tries to solve problems	P	H	I	S	P	H	I	S	P	H	I	S	P	H	I	S
9. Shows preferences	P	H	I	S	P	H	I	S	P	H	I	S	P	H	I	S
10. Pursues activity to completion/ accomplishment	P	H	I	S	P	H	I	S	P	H	I	S	P	H	I	S
11. Stays engaged	P	H	I	S	P	H	I	S	P	H	I	S	P	H	I	S
12. Invests additional energy/ emotion/attention	P	H	I	S	P	H	I	S	P	H	I	S	P	H	I	S
13. Indicates goals	P	H	I	S	P	H	I	S	P	H	I	S	P	H	I	S
14. Shows that an activity is special or significant	P	H	I	S	P	H	I	S	P	H	I	S	P	H	I	S

Rating Key : **P** = Passive, **H** = Hesitant, **I** = Involved, **S** = Spontaneous

Once again her dominant score on the VQ was hesitant.

In session 4, her volition was much different from that in other sessions. She was invited to the group to make rice cake balls that are traditional work at the end of the year in Japan. She chose to sit at a table with other clients and immediately started making rice cake balls without encouragement by the therapist. She continued working until the task was done. During the task she smiled, communicated with others, and was very lively. She clearly enjoyed the activity. In this observation her VQ scores were mainly involved.

The four VQ observations revealed volitional strengths and weaknesses as well as critical information about how the environment influenced Reiko. Her strengths included:

- Reiko was very motivated when presented with a familiar, relatively simple, and culturally meaningful occupational form
- Reiko was very responsive to her therapist's encouragement.

Some of Reiko's volitional weaknesses were:

- When she perceived a task as too complex she became totally passive, relying on the therapist to guide her
- She appeared not to feel in control of her own performance much of the time
- She did not take an interest in therapeutic or self-care activities; this seemed linked to generalized feelings of being out of control and her lack of awareness of the purpose of doing these things
- Unless she had a context that encouraged joining others, she tended to isolate herself.

It was also clear that while Reiko passively acquiesced to the therapist's instructions, she was not invested in, nor did she pay attention to, the activity sufficiently to benefit. Giving a lot of verbal instructions actually made Reiko more confused and passive. Consequently, she was not really gaining anything in the activities of daily living training or activities designed to address her neglect. Although very compliant, she was not really benefiting from the therapy. Also, she appeared to lack interest generally because activities of daily living were so difficult for her. It was not apparent from her performance how she would ever be able to do them.

The factors in the environment that appeared to most affect her volition were:

- Whether the occupational form and social group were meaningful and understood
- How complex the occupational form, objects, and space were (if too complex, she became overwhelmed and passive)
- Whether there was social support and encouragement.

Resulting Changes in the Therapeutic Environment

The insights to Reiko's volition and the environmental impact on it indicated the following changes in her therapy:

- There were increased opportunities for Reiko to do familiar/traditional Japanese occupational forms with her peers and to do things in which she was previously interested. These volitionally relevant occupational forms clearly motivated her and stimulated her to engage in social interaction. Within such activities she could be encouraged and coached to attend the neglected side.
- Given Reiko's neglect and mild dementia, the physical environment for any performance was simplified so that doing things was not so overwhelming
- When practicing activities of daily living, she was to do only small components that she could successfully complete (e.g., only putting on one piece of clothing at a time) so she could feel a sense of accomplishment
- Challenging occupational forms were done individually, so Reiko could receive constant encouragement and support from the therapist. They were done slowly and one step at a time, so Reiko was not overwhelmed with instructions
- When she tried new things that were harder, the therapist took extra time to explain what they were doing and why, as well as to remind her throughout of their purpose
- Her accomplishment was acknowledged when she completed each step in a task to provide constant positive feedback.

In sum, the VQ gave important insights into Reiko's volition that informed better strategies for therapy. As the case illustrates, the VQ can be useful in discovering the kind of therapeutic strategies that will be most meaningful for a client. Notably, these strategies are useful not only to address motivation, but also to enhance the efficacy of therapy in increasing occupational participation.

Pediatric Volitional Questionnaire

The Pediatric Volitional Questionnaire (PVQ) (Geist et al. 2002) is an observational assessment that is similar to the VQ and intends to capture a younger child's volition. The PVQ was originally developed for and studied on children aged 2–6 years. In practice, many clinicians find it useful for older children and even adolescents who have significant developmental delays.

The items on the PVQ parallel many of those on the VQ, but the items are designed to be developmentally appropriate to younger children. This accounts for the practical relevance of the tool to clients who are chronologically older than 6 years but developmentally suited for the assessment. Like the VQ, the items are rated on a four-point scale (passive, hesitant, involved, and spontaneous). By systematically capturing how children react to and act within their environments, the PVQ provides both insight into the child's motivation and information about how the environment supports or constrains the child's volition.

Children with cognitive or motor problems that limit their ability to act on the world need support and development of their volition. However, their volition is ordinarily the most difficult to understand. When children are unable to express their likes, dislikes, confidence, or fears, there is a greater challenge to understand how they are motivated. Nonetheless, a great deal can be learned about children's motives by observing how they go about doing things. Withdrawal, enthusiasm, hesitation, and persistence are all examples of observable behavior patterns that reveal important things about a child's volition. By providing a means of systematically observing such behavior patterns, the PVQ yields a picture of a child's volition.

The PVQ is also designed to gather information on how the environment influences the child's volition. An environmental form is used to systematically record in-

formation on the environments in which the child is observed. Use of the PVQ ordinarily involves observation of the child in different contexts to determine environmental impacts on volition. Alternatively, the therapist may create different conditions within therapy to examine how different conditions in the environment affect the child's volition. With such information, the therapist can alter or make recommendations for altering the physical and social environment to maximize the child's desire for action and his or her feeling of accomplishment and enjoyment. The PVQ also provides qualitative information that can be used in designing treatment programs and interventions as well as for providing feedback and suggestions to parents, teachers, or other caregivers.

ADMINISTRATION

The PVQ is explained in a detailed manual that discusses its purpose, uses, and administration protocol (Geist et al. 2002). Each of the items on the PVQ scale is explained in terms of what it is intended to capture. Guidelines for rating each item are supported by examples. Notably, the examples in this manual include children with a wide range of functioning. Therefore, the PVQ can readily be applied to children with a wide array of impairments. The manual is designed for therapists who wish to learn administration of the PVQ through self-study. A videotape is also available for therapists to observe and practice the rating procedure.

The PVQ consists of a 14-item rating scale that systematically captures information about the child's volition. In addition to the rating scale, there are forms for collecting information on features of the environment that impact volition and on the child's volitionally influenced style of interacting with the environment.

The therapist begins application of the assessment with observation of the child in play and/or self-care. It is recommended that the therapist observe the child in different contexts to determine how different environmental factors affect the child's volition. Appropriate settings include the classroom, home, playroom, playground, and clinic. The therapist ordinarily observes the child for 15–30 minutes in each context.

After the observation, the therapist completes the rating scale and, if desired, adds qualitative comments to this scale. These comments ordinarily explain the rationale for or elaborate the ratings that were assigned to the child. At the bottom of the PVQ scale, the therapist summarizes main issues relevant to the child's volition. The PVQ includes forms to systematically consider how different contexts influence the child's volition.

DEPENDABILITY

Geist (1998) first examined the PVQ using 13 occupational therapists who learned the PVQ through study of the manual. These therapists rated videotapes of nondisabled children. The study indicated that all the items of the scale worked well together to capture volition. The arrangement of the items from more to less volition also supported the validity of the scale. That is, they paralleled the continuum found in the VQ. As expected, there was a difference of volition in the two environments examined (classroom and playground), with children exhibiting higher volition in the playground. All the raters were able to use the PVQ in a valid manner, indicating that the assessment can be learned adequately from the supporting manual.

In a subsequent study, Anderson (1998) added ratings based on children with a wide range of disabilities to the pool of ratings based on children without disabilities. Once again, the items were shown to work well together to capture the intended construct of volition. Grouping of the items from less to more volition also paralleled findings with the VQ and from the first study. At the lowest end were behaviors such as exploring novelty, initiating actions, and producing effects. At the next level were behaviors such as practicing skills and trying to solve problems. At the highest level were behaviors such as organizing/modifying the environment and seeking challenges. These findings are particularly useful in interpreting the pattern of scores a child receives on the PVQ. As with the VQ, increasing volition is reflected in the client exhibiting increasingly higher-level volitional behaviors.

All the children were validly assessed in the study, indicating that the PVQ can be used to assess children with a wide range of disabilities as well as typically developing children. The findings of this study also strongly suggest that children with disabilities are at risk for decreased volition. Once again therapists consistently used the PVQ in a valid manner, indicating that study of the manual is adequate preparation for using the assessment. At the time of this writing, further revisions and refinements have been made to the PVQ and additional research on these changes is underway. As with the VQ, long-term plans include development of a paper-and-pencil method of determining a measure of volition.

Kenny

Using the PVQ as a Consulting Tool

Kenny is a 7-year-old boy who has lived in a pediatric residential facility since age 3. He has been diagnosed with spastic quadriplegic cerebral palsy. He has some hearing loss. Although diagnosed with cortical blindness, Kenny is able to see some things.

Following gentle handling and relaxation, Kenny exhibits full passive range of motion in his upper extremities. His active movement capacities are severely limited. Kenny enjoys gentle handling and tactile play with soft textures. His enjoyment is evidenced by orienting, smiling, laughing, and reaching. Kenny consistently turns his face and body toward the direction of sounds. He alerts to novel sounds and smiles when he hears familiar sounds or voices. He is able to reach for objects of interest when placed in supported sitting, supine lying, and side lying positions and when the objects are placed in close proximity to his hands and within his residual visual field. Kenny can open either hand volitionally to bat at or to attempt to grasp desired objects or toys. He requires occasional physical assistance to contact objects but will volitionally open/close his fingers in an apparent attempt to grasp them.

Kenny has received direct and consultative occupational therapy services a minimum of 30 minutes per week since his admission to school at age 3. Therapy has aimed to enhance Kenny's repertoire of sensory tolerance, mobility, and upper extremity function, especially visually directed reach. The long-term aim of Kenny's therapy is to enhance his ability to interact with the environment and derive satisfaction from it.

Rationale for Use of the PVQ

When evaluated on traditional developmental assessments, children like Kenny tend to demonstrate the same age level scores from year to year. These assessments have limited value for developing meaningful classroom programs and therapeutic intervention strategies. Given Kenny's visual impairment combined with his multiple physical and cognitive challenges, traditional developmental assessments reveal little about him. Therefore, in preparation for his annual review, the PVQ was used to gather information on Kenny's volition to identify relevant and functional goals and intervention strategies within his day school program.

Administration

The PVQ was administered on two separate occasions, each of which involved approximately 20 minutes of observation. On each occasion the observations were of Kenny's participation in three separate classroom activities. The first activity involved "sensory time," during which Kenny was exposed to touch/handling of a new sensory material. The second activity consisted of using an adaptive switch to respond to a simple story during the first session and to activate music during the second session. The third activity involved free movement experiences on the classroom mat. Kenny's performance ratings for the two PVQ administration sessions are shown in *Figures 13-4* and *13-5*.

Because of their brevity and Kenny's limited repertoire for expressing volition, the three classroom activities were treated as a single observation session, although unique features of each activity that impacted his volition were noted. Additionally, brief interviews were also done with the teacher and classroom aide to verify that the volitional observations were typical of Kenny.

The first observation was done primarily to establish a baseline and a better understanding of Kenny's volition within typical school contexts. Due to scheduling disruptions, three weeks lapsed between the first and second administration of the PVQ. Although unplanned, this hiatus allowed the therapist to make some recommendations for adapting the classroom environment based on the initial observations of Kenny's volition and how the environment impacted it.

FIGURE 13-4 Kenny's First PVQ.

Behavioral Indicators	Rating Scale				Comments
Explores Novelty	P	**H**	I	S	Requires multiple verbal cues/physical prompts to touch textures
Initiates Actions	P	H	**I**	S	Initiates switch activation
Task Directed	P	H	**I**	S	Stays on task with familiar activity
Shows Preferences	P	H	**I**	S	Can make choices given familiar routine
Tries New Things	P	**H**	I	S	Requires multiple cues during unfamiliar activities
Stays Engaged	P	**H**	I	S	Requires multiple cues to maintain engagement/focus
Expresses Mastery Pleasure	**P**	H	I	S	No overt expression of pleasure
Tries to Solve Problems	**P**	H	I	S	
Tries to Produce Effects	**P**	H	I	S	
Practices Skills	**P**	H	I	S	
Seeks Challenges	**P**	H	I	S	
Organizes/Modifies Environment	**P**	H	I	S	
Pursues Activity To Completion	P	**H**	I	S	Requires multiple cues and prompts to remain on task for the duration of the activity
Use Imagination/Symbolism	**P**	H	I	S	No opportunity
Rating Key : **P** = Passive, **H** = Hesitant, **I** = Involved, **S** = Spontaneous					

FIGURE 13-5   Kenny's Second PVQ.

Behavioral Indicators	Rating Scale				Comments
Explores Novelty	P	H	I	S	Requires multiple physical prompts to remain engaged
Initiates Actions	P	H	I	S	Requires one physical prompt paired with verbal cue to initiate interaction with a known "liked" activity
Task Directed	P	H	I	S	Simple tasks, requires one verbal cue to remain attentive to task for short time period
Shows Preferences	P	H	I	S	Exhibits noticeable affect change to people and activities he likes
Tries New Things	P	H	I	S	Requires multiple physical prompts and verbal cues to initiate and sustain engagement.
Stays Engaged	P	H	I	S	Variation in score relative to specific tasks used (e.g. music)
Expresses Mastery Pleasure	P	H	I	S	Given repetitive input for a simple, familiar activity, Kenny smiled and oriented to the item
Tries To Solve Problems	P	H	I	S	Variation in score relative to specific tasks observed
Tries To Produce Effects	P	H	I	S	Engaged but requires multiple cues and prompts within this context
Practices Skills	P	H	I	S	Activity context changed from one session to the next
Seeks Challenges	P	H	I	S	
Organizes/Modifies Environment	P	H	I	S	Observable changes relative to activity/context change and level of involvement
Pursues Activity To Completion	P	H	I	S	Requires multiple cues and prompts to remain on task for the duration of the activity
Uses Imagination/Symbolism	P	H	I	S	Most significant area for change between administration sessions. Variations in scores relative to specific activity observed

Rating Key: **P** = Passive, **H** = Hesitant, **I** = Involved, **S** = Spontaneous

The therapist and teaching staff developed a greater appreciation for Kenny's inner experiences from the systematic observation of his behavior that the PVQ provided. This prompted the therapist and classroom personnel to pay closer attention to discreet changes in Kenny's affect or attention. Any such changes guided the timing and grading of cues and other events in Kenny's environment. Consequently, Kenny's environment was subtly refined to be more responsive to Kenny. Some of the specific modifications that were made included:

- Providing verbal cues/prompts to Kenny at close range, whereas the teacher had previously given these cues from a group instructional distance
- Combining a physical prompt with the close-range verbal cue

- Providing different placement of objects for optimal access; close observation indicated that subtle changes in positioning of objects made a difference in Kenny's willingness to interact with them.

In addition to these strategies, the initial PVQ lead to rethinking of how to incorporate Kenny into classroom events. By systematically considering what Kenny was capable of doing and creating contexts that incorporated those actions into simple routines, his actions were given purpose or meaning, and they could have clearer consequences.

Moreover, Kenny was observed during the PVQ assessment to be very attentive to others' emotions. Therefore, the therapist guided the teacher and aide to offer clear indications of approval and pleasure at Kenny's exhibiting desired behaviors, so that he could recognize that others were responding to his actions.

Finally, whenever an action was being solicited from Kenny, the motor or cognitive demand was matched to the kinds of things his behavior indicated that he liked doing. Then the physical or social environment was modified so that the action required matched Kenny's capacity and preference for doing.

As a result of these subtle changes, Kenny exhibited improvements in the ratings he obtained between the first and second session for 6 of the 14 behavioral indicators as shown in Figures 13-4 and 13-5. We will discuss each of these changes, illustrating the value of information obtained in the PVQ for guiding intervention strategies that elicited these changes.

The rating for the item "Stays Engaged" changed from "hesitant" to "involved." The first administration session included observing Kenny using a switch during a classroom story time. Each child in the group had a portion of the story recorded on voice output. When given cues, the children were expected to activate their portion of the story. Kenny required repeated verbal cues and physical prompts to activate his switch each time it was his turn to participate in the story. He received a score of "hesitant" for his responses in this group because of the extensive input he required to activate the switch. It was decided that this occupational form presented too much of a challenge for Kenny. He could not follow the story, and the time gaps between his turns were too long.

The second session included observation of Kenny using a similar switch to turn on music during group music time. Kenny's job was to activate the switch each time the music turned off. The occupational form had been modified in several ways to more nearly match Kenny's abilities. Music required less cognition than the story. Also, turn taking was eliminated and Kenny was put in charge of activating the music. The cues were simpler (i.e., the music stopped combined with verbal prompts presented in close proximity). Finally, Kenny likes music and thus the occupational form is more naturally motivating for him. Kenny exhibited greater involve-

ment and relatedness within this context, earning him a rating of "involved" for staying engaged.

During the first administration session, Kenny did not exhibit any affect change (perceived as pride) on completion of a task, resulting in a rating of "passive" for the item "Expresses Mastery Pleasure." Teacher interview confirmed that Kenny typically did not exhibit any semblance of mastery pleasure. Based on this observation the therapist recommended that the teacher display a large affective response (e.g., clapping and cheering) whenever Kenny managed to do the behavior. During the second administration session, Kenny consistently exhibited smiling and laughter on successful activation of the music switch when this activation was combined with high affect praise from his teacher. Consequently, Kenny received a higher rating of "hesitant" for his performance during the second session.

For the items "Tries to Solve Problems" and "Organizes/Modifies Environment," Kenny initially received a rating of "passive." When faced with barriers preventing easy access to objects/toys he appears to enjoy, Kenny made no attempt to move barriers to gain access to these items even after extensive verbal coaching and physical demonstration. During the second observation, once Kenny exhibited three to four involved attempts at activating the music switch, the therapist and teachers modified the environment by moving the switch. This required Kenny to reach further. When he was able to adapt to this challenge, they begin placing barriers (e.g., small toy in front of the switch) and encouraged him to "get his switch." These alterations were designed to prompt Kenny to engage problem-solving and environmental modification. Given repeated verbal cues and physical prompts Kenny eventually batted the toy out of the way to clearly gain access to the switch. Consequently, the problem-solving and environmental modification items were rated as "hesitant" for this session.

Kenny initially received a rating of "passive" for "Practices Skills" and "Uses Imagination/Symbolism." He did not repeat actions (which would indicate practice). Kenny typically did not indicate any sense of symbolic awareness or imaginative expansion of any of the activity/play scenarios available to him throughout his school day. During the free movement mat experience within the first session, Kenny displayed his usual behavior of kicking and rolling from side to side while on his back; this behavior inches him forward on the mat. However, Kenny did not appear to intend this action to move himself in a particular direction. He has never used it as a means for retrieving a desired item or to move to a more desired place in the room.

Based on this observation from the first administration, the therapist recommended that the movement pattern be incorporated into a dressing/diaper change routine as a means for promoting active participation in self-care tasks. This strategy had been implemented during the period after the first administration upon recommendation by the therapist. During the second session Kenny exhibited the ability to roll to either side and to raise his hips off the mat or to change table surface when given tactile cues that had been used consistently as part of the new routine. He was also observed performing these specific movement sequences after the diaper change occurred, indicating that Kenny was intentionally practicing the routine. Consequently, Kenny received a rating of "involved" for both items during the second session.

Summary

The use of the PVQ with Kenny enhanced the understanding of his volition and helped generate strategies to further support his motivation to do things. Even in the short period between the two administrations of the PVQ, changes in Kenny's environment yielded notable changes in his volition that also translated into more functional behavior.

The PVQ provided the opportunity to view and formally record Kenny's volitionally relevant behavior and note changes in his volition. Moreover, it provided new insights into how Kenny was motivated and how the environment impacted on his volition. The information gained from both administrations of the PVQ resulted in several new goals. The following are two examples of kinds of functional goals that were added to Kenny's program based on the PVQ:

- Kenny will participate in a group activity by spontaneously activating the music switch during group music 100% of the time (each time the music stops)
- Kenny will participate in self-care by rolling to either side to assist with lower extremity dressing and diapering when given a tactile cue to either hip.

In summary, the PVQ provided the therapist with information to recommend to the classroom staff new strategies of organizing Kenny's environment that enhanced Kenny's volition and expanded his repertoire of participation. As this case illustrates, when a therapist (or other caretaker) understands the child's volition and appreciates how the environment influences it, strategies can be developed that support new learning and development. The physical and social environments can be shaped to maximize children's desires for action and their feelings of accomplishment and enjoyment.

Conclusion

This chapter presented four assessments that use observation as a means of collecting information about clients. Two assessments provide important information about clients' motor, process, and communication/interaction skills. The two volitional assessments provide information about the client's motivation. All four assessments use rating scales to record the observations and allow qualitative information to be gathered as well. Although they do so in different ways, each of the assessments takes into consideration the effects of the environment on the observed skill or volition, thus incorporating an assessment strategy consistent with the systems concepts discussed in Chapter 3.

References

Anderson, S. P. (1998). *Using the Pediatric Volitional Questionnaire to assess children with disabilities.* Unpublished master's thesis, University of Illinois at Chicago, Chicago, IL.

Atchison, B. T., Fisher, A. G., & Bryze, K. (1998). Rater reliability and internal scale and person response validity of the School Assessment of Motor and Process skills. *American Journal of Occupational therapy, 52,* 843–850.

Baron, K. B. (1994). Clinical interpretation of "The assessment of motor and process skills of persons with psychiatric disorders." *American Journal of Occupational Therapy, 48,* 781–782.

Bernspång, B., & Fisher, A. G. (1995). Differences between persons with right or left cerebral vascular accident on the assessment of motor and process skills. *Archives of Physical Medicine and Rehabilitation, 76,* 1144–1151.

Bernspång, B., & Fisher, A. G. (1999). Rater calibration stability for the assessment of motor and process skills. *Scandinavian Journal of Occupational Therapy, 6,* 101–109.

Chern, J., Kielhofner, G., de las Heras, C. G., & Magalhaer, L. C. (1996). The Volitional Questionnaire: Psychometric development and practical use. *American Journal of Occupational Therapy, 50* (7), 515–525.

Darragh, A. R., Sample, P. L., & Fisher, A. G. (1998). Environment effect on functional task performance in adults with acquired brain injuries: Use of the assessment of motor and process skills. *Archives of Physical Medicine and Rehabilitation, 79,* 418–423.

de las Heras, C. G. (1993a). *Validity and reliability of the Volitional Questionnaire.* Unpublished master's thesis, Tufts University, Boston, MA.

de las Heras, C. G. (1993b). *The Volitional Questionnaire.* Unpublished manual, Santiago, Chile.

de las Heras, C. G., Geist, R., Kielhofner, G., & Li, Y. (2002). *The Volitional Questionnaire (VQ) (Version 4.0).* Chicago: Model of Human Occupation Clearinghouse, Department of Occupational Therapy, College of Applied Health Sciences, University of Illinois at Chicago

de las Heras, C. G., Llerena, V., & Kielhofner, G. (2002). *Remotivation process: Progressive intervention for individuals with severe volitional challenges. (Version 1.0)* Chicago: Department of Occupational Therapy, University of Illinois at Chicago.

Dickerson, A. E., & Fisher, A. G. (1993). Age differences in functional performance. *American Journal of Occupational Therapy, 47,* 686–692.

Doble, S. E., Fisk, J. D., Fisher, A. G., Ritvo, P. G., & Murray, T. J. (1994). Evaluating the functional competence of community-dwelling persons with multiple sclerosis using the Assessment of Motor and Process Skills. *Archives of Physical Medicine and Rehabilitation, 75,* 843–851.

Doble, S. E., Fisk, J. D., Lewis, N., & Rockwood, K. (1999). Test-retest reliability of the Assessment of Motor and Process skills in elderly adults. *Occupational Therapy Journal of Research, 19,* 203–215.

Duran, L. J., & Fisher A.G. (1996). Male and female performance on the assessment of motor and process skills. *Archives of Physical Medicine and Rehabilitation, 77,* 1019–1024.

Fisher, A. G. (1993). The assessment of IADL motor skills: An application of many-faceted Rasch analysis. *American Journal of Occupational Therapy, 47,* 319–338.

Fisher, A. G. (1997). Multifaceted measurement of daily life task performance: Conceptualizing a test of instrumental ADL and validating the addition of personal ADL tasks. *Archives of Physical Medicine and Rehabilitation: State of the Art Reviews, 11,* 289–303.

Fisher A. G. (1999). *Assessment of motor and process skills* (3rd ed.). Ft. Collins, CO: Three Star Press.

Fisher, A. G., Liu, Y., Velozo, C. A., & Pan, A. W. (1992). Cross-cultural assessment of process skills. *American Journal of Occupational Therapy, 46,* 876–885.

Fisher, W. P., & Fisher, A. G. (1993). Applications of Rasch analysis to studies in occupational therapy. *Physical Medicine and Rehabilitation Clinics of North America: New Developments in Functional Assessment, 4,* 551–569.

Forsyth, K. (1996). *Measurement properties of the Assessment of Communication and Interaction Skills (ACIS).* Unpublished master's thesis, University of Illinois at Chicago, Chicago, IL.

Forsyth, K., Lai, J., & Kielhofner, G. (1999). The Assessment of Communication and Interaction Skills (ACIS): Measurement properties. *British Journal of Occupational Therapy, 62* (2), 69–74.

Forsyth, K., Salamy, M., Simon, S., & Kielhofner, G. (1998). *The Assessment of Communication and Interaction Skills (version 4.0).* Chicago: Department of Occupational Therapy, University of Illinois at Chicago.

Geist, R. (1998). *The validity study of the pediatric volitional questionnaire.* Unpublished master's thesis, University of Illinois at Chicago, Chicago, IL.

Geist, R., & Kielhofner, G., Basu, S., & Kafkes, A. (2002). *The Pediatric Volitional Questionnaire (PVQ) (Version 2.0).* Chicago: Model of Human Occupation Clearinghouse, Department of Occupational Therapy, College of Applied Health Sciences, University of Illinois at Chicago.

Goto, S., Fisher, A. G., Mayberry, W. L. (1996). The assessment of motor and process skills applied cross-culturally to the Japanese. *American Journal of Occupational Therapy, 50,* 798–806.

Nygård, L., Bernspång, B., Fisher, A. G., & Winblad, B. (1994). Comparing motor and process ability of persons with suspected dementia in home and clinic settings. *American Journal of Occupational Therapy, 48,* 689–696.

Pan, A. W., & Fisher, A. G. (1994). The assessment of motor and process skills of persons with psychiatric disorders. *American Journal of Occupational Therapy, 48,* 775–780.

Park, S., Fisher, A. G., & Velozo, C. A. (1994). Using the Assessment of Motor and Process Skills to compare occupational performance between clinic and home settings. *American Journal of Occupational Therapy, 48,* 697–709.

Puderbaugh, J. L., & Fisher, A. G. (1992). Assessment of motor and process skills in normal young children and children with dyspraxia. *Occupational Therapy Journal of Research, 12,* 195–216.

Robinson, S. E., & Fisher, A. G. (1996). A study to examine the relationship of the Assessment of Motor and Process Skills (AMPS) to other tests of cognition and function. *British Journal of Occupational Therapy, 59,* 260–263.

Salamy, M. (1993). *Construct validity of the Assessment for Communication and Interaction Skills.* Unpublished master's thesis, University of Illinois at Chicago, Chicago, IL.

Simon, S. (1989). *The development of an assessment for communication and interaction skills.* Unpublished master's thesis, University of Illinois at Chicago, Chicago, IL.

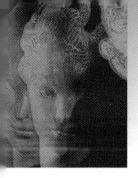

14

Self-Report Assessments

- **Gary Kielhofner**
- **Kirsty Forsyth**
- **Jeanne Federico**
- **Alexis Henry**
- **Riitta Keponen**
- **Frances Oakley**
- **Ay Woan Pan**

The assessments discussed in this chapter have been designed for clients to record information about themselves, their life circumstances, and their environments. These assessments give clients a voice in characterizing their lives and desires. The very process of filling out these assessments often helps clients clarify their own thoughts and feelings about their circumstances. Moreover, they have the virtue of actively engaging clients in generating information that will influence the therapeutic process. Hence, the proper use of these assessments can help generate a client-centered and client-empowering therapeutic process.

These self-report assessments are designed so that clients can readily comprehend the meaning of what is reported in them. Having completed one or more of these assessments, clients often see revealing patterns in their own responses that augment insight and support problem-solving and planning. Secondly, the assessments are designed to be used as part of a dialogue between therapist and client that aims to generate a deeper understanding of the client's circumstances and to determine directions and strategies for therapy. Consequently, therapists always discuss the responses with the client to clarify both their meaning for the client and their significance for the direction therapy should take.

While these assessments are designed as forms to be filled out independently by the client, therapists can administer them in different ways to accommodate

needs of clients. For example, they are sometimes given verbally when clients have difficulty reading or writing. Sometimes the assessments are used as part of a group planning or problem-solving exercise. On other occasions, family members may report the information on the client's behalf when the client is incapable of doing so.

The self-report instruments discussed in this chapter are:

- The Modified Interest Checklist
- The Occupational Questionnaire and Activity Record
- The Occupational Self Assessment and Child Occupational Self Assessment
- The Pediatric Interest Profiles
- The Role Checklist.

With the exception of the Interest Checklist, which existed before the introduction of MOHO and was later modified, these assessments were developed as part of efforts to apply concepts from MOHO in practice and research.

Modified Interest Checklist

The Interest Checklist was originally developed by Matsutsuyu (1969). Later, when the checklist was being used routinely in association with MOHO, it was modified by Scaffa (1981) and then by Kielhofner and

FIGURE 14-1 Format of the Modified Interest Checklist.

Activity	What has been your level of interest?						Do you curently participate in this activity?		Would you like to pursue this in the future?	
	In the past 10 years			In the past year						
	Strong	Some	No	Strong	Some	No	Yes	No	Yes	No
Gardening/yardwork										
Sewing/needlework										
Playing cards										
Foreign languages										
Church activities										
Radio										
Walking										
Car repair										
Writing										
Dancing										
Golf										
Football										
Listening to popular music										

Neville (1983). They retained its 68 interests, but altered how clients responded to them to gather more detailed information. The Modified Interest Checklist (Kielhofner & Neville, 1983) also includes opportunity to indicate what current interests are, how interests have changed, and whether one participates or wishes to participate in an interest in the future.

The Modified Interest Checklist is a leisure interest inventory appropriate for adolescents. Although it can be used to gather information relevant to a person's overall occupational interests, its main focus is on avocational interests that influence activity choices. This checklist is interpreted by examining the pattern of interests. Originally, it was thought that the checklist would be useful in determining clusters of interests (e.g., whether a person's interests were manual versus intellectual or cultural). Research failed to establish the validity of such clusters of interests (Rogers, Weinstein, & Figone, 1978), and practical use suggests that the main value of the checklist is in what it reveals about each individual's unique pattern of interests.

Modified Interest Checklist	Gathers information on strength of interest and present and future engagement in 68 activities	Can be printed out from the Model of Human Occupation Clearinghouse web site at: http://www.uic.edu/hsc/acad/cahp/OT/MOHOC Or go to: http://www.uic.edu Link to: 1) Academic Departments 2) Applied Health Sciences 3) Occupational Therapy 4) MOHO

Administration

As shown in *Figure 14-1,* clients indicate their level of interest in each of the items over the past 10 years and the past 1 year. Further, clients indicate whether they actively participate in and would like to pursue each potential interest in the future. After completion of the checklist, the occupational therapist and client discuss the client's responses. This is particularly useful for appreciating the impact that disability has had on how the client is experiencing pleasure from an activity or the significance disability has had in altering a client's attraction to particular kinds of activities.

Dependability

Factor-analytic studies aimed at establishing the validity of interest patterns identified by the instrument do not support the practice of formal scoring of activities by category of interests (Katz, Giladi, & Peretz, 1988; Rogers et al., 1978). Other studies that compare disabled and nondisabled populations show the instrument can discriminate and indicate that persons with disabilities exhibit fewer interests and less participation in things of interest (Ebb, Coster, & Duncombe, 1989; Katz et al., 1988). Research also suggests that comparing information on the extent of interest and the degree of participation is also an important strategy. For example, Scaffa (1991) found that clients beginning rehabilitation for alcoholism and those with extended periods of sobriety recorded similar numbers of strong interests. However, clients with longer periods of sobriety had more frequent participation in pleasurable activities.

Erik

An Illustration of Use of the Interest Checklist

Erik, a young adult with a diagnosis of schizophrenia, indicated the following strong interests on the checklist: radio, walking, listening to popular music, movies, listening to classical music, attending lectures, and reading. He pursued all these interests alone, even though he complained of being lonely. The only strong interests that involved interaction with others were holiday activities that his family organized and bowling, which was an activity organized by the day hospital he attended.

What the pattern illustrated was that Erik's interest pattern influenced him to make activity choices that kept him isolated from others. Erik's interest checklist and the clarification his occupational therapist received when discussing it with him provided necessary information to develop a conclusion that his interest pattern led to dissatisfying activity choices. This discussion also helped to develop treatment objectives that helped Erik find ways to pursue some of his current interests with others and of developing new, more socially oriented interests.

Occupational Questionnaire and the NIH Activity Record

The NIH Activity Record (ACTRE) (Furst, Gerber, Smith, Fisher, & Shulman, 1987; Gerber & Furst, 1992) and the Occupational Questionnaire (OQ) (Smith, Kielhofner, & Watts, 1986) are self-report forms that ask the client to indicate what activity he or she engages in over the course of a weekday and weekend day. The OQ and ACTRE are appropriate for use with adolescents and adults.

The OQ, on which the ACTRE is based, is the simpler form. It asks persons to report what they are doing during each half-hour waking period of their day. Then they indicate:

- Whether he or she considers it to be work, leisure, a daily living task, or rest
- How much he or she enjoys it
- How important it is
- How well he or she does it.

The latter three questions give insight into the volitional characteristics of the activity pattern. That is, they reveal the personal causation, interest, and value experienced in the activity. The questionnaire also provides information about the person's habit patterns (i.e., the typical use of time) and about occupational participation (i.e., the kind of work, leisure, and self-care that make up a person's current life).

The ACTRE, developed for use with persons who have physical disabilities, asks additional questions per-

NIH Activity Record (ACTRE)	Records information in half-hour intervals throughout the day Information includes a person's perception of competence, value of activity, enjoyment of activity, difficulty, pain, and rest	Copies of the NIH ACTRE and a method of scoring with a computer spreadsheet can be obtained from: Gloria Furst OTR/L, MPH National Institutes of Health Rehabilitation Medicine Department 10 Center Drive MSC 1604 Room 6S235 Bethesda, MD 20892-1604 Fax: 301-480-0669 E-mail: gfurst@nih.gov
Occupational Questionnaire (OQ)	Records information in half-hour intervals throughout the day Information includes a person's perception of competence, value of activity, and enjoyment of activity	Can be printed out from the Model of Human Occupation Clearinghouse web site at: http://www.uic.edu/hsc/acad/cahp/OT/MOHOC Or go to: http://www.uic.edu Link to: 1) Academic Departments 2) Applied Health Sciences 3) Occupational Therapy 4) MOHO

taining to pain, fatigue, difficulty of performance, and whether one rests during the activity *(Fig. 14-2)*. Consequently, in addition to the information provided by the OQ, the ACTRE provides detailed information about how a disability influences performance of everyday activities (e.g., it asks about the level of energy required, the amount of pain and fatigue experienced, and whether rest was taken during the activity). The ACTRE is designed to be used primarily as a 24-hour time log completed at three points during each day. This method helps improve the accuracy of the instrument, since recall is of a very recent past.

Although both forms are designed to be used as self-reports, they can be administered as semistructured interviews. The forms are ordinarily used to report on an actual period of time, being filled out as diaries during the reporting period. However, it is sometimes more practical to ask clients to report on what is a typical day. Each of these methods has its advantages (e.g., diaries tend to be more accurate but may reflect an unusual day). Actual use depends on the purpose and circumstances of therapy. Ordinarily, therapists minimally ask clients to report on a weekday and a weekend day, but this also depends on the circumstances in which the instruments are being used.

In addition to providing details about a client's use and experience of time, these instruments potentially give the occupational therapist important information about the following kinds of problems:

- Particularly troublesome times or activities in the daily schedule
- Disorganization in the person's use of time
- Lack of balance in time use
- Problems such as a lack of feeling competent, a lack of interest, or a lack of value in daily activities.

The instruments can be used to produce scores that represent the amount of value, interest, personal causation, pain, and fatigue experienced in a day. In addition to the possibility of generating such numbers from the instruments, the results of the instruments can be graphically portrayed for or by the client. For example, the time spent in any area (e.g., work, play, or rest) can be portrayed as the portion of the day devoted to each of these life spaces, the portion spent doing things not valued, and so on. This can be done as an individual or group exercise. It provides clients a new way to examine their patterns of doing things and identify changes they would like to make. Used in this way, these instruments can help to establish therapeutic goals in col-

FIGURE 14-2 Format of the NIH Activity Record.

Name		Age		Day/Date		I.D.#			
Day 1	Afternoon		Question 1	Question 2	Question 3	Question 4	Question 5	Question 6	Question 7	Question 8

Key	Half-Hour Beginning At	Activity	C a t e g o r y*	During This Time Felt Pain 1=Not at All 2=Very Little 3=Some 4=A Lot	At the Beginning Of This-Half-Hour I Felt Fatigue 1=Not at All 2=Very Little 3=Some 4=A Lot	I Think That I Do This 1=Very Difficult 2=Poorly 3=Average 4=Well	I Find This Activity To Be 1=Very Difficult 2=Difficult 3=Slightly Difficult 4=Not Difficult	For Me This Activity is 1=Not Meaningful 2=Slightly Meaningful 3=Meaningful 4=Very Meaningful	This Activity Causes Fatigue 1=Not at All 2=Very Little 3=Some 4=A Lot	I Enjoy This Activity 1=Not at All 2=Very Little 3=Some 4=A Lot	I Stopped To Rest During The Activity 1=Yes 2=No
	12:30 PM			1 2 3 4	1 2 3 4	1 2 3 4	1 2 3 4	1 2 3 4	1 2 3 4	1 2 3 4	1 2
	1:00 PM			1 2 3 4	1 2 3 4	1 2 3 4	1 2 3 4	1 2 3 4	1 2 3 4	1 2 3 4	1 2
	1:30 PM			1 2 3 4	1 2 3 4	1 2 3 4	1 2 3 4	1 2 3 4	1 2 3 4	1 2 3 4	1 2
	2:00 PM			1 2 3 4	1 2 3 4	1 2 3 4	1 2 3 4	1 2 3 4	1 2 3 4	1 2 3 4	1 2

*Key to Category:

Rest (RE) - rest periods taking one-half hour or longer

Self-Care (SC) - personal care activities including dressing, grooming, exercises, normal meals, showering, or other similar activities

Preparation or Planning (PP) - time spent preparing to do an activity or planning when and how to do your daily or weekly activities

Household Activities (HA) - cooking, cleaning, mending, shopping for or putting away groceries, gardening, or other similar activities

Work (WK) - paid or volunteer activities in or out of the home, school work, writing papers, attending classes, studying, or other similar activities

Recreation or Leisure (RL) - hobbies, TV, games, reading (unless done during short rest breaks), sports, out-for-meals, movies, adult education classes, shopping, gardening, talking with friends, or other similar activities

Transportation (TR) - traveling to and from activities

Treatment (RX) - doctor or therapy appointments, home exercise, etc.

Sleep (SL) - when you go to bed for the night

laboration with the client. Like all self-report assessments, they are best supplemented with an in-depth discussion with the client.

Dependability of the OQ and ACTRE

The OQ was pilot tested in a study by Riopel (1982) that examined how patterns of daily activity affected volition and life satisfaction. This preliminary evidence suggested the OQ had adequate test-retest reliability and concurrent validity. Validity is further supported by findings from studies in which the instrument identified differences between persons with and without disabilities (Barris, Dickie, & Baron, 1988; Ebb et al., 1989; Kielhofner & Brinson, 1989; Smyntek, Barris, & Kielhofner, 1985).

The initial validation of the ACTRE was undertaken with a group of clients with rheumatoid arthritis (Gerber & Furst, 1992). The validity of the ACTRE is supported by the fact that it correlates well with other measures of pain, fatigue, and activities of daily living performance. This instrument also is able to discriminate between different patient groups.

Lin

An Illustration of the Use of the OQ

Lin is a 25-year-old man who lived in Taipei. He was diagnosed as having obsessive-compulsive disorder with a suspected schizoid personality. Lin was admitted to a psychiatric ward due to emotional difficulties that stemmed from his army training. He had displayed compulsive behaviors since his first year in college. Lin spent a great amount of time washing himself, washing his hands, and folding his clothes. However, he was able to adjust to the requirements of college life and to graduate with a Bachelor's degree in accounting.

After graduation, he enlisted in the Taiwanese army. However, he was unable to cope with the army routines. He spent too much time washing himself and his hands, and he was disciplined for these behaviors. He was sent to the army-affiliated hospital for screening and was diagnosed as having an adjustment disorder. Eventually, he was dismissed from the army due to his inability to cope

with army life. Since that time, he has been living alone in an apartment in Taipei, relatively isolated from others and without employment.

Lin was referred to occupational therapy for evaluation of his communication and interaction skills, roles, and habits. In addition to other assessments, the occupational therapist asked Lin to complete the OQ to assess his daily routines and role performance. Lin was very serious about filling out the questionnaire and took a great deal of time deciding how to respond, making several corrections.

The OQ (Fig. 14-3) highlighted that Lin spent about 10.5 hours in mainly passive and solitary leisure things, 3.5 hours in activities of daily living, and 4 hours doing work-related things. The way in which he rated activities was revealing for both the therapist and Lin. Together they identified the following patterns. The only thing Lin indicated doing very well was eating meals, which along with sleep, were the only things that he rated as extremely important. Similarly, these and mainly passive leisure things were what he indicated liking most. While he did not see himself as having a problem doing anything, or find anything he did to be a waste of time or distasteful, he also did not indicate that he valued or derived a high level of competence or enjoyment from anything productive. Moreover, his response to activities sometimes appeared to be as related to the time of day as to what he was doing, suggesting that he was not deriving a specific sense of value, competence, or interest from what he did.

Lin found the information derived from the OQ to be very revealing. It made him more aware of features of his daily routine. He indicated that his routine "just sort of happened." He did not actively choose it. Moreover, he indicated that it was a sad thing that the highlight of his day was when he ate meals. Thus, he was very motivated to try to improve his daily life.

After the evaluation, Lin collaborated with the therapist to identify goals for himself. Since his length of hospital stay was anticipated to be only a few days, Lin and his therapist decided to focus on goals and plans that he could work on implementing in his community life. Using information from the OQ, Lin identified the goals of redesigning his life style according to the major roles he wanted in his

FIGURE 14-3 Lin's Responses on the Occupational Questionnaire.

Time	Typical activities	Question 1 — I consider this activity to be: (W: Work, D: Daily living task, R: Recreation, RT: Rest)	Question 2 — I think that I do this: (VW: Very well, W: Well, AA: About average, P: Poorly, VP: Very poorly)	Question 3 — For me this activity is: (EI: Extremely important, I: Important, TL: Take it or leave it, RN: Rather not do it, TW: Total waste of time)	Question 4 — How much do you enjoy this activity? (LVM: Like it much, L: Like it, NLD: Neither like nor dislike, D: Dislike it, SD: Strongly dislike)
06:30–07:00	Sleep	W D R [RT]	VW [W] AA P VP	[EI] I RN TW	[LVM] L NLD D SD
07:00–07:30	Breakfast	W [D] R RT	[VW] W AA P VP	[EI] I RN TW	[LVM] L NLD D SD
07:30–08:00	Computer	[W] D R RT	VW [W] AA P VP	[EI] I TL RN TW	[LVM] L NLD D SD
08:00–08:30	Computer	[W] D R RT	[VW] W AA P VP	[EI] I TL RN TW	[LVM] L NLD D SD
08:30–09:00	Read Newspaper	[W] D R RT	[VW] W AA P VP	[EI] I TL RN TW	[LVM] L NLD D SD
09:00–09:30	Reading	[W] D R RT	VW [W] AA P VP	EI [I] TL RN TW	[LVM] L NLD D SD
09:30–10:00	Reading	[W] D R RT	VW [W] AA P VP	EI [I] TL RN TW	[LVM] L NLD D SD
10:00–10:30	Listen to Music	[W] D R RT	VW [W] AA P VP	EI [I] TL RN TW	[LVM] L NLD D SD
10:30–11:00	Music	[W] D R RT	VW [W] AA P VP	EI [I] TL RN TW	[LVM] L NLD D SD
11:00–11:30	Music	[W] D R RT	VW [W] AA P VP	EI [I] TL RN TW	[LVM] L NLD D SD
11:30–12:00	Lunch	W [D] R RT	[VW] W AA P VP	[EI] I TL RN TW	[LVM] L NLD D SD
12:00–12:30	Lunch	W [D] R RT	[VW] W AA P VP	[EI] I TL RN TW	[LVM] L NLD D SD
12:30–01:00	Computer	W D [R] RT	VW [W] AA P VP	EI I [TL] RN TW	LVM L [NLD] D SD
01:00–01:30	Computer	W D [R] RT	VW [W] AA P VP	EI I [TL] RN TW	LVM L [NLD] D SD
01:30–02:00	Go to Library	W D [R] RT	VW [W] AA P VP	EI I [TL] RN TW	LVM L [NLD] D SD
02:00–02:30	Library	W D [R] RT	VW [W] AA P VP	EI I [TL] RN TW	LVM L [NLD] D SD
02:30–03:00	Exercise	W D [R] RT	[VW] W AA P VP	EI I [TL] RN TW	LVM L [NLD] D SD
03:00–03:30	Exercise	W D [R] RT	[VW] W AA P VP	EI I [TL] RN TW	LVM L [NLD] D SD
03:30–04:00	Play ball	W D [R] RT	[VW] W AA P VP	EI I [TL] RN TW	LVM L [NLD] D SD
04:00–04:30	Play ball	W D [R] RT	VW [W] AA P VP	EI I [TL] RN TW	LVM L [NLD] D SD
04:30–05:00	Play ball	W D [R] RT	VW [W] AA P VP	EI I [TL] RN TW	LVM L [NLD] D SD
05:00–05:30	Dinner	W [D] R RT	[VW] W AA P VP	EI I TL RN TW	[LVM] L NLD D SD
05:30–06:00	Dinner	W [D] R RT	[VW] W AA P VP	[EI] I TL RN TW	[LVM] L NLD D SD

(continued)

FIGURE 14-3 (Continued)

Time	Typical activities	Question 1: I consider this activity to be: (W: Work, D: Daily living task, R: Recreation, RT: Rest)	Question 2: I think that I do this: (VW: Very well, W: Well, AA: About average, P: Poorly, VP: Very poorly)	Question 3: For me this activity is: (EI: Extremely important, I: Important, TL: Take it or leave it, RN: Rather not do it, TW: Total waste of time)	Question 4: How much do you enjoy this activity? (LVM: Like it much, L: Like it, NLD: Neither like nor dislike, D: Dislike it, SD: Strongly dislike)
06:00-06:30	Watching	W D [R] RT	VW [W] AA P VP	EI I TL [RN] TW	LVM [L] NLD D SD
06:30-07:00	TV	W D [R] RT	VW [W] AA P VP	EI I TL [RN] TW	LVM [L] NLD D SD
07:00-07:30	&	W D [R] RT	VW [W] AA P VP	EI I TL [RN] TW	LVM [L] NLD D SD
07:30-08:00	Phone	W D [R] RT	VW [W] AA P VP	EI I TL [RN] TW	LVM [L] NLD D SD
08:00-08:30	-Call to-	W D [R] RT	VW [W] AA P VP	EI I TL [RN] TW	LVM [L] NLD D SD
08:30-09:00	-Friend	W D [R] RT	VW [W] AA P VP	EI I TL [RN] TW	LVM [L] NLD D SD
09:00-09:30	Bathing	W D [R] RT	VW [W] AA P VP	EI I TL [RN] TW	LVM [L] NLD D SD
09:30-10:00	&	W D [R] RT	VW [W] AA P VP	EI I TL [RN] TW	LVM [L] NLD D SD
10:00-0:30	Washing	W D [R] RT	VW [W] AA P VP	EI I TL [RN] TW	LVM [L] NLD D SD
10:30-11:00	Clean	W D [R] RT	VW [W] AA P VP	EI I TL [RN] TW	LVM [L] NLD D SD
11:00-11:30	-Up-	W D [R] RT	VW [W] AA P VP	EI I TL [RN] TW	LVM [L] NLD D SD
11:30-00:00	-Room	W D [R] RT	VW [W] AA P VP	EI I TL [RN] TW	LVM [L] NLD D SD
00:00-00:30	Go to sleep	W D R [RT]	VW [W] AA P VP	[EI] I TL RN TW	[LVM] L NLD D SD

life. He planned how to reduce the time he spent in leisure and self-care in order to have more time to engage in productive things. He systematically examined each of the things he did in the course of the day, deciding what kinds of changes he would like to make to feel more productive and involved. He was then able to choose things he wanted to do and plan for how to integrate these into his daily routines. This planning process, of itself, helped Lin feel much more like he could control and improve his daily life.

Occupational Self Assessment and Child Occupational Self Assessment

The Occupational Self Assessment (OSA) (Baron, Kielhofner, Iyenger, Goldhammer, & Wolenski, 2002) and the Child Occupational Self Assessment (COSA) (Federico & Kielhofner, 2002) are designed to capture clients' perceptions of their own occupational competence and of the impact of their environments on their occupational adaptation. They also allow clients to indicate personal values and to set priorities for change. Thus, the OSA and COSA are designed to give voice to the client's perspective and to give the client a role in determining the goals and strategies of therapy.

The OSA and COSA are also designed to be outcomes measures that capture self-reported client change. To be used as outcomes measures, the OSA and COSA are administered at the beginning and at the end of therapy.

Administration

The OSA is a two-part self-rating form. *Figure 14-4* shows the format of the OSA. Section one includes a series of statements about occupational functioning, to which clients respond by labeling each in terms of how well they do it using a four-point scale. Clients then respond to these same statements, indicating the importance of each on a four-point scale. Section two includes a series of statements about the client's environment, to which similar responses are given. On the OSA, once clients have completed the ratings, they establish priorities for change. There is a column on the form in which the client selects and ranks the areas for change related to self and environment. When completing the OSA, some clients independently determine their priorities for change and then discuss them with the therapist. Other clients, who need or wish more structure, do this with the therapist. The OSA also includes a form on which the therapist and client together may formally record and review therapy goals and strategies.

The COSA is similar to the OSA but has the following differences. It does not include a second section on the environment. It uses three-point scales for both ratings (of how well the child does the item and how important it is). To facilitate children's responses, the COSA uses happy faces and stars to indicate the rating choices as shown in *Figure 14-5*. The COSA form does not include a third step for selecting areas of priorities for change. Instead, the therapist structures the process, helping the child review the items and select priorities for change.

| Occupational Self Assessment (OSA)

Child Occupational Self Assessment (COSA) | *Provide information on clients perceptions of their own occupational competence (OSA and COSA) and of the impact of their environments (OSA only)*

Allow clients to indicate personal values and to set priorities for change | *Information on ordering can be found on the Model of Human Occupation Clearinghouse web site at:*
http://www.uic.edu/hsc/acad/cahp/OT/MOHOC
Or go to: uic.edu
Link to:
1) Academic Departments
2) Applied Health Sciences
3) Occupational Therapy
4) MOHO |

FIGURE 14-4   Sample Portion From the OSA.

Step 1: Below are statements about things you do in everyday life. For each statement, circle how well you do it. If an item does not apply to you, cross it out and move on to the next item.					Step 2: Next, for each statement circle how important this is to you.				Step 3: Choose up to 4 things about yourself that you would like to change.
	I have lot of problems doing this	I have some difficulty doing this	I do this well	I do this extremely well	This is not so important to me	This is important to me	This is more important to me	This is most important to me	I would like to change
Concentrating on my tasks	lot of problem	some difficulty	well	extremely well	not so important	important	more important	most important	
Physically doing what I need to do	lot of problem	some difficulty	well	extremely well	not so important	important	more important	most important	

When therapy is terminated (or when progress or follow-up information is desired), the OSA or COSA follow-up forms can be administered. Comparing the initial OSA and COSA raw scores with follow-up raw scores provides a visual representation of how the client has changed on each item. In the future, paper-and-pencil forms that allow a measure to be derived from the raw scores will be developed.

Dependability

Two international studies of the OSA have been completed (Iyenger, 2001; Kielhofner & Forsyth, 2001). These studies, which examined the OSA in multiple languages, indicated that the items that made up the four scales (competence, values about competence, environmental impact, and values about environment) worked well to define the intended constructs. Findings support the conclusion that the scale works well across the cultural, language, and diagnostic differences represented in the subjects. Following each

study, revisions were made in the OSA form to enhance its sensitivity. Further research on the OSA is currently underway. A future revision of the environment scale of the OSA is planned to increase its sensitivity. The COSA has been piloted, and future psychometric studies are planned.

Sinikka

Using the OSA to Support Client Collaboration in Therapy

Sinikka is a 30-year-old catering worker who lives in Helsinki. She has had complex regional pain syndrome for the past 2.5 years, since she experienced a workplace accident in which she sustained an electrical shock from a food processor to her right, dominant hand. Sinikka had sought a variety of interventions to no avail. These included undergoing previous occupational therapy that emphasized assessment of her hand function and learning to use a wrist support.

FIGURE 14-5   Sample Portion From the COSA.

MYSELF	I HAVE A BIG PROBLEM DOING THIS	I HAVE A LITTLE PROBLEM DOING THIS	I DO THIS	NOT SO IMPORTANT	IMPORTANT	REALLY IMPORTANT
Keep my mind on what I am doing	☹	😐	☺	★	★★	★★★
Make my body do what I want in to do	☹	😐	☺	★	★★	★★★

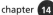

Sinikka recently began a pain rehabilitation program that consists of group treatment followed by outpatient, individualized therapy. Sinikka is anxious about her condition and symptoms and angry about the lack of efficacy of the previous care she received. She indicates that she feels like her hand and arm are living a life of their own, over which she has little control.

She feels that everything seems to be closing down on her. To maintain some measure of control, she has organized a structured daily routine aimed at minimizing her chronic pain. For example, at home she uses electronic equipment to reduce work demands, spaces her workload, and uses her left hand whenever possible. She frequently wakes up during the nighttime because of pain. When she tries activities that are not part of her current routine, she is hesitant, fearful of evoking pain, and has difficulty making decisions. She was very dependent on the therapist to guide her in doing anything new. Still, Sinikka expressed doubt over whether therapy would be able to help her in the long run.

The therapist introduced the OSA to Sinikka as a means of giving her an opportunity to take more control over her life and the therapeutic process. Sinikka's initial responses on the OSA are shown on *Figure 14-6*. The therapist discussed the responses with Sinikka. Sinikka indicated that the chronic pain

FIGURE 14-6   Sinikka's Initial Responses on the Myself Section of the OSA.

Myself	Competence				Values			
	Lot of problems	Some difficulty	Well	Extremely well	Not so important	Important	More Important	Most Important
Concentrating on my tasks		▓				▓		
Physically doing what I need to do		▓					▓	
Taking care of the place where I live	▓							▓
Taking care of myself			▓			▓		
Taking care of others for whom I am responsible		▓				▓		
Getting where I need to go		▓						▓
Managing my finances			▓					▓
Managing my basic needs (food, medicine)			▓			▓		
Expressing myself to others			▓			▓		
Getting along with others			▓				▓	
Identifying and solving problems				▓		▓		
Relaxing and enjoying myself		▓			▓			
Getting done what I need to do		▓				▓		
Having a satisfying routine		▓			▓			
Handling my responsibilities		▓					▓	
Being involved as a student, worker, volunteer, and/or family member		▓				▓		
Doing activities I like		▓				▓		
Working towards my goals		▓					▓	
Making decisions based on what I think is important		▓						▓
Accomplishing what I set out to do			▓				▓	
Effectively using my abilities			▓			▓		

had made many negative changes in her ability to do things she valued. These included difficulties in her roles as daughter-in-law, spouse, sister, home maintainer, caregiver, and worker. She explained that before her injury, she saw herself as a woman who was able to do anything she undertook and was recognized by others as resourceful and self-reliant. Now even the people closest to her could not comprehend her situation. She had very high standards for her performance, and the problems of pain and inability to use her dominant hand effectively left her feeling ineffective and helpless at times. Also, asking for help was not something Sinikka felt comfortable doing. She summed up her experience as being like floating paralyzed in a big lake, unable to move or swim.

During the next therapy session, the therapist asked Sinikka about their previous session, thinking that she might want to add something or continue the conversation they had begun after Sinikka completed the assessment. Sinikka told the therapist that doing the OSA had a profound effect on her. She found herself many times during the day just sitting deep in her thoughts. She told the therapist that she had started to think about what she really wanted in her life and what kind of options she would have in the future.

At this point she decided to choose the following priorities from the OSA statements to work on in therapy:

- Being involved as a student, worker, volunteer, and/or family member
- Handling my responsibilities
- Making decisions based on what I think is important.

Consequently, therapy sessions were organized to address these as goals. The therapist supported Sinikka to choose occupational forms for therapy that were linked to her roles and habits. Her ability to make decisions both for what to do and how to proceed in doing things quickly progressed. She resumed cooking, because this was an important part of her homemaker role. She worked at the computer to be productive by doing some of the bookkeeping for her husband's business. Lastly, she reengaged in an old hobby of silk painting. She did these things in therapy to get support for any adaptation

and problem-solving. She then carried them out at home routinely.

Sinikka had to drive her car quite a distance to come to therapy. This was hard because the rough road near her house made driving a challenge and precipitated pain. The therapist discussed with her the possibility of looking into a car with an armrest, wondering if the support for the arm would make any difference. Sinikka responded by renting such a car from a dealer to try it out and went on to trade cars. She managed to get her personal insurance to pay for aids she found useful in kitchen tasks as well as for a movable armrest for the computer she used at home.

She gave one of the silk scarves she decorated to her mother-in-law, which was very symbolic for Sinikka. Then, when her mother-in-law became ill, Sinikka took responsibility for driving her to appointments at the hospital. During therapy, Sinikka also spent time discussing future work plans. She decided to explore how she might build on her experience in catering by becoming employed in the hotel industry. A few months after therapy ended, the therapist received an e-mail message from Sinikka. She was excited because she had secured a work-training position in a high-class hotel.

John

Using the COSA to Engage a Student in Overcoming Challenges

John was 10 years old and in fourth grade. He had diagnoses of attention deficit disorder and anxiety disorder and had been identified as having sensory integrative dysfunction. John had been receiving school-based occupational, physical, and speech therapy since first grade. At the time, he also received private occupational therapy to address his sensory integration problems.

John had experienced little success at school. He was hesitant to attempt anything new in school, afraid that it would be too difficult. He went to great lengths to avoid tasks and interactions that threatened failure. Due to his sensory needs, John had many adaptations that made him stand out from his peers. In addition, his difficulty with handwriting was interfering with his academic performance. Overall, his school experience was negative and complicated by the fact that John had grown not to trust adults in the school environment.

Recognizing that John needed a voice and a sense of control, the new school occupational therapist began the school year by asking John to complete the COSA. The therapist explained to John that he was the expert on his own situation and that completing the COSA would allow him to tell the therapist about how he saw his situation. She also indicated to him that when he filled it out, he would have an opportunity to give her advice about how his therapy might be improved to better suit what he needed.

John was originally taken back by the idea that the therapist saw him as the expert on his problems. Nevertheless, as she reassured him, John immediately warmed to the idea of the assessment. He carefully read every item, completing all the responses. The competence responses he chose are shown in *Figure 14-7*. John paused several times to ask if the therapist really wanted to know what he thought. She reassured him that she considered it very important to know his opinion. When John finished, the therapist and he together reviewed each item and John's responses. This allowed the therapist to clarify John's responses to each item and gave them an opportunity to discuss what contributed to each problem he identified. They concluded by having John identify the areas from the COSA that he wanted to work on the most. John indicated that having more free time to engage in things he enjoyed was most important to him. Following that, he wanted to have better relationships with his peers.

They next discussed the kinds of problems John was having in completing his schoolwork and getting necessary things done at home, since these were what interfered with his free time. For example, John identified cursive writing as something that caused him extreme anxiety and problems in completing schoolwork. He also identified that he had problems with his morning routine. They also discussed getting along with peers. John identified that he felt the adaptations he used to meet his sensory needs (e.g., adaptive cushions) made him stand

out and interfered with his developing friendships. Finally, they discussed strategies that could be used to accomplish John's goals. These strategies, which were also shared with and agreed to by John's parents and the school team, were:

The need for John to complete his schoolwork with cursive writing was to be eliminated as much as possible. It was important to John and his parents that he read cursive, but given the extreme difficulty he had with handwriting, it was decided that this was less important. John was particularly pleased that his frustrations with cursive writing were heard and built into the plan.

John was to learn computer keyboarding as a means of writing. This strategy appealed to John very much. He worked hard at it and demonstrated good skill in learning letter position and using a modified two-handed keyboarding technique. He had access to both classroom and home computers as needed and soon became good at using the computer to write.

Written assignments were also scanned into the computer, so John could complete them. John was also given the possibility of dictating answers to some assignments into a tape recorder.

John was provided visual cues to help him organize his daily tasks at home and at school. He and the therapist worked out a pictorial schedule for home and a one-word schedule for school. The one at home was put up in his room. The one at school was taped inside his desk so it would not be so visible to other students.

Together the therapist and John explored more age-appropriate ways for him to fulfill his sensory needs at home and in the classroom. John took an active part in this process, as he was highly motivated to be better accepted by his peers. For example, John frequently raised his hand and asked permission to use the bathroom as a means of being able to get up and move around. These frequent bathroom requests were the target of jokes from his classmates, which embarrassed John. Because John needed to be able to move around, a system was developed whereby he would discreetly indicate his need to get up and the teacher would give him permission by nodding.

These interventions were implemented over the course of an academic year.

FIGURE 14-7   Changes in John's Responses on the COSA From Beginning to End of School Year.

	Beginning of school year	End of school year		Beginning of school year	End of school year
Keep my mind on what I am doing	☹	😐	Think of other ways to do things when I have a problem	☹	😐
Make my body do what I want it to do	☹	😐	Calm down when I am having a problem	☹	😐
Dress myself	☹	😐	Do things that make me happy	☹	☺
Brush my teeth	😐	😐	Do things I am good at	😐	☺
Bathe myself	😐	😐	Finish my work in school on time	☹	☺
Get my homework done	☹	☺	Have enough time to do things I like	☹	😐
Get myself a snack	☹	☺	Follow classroom rules	☹	😐
Keep my room clean	☹	☹	Be a good friend	☹	☺
Keep my desk neat	☹	☹	Do what my parents ask	☹	☺
Get my chores done	☹	☺	Do activities in school	☹	😐
Get around in my neighborhood	😐	😐	Do activities in my neighborhood	☹	😐
Buy things by myself	😐	😐	Do things with friends	☹	☺
Answer questions in school	☹	☺	Keep working on something even when it gets hard	☹	😐
Tell others my ideas and they understand	☹	😐	Make up my mind on important things	☹	😐
Get along with my classmates	☹	😐	Try my best	☹	☺
Ask the teacher questions when I do not understand something	☹	😐			

By the end of the year, John had made significant progress in being able to keep up with his schoolwork. Moreover, he had gained control over how he would do it. For example, when he got a written assignment, he would choose whether he would complete it by dictating, writing in cursive, or using the computer. Often he decided to handwrite shorter assignments and use the computer for longer ones. He mostly used dictating on audiotape as a backup if he felt anxious or pressured.

John no longer used adaptive cushions in the classroom. As in the example given above, he had established a number of ways to get his sensory needs met that blended naturally into the classroom. At midyear, John was still having some difficulty interacting with peers so the therapist administered the

Assessment of Communication and Interaction Skills (see Chapter 13) with John. The assessment revealed that John had difficulty with gazing (making eye contact), orienting his body to others, asking for information, asserting himself, expressing his feelings, modulating his speech, sharing information, collaborating with peers, conforming to implicit social norms, focusing, relating to others, and respecting others' requests. These results were shared with the speech therapist who collaborated with the occupational therapist and John to develop a joint intervention for improving John's communication/interaction skills. With this intervention, John's social interaction with peers began to improve.

John completed the COSA again near the end of the school year. As Figure 14-7 indicates, John felt he had made significant progress during the academic year. The therapist discussed the items that had changed with John to see why and how they had changed. For example, John stated that the visual schedules he and the therapist constructed helped him in his morning routine and at school. By using them as reminders of the steps of his routine, he needed fewer verbal prompts from his parents and teacher. At home, because he demonstrated improved ability to complete basic self-care tasks, his parents began to let him select and help prepare his lunch. He was very pleased about this.

John stated that he had developed a good routine for completing his homework. He liked doing his work on a computer as it required much less effort than handwriting. He even had begun to e-mail his homework assignments to his teachers.

He indicated that he was doing well with having friends to do things with and felt that he got along well with his classmates. The therapist asked why he did not report as much improvement in the item "Tell Others My Ideas and They Understand." He indicated that getting along and doing things was different than telling things. It was not a problem, but John felt that that they had not been friends long enough to tell them everything.

As Figure 14-7 shows, John continued to identify the following items as problem areas:

- Keep my mind on what I am doing
- Keep my room clean
- Keep my desk clean.

The therapist discussed these items to establish their level of importance to John. He did not feel that keeping his room clean was a priority for him. However, he did feel that keeping his desk neat was important. When the therapist asked about the difference, he explained that in school there is less time to find things. If he could keep his desk neat then he would not waste time locating things and could complete his schoolwork sooner. He honestly replied that keeping his mind on what he was doing was important but still difficult for him. The therapist praised John for what he had accomplished, acknowledged his views on what was important, and suggested they plan for one last goal of keeping his desk neat before the year ended. John agreed.

As these two cases illustrate, the OSA and COSA provide an excellent means of giving clients a voice about their own problems, strengths, and desires. The instruments also begin a process that can empower and enable clients to achieve more control over their situations and over the objectives and courses of their therapy. Finally, as the case of John illustrates, the instruments can serve as a concrete means to demonstrate change achieved in therapy. This is helpful not only to document change but also for clients to concretely see and be reinforced by the changes they accomplish.

The Pediatric Interest Profiles

The Pediatric Interest Profiles (PIP) (Henry, 2000) are three age-appropriate profiles of play and leisure interests and participation that can be used with children and adolescents. The three profiles are:

- Kid Play Profile, which is designed for use with children from 6–9 years of age
- The Preteen Play Profile, which is for children from the ages of 9–12 years
- Adolescent Leisure Interest Profile, which can be used with adolescents from 12–21 years of age.

The items, the questions about them, and the response formats of each version of the PIP have been designed to be appropriate for and easily understood by clients within the targeted age range.

In the Kid Play Profile, the child answers up to 3 questions about each of 50 activity items. For each activity

Pediatric Interest Profiles (PIP)	Includes three age-appropriate profiles of play and leisure interests and participation: Kid Play Profile (ages 6–9) The Preteen Play Profile (ages 9–12) Adolescent Leisure Interest Profile (ages 12–21)	PIP can be ordered from: Therapy Skill Builders 555 Academic Court San Antonio, TX 78204-2498 Tel: 800-228-0752 www.tpcweb.com

item, the child is asked, "Do you do this activity?" If the answer is yes, the child is also asked, "Do you like this activity?" and "Who do you do this activity with?" The child answers the questions by circling or coloring in a response. As shown in *Figure 14-8*, simple stick-figure drawings and words are used to depict each item. In addition, simple drawings and words are used to represent each possible response. The Kid Play Profile activity items are grouped into eight categories: sports activities, outside activities, summer activities, winter activities, indoor activities, creative activities, lessons/classes, and socializing.

In the Preteen Play Profile, the child answers up to 5 questions about each of 59 activity items. For each activity item, the child is asked, "Do you do this activity?" If the answer is yes, the child is also asked:

- How often do you do this activity?
- How much do you like this activity?
- How good are you at this activity?
- Who do you do this activity with?

The child answers the questions by circling a response. As with the Kid Play Profile, stick figure drawings are used to depict each activity. The Preteen Play Profile activity items are grouped into eight categories: sports activities, outside activities, summer activities, winter activities, indoor activities, creative activities, lessons/classes, and socializing.

In the Adolescent Leisure Interest Profile, the adolescent answers up to 5 questions about each of 83 activity items. For each activity item, the adolescent is asked, "How interested are you in this activity?" and "How often do you do this activity?" If the adolescent does the activity, he or she is also asked:

- How well do you do this activity?
- How much do you enjoy this activity?
- Who do you do this activity with?

The adolescent is instructed to place a checkmark beside one of the responses to each question. No drawings are used in the adolescent profile. The Adolescent Leisure Interest Profile activity items are grouped into eight categories: sports activities, outside activities, exercise activities, relaxation activities, intellectual activities, creative activities, socializing, and club/community organizations.

Therapists can use the information gathered with the PIP to identify children or adolescents who may be at risk for play-related problems. The PIP can also be used to identify specific play activities that are of interest to an individual child or adolescent so that those activities can be used to engage the child in therapeutic or educational interventions.

Administration

These three paper-and-pencil self-report assessments are quick and easy to administer. Each profile lists and/or depicts via pictures a variety of play and leisure activities and asks the child or adolescent to respond to multiple questions about the activities. As noted above, these questions focus on the child's participation in the activities, feelings of enjoyment and/or competence in the activities, and whether the activities are done alone or with others.

It is recommended that the PIP be used to facilitate a conversation between the therapist and the child or adolescent. The PIP can provide a means to engage children or adolescents in a more detailed interview about their play experiences. Children, in particular, seem to enjoy telling stories about their play. Such interviews can enhance rapport between the client and provider and can give a more detailed picture of any play/leisure-related problems.

Dependability

The impetus for developing these profiles came from Henry's follow-up study of adolescents hospitalized for a first episode of psychosis (Henry, 1994). This study

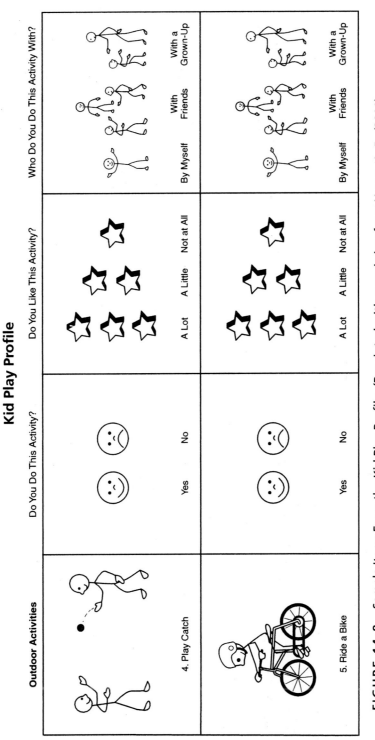

FIGURE 14-8 Sample Items From the Kid Play Profile. (Reprinted with permission from Henry, A. D. (2000). *Pediatric interest profiles*. San Antonio, TX: Therapy Skill Builders, p. 44.)

showed social-recreational activities to be good predictors of the person's functioning 6 months after discharge. Existing assessments were insufficient to adequately assess leisure interests in children and adolescents. Consequently, more appropriate age-targeted measures of leisure interests were needed.

Initial studies were conducted to develop items and test reliability testing of a pilot version of the adolescent measure (Brophy et al.,1995). After further refinement, an additional reliability study of the Adolescent Leisure Interest Profile was undertaken (Henry, 1994), indicating good test-retest reliability. Next, studies were undertaken for item development and pilot testing of preliminary versions of the Kid Play Profile and the Preteen Play Profile (Andrews et al., 1995; Beck et al., 1996; Budd et al., 1994; Henry, 2000). The results of these studies indicated that young children (ages 6–12) can comprehend and respond appropriately to the format of the profiles. In addition, these studies showed that total scores on the Kid Play Profile and the Preteen Play Profile have acceptable internal consistency and test-retest reliabilities.

Jerome

An Illustration of Use of the Kid Play Profile

Jerome was 6 years old and attended first grade at an urban, public elementary school in Maryland. He lived with his mother, maternal grandmother, and 8-year-old brother Joe. Jerome's mother worked full-time in a manufacturing plant and attended school one evening a week. Jerome's parents were divorced. Jerome and his brother visited their father in Pennsylvania one weekend each month, and for three week-long vacations each year. Jerome's grandmother provided childcare for Jerome and his brother when their mother was working or at school.

His mother reported that Jerome had always been more difficult than her other son. As a baby he was not easily soothed, was a picky eater, and rarely slept through the night. She felt that she had to carry him all the time. As a toddler, he was very physically active and frequently got bumps and bruises. His high level of physical activity continued. At the end of the day, Jerome's mother noted, he

was "literally bouncing off the walls." In addition, since toddlerhood, he had been very particular about his clothing, disliking most types of underwear, socks, turtleneck shirts, and jeans. His mother reported, "Sometimes we go through five shirts in the morning before he is ready for school."

Jerome enjoyed kindergarten, but his progress in developing pre-academic skills such as letter recognition and writing was slower than most of his classmates. First grade had been more difficult. Jerome had trouble attending in class, was often disruptive because he could not sit still, and was falling further behind in developing reading-readiness skills. He was having difficulty with handwriting and other fine-motor tasks. While his teacher was very supportive and patient, she was beginning to feel frustrated with her ability to manage his behavior in the classroom and worried about his ability to keep up with the pace of classroom activities. He interacted only minimally with classmates, and on the playground spent most of his time on the swings or running in circles. Since the middle of the school year, Jerome had been receiving resource-room help for language arts and classroom-based occupational therapy for fine-motor activities and handwriting.

At a recent parent meeting, Jerome's mother expressed concern about his increasing social isolation. She was concerned because Jerome told her that he ate lunch alone, usually played by himself during recess, and did not get included in most social activities. Jerome's classroom teacher confirmed this.

The occupational therapist administered the Kid Play Profile to gain Jerome's perspective on his play participation and interviewed Jerome's mother and teacher about his behavior at home and school. Jerome was able to complete the Kid Play Profile with considerable assistance from the occupational therapist. His responses on the Kid Play Profile indicate that he primarily enjoyed outdoor, gross motor activities such as biking, roller-blading, swimming, sledding, going to the playground, and playing "superheroes." He seemed to enjoy few indoor or fine-motor activities but indicated that he liked to build things. He told the occupational therapist that his favorite play activities are riding his bike and climbing on the jungle gym at the playground. He reported that he most often plays by himself or sometimes with his older brother, but said that his brother "doesn't always like to do stuff with me." He indicated that he had a few friends at school, but could name only one boy in his class (Andrew) with whom he plays during recess. When asked if he has any other friends, he stated, "Well, they don't really like me." He reported that there are no kids in the neighborhood with whom he can play. His mother confirmed that Jerome and his older brother do not always play together. She indicated that Jerome was actually more skilled at gross motor activities such as biking and roller-blading than his older brother and that the older brother preferred more creative or indoor activities such as drawing, listening to music, reading, or watching TV. She noted, "They are like night and day." Her biggest concern about Jerome was his academic performance and the fact that he did not seem to know how to make friends.

The classroom teacher confirmed that Jerome did not seem to be making friends in school. She was concerned that his disruptive behavior was causing him to be marginalized by other classmates. On the playground, she had observed that he had difficulty following the rules of organized games such as soccer and kickball and was often not invited to play by the other children.

The interventions recommended by the occupational therapist primarily addressed Jerome's social skills and his actions in the classroom. She referred Jerome to the Friendship Group, jointly run by herself and the school psychologist. The goals of this group are to help referred children develop appropriate social-interaction skills in the context of structured dyadic play with one other child. Jerome was encouraged to invite one classmate to partici-pate in the Friendship Group with him. The play activities used in the group require cooperation, turn-taking, and negotiation. The group teaches skills in communication and self-regulation.

The occupational therapist also encouraged Jerome's mother to foster more play between Jerome and his brother. She suggested that Joe might be encouraged to share with Jerome his interest in drawing or building things with construction toys such as Lego or K-Nex. Such activities would also help the development of Jerome's fine motor skills. Because Jerome enjoyed and was good at a variety of gross motor activities, the occupational therapist encouraged his mom to help him develop friendships building on these interests. The occupational therapist suggested that participating in recreational programs at the local community center might help Jerome find friends with similar interests, and that his mom could help Jerome arrange occasional "play dates" with one other child.

The Role Checklist

The Role Checklist (Oakley, Kielhofner, & Barris, 1985) was developed to obtain information on clients' perceptions of their participation in occupational roles throughout their life and on the value they place on those occupational roles. The checklist can be used with adolescents or adults. Respondents indicate for each of the 10 occupational roles listed:

- Whether they have held the role in the past
- Whether they are currently in the role
- Whether they expect to be in the role in the future
- How much they value the role.

Role Checklist	*Provides information on what roles a person values and perceived participation in roles in the past, present, and future*	*Copies of the Role Checklist can be obtained from NIH:* *Frances Oakley, MS, OTR/L, BCN, BCG, FAOTA* *National Institutes of Health* *Building 10 Room 6S235 10 Center Drive MSC 1604* *Bethesda, MD 20892-1604* *E-mail: foakley@nih.gov*

Brief lay-oriented definitions of each role are provided, followed by examples of that particular role.

Since MOHO is concerned with how roles structure occupational participation, the definitions employ the criteria of at least weekly involvement in each role. Thus, for example, being a family member is defined not merely as a kinship but as doing something with a family member such as a child, parent, spouse, or other relative at least once a week. In this way, when persons indicate they are in a role, it also means that the role influences what the person does.

The Role Checklist can be filled out in a few minutes either independently or with the assistance of the therapist. Occupational therapists have reported that it is important to discuss the pattern of responses with clients to obtain more detailed information about their role-pattern and its meaning for occupational participation. Some therapists have clients fill it out along with several other persons in a group, where discussion can be used to search for the meaning of each person's responses. In this context, the checklist can facilitate planning future role-behavior.

The Role Checklist is interpreted by examining the pattern of responses; a summary sheet aids in the visual examination and interpretation of the response pattern. For example, it may reveal the following kinds of patterns:

- Loss of many or all occupational roles
- Lack of involvement in roles that are valued
- Overcommitment and difficulty discriminating between the importance of roles
- Desires for future roles that are incompatible with capacities or other role responsibilities.

Occupational therapists find that sharing such interpretations of the Role Checklist with clients is critical both to give information to the client and to validate whether the therapist's interpretation fits with the client's experience.

Dependability

The majority of the psychometric work on the Role Checklist was carried out during the development of the instrument. Content validity was established by an extensive review of the literature and a review by a panel of occupational therapists, which resulted in revisions to some aspects of the checklist. Initial measures of test-retest reliability indicated that the instrument was stable over time with adolescents and adults (Oakley, Kielhofner, Barris, & Reichler, 1986; Pezzulli, 1988). The Role Checklist has been used frequently in research (Barris et al., 1986; Barris, Dickie, & Baron, 1988; Bränholm & Fugl-Meyer, 1992; Duellman, Barris, & Kielhofner,1986; Ebb et al., 1989; Egan, Warren, Hessel, & Gilewich, 1992; Elliott & Barris, 1987; Lerder, Kielhofner, & Watts, 1985). Many of these studies use the checklist as a measure of role performance or value that was shown to be associated with future orientation and life satisfaction. Studies also showed differences in roles between persons with and without disabilities, examined the impact of a child's disability on the mother's role, and investigated the long-term effects of traumatic brain injury on the roles of caregivers.

Administration

The therapist begins by explaining the purpose of the checklist and informing the client that they will discuss responses together. The checklist is relatively simple in format and ordinarily easy for clients to complete. The client considers each of 10 occupational roles described on the checklist, which is divided into 2 parts. In part one, clients check those roles they have performed in the past, are currently performing, and/or plan to perform in the future. For example, if a client volunteered in the past, does not volunteer at present, but anticipates volunteering in the future, he or she would check the role "Volunteer" in both the past and future columns. "Past" refers to anytime up to the preceding week. "Present" includes the week prior, up to and including the day of administration of the checklist. "Future" refers to tomorrow onward. These instructions are on the checklist, and the therapist can review them at the beginning of administration if it is deemed useful to the client.

In part two of the checklist, the client rates each role as to whether he or she finds it not at all valuable, somewhat valuable, or very valuable. Value refers to the personal worth or importance of the role.

The occupational therapist ordinarily remains with the client to answer or clarify questions. When followed up with an interview, the Role Checklist further helps the occupational therapist and client identify

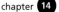

patterns in role selection, preference, and performance. For example, they can examine:

- The kinds of roles persons have been successful at over the course of their lives
- The kinds of roles they have avoided or given up
- Whether roles focus around particular kinds of occupational forms (e.g., social relationships, service delivery)
- If they have a balance among roles
- If they are performing roles they consider not at all valuable.

Such discussions are helpful to both the client and therapist in providing insights into the client's life.

Mary

Using the Role Checklist to Identify Priorities for Maintaining Roles

Mary is a 78-year-old retired widow diagnosed with early-stage dementia of the Alzheimer's type who lives in her family's home. She has a very supportive and loving family. Because of her short-term memory impairment, her grandson recently moved in to help out, keep an eye on her, and manage her financial affairs.

Mary filled out the Role Checklist with assistance from the occupational therapist. To gain a compre-

hensive picture, her grandson also provided information related to her role behavior. The occupational therapist used the results from the completed checklist to begin a dialogue with Mary and her grandson about her occupational role functioning.

Mary's pattern of role identification and value *(Fig. 14-9)* reflects involvement throughout her life in a variety of very valuable roles. This pattern reflects Mary's view that, at 78 years of age, she has lived a full life. Despite identifying all roles as very valuable, Mary currently identifies participation in four roles: home maintainer, friend, family member, and hobbyist. She indicated that she would like to continue involvement in those four roles and resume involvement in the future in four additional roles: worker, volunteer, caregiver, and religious participant.

The therapist, in collaboration with Mary and her grandson, decided to concentrate on Mary's present roles and to forgo pursuit of future roles. Coming to this collaborative decision precipitated some of the first frank discussion of the functional implications of Mary's dementia and its expected future course. The therapist discussed with Mary and her grandson her current impairment and the degenerative nature of Mary's disease. After discussion, they all agreed it was unlikely that Mary would be able to independently resume participation in some of her

FIGURE 14-9   Mary's Responses on the Role Checklist.

Role	Role Identity			Value Designation		
	Past	Present	Future	Not at all	Some what	Very
Student						
Worker						
Volunteer						
Care Giver						
Home Maintainer						
Friend						
Family Member						
Religious Participant						
Hobbyist/Amateur						
Participant in Organizations						
Other						

desired future roles such as worker and caregiver. As part of the discussion, they all affirmed the value of the life Mary had led to date and the importance of continuing to live as full a life as possible. The discussion also revealed that when Mary checked the future role of religious participant she meant that she wanted to continue to attend church on a regular basis. Mary had been unable to do so because she had to give up driving, which was her means of getting to church. Mary's grandson is in the process of making other arrangements to ensure that Mary is able to attend church on Sundays.

In discussion with the therapist, Mary was able to identify the responsibilities of her roles, but admitted that at times her forgetfulness constrained her ability to fully meet her role expectations. Thus, the therapist proposed that they together identify the present role responsibilities Mary could continue to safely perform and those for which she would need assistance. They then devised adaptive strategies in collaboration with Mary and her grandson to assure her continued participation in the roles she valued. The following are some examples of how they accomplished this.

As part of the home maintainer role, Mary vacuumed the rooms in the house. However, she often forgets whether or not she vacuumed a particular room. To aid her, Mary, the therapist, and her grandson made a sign that said, "This room has been vacuumed." They agreed that, once Mary vacuumed the room, her grandson would place the sign on the doorknob.

As part of her hobbyist role, Mary loved to crochet afghans, which over the years she made for family and friends. However, she often misplaced her crocheting supplies. To aid her in finding her supplies they agreed that her grandson would purchase a large but manageable, brightly colored basket in which he and Mary could place all her supplies.

As this case illustrates, the information gleaned from the checklist along with the resulting dialogue with Mary and her grandson helped to:

- Validate Mary's past pattern of roles that affirmed her full life
- Identify what was important to Mary now
- Serve as a basis for discussion of what roles were realistic for Mary to maintain in light of her disability.

As with this case, the Role Checklist often serves as a catalyst for discussion of realistic priorities with clients. Also, as with Mary, clients often find the checklist to be affirming since it gives them a concrete representation of their life pattern. For example, one depressed patient, having filled out the form, noted his several past roles. He reflected that he had been feeling very incompetent, but when he saw how many roles he was able to fill in the past, he felt better about his abilities and more hopeful for the future. Finally, as with the case of Mary's desire to reinstate her religious participant role, discussing responses on the checklist is always important for understanding what clients meant when filling out the form.

Conclusion: Self-Report Assessments in Perspective

This chapter presented assessments based on the method of self-report and illustrated their use through case examples. All these assessments allow clients to provide information about themselves by completing paper-and-pencil forms. The assessments can be administered verbally when necessary. These methods have many virtues including efficiency and the opportunity for the client to become actively engaged in the process of gathering information and influencing what goes on in therapy. As noted throughout the chapter, these assessments should always be used in the context of a discussion between the therapist and client to clarify responses and validate interpretations, as well as to achieve mutual agreement about their implications for therapy.

References

Andrews, P. M., Bleecher, R., Genoa, A. M., Molloy, P., Monahan, K., & Sargent, J. (1995). *Leisure interests of children.* Unpublished manuscript, Worcester State College, Worcester, MA.

Baron, K., Kielhofner, G., Iyenger, A., Goldhammer, V., & Wolenski, J. (2002). *The Occupational Self Assessment(OSA) (Version 2.0).* Chicago: Model of Human Occupation Clearinghouse, Department of Occupational

Therapy, College of Applied Health Sciences, University of Illinois at Chicago.

Barris, R., Dickie, V., & Baron, K. (1988). A comparison of psychiatric patients and normal subjects based on the model of human occupation. *Occupational Therapy Journal of Research, 8*, 3–23.

Barris, R., Kielhofner, G., Burch, R. M., Gelinas, I., Klement, M., & Schultz, B. (1986). Occupational function and dysfunction in three groups of adolescents. *Occupational Therapy Journal of Research, 6*, 301–317.

Beck, D., Benson, S., Curet, J., Froehlich, D., McCrary, L., Rasmussen, L., & Skowyra, K. (1996). *Pilot study of a child's play interest profile.* Unpublished manuscript, Worcester State College, Worcester, MA.

Bränholm, I., & Fugl-Meyer, A. R. (1992). Occupational role preferences and life satisfaction. *Occupational Therapy Journal of Research, 12*, 159–171.

Brophy, P., Caizzi, D., Crete, B., Jachym, T., Kobus, M., & Sainz, C. (1995). *Preliminary reliability study of the Adolescent Leisure Interest Profile.* Unpublished manuscript, Worcester State College, Worcester, MA.

Budd, P., Ferraro, D., Lovely, A., McNeil, T., Owanisian, L., Parker, J., Peters, M., Hann, J., Regele, K., Walsh, C., Fontana, L., & Bentley, R. (1994). *Item development for a new measure of adolescent leisure interests.* Unpublished manuscript, Worcester State College, Worcester, MA.

Duellman, M. K., Barris, R., & Kielhofner, G. (1986). Organized activity and the adaptive status of nursing home residents. *American Journal of Occupational Therapy, 40*, 618–622.

Ebb, E. W., Coster, W., & Duncombe, L. (1989). Comparison of normal and psychosocially dysfunctional male adolescents. *Occupational Therapy in Mental Health, 9*(2), 53–74.

Egan, M., Warren, S. A., Hessel, P. A., & Gilewich, G. (1992). Activities of daily living after hip fracture: Pre- and post discharge. *Occupational Therapy Journal of Research, 12*, 342–356.

Elliott, M., & Barris, R. (1987). Occupational role performance and life satisfaction in elderly persons. *Occupational Therapy Journal of Research, 7*, 215–224.

Federico, J., & Kielhofner, G. (2002). *The Child Occupational Self Assessment (COSA)(Version 1.0).* Chicago: Model of Human Occupation Clearinghouse, Department of Occupational Therapy, College of Applied Health Sciences, University of Illinois at Chicago.

Furst, G., Gerber, L., Smith, C., Fisher, S., & Shulman, B. (1987). A program for improving energy conservation behaviors in adults with rheumatoid arthritis. *American Journal of Occupational Therapy, 41*, 102–111.

Gerber, L., & Furst, G. (1992). Scoring methods and application of the Activity Record (ACTRE) for patients with musculoskeletal disorders. *Arthritis Care and Research, 5*, 151–156.

Henry, A. D. (1994). *Predicting psychosocial functioning and symptomatic recovery of adolescents and young adults with a first psychotic episode: A six-month follow-up study.* Unpublished doctoral dissertation, Boston University, Boston, MA.

Henry, A. D. (2000). *The Pediatric Interest Profiles: Surveys of play for children and adolescents.* San Antonio, TX: Therapy Skill Builders.

Iyenger, A. (2001). *A study of the psychometric properties of the OSA.* Unpublished master's thesis, University of Illinois at Chicago, Chicago, IL.

Katz, N., Giladi, N., & Peretz, C. (1988). Cross-cultural application of occupational therapy assessments: Human occupation with psychiatric inpatients and controls in Israel. *Occupational Therapy in Mental Health, 8* (1), 7–30.

Kielhofner, G., & Brinson, M. (1989). Development and evaluation of an aftercare program for young and chronic psychiatrically disabled adults. *Occupational Therapy in Mental Health, 9* (2), 1–25.

Kielhofner, G., & Forsyth, K. (2001). Development of a client self-report for treatment planning and documenting therapy outcomes. *Scandinavian Journal of Occupational Therapy. 8* (3), 131–139.

Kielhofner, G., & Neville, A. (1983). *The modified interest checklist.* Unpublished manuscript, University of Illinois at Chicago, Chicago, IL.

Lerder, J., Kielhofner, G., & Watts, J. (1985). Values, personal causation and skills of delinquents of the acute hand injured patient. *Occupational Therapy in Mental Health, 5*, 59–77.

Matsutsuyu, J. (1969). The Interest Check List. *American Journal of Occupational Therapy, 23*, 323–328.

Oakley, F., Kielhofner, G., & Barris, R. (1985). An occupational therapy approach to assessing psychiatric patients' adaptive functioning. *American Journal of Occupational Therapy, 39*, 147–154.

Oakley, F., Kielhofner, G., Barris, R., & Reichler, R. K. (1986). The Role Checklist: Development and empirical assessment of reliability. *Occupational Therapy Journal of Research, 6*, 157–170.

Pezzulli, T. (1988). *Test-retest reliability of the role checklist with depressed adolescents in short term psychiatric hospitals.* Unpublished master's thesis, Virginia Commonwealth University, Richmond, VA.

Riopel, N. J. (1982). *An examination of the occupational behavior and life satisfaction of the elderly.* Unpublished master's thesis, University of Illinois at Chicago, Chicago, IL.

Rogers, J., Weinstein, J., & Figone, J. (1978). The Interest Check List: An empirical assessment. *American Journal of Occupational Therapy, 32, 628–630.*

Scaffa, M. (1981). *Temporal adaptations and alcoholism.* Unpublished master's thesis, Virginia Commonwealth University, Richmond, VA.

Scaffa, M. (1991). Alcoholism: An occupational behavior perspective. *Occupational Therapy in Mental Health, 11* (2/3), 99–111.

Smith, N. R., Kielhofner, G., & Watts, J. (1986). The relationship between volition, activity pattern, and life satisfaction in the elderly. *American Journal of Occupational Therapy, 40,* 278–283.

Smyntek, L., Barris, R., & Kielhofner, G. (1985). The model of human occupation applied to psychosocially functional and dysfunctional adolescents. *Occupational Therapy in Mental Health, 5* (1), 21–40.

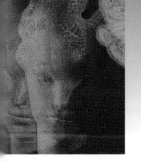

15

Talking With Clients: Assessments That Collect Information Through Interviews

- Gary Kielhofner
- Kirsty Forsyth
- Christine Clay
- Elin Ekbladh
- Lena Haglund
- Helena Hemmingsson
- Riitta Keponen
- Linda Olson

Whether formal or informal, client interviews provide a large portion of the information through which therapists come to know their clients. Five assessments that use interviews have been developed for use with MOHO:

- Occupational Circumstances Assessment-Interview and Rating Scale
- Occupational Performance History Interview-Second Version
- School Setting Interview
- Worker Role Interview
- Work Environment Impact Scale.

Each of these assessments has a distinct format and purpose. The Occupational Circumstances Assessment-Interview and Rating Scale (OCAIRS) (Haglund, Henriksson, Crisp, Freidheim, & Kielhofner, 2001) is based on the Occupational Case Analysis Interview and Rating Scale (Kaplan & Kielhofner, 1989). This assessment focuses primarily on present functioning. The Occupational Performance History Interview-Second Version (OPHI-II) (Kielhofner et al., 1998) is a life

history interview. The Worker Role Interview (WRI) (Velozo, Kielhofner, & Fisher, 1998) is designed for use with injured or disabled workers. The Work Environment Impact Scale (WEIS) (Moore-Corner, Kielhofner, & Olson, 1998) was developed to examine the impact of the work environment on the worker. The School Setting Interview (SSI) (Hoffman, Hemmingsson, & Kielhofner, 2000) is a semi-structured interview designed to assess school environment impact and identify the need for accommodations for students with disabilities.

These assessments all share some common features. Each has a semi-structured interview that the therapist adapts to fit the unique circumstances of each client. After the interview is conducted, the therapist must have some means of analyzing the information. Each assessment has a rating scale or checklist that when completed represents what was learned in the interview. Each of these assessments also has a means of recording qualitative information gathered during the interview.

Occupational Circumstances Assessment-Interview and Rating Scale

The Occupational Circumstances Assessment Interview and Rating Scale (OCAIRS) (Haglund et al., 2001) is based the Occupational Case Analysis Interview and Rating Scale (Kaplan, 1984; Kaplan & Kielhofner, 1989).

The OCAIRS provides a structure for gathering, analyzing, and reporting data on the extent and nature of an individual's occupational adaptation. The interview is used to collect information on occupational adaptation and participation, personal causation, values and goals, interests, roles, habits, skills, and the environment. The OCAIRS is designed to be relevant to adolescent and adult clients with a wide range of backgrounds and impairments.

Administration

A manual details the OCAIRS, providing information on conducting the interview and completing the scale (Haglund et al., 2001). The OCAIRS consists of a semi-structured interview that can be adapted to each unique client. After conducting the interview, the therapist completes a rating scale and records comments regarding the client's occupational functioning. The interview averages 40 minutes, and completion of the scale with comments takes 15 minutes.

The rating scale is completed by checking off criteria that best describe the client and then using them as a guide to selecting the appropriate rating. A sample item is shown in *Figure 15-1*. The rating scale provides a profile of strengths and weaknesses, which is useful for therapy and discharge planning. As with other assessments, a measure may be calculated by computer for research purposes. Long-term plans are to develop a paper-and-pencil method of obtaining a measure.

Dependability

The OCAIRS is in the process of being investigated. Its format and content reflect findings from substantial research concerning the previous assessment on which it is based (Brollier, Watts, Bauer, & Schmidt, 1989; Haglund & Henriksson, 1994; Haglund, Thorell, & Wålinder, 1998a, 1998b; Kaplan, 1984; Lai, Haglund, & Kielhofner, 1999). Collectively, these studies found evidence of good interrater reliability and the ability to effectively discriminate between clients with different severities of psychiatric illness. These studies also pointed to weaknesses in the previous instrument that were used as a basis for constructing the OCAIRS.

Olaf

Using the OCAIRS to Guide Intervention and Discharge Planning

At the age of 23, Olaf was hospitalized for the first time in an acute psychiatric ward. His older sister, younger brother, and parents (who are professors) live in the same town in Sweden. Olaf moved to his own apartment 2 years earlier when he began studying nursing at the local university. When he was younger, Olaf always had many friends. However, in the past 4 years he had been very isolated, spending most of his time studying. For 6 months, Olaf experienced increasing difficulty keeping up with his studies. Most recently, he complained of hearing a voice that told him to hurt himself because he is not good enough.

Occupational Circumstances Assessment-Interview and Rating Scale (OCAIRS)	*Gathers information on values, goals, personal causation, interests, habits, roles, skills, environmental impact, participation, and adaptation*	*Information on ordering can be found on the Model of Human Occupation Clearinghouse web site at:* *http://www.uic.edu/hsc/acad/cahp/OT/MOHOC* *Or go to: http://www.uic.edu* *Link to:* *1) Academic Departments* *2) Applied Health Sciences* *3) Occupational Therapy* *4) MOHO*

FIGURE 15-1 Sample Item (Interests) From the OCAIRS.

RATING	DESCRIPTION	COMMENTS
4	Identifies and participates in 3 or more varied interests outside of work	
	Expresses a high level of interest in primary occupation	
	Expresses a high level of satisfaction with both the interests and level of participation	
3	Identifies and participates in 2 interests regularly outside of work	
	Is somewhat interested in primary occupation	
	Expresses satisfaction with either interests and/or level of participation	
2	Identifies 1-2 interests outside of work with inconsistent participation	
	Has little interest in primary occupation	
	Expresses some dissatisfaction with both the interests and/or level of participation	
1	Does not identfy or does not participate in any interests	
	Has no interest in primary occupation	
	Expresses strong dissatisfaction with both interests and level of participation	
IM	Unable to obtain information regarding	

Key:
Adaptive **4** **3** **2** **1** Maladaptive
IM = Information Missing

during the interview he asked, "Do you think I'm schizophrenic?" Despite his confusion and fear, he was able to participate effectively in the interview. Olaf's scores on the OCAIRS are shown in *Figure 15-2*. The following qualitative information was also gathered during the interview.

When asked about his interests, Olaf noted that he used to like to listen to hard rock music, study, and read science literature, but he had not been able to do these things for some time. He did have some goals. In particular, he wanted to begin his studies again. After finishing the nursing program, he wanted to enroll in management courses at the university and then start his own business. He

FIGURE 15-2 Olaf's Ratings on the OCAIRS.

	4	3	2	1	IM
Interests		■			
Personal causation				■	
Values			■		
Short-term goals				■	
Long-term goals			■		
Habits				■	
Roles	·			■	
Motor skills	■				
Process skills				■	
Communication/interaction skills				■	
Previous experiences			■		
Physical environment supports	■				
Physical environment opportunities	■				
Physical environment demands/constraints				■	
Physical environment fit			■		
Social environment supports			■		
Social environment opportunities					✕
Social environment demands/constraints			■		
Social environment fit				■	
Occupational participation				■	
Occupational adaptation				■	

Key:
Adaptive **4** **3** **2** **1** Maladaptive
IM = Information Missing

The occupational therapist used the OCAIRS to gather information about Olaf's occupational adaptation to help with planning during his anticipated 4-week hospitalization. Olaf was quite confused about what was happening to him. Several times said that it was very important to him to be smart and successful.

In contrast to his goal of beginning school again, Olaf's sense of personal causation was extremely low. He felt very out of control. He feared that the voice he heard would control him. Although he felt compelled to return to his studies, he did not see how he could possibly succeed. Olaf indicated that he was no longer able to do anything well and he could not point out any skills of which he was proud. He complained that he could not plan or organize his behavior to accomplish even everyday activities.

Olaf previously was able to maintain a daily routine as follows. He attended the university in the morning and studied in the evening. He carried out his routine alone, remaining isolated during the weekend. He disliked cooking, so he mostly ate at the university canteen or a local restaurant. He noted that each day had been more or less the same for him for the past 4 years. He indicated, "I'm not a sociable person anymore." During the previous 6 months, Olaf had difficulty completing daily routines and concentrating on tasks. In the 3 weeks before being hospitalized, he remained in his flat alone, drinking tea and eating sandwiches, ignoring everything else including his personal hygiene.

Olaf described actively avoiding other people, noting that he was very shy and felt uncomfortable initiating conversation. When asked about important people in his life, he hesitated and then finally mentioned his sister. He recalled that he had a girlfriend some years before. However, at the time, there was no person that he considered a significant support. While Olaf recalled a happy family life during childhood and adolescence, he felt that he no longer had anything to say to his parents. He admitted feeling very lonely and longed for more social contact.

Olaf liked his flat and very much wanted to return to it. He received a substantial amount of money from his grandmother when he bought his flat so he could furnish it the way he wanted. The flat is in the central part of the town, a location that he liked.

The interview helped the occupational therapist identify Olaf's strengths and weaknesses as shown in Figure 15-2. Although many aspects of his occupational life were quite eroded, his long-term goals and his physical environment were strong points. It was apparent in the interview that Olaf's greatest priorities were to:

- Engage in his studies again
- Take part in some social occupations
- Move back to his flat as soon as possible.

The OCAIRS also provided a structured way of helping the therapist start to plan Olaf's intervention. She planned to address his volitional status through structured graded occupations. Information about Olaf's occupational lifestyle gained from the OCAIRS was used to select the specific occupational forms used in intervention. These were things he indicated an interest in and that related to his long-term goals. She also chose occupational forms that were within his skill level so that he could experience success and thereby begin to rebuild personal causation. Given that Olaf felt he could not do anything, the therapist routinely provided Olaf with concrete feedback aimed at shaping his experience of doing things. Therefore, whenever he completed an occupational form, the therapist took time to review what he had accomplished and highlighted his strengths. She also carefully pointed out how his successes in therapy related to his long-term aims.

As Olaf gained some confidence, the therapist and he started to work together on his goal of returning to independent living in his own flat. He began by taking increased responsibility for self-care and care of his immediate environment. Since Olaf stated he was having difficulties maintaining a daily routine and completing his homemaker tasks, they developed a routine that included some of these tasks in the inpatient setting. Olaf followed this routine and reviewed it twice a week with the therapist. As he approached time for discharge, the therapist accompanied Olaf to his apartment several times to identify and practice homemaking tasks. Finally, Olaf was enrolled in several inpatient groups to increase his level of social interaction. While he remained quiet, his level of skill became adequate for social interaction once he regained some of his confidence for interacting with others.

The OCAIRS was also useful in planning for Olaf's discharge. His level of functioning was still not consistent with the demands of returning to university studies. However, given the importance for Olaf of being involved in studies, the therapist arranged for him to attend a supported educational facility for persons with psychosocial impairments. She worked with him to make choices for courses, focusing on those related to his long-term goals. She also helped Olaf plan a daily routine to accommodate attending the courses. Because of his poor sense of efficacy, she accompanied him to the school to sign up for the first day of classes. She also guided him to identify some groups at the school that he could join to have social contact. The therapist continued to make home visits with Olaf in his apartment after discharge to monitor the routine they had planned together so that he could manage his self-care and maintain the apartment.

In sum, the OCAIRS provided the therapist with information to gain an understanding of Olaf's occupational life, the challenges he faced, and his goals for the future. This information helped in identifying therapeutic goals and strategies and assured that therapy addressed what mattered to Olaf.

Occupational Performance History Interview-Second Version

As a historical interview, the Occupational Performance History Interview-Second Version (OPHI-II) (Kielhofner et al., 1998) gathers information about a client's past and present occupational adaptation. The OPHI-II is a three-part assessment that includes:

- A semi-structured interview that explores a client's occupational life history
- Rating scales that provide a measure of the client's occupational identity, occupational competence, and the impact of the client's occupational behavior settings
- A life history narrative designed to capture salient qualitative features of the occupational life history.

It is designed to give the interviewer a means of understanding the way a client perceives her or his life to be unfolding. The OPHI-II can be used with adolescents and adults who have a range of impairments.

As a semi-structured interview, the OPHI-II provides a framework and recommended questions for conducting the interview to assure that the necessary information is obtained. The interview is organized into the following thematic areas:

- Activity/occupational choices
- Critical life events
- Daily routine
- Occupational roles
- Occupational behavior settings.

Within each of these thematic areas, a possible sequence of interview questions is provided. The interview is designed to be very flexible so that therapists can cover the areas in any sequence or move back and forth between them.

The second part of the OPHI-II is composed of the three rating scales:

- Occupational identity scale
- Occupational competence scale
- Occupational behavior settings scale.

Occupational Performance History Interview-Second Version (OPHI-II)	*Gathers information on client's life history with a focus on identity, competence, and environment*	*Information on ordering can be found on the Model of Human Occupation Clearinghouse web site at: http://www.uic.edu/hsc/acad/cahp/OT/MOHOC Or go to: http://www.uic.edu Link to:* *1) Academic Departments* *2) Applied Health Sciences* *3) Occupational Therapy* *4) MOHO*

The three scales provide a means of converting the information gathered in the interview into three measures. The occupational identity scale measures the degree to which persons have values, interests, and confidence; see themselves in various occupational roles; and hold an image of the kind of life they want. The occupational competence scale measures the degree to which a person is able to sustain a pattern of occupational participation that is productive and satisfying. The occupational behavior settings scale measures the impact of the environment on the client's occupational life.

Administration

The OPHI-II is presented in a detailed manual designed to allow the therapist to learn how to administer the assessment. It includes detailed guidelines for conducting the interview and provides several resources for supporting the interview process. It also gives detailed instructions and examples for completing the rating scales and life history narrative.

The therapist begins by conducting the interview, which takes approximately 45–60 minutes to complete. Although the OPHI-II is designed so that it can be completed as a single interview, therapists may conduct the interview in more than one part. Following the interview, the therapist scores the 3 rating scales consisting of a total of 29 items. The therapist rates each item with a 4-point rating that indicates the client's level of occupational adaptation/environmental impact. The rating is completed by first noting criteria that describe the client for each item and then selecting the corresponding rating, as shown in Figure 15-3. Each of the three scales provides a profile of strengths and weaknesses related to identity, competence, and environmental impact, which is useful to planning therapy. As with other assessments, a measure may be calculated for each scale by computer. Paper-and-pencil methods of generating measures from each scale have been developed.

Finally, the therapist completes the life history narrative form that is used to report qualitative information from the interview. As part of this process, the therapist graphically plots the client's life story, thereby indicating the narrative slope, as discussed in Chapter 9. This allows the therapist to develop an ap-

FIGURE 15-3   An Example of Scoring the OPHI-II Scale: Criteria Are Checked and the Rating Indicated by the Criteria Selected.

Item	Rating	Criteria
Has personal goals and projects	4	☐ Goals/personal projects challenge/extend/require effort
		☐ Feels energized/excited about future goals/personal projects
	3	☐ Goals/personal projects fit strengths/limitations
		☐ Enough desire for future to overcome doubt/challenges
		☐ Motivated to work on goals/personal projects
	2	☐ Goals/anticipated projects under/overestimate abilities
		☐ Not very motivated to work on goals/personal projects
		☒ Difficulty thinking about goals/personal projects/future
		☒ Limited commitment/excitement/ motivation
	1	☐ Cannot identify goals/personal projects
		☐ Personal goals/desired projects are unattainable given abilities
		☐ Goals bear little/no relationship to strengths/limitations
		☐ Lacks commitment or motivation to the future
		☐ Unmotivated due to conflicting/ excessive goals/personal projects

Key: **4** = Exceptionally competent occupational functioning; **3** = Appropriate satisfactory occupational functioning; **2** = Some occupational dysfunction; **1** = Extremely occupationally dysfunctional

preciation of the plot of the occupational narrative underlying the client's identity and competence.

Dependability

Kielhofner and Henry (1988) found that a total score obtained from the original OPHI rating scale was only marginally stable across raters and time. A second study (Kielhofner, Henry, Walens, & Rogers, 1991) sought to improve reliability by developing more specific guidelines for rating. This study found that the total score on the scale was acceptably stable. Gutkowski (1992) devised and studied a revised OPHI scale but failed to improve reliability further.

Two studies provided evidence of the concurrent and predictive validity of the OPHI (Henry, Tohen, Coster, & Tickle-Degnen, 1995; Lynch & Bridle, 1993). Mallinson, Mahaffey, and Kielhofner (1998) examined internal validity and found that the items of the revised OPHI scale revealed three underlying constructs: competence, identity, and environmental impact. This finding provided the basis for creating the three scales that comprise the OPHI-II.

Two studies examined the qualitative information gained from the OPHI. Kielhofner and Mallinson (1995) found that the types of questions recommended in the original OPHI and used by therapists often prevented interviewees from giving richer narrative data. Based on this, they recommended changes that were incorporated into the OPHI-II interview. Mallinson, Kielhofner, and Mattingly (1996) found that interviewees often narrated their life histories by evoking metaphors as a way of making sense of their life situations. These findings are reflected in the OPHI-II narrative analysis. Cumulative findings from previous studies of the OPHI provided a substantial foundation for creating the OPHI-II.

Kielhofner, Mallinson, Forsyth, and Lai (2001) conducted an international study using six different language versions of the OPHI-II. They found that all three scales validly and sensitively assessed a wide range of persons who varied by nationality, culture, age, and diagnostic status. Raters in this study, who learned the OPHI-II in a variety of ways including study of the manual, were able to validly rate clients.

Christine

The OPHI-II as the Beginning of a Way Out

Christine is an African-American woman in her mid-30s. Over the past several years, she has had a series of surgeries for recurrent, nonmalignant brain tumors. In addition to repeated surgical removal of the tumors over a several-year period, she has also received a shunt to alleviate elevated intraventricular pressure. As a consequence of her tumors and surgery, Christine has both mild cognitive impairments (mostly difficulty with short-term memory) and low vision impairment.

Following her most recent surgery, Christine was hospitalized in a short-term rehabilitation unit. During her stay, the occupational therapist focused on supporting Christine to use adaptive strategies to more effectively perform activities of daily living. As Christine neared discharge, she indicated to her therapist a desire to make some major changes in her life, specifically to return to work and live on her own.

The therapist referred Christine to an outpatient occupational therapy program, Work Readiness, that was designed to support clients who wished to achieve greater independence and move toward employment. As part of the entrance into this program, Christine participated in the OPHI-II interview. Because the program was designed to assist clients in making major life changes, this historical interview was especially appropriate. It was routinely used both to help clients and therapists together decide whether the program was appropriate for the client and to help determine long-term goals and approaches.

The results of Christine's interview on the three rating scales are shown in *Figure 15-4*. Christine related a life story in which her strong occupational identity had been partly eroded by her prolonged illness, impairments, and consequent loss of major occupational roles. Christine grew up on the south side of Chicago in a working class family. She described her parents as warm and proud individuals with strong values. They instilled in their children a sense that they should make something of their lives, be leaders, and give something back to their community. As Christine put it, her parents not only expected that their children have a vision of their goals in life, but also be able to "have a concrete plan for getting there."

Christine's father died when she was 12, which left the family in financial jeopardy. Christine recalls her father's death as both a tragic and defining moment in her life. According to her, "I walked to my father's coffin and looked down at him, pledging that I would never let my mother and sister go hun-

FIGURE 15-4 Summary of Christine's Scores on the OPHI-II.

Occupational Identity Scale	1	2	3	4
Has personal goals and projects		■		
Identifies a desired occupational lifestyle				■
Expects success	■			
Accepts responsibility		■		
Appraises abilities and limitations		■		
Has commitments and values				■
Recognizes identity and obligations				■
Has interests				■
Felt effective (past)				■
Found meaning and satisfaction in lifestyle (past)				■
Made occupational choices (past)				■

Occupational Competence Scale	1	2	3	4
Maintains satisfying lifestyle	■			
Fulfills role expectations	■			
Works toward goals	■			
Meets personal performance standards	■			
Organizes time for responsibilities	■			
Participates in interests	■			
Fulfilled roles (past)				■
Maintained habits (past)				■
Achieved satisfaction (past)				■

Occupational Behavior Settings Scale	1	2	3	4
Home-life occupational forms			■	
Major productive role occupational forms	Not applicable			
Leisure occupational forms		■		
Home-life social group			■	
Major productive social group	Not applicable			
Leisure social group		■		
Home-life physical spaces, objects, and resources			■	
Major productive role physical spaces, objects, and resources	Not applicable			
Leisure physical spaces, objects, and resources		■		

Key: **4** = Exceptionally competent occupational functioning; **3** = Appropriate satisfactory occupational functioning; **2** = Some occupational dysfunction; **1** = Extremely occupationally dysfunctional

gry . . . or have to live on the streets." Christine was true to her vow. After earning a college degree in teaching, she still had part-time jobs in addition to being a full-time teacher in an inner city Head Start program. This she did to provide extra income for her mother and younger sister.

Despite the family challenges, Christine still remembers her adolescence fondly. She recalls that she, her sister, and mother "found ways to be happy." For Christine, one of the key factors was her involvement in amateur acting. She became part of a group that put on regular performances in a local community theater.

Whether in pursuing education, supporting her mother or sister, or finding ways to be happy, resourcefulness and self-reliance were key elements of Christine's experience during that early period. Then, one day in the classroom, everything changed. A peer teacher observed Christine do something strange. She attempted to pick up an object pictured on the page of a book she was reading to the children. Christine remembers that she saw it as three-dimensional and real. This perceptual error, which led Christine to seek medical attention, and increasing headaches were the first signs of something awry in her brain. Christine still remembers the classroom incident both as her last day of teaching and as the turning point where the life she had crafted began to disintegrate.

Surgery to remove a tumor swiftly followed and left Christine with short-term memory loss and visual restrictions. Her job was gone and she moved from her apartment back to her mother's house. The mother and sister, to whom Christine had offered financial support, now helped Christine through even her most basic daily routines. During several ensuing years, recurring surgeries and their cumulative sequelae left Christine increasingly impaired and more and more distanced from the life she once lived.

Christine was afraid to have others "see what she had become." She describes how, when people came to the house, she ran to the basement to "hide herself away." While Christine realized her incarceration was self-imposed, she saw "no way out." The person she once was and the life she once lived were gone forever. She described herself as "boxed in" by the fear of what others may see in her. She described the deep and painful frustration of being unable to pull out of herself what she used to be able to do. She had no other way to sum her life than the feeling of being "locked away."

Christine's daily routine reflected both her difficulties with short-term memory and her complete demoralization. She noted that the first big chore of the day was getting out of bed. This did not ordinarily occur without repeated entreaties from her mother. When she did finally manage to emerge from bed, the routines of daily life unfolded with excruciating slowness. Christine explained that the reason for her pace of performing was that she could not remember what she has just done. Things as simple as bathing became long, confusing trials in which she tried to tally each completed step and inevitably repeated herself several times to allay the anxiety that she has forgotten something. Christine was able to do little beyond self-care and helping out with chores around the house. She left the house only for necessary medical appointments. Her former roles and routines were things of the past.

Christine still had a vivid image of the kind of life she wanted, even if she did not dare to hope for it. Christine longed to return to teaching children. She wanted to go back to a time when she was supporting her mother and sister instead of them guiding her through her day. She was explicit and articulate in expressing her desire to still make a difference. At the same time, Christine could not reconcile the image of who she wanted to be with the impairments she experienced. So she was stuck, unable to get, in her words, "out of the box" in which she found herself. She longed for but could not see a "way out." Thus, while her goals were clear, they were not attainable.

As reflected in the OPHI-II ratings from Figure 15-4, Christine's identity had many strengths, along with the challenges of her compromised personal causation and her difficulty in formulating a realistic goal. The therapist recognized and built on these strengths and weaknesses in the course of Christine's involvement in the Work Readiness program. As will be discussed below, therapy focused on rebuilding her sense of capacity and efficacy and her selecting realistic goals for the future. Her compe-

tence was more severely affected in all aspects. Being "locked away," she did not pursue goals, enact roles and routines, or take on responsibilities as in the past. Finally, as Christine noted, she existed a long way from the high standards of performance that she inherited from her family. The course of therapy was designed to enable Christine to gradually rebuild these aspects of her competence.

Christine's removal from the world of work and her narrowed world of everyday life and recreation are reflected in the ratings on the occupational behavior settings scale. Her mother and sister were sources of guidance and comfort for her. As she notes, they kept her going and helped her "remember where she came from."

Christine's narrative slope, as depicted in *Figure 15-5,* has all the features of a tragedy. This woman, who drew strength from and rose out of the challenges of her early life to earn a college degree and take on a professional role, found herself sliding steadily downward. Christine's narrative also reveals a strong metaphor of entrapment (see discussion of metaphors in Chapter 9). Her feelings of being "locked away" found expression in her being house-bound and in hiding from others.

When the therapist shared these interpretations of Christine's life with her, she agreed that they were accurate. The metaphor of being locked away and its implied solution of needing to find a way out served as both an incentive for Christine to join the Work Readiness program and a recurrent theme in Christine's therapy. Through the course of therapy, Christine slowly rebuilt a routine by attending the program with increasing frequency. She learned with ongoing support how to monitor her performance and check for mistakes without repeating herself endlessly. After a couple of months, Christine attended the program daily and was able to join and perform in the presence of others. As she noted, she had found a "way out" through therapy.

When Christine progressed to the point of considering a return to work, she had to find out for herself whether teaching was still a possibility. The therapist arranged a placement for Christine as a classroom volunteer. It was quickly apparent to Christine that her residual impairments made teaching unrealistic. Instead, in making her first foray into

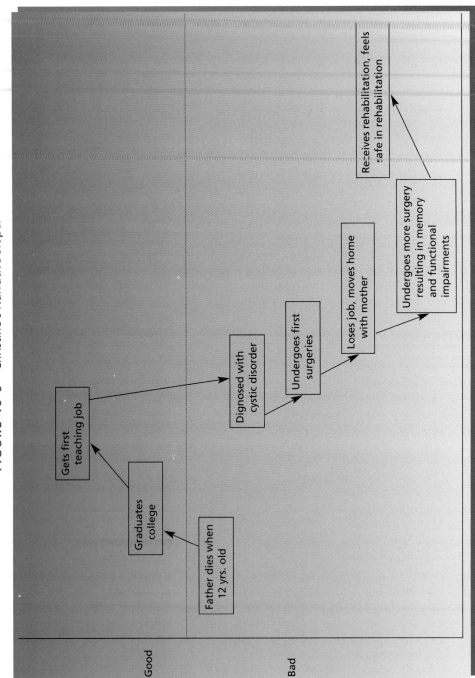

FIGURE 15-5   Christine's Narrative Slope.

the world of work, Christine reached back to her old experiences of theatrical performance and secured a job in a gambling casino where her responsibilities included entertaining customers with a little "soft shoe." Christine had traversed the wide gulf from hiding away to presenting herself in a most public way. For her, this was an important journey.

Nevertheless, after a period of working in the casino, Christine longed for work that would more nearly match her value system. Taking advantage of the program's long-term follow-up services, she received support for a job search and eventually became an intake counselor in a program serving people with visual impairments. Having a visual disability herself, Christine found that she was able to put new clients at ease and to serve as a role model for what could be achieved despite impairments.

Christine also found her way back into the role of teaching as a lecturer in occupational therapy, speaking to students about the experience of disability and the client's perspective in undergoing therapy. She has gone on to create, in poetry, visual imagery, and film, teaching tools aimed at a variety of audiences to encourage the understanding of disability and how to cope with it. Her most recent accomplishment is becoming one of the authors of this chapter!

As this case illustrates, the OPHI-II provides a detailed chronicle of the salient features of a client's life and the impact of events and environment on identity and competence. It also provides insight into how the client interprets his or her life by evoking the client's occupational narrative. This information, as illustrated through the previous case, provides a foundation for determining the focus of therapy and negotiating its meaning with the client. In this regard, the OPHI-II is a powerful tool to assure that therapy is client-centered. More specifically, it can allow therapy to address and effectively become part of the lives clients want to craft for themselves.

The School Setting Interview

The School Setting Interview (SSI) (Hoffman et al., 2000) is a semi-structured interview designed to assess the impact of the school environment on the student. The SSI uses MOHO's conceptualization of the social and physical environment as a framework for the assessment.

The SSI is used to identify the need for school setting accommodations for students with disabilities. It is a client-centered interview that examines the student's interaction with the physical and social environments at school. It covers 14 content areas that make up a student's participation in school (writing; reading; speaking; remembering things; doing mathematics; doing homework; taking examinations; going to art, gym, and music; getting around the classrooms; taking breaks; going on field trips; getting assistance; accessing the school; and interacting with the staff). The SSI is intended for students who are able to communicate adequately enough to discuss their experiences. This assessment is administered as a collaborative discussion that examines the student's

School Setting Interview (SSI)	*Gathers information on school environment impact and identifies need for accommodations*	*Information on ordering can be found on the Model of Human Occupation Clearinghouse web site at:* http://www.uic.edu/hsc/acad/cahp/OT/MOHOC *Or go to:* http://www.uic.edu *Link to:* *1) Academic Departments* *2) Applied Health Sciences* *3) Occupational Therapy* *4) MOHO*

performance with a specific focus on how the school setting impacts on the student. Whereas it was originally designed for students who had physical impairments, the instrument has been successfully used with students who have emotional, developmental, and behavioral impairments.

The SSI considers the student's occupational performance in all aspects of the school environment, such as the classroom, playground, toilets, lockers, gymnasium, corridors, and field trips. In addition to determining whether accommodations are necessary, the therapist gains a qualitative understanding of the student's experiences. Furthermore, the SSI guides the therapist to discuss with the students how they want to manage in school. The SSI empowers students to collaborate with the therapist in determining the types of accommodations they may need. It reflects the assumption that determining the student's preferences, values, needs, and interests is crucial to successful physical and social accommodations in the school setting.

Administration

Before beginning the interview, the therapist stresses to the student that the SSI is not designed to identify the student's weaknesses. The therapist explains that instead, the purpose of this assessment is to make sure the school setting is doing its best to assist the student to do well in school. In conducting the interview, the therapist explores each of the 14 content areas, asking the student:

- How he or she has functioned and currently functions in the area
- Whether the student perceives a need for accommodation to perform in the area
- Whether the student currently has an accommodation in this area.

The SSI interview takes about 40 minutes to complete, and the therapist records necessary information during the interview. A form allows identification of whether there are accommodation needs in each area and whether they are met. Another form allows recording of accommodation recommendations. This form indicates recommended changes to be made in objects, spaces, occupational forms, and social groups. It also records who will be responsible for each accommodation and how it will be implemented.

Dependability

The SSI was originally developed in Sweden and then translated into English. One study provided evidence of good test-retest reliability and indicated that the SSI identified previously unacknowledged and unmet need for accommodations for more than 80% of students (Hemmingsson & Borell, 1996). Additional studies have used the SSI in investigations of how environments impacted on students in special schools (Hemmingsson & Borell, 2000) and in regular schools (Prellwitz & Tham, 2000). These studies also identified the need to add 3 areas to the original SSI that only examined 11 areas of student functioning. Further psychometric research on the SSI is ongoing in Sweden.

Thomas

Use of the SSI to Give Voice to a Student's Experiences and Needs

The principal of a high school in a Stockholm suburb invited the school occupational therapist to a routine planning meeting concerning Thomas, a first-year high school student. Thomas' parents, the school nurse, a special education teacher, and his language, physical education, and math teachers were also invited to attend. The therapist had known Thomas and his family for nearly 10 years.

At the age of 4, Thomas was diagnosed with muscular dystrophy. He had always attended a regular school, and most things had gone well. Throughout primary school, he had a couple of good friends in his class. He also had a teacher who was empathic, flexible, and adept at including Thomas in class activities with the other children. The therapist had previously worked with Thomas and occasionally consulted with Thomas' mother by telephone.

Thomas' mother called the therapist, indicating that Thomas had asked her to make the call. The mother explained that, as far as she knew, everything was going fine with Thomas in his new school. Thomas then took the telephone and explained that he had heard of the upcoming meeting from his mother. As far Thomas knew, he was not invited, and none of the teachers had spoken to him about it. He wanted to know what the meeting was about. So, the therapist explained that she understood the meeting to be a routine review meeting to assure Thomas was doing fine. When the therapist asked Thomas how he liked the new school, he responded, "It's okay, I suppose." Thomas' tone suggested otherwise, so the therapist made an appointment to meet Thomas after school that week.

The therapist then called the principal back to ask if there was some special preparation that he wanted her to do before the meeting. He explained again that it was a routine meeting. The principal was not aware of any problems. Thomas appeared to be doing fine and had not complained of anything. He expected the meeting to affirm that Thomas was performing well and adjusting to the new school.

Thomas' school was big and rather traditional, having been built in the beginning of the century. When the therapist arrived for the appointment, Thomas was waiting at the entrance and appeared to be the only student present. He explained that it was the day of a sports outing. Thomas was not capable of going along, so he was there alone.

The therapist explained that since she was invited to the planning meeting next week, she wanted to interview Thomas to get his opinion about the school situation and how it affected his participation in school activities. As the interview progressed, it was obvious that Thomas found being in the new school a negative experience. Things that he readily did in his former school were now difficult or impossible for him. He had tried hard to adapt to the new circumstances and he had not wanted to complain, as he was afraid of drawing too much attention to himself. During the SSI interview, Thomas identified unmet needs for changes to his school environment in 8 of the 14 content areas as shown in *Figure 15-6*.

In his previous school, Thomas' homeroom teacher had taught the students in nearly all subjects. Therefore, she had come to know his special needs and was able to integrate the accommodations he needed into her plans for the class. For example, in the area of writing, she always made a paper copy of any visual aids she used in class. She gave a copy of these to Thomas since he wrote slowly and

FIGURE 15-6 Thomas' Identified Needs for Accommodations on the SSI.

Content Areas	Student Identified Need for Accommodations		
	Needs New	Already Has	No Need For
Writing	▨		
Reading		▨	
Speaking			▨
Remembering things			▨
Doing mathematics			▨
Doing homework			▨
Taking exams	▨		
Going to art, gym, music			▨
Getting around the classrooms	▨		
Taking breaks	▨		
Going on field trips	▨		
Getting assistance	▨		
Accessing the school	▨		
Interacting with staff	▨		

needed additional time to take notes. Now, in secondary school, Thomas had different teachers in nearly all subjects. He had informed some of his teachers about his need for paper copies of slides and overheads. However, the information had not reached some teachers or they had forgotten. Consequently, he rarely got paper copies of class audiovisuals. Thomas also needed more time for writing in exams, but no such arrangements had been made in the new school.

Thomas was used to being able to participate in activities like field trips or outdoor activities, as his teacher always tried to include his needs in her planning. He had a powered wheelchair he could use on outings, since his ambulation was too labored for such events. There had already been several occasions in the new school when plans for special events were made without consideration of his needs. This meant that he was excluded. On the other hand, Thomas was very happy that he did not have to participate in gym as he found it embarrassing that he could not dress himself.

Another big difference was that, in his former school, all of Thomas' classes were held in his home classroom. Now, in secondary school, he had to travel between classrooms. During the short breaks between classes, Thomas often had go to a different floor or a different building. Ambulating made it difficult for him to carry books and other things that he needed in the next classroom. Neither his balance nor his strength was good enough to walk when carrying a heavy bag. Of his own accord, Thomas had decided to start using his wheelchair at school, which made it possible for him to carry his things between classrooms. Using a wheelchair in school had also made lunchtime easier, as he had experienced difficulty standing in line in the lunchroom.

Using the wheelchair, however, created new problems. The organization of the school day required rather quick transfer between different classrooms. To use the elevator was time-consuming and he had difficulty opening the manual elevator door. Moreover, there was only one wheelchair-accessible toilet on the second floor of one building. Finally, there were only steps to the entrance of school, forcing him to take an otherwise unused side entrance that also increased the distance he had to travel when entering and exiting the building. Another problem related to frequent classroom changes was that Thomas and his personal equipment (e.g., assistive devices, special chair, special desk, and personal computer) were, unfortunately, seldom in the same classroom.

Finally, as part of the SSI interview, the therapist and Thomas collaboratively discussed ways that the school might address his unmet needs in each content area. The therapist suggested that Thomas be given an assistant who would carry his bag and take notes when needed, or that he request a home classroom. However, Thomas did not want a personal assistant. He preferred to ask some classmates who were friends to assist him. He noted that they already helped him voluntarily sometimes, without him even asking. He also did not want to ask for a home classroom as he thought it would adversely affect his relationships with classmates who would find it childish. He was most satisfied with the idea that the school be asked to schedule as many of his courses on the ground floor as possible to minimize his need to use the elevator.

The therapist then brought up to Thomas the risk of immobilization. She explained that if he constantly used the wheelchair, he increased the risk of contractures in his hip flexors. She pointed out that, with his diagnosis, immobilization even for short periods may cause permanent loss of ambulation. She pointed out that his use of the wheelchair in school, in combination with avoiding gym, was a serious risk. It was obvious that Thomas did not want to think about this. However, the therapist got his permission to talk with the physical therapist and with the gym teacher about arranging an individual gym program for Thomas.

Finally, they discussed ways that the school could become more aware of and attentive to Thomas' special needs. Thomas and the therapist decided together that the therapist should share the information from the SSI with the other team members at the planning meeting. She would be responsible to report back to Thomas what happened.

Recommendations for Accommodation

At the staff meeting, the therapist presented the SSI results and discussed necessary accommodations for Thomas with the team. The therapist recorded the results of this meeting on the SSI Environmental Accommodations and Interventions Form that is shown on *Figure 15-7* and discussed below. The therapist began with presenting Thomas' need for classroom scheduling to keep him mostly on one floor. Secondly, she emphasized that all of Thomas' teachers needed better information about his special needs. She recommended that there be a written document about Thomas' needs (i.e., copies of slides, a desk suitable for a wheelchair, extra time in examinations, and consideration of his physical limitations when planning outdoor activities and field trips). The therapist recommended that the principal give this document to any new teacher. In addition, Thomas would receive copies that he could give to teachers as a reminder.

The therapist also requested on Thomas' behalf:

- Adapting one of the toilets on the ground floor
- A ramp at the entrance
- An automatic door opener to the elevator.

FIGURE 15-7 Thomas' Environmental Accommodations and Interventions Form.

Content Area	Necessary Environmental Accommodations				Team Members	Intervention: Steps for Implementation of Accommodations
	Modified or Special Objects	Space Modifications	Changes in How Task is Performed	Alterations In Social Groups		
1. Writing			Thomas is given photocopies of visual aides		• OT • Teacher • Thomas • Principal	• OT and Thomas write his special needs report • Principal informs Thomas' teacher about helpful strategies decided in the planning meeting
7. Taking exams			Thomas is given more time to take exams		• Same as above	• Same as above • PT consults with PE instructor and parents
8. Going to art, gym, music			Alternative P E activities at school and home		• PT • Teacher • Thomas • Parents	• PT, parents, and PE instructor regularly remind Thomas of contracture risks • Regular assessment of Thomas' mobility by PT
9. Getting around the classrooms	Desk adjusted to fit wheelchair in more than one classroom		Minimize the use of different classrooms		• Principal • Thomas • Teachers • OT	• Principal, Thomas, and teachers discuss how to minimize the use of different classrooms • OT orders appropriate desks
10. Taking breaks	Raised toilet seat in bathroom at ground floor				• OT • Thomas	• Decide on type of toilet seat and OT to order
11. Going on field trips			Select field trip sites that are accessible to powered wheelchair	Thomas will be included in class field trip	• OT • Thomas • Teacher • Parents	• OT consults on selections of field trip sites • Prior information from school to Thomas and parents to provide powered wheelchair

continued

FIGURE 15-7 (continued)

| Content Area | Necessary Environmental Accommodations | | | | Team Members | Intervention: Steps for Implementation of Accommodations |
	Modified or Special Objects	Space Modifications	Changes in How Task is Performed	Alterations In Social Groups		
13. Accessing the school		Ramp to the main door entrance Automatic door opener to elevator	Reduce transfer between different classrooms		• OT • Thomas • Principal	• OT to provide temporary ramp • Principal arranges for permanent ramp
14. Interacting with staff				The school nurse provides mentorship to Thomas	• Thomas • School nurse • OT	• School nurse to advocate on behalf of Thomas when needed • The school nurse to cooperate with OT when needed

Finally, she brought up the serious risk of immobilization from constant use of the wheelchair in combination with not attending gym lessons.

Thomas' parents, teachers, and principal were surprised when the therapist described the results from the SSI. They had assumed that everything was fine, as Thomas had never complained. However, they appreciated the information and supported doing everything reasonable to adapt his learning environment. After discussion, the following decisions were made:

- The principal would investigate the logistics of reducing the number of classrooms and the number of teachers who taught in Thomas' classes. He was to consult with Thomas before he made any final decisions
- The team agreed that a written document about Thomas' special needs was a good idea. The therapist agreed to write the document in cooperation with Thomas
- The principal agreed to install a ramp at the entrance. As a ramp was needed immediately, the therapist offered to obtain for the school a borrowed ramp from a rehabilitation center until the school installed something more stationary at the entrance. The principal believed that the elevator alterations were cost-prohibitive
- The gym teacher indicated that since he had limited experience with students who had physical impairments, he would need support to meet Thomas' needs. The physiotherapist was identified as the best person to consult with him
- The physiotherapist agreed to regularly assess Thomas' locomotion as well as consult with the school, Thomas, and his parents on how to avoid contractures
- The school nurse was assigned the responsibility to serve as an advocate and coordinator to assure that Thomas' needs were being met.

Finally, they decided to invite Thomas to the next planning meeting.

As this case illustrates, the SSI can be particularly helpful in identifying unmet needs for accommodation in the school setting. The framework of the interview, which gives students opportunity to talk about their experiences, preferences, and needs, is well suited to this end.

Worker Role Interview

The Worker Role Interview (WRI) (Velozo et al., 1998) was first developed as part of a study designed to determine psychosocial variables influencing work suc-

Worker Role Interview (WRI)	Gathers information on values, interests, personal causation, habits, roles, and environmental perceptions as they affect work success	Information on ordering can be found on the Model of Human Occupation Clearinghouse web site at: http://www.uic.edu/hsc/acad/cahp/OT/MOHOC Or go to: http://www.uic.edu Link to: 1) Academic Departments 2) Applied Health Sciences 3) Occupational Therapy 4) MOHO

cess. Its usefulness as a client assessment quickly became apparent, and the instrument was further adapted for such use. The WRI is a semi-structured interview with an accompanying rating scale. The 17-item scale is rated according to the implications of each item for the client's likelihood of work success (either returning to a specific job or employment in general). The WRI is designed to collect data on six content areas:

- Personal causation
- Values
- Interests
- Roles
- Habits
- Perception of the environment.

The WRI was originally designed to gather data from an injured worker (Velozo et al., 1998). A modified version was designed to be relevant to any person with a disability and relatively recent work experience. The interview provides a solid foundation for planning intervention with a worker whose impairments are interfering with work (Fisher, 1999).

Administration

The WRI is presented in a manual (Velozo et al., 1998) that provides background information as well as detailed instructions and guidelines for administration. An accompanying videotape provides an opportunity to see the WRI administered and to practice scoring the scale.

Therapists use the assessment by first administering a semi-structured interview that takes approximately 30–60 minutes. They then complete the rating scale, entering comments as appropriate. This instrument is designed for concurrent use with other assessments that provide information on work-related capacity. Because the WRI identifies psychosocial factors related to work that are not considered by most work assessments, it often reveals unique strengths and weaknesses that should be considered in therapeutic services aimed at enabling the client to achieve employment.

Dependability

Studies support the internal validity of the instrument as well as test-retest and interrater reliability (Biernacki, 1993; Velozo et al., 1999). Velozo et al. (1999) found that the WRI items work well to measure psychosocial capacity for work and that the WRI effectively separated clients into distinct groups with good reliability. Haglund, Karlsson, Kielhofner, and Lai (1997) translated the WRI into Swedish and studied its use with persons who had psychiatric disabilities. They found the WRI to be valid across culture, language, and populations. Studies currently underway examine the ability of the WRI to predict success in employment.

Peter

An Illustration of Use of the Worker Role Interview

Peter was a middle-aged man who lived in Gothenberg, Sweden. He was married and had a teenage son. Peter worked in a large company that made technological products. He had been employed in the company his entire working career. Previously, he worked with engineers in the product development department, work that Peter found very stimulating.

When the product development part of the company moved to another town, Peter's work responsibilities were changed. He began working as an assembly line worker, doing piecework together with others. Peter did not find this type of work challenging or satisfying. After working for 5 years in this job, he started to suffer from low back pain due to degeneration in his lumbar discs. Nearly 3 years ago, the pain increased to the point that he was absent from work for 6 months. Following this, he was able to work part time for 1.5 years. Seven months ago, he had a recurrence of back pain and had been absent from work since then.

The Worker Role Interview was administered to Peter to assess his potential for return to work. Results of the interview are shown in *Figure 15-8*. The following qualitative information was gathered in the interview.

Peter felt as though he could not manage to do anything anymore, either at work or at home. When asked, he could not identify any tasks that he felt able to do at work. He had completely lost belief in his capabilities. Peter also could not see any solution to his problems as long as the doctors could not help his back pain. He did not see that there was anything he could do for himself. He felt that he would not be able to work again. Because Peter felt so out of control, he did not assume any responsibility for his situation. His only hope, as he saw it, was that some medical intervention would alleviate his pain.

It had always been important for Peter to do his share. By working, he had been able to achieve this and provide for his family, which was extremely important for Peter. That he had not worked made him feel ashamed. He stated, "I can't look other people in the eyes anymore." For Peter, it was also important to have a job that he could be proud of, where his skills as a craftsman were of use. When Peter worked at the product development department, he had many work-oriented goals. However, when he changed work responsibilities, much of his enthusiasm for the future of his career was lost. The only thing that was important for Peter at his present job was being able to do his fair share of work.

Working with the product development team had been interesting and involved exciting work tasks. He appreciated the freedom he had in his work and enjoyed working with the engineers. He had been expected to creatively contribute ideas which he really enjoyed doing and he felt very supported by his supervisors. He found his present job responsibilities boring and described it as "a job that anyone could do." One of Peter's major leisure interests was sailing, an interest he shared with his family. Before the back pain started, he spent much time at the boat club. Peter was still often at the boat club. His boat was old and made of wood, which demanded upkeep that he found hard to manage because of his back. "At least I have the boat in the sea every year," he said. Nevertheless, he and his family did not sail much anymore.

Peter knew what was expected of him at work but did not like his current job. Despite being out of work, he still identified himself with being a worker. He noted, "I'd rather work than watch TV all day." He also saw himself in the role of the family provider, despite not being able to do so. Peter had also lost several other past roles. Before, he and his wife shared the responsibilities of taking care of the household (e.g., cooking, cleaning, and washing). The only thing that Peter still did in the household was taking care of the car. Peter also had taken on the sick role in that he spent a great deal of time seeking medical care, focusing on his symptoms, and looking to medical providers to find a solution to his pain.

Before Peter's back pain began, he had well-organized habits. His days were well ordered and his work, family, household, and sailing involvements constituted a full and satisfying routine. Peter's routine had changed dramatically since he has been absent from work. Watching TV was his main current daily activity. The only strategy Peter had for managing his pain was to lie down. He felt that the need to lie down regularly had restricted him socially. Previously, Peter and his wife often had friends over for dinner, but they seldom saw their friends anymore because he might have to lie down.

Peter described the physical work environment as "impossible to adjust to my needs." He needed

FIGURE 15-8 Results of Peter's Worker Role Interview (WRI).

	Rating					Comments
PERSONAL CAUSATION						
1 ASSESSES ABILITIES AND LIMITATIONS	**1**	2	3	4	NA	Can't identify any tasks he can perform Is not aware of his strengths
2 EXPECTATIONS OF JOB SUCCESS	1	**2**	3	4	NA	Doesn't think he can work at his present job anymore
3 TAKES RESPONSIBILITY	**1**	2	3	4	NA	The problem is beyond his control The doctors have to make him well and he can't do anything before that
VALUES						
4 COMMITMENT TO WORK	1	2	3	**4**	NA	To work and provide for the family has been and is important for Peter
5 WORK RELATED GOALS	1	**2**	3	4	NA	Previously, Peter had work related goals, but not any longer
INTERESTS						
6 ENJOYS WORK	**1**	2	3	4	NA	The present work isn't challenging at all Peter doesn't get any opportunities to use his skills
7 PURSUES INTERESTS	1	**2**	3	4	NA	Can't perform his interest on a satisfactory level
ROLES						
8 IDENTIFIES WITH BEING A WORKER	1	2	3	**4**	NA	The work has been an important part in Peter's life. Today he would rather work than watch TV all day
9 APPRAISES WORK EXPECTATIONS	1	2	**3**	4	NA	Peter can't identify what is expected of him at work
10 INFLUENCE OF OTHER ROLES	**1**	2	3	4	NA	Strong sick role
HABITS						
11 WORK HABITS	1	2	**3**	4	NA	Peter's work habits went along well when he was working
12 DAILY ROUTINES	**1**	2	3	4	NA	Has lost his structure Daily routines are not functional
13 ADAPTS ROUTINE TO MINIMIZE DIFFICULTIES	**1**	2	3	4	NA	Only solution when he has pain is to go and lay down. It's his only strategy and he has not tried anything else
ENVIRONMENT						
14 PERCEPTION OF WORK SETTING	1	**2**	3	4	NA	Peter thinks that work environment is impossible to adjust for his needs Can't change working position enough in his work tasks
15 FAMILY AND PEERS	1	2	3	4	**NA**	Not enough information
16 PERCEPTION OF CO-WORKERS	1	**2**	3	4	NA	Doesn't want to make trouble for his co- workers and "destroy" their piecework

Key: **4** = Srongly supports return to job; **3** = Supports return to job; **2** = Interferes with return to job; **1** = Strongly interferes with return to job; **NA** = Not applicable to vary his body position more than was possible at work. Peter's boss had been supportive. However, Peter said that he knew that the boss must have someone, unlike himself, who could do the job completely. Peter had always gotten along well with his coworkers. However, with the onset of his back pain, he had not been able to "pull his weight," which adversely affected his coworkers' ability to get bonuses for team productivity. Consequently, he felt that, while they did not say so, his coworkers would have preferred someone else in his position.

The interview revealed that Peter had both strengths and weaknesses related to work. His greatest liability was that he had lost control over his situation and confidence in himself and his capabilities. To work was important for Peter; therefore, therapy needed to restore his conviction that he could work. It also became apparent from the interview that the lack of enjoyment in his work was likely abetting the interference of his pain with working. The rote work of his assembly line task encouraged him to concentrate on his pain. The therapist felt, therefore, that he should try a new form of work that required more problem-solving. His lowered personal causation combined with taking on the sick role had also made Peter so passive that he was not applying his own natural ability and enjoyment of problem-solving to figure out how to manage his pain. Therefore, the therapist planned to engage Peter more actively in coming up with solutions for being able to work and to manage his pain. Since Peter had lost his old routine and habits, the therapist also wanted to intervene in such a way that he could begin to reinstate a routine.

With the results from the WRI as the starting-point, the therapist and Peter discussed how to go further with his situation. The therapist shared with Peter her understanding of his situation and what she thought he needed to do. She further recommended that Peter test out his work capability in a realistic environment that would also better match his interests. With support, Peter agreed to begin work-practice at a company that contracted to maintain apartment buildings. The span of work included a wide variety of repair, grounds maintenance, and oversight of the general conditions and needs of the properties. Peter and the therapist together chose this particular workplace because the work there matched Peter's interest in being able to engage in planning and problem-solving.

At first, he worked 2 hours per day. At the end of each week, Peter, his therapist, and the foreman met briefly to find out how the work was going for Peter and to make any necessary adjustments in how Peter did his job. By the end of 12 weeks, Peter had increased to working 4 hours per day.

This work-practice period also helped Peter to redevelop his habits and structure his daily routines. Peter also developed a more realistic view of his work abilities and limitations. In the beginning of the work-practice period, the occupational therapist educated Peter and his colleagues in lifting techniques and ergonomics. Although Peter still experienced pain in his back and had difficulty managing some work tasks (e.g., heavy lifting), he displayed an increasing confidence in his work capabilities.

He also learned new strategies for handling his pain. When he was at work, there were hardly any opportunities to lie down. Instead, Peter found out that by varying his work tasks, he could reduce his pain. Working as a building caretaker suited Peter well, since he was able to use his technical and practical skills. He felt responsible to exercise judgment and able to intervene when problems arose in the buildings—a role that he liked. Consequently, his belief in his capabilities grew stronger. That he had found new strategies to handle the pain at work and home increased his sense of efficacy in both managing the pain and being able to be productive. At a final meeting of Peter and his rehabilitation team, it was concluded that he had a 50% work capacity and that he would receive a disability benefit for the other 50%.

As this case illustrates, the WRI provides information on volition, habituation, and perceptions of environment that influence work success and satisfaction. Thus, it is a useful complement to the performance-capacity–oriented assessments that are often used in a work rehabilitation context. It identifies unique factors that influence a person's work success.

Work Environment Impact Scale

The Work Environment Impact Scale (WEIS) (Moore-Corner et al., 1998) is a semi-structured interview and rating scale designed to gather information on how individuals with physical or psychosocial disabilities experience their work environments. The WEIS is recommended for use with individuals who are currently employed and for individuals who are not currently working but are anticipating return to a specific job or type of work. Typical candidates for this assessment are persons who are experiencing difficulty on the job and persons whose work is interrupted by an injury or episode of illness.

The interview questions were not developed to be used with individuals who have been chronically unemployed because they ask respondents to reflect on how a given work environment affects them. Nonetheless, there may be times when the WEIS may be useful to identify how past work environments impacted on work productivity and satisfaction. In the end, the therapist must decide whether the instrument is appropriate to use with a given client.

The WEIS is designed to provide a comprehensive assessment of how the qualities and characteristics of the work environment affect a worker. An important concept underlying this scale is that workers are most productive and satisfied when there is a fit or match between the worker's environment and the needs and skills of the worker. Hence, the same work environment may have a different impact on different workers. It is important to remember that the WEIS does not assess the environment. Rather, it assesses how the work environment impacts a given worker.

The WEIS is organized around 17 environmental factors such as the physical space, social contacts and supports, temporal demands, objects utilized, and daily job functions. Consequently, it seeks to gain a comprehensive picture of how a wide range of features of the work environment affect a worker. These 17 factors are reflected in 17 items on the rating scale. Each of the items is scored with a four-point rating that indicates how the environmental factor impacts the worker's performance, satisfaction, and physical, social, and emotional well-being. The scale provides a profile of which aspects of the environment negatively or positively affect the worker.

Administration

The WEIS is described in a detailed manual that provides background as well as detailed guidelines for completing the interview and rating scale. The manual also discusses how the WEIS can be used to identify the need for workplace modification to accommodate a disabled worker.

The therapist begins by administering a semi-structured interview. The interview must be done so as to capture the unique characteristics of the client's workplace and how they affect the client. After the interview, the therapist completes the rating scale and enters appropriate qualitative data. There is an optional summary sheet to identify environmental characteristics that facilitate as well as those that inhibit worker performance and satisfaction and may require accommodation. The summary sheet is a useful way to communicate the results and implications of the WEIS to other disciplines, the client, and the workplace.

| Work Environment Impact Scale (WEIS) | *Gathers information on work environment impact and identifies need for accommodations* | *Information on ordering can be found on the Model of Human Occupation Clearinghouse web site at: http://www.uic.edu/hsc/acad/cahp/OT/MOHOC Or go to: http://www.uic.edu Link to:*
 1) Academic Departments
 2) Applied Health Sciences
 3) Occupational Therapy
 4) MOHO |

The WEIS may be used as an independent tool when the work environment is of concern. However, the WEIS is often used in conjunction with the WRI. The two interviews can be combined, saving time in administration.

Dependability

Two studies have been completed on the WEIS. The first by Corner, Kielhofner, and Lin (1997) found evidence for the overall construct validity of the WEIS. Kielhofner et al. (1999) examined the psychometric properties of the WEIS in the United States and Sweden and found that the items work well together to measure the construct of work environment impact. The scale also effectively discriminated different levels of work environment impact. The findings also suggest that the scale is free of cultural biases.

Samantha

Using the WEIS to Identify Needed Workplace Accommodations

Samantha was a 36-year-old woman who was admitted to an acute care, inpatient unit with a diagnosis of major depression. She was admitted due to noncompliance with medication which resulted in increased isolation, decreased ability to care for self, and increased flashbacks from earlier sexual abuse. This was her second admission to this unit in less than 1 year.

In the course of responding to the OCAIRS interview, Samantha indicated that she was working and that stress on the job had resulted in her current decompensation and need for hospitalization. She was unable to pinpoint the cause of her stress on the job to either the occupational therapist or the treatment team. Consequently, the therapist decided that the WEIS would be useful to gain further information about Samantha's perception of her workplace. The therapist anticipated that the WEIS could be used to work with Samantha to identify specific areas on the job that were stressful and to determine if changes/accommodations could be made to decrease the stress and increase her success in the worker role.

The WEIS was conducted approximately 1 week after her admission to the unit. Samantha was willing to engage in the interview and spoke openly. The WEIS rating scale as shown in Figure 15-9 indicated that the majority of factors in the work environment either supported or strongly supported Samantha's work performance and well-being. The primary negative impacts of her work environment were her supervisor, the unclear performance expectations and rewards, and her work schedule. The interview elicited the following qualitative information about Samantha's workplace.

Samantha worked in a corporate distribution center. Her three primary work responsibilities were gathering and packing ordered items, replenishing inventory, and confirming orders. Overall, she reported that she enjoyed the work tasks, that she was able to complete tasks in a timely manner, and that she consistently exceeded productivity quotas. She reported some dissatisfaction in learning new jobs and equipment.

Samantha indicated that she was required to learn new tasks and equipment on her own because her supervisor and coworkers were not helpful in this area. Samantha had no need for regular contact with her coworkers to complete her job. This was something she found supportive for herself as she valued her independence and autonomy.

Samantha reported difficulty with her immediate supervisor. She perceived that his expectations and requests were unclear and that he did not communicate with her effectively. She also felt that he did not appropriately support her in the performance of her work tasks. Samantha indicated that the day before being admitted, she had to work late at her supervisor's request. When she went to ask her supervisor a question, he had gone home without indicating to her that he was leaving. She became tearful during the interview and kept saying, "I can't believe he went home." Samantha saw this event as typical of his increasing lack of support.

She also expressed dissatisfaction with her work hours. The company was willing to decrease her work to 4–6 hours a day but indicated she could not work less. Samantha felt that her work schedule negatively affected other aspects of her life. She was able to accomplish little outside of work.

FIGURE 15-9 Results of Samantha's Work Environment Impact Scale (WEIS).

	1	2	3	4	N/A	Comments
Time Demands: Time allotted for available/expected amount of work			■			Able to complete things on time
Task Demands: The physical, cognitive, and/or emotional demands/opportunities of work tasks			■			Limited support from others to learn work tasks
Appeal of Work Tasks: The appeal/ enjoyableness or status/value of work tasks			■			She enjoys the work
Work Schdedule: The influence of work hours upon other valued roles, activities, transportation, and basic self-care needs		■				Ambivalent about work schedule
Coworker Interaction: Interaction/collaboration with coworkers required for job responsibilities					■	Not required to interact with others
Work Group Membership: Social involvement with coworkers at work/outside of work					■	Chooses not to interact
Supervisor Interaction: Feedback, guidance, and/or other communication/interaction with supervisor(s)		■				Strained relationship with boss whom she does not see as supportive
Work Role Standards: Overall climate of work setting expressed in expectations for quality, excellence, commitment, achievement, and/or efficiency		■				She routinely exceeds production goals, but receives no recognition or rewards. Expectations not clear
Work Role Style: Opportunity/expectations for autonomy/compliance when organizing, making requests, negotiating, and choosing how and what work tasks will be done daily			■			Enjoys the autonomy
Interaction with Others: Interaction/ communication with subordinates, customers, clients, audiences, students or others, excluding supervisor or coworkers					■	
Rewards: Opportunities for job security, recognition/advancement in position, and/ or compensation in salary or benefits		■				Feels she has poor job security because of disability
Sensory Qualities: Properties of the work place such as noise, smell, visual, or tactile properties, temperature/climate, or air quality and ventilation			■			Environment is noisy but it doesn't affect her
Architecture/Arrangement: Architecture or physical arrangements of and between work spaces and environments			■			Has decreased negative effects

continued

FIGURE 15-9 *(continued)*

Ambience/Mood. the feeling/mood associated with the degree of privacy, friendliness, morale, excitement, anxiety, frustration in the work place					Generally positive atmosphere of cooperation
Properties of Objects: The physical, cognitive, or emotional demands/opportunities of tools, equipment, materials, and supplies					
Physical Amenities: Non-work-specific facilities necessary to meet personal needs at work such as restrooms, lunchrooms, or break rooms					Adequate, although she doesn't frequently use
Meaning of Objects: What objects signify to a person					

Key: **4** = Strongly supports return to job; **3** = Supports return to job; **2** = Interferes with return to job; **1** = Strongly interferes with return to job; **NA** = Not applicable

Following the interview, the therapist shared her perceptions of the impact of Samantha's work environment with her. Together, they agreed that the two main problems that needed attention were:

- Decreasing her work hours
- Clarifying her relationship with her supervisor.

The therapist shared with Samantha that shorter work hours could be considered a reasonable accommodation and that it was within her rights under the Americans with Disabilities Act to request it. The therapist also recommended that she work with Samantha to identify what changes she wanted to occur in her supervision and how she would present these requests for changes to her supervisor. The therapist gave her an opportunity to role-play making the request.

The therapist also engaged Samantha in time management exercises. These were designed to assist her in prioritizing activities outside of work to increase her sense of efficacy and decrease feelings of being overwhelmed. Samantha also attended a stress management group at the therapist's recommendation.

The therapist shared the information that came from the WEIS with Samantha's outside case manager. The therapist recommended that if Samantha was unable to communicate her needs to her supervisor, the case manager should assist in this dialogue with the supervisor or with the employee assistance program at Samantha's workplace.

Samantha was able to act on these recommendations. She requested and was granted a shorter workday. This change helped her to manage her other responsibilities. Samantha had less success in obtaining more direct support and clarity from her supervisor. This was an issue that she continued to work on with her case manager. Nonetheless, Samantha demonstrated an increased ability to adapt to her job demands and has not required another inpatient hospitalization in the past 18 months.

Conclusion: Interviews in Perspective

This chapter presented and illustrated five interviews that have been developed for different clients and different contexts. The variety of interviews allows the therapist to select which one will be most appropriate in a given setting or for a given client. These interviews are also designed to be flexible in use so that they can be adapted to each client.

Although interviews will not be feasible for use with all clients, they do present opportunities to gather important information to achieve a client-centered focus. Hence, their use whenever possible is strongly encouraged. Interviews also actively engage clients in discussing and giving perspectives on their own situations, which helps them begin a collaborative role in their own therapy. Finally, they serve as important opportunities to build rapport. Although interviews take time, the time is well spent, given the kinds of information they yield and the opportunities they represent for beginning true collaboration with the client.

References

Biernacki, S. D. (1993). Reliability of the Worker Role Interview. *American Journal of Occupational Therapy, 47,* 797–803.

Brollier, C., Watts, J. H., Bauer, D., & Schmidt, W. (1989). A concurrent validity study of two occupational therapy evaluation instruments: The AOF and OCAIRS. *Occupational Therapy in Mental Health, 8* (4), 49–59.

Corner, R., Kielhofner, G., & Lin, F. L. (1997). Construct validity of a work environment impact scale. *Work, 9,* 21–34.

Fisher, G. S. (1999). Administration and application of the Worker Role Interview: Looking beyond functional capacity. *Work: A Journal of Prevention, Assessment & Rehabilitation, 12* (1), 25–36.

Gutkowski, L. (1992). *A generalized study of the revised Occupational Performance History Interview.* Unpublished master's thesis, University of Illinois at Chicago, Chicago, IL.

Haglund, L., & Henriksson, C. (1994). Testing a Swedish version of OCAIRS on two different patient groups. *Scandinavian Journal of Caring Sciences, 8,* 223–230.

Haglund, L., Henriksson, C., Crisp, M., Freidheim, L., & Kielhofner, G. (2001). The *Occupational Circumstances Assessment-Interview and Rating Scale (OCAIRS) (version 2.0).* Chicago: Model of Human Occupation Clearinghouse, Department of Occupational Therapy, College of Applied Health Sciences, University of Illinois at Chicago.

Haglund, L., Karlsson, G., Kielhofner, G., & Lai, J-S. (1997). Validity of the Swedish version of the Worker Role Interview. *Scandinavian Journal of Occupational Therapy, 4* (1-4), 23–29.

Haglund, L., Thorell, L., & Walinder, J. (1998a). Assessment of occupational functioning for screening of patients to occupational therapy in general psychiatric care. *Occupational Therapy Journal of Research, 4,* 193–206.

Haglund, L., Thorell, L., & Walinder, J. (1998b). Occupational functioning in relation to psychiatric diagnoses: Schizophrenia and mood disorders. *Nordic Journal of Psychiatry, 52(3),* 223-229.

Hemmingsson, H., & Borell, L. (1996). The development of an assessment of adjustment needs in the school setting for use with physically disabled students. *Scandinavian Journal of Occupational Therapy, 3,* 156–162.

Hemmingsson, H., & Borell, L. (2000). Accommodation needs and student-environment fit in upper secondary school for students with severe physical disabilities. *Canadian Journal of Occupational Therapy, 67,* 162–173.

Henry, A. D., Tohen, M., Coster, W. J., & Tickle-Degnen, L. (1995). *Predicting psychosocial functioning and symptomatic recovery of young adolescents and young adults following a first psychotic episode.* Unpublished manuscript.

Hoffman, O. R., Hemmingsson, H., & Kielhofner, G. (2000). *A User's manual for the School Setting Interview (SSI) (version 1.0).* Chicago: Model of Human Occupation Clearinghouse, Department of Occupational Therapy, College of Applied Health Sciences, University of Illinois at Chicago.

Kaplan, K. (1984). Short-term assessment: The need and a response. *Occupational Therapy in Mental Health, 4* (3), 29–45.

Kaplan, K., & Kielhofner, G. (1989). *The Occupational Case Analysis Interview and Rating Scale.* Thorofare, NJ: Slack.

Kielhofner, G., & Henry, A. D. (1988). Development and investigation of the Occupational Performance History Interview. *American Journal of Occupational Therapy, 42,* 489–498.

Kielhofner, G., Henry, A., Walens, D., & Rogers, E. S. (1991). A generalizability study of the Occupational Performance History Interview. *Occupational Therapy Journal of Research, 11,* 292–306.

Kielhofner, G., Lai, J-S., Olson, L., Haglund, L., Ekbladh, E., & Hedlund, M. (1999). Psychometric properties of the Work Environment Impact Scale: A cross-cultural study. *Work: A Journal of Prevention, Assessment & Rehabilitation, 12,* 71–78.

Kielhofner, G., & Mallinson, T. (1995). Gathering narrative data through interviews: Empirical observations and suggested guidelines. *Scandinavian Journal of Occupational Therapy, 2,* 63–68.

Kielhofner, G, Mallinson, T., Crawford, C., Nowak, M., Rigby, M., Henry, A., & Walens, D. (1997). *A user's guide to the Occupational Performance History Interview-II (OPHI-II) (version 2.0).* Chicago: Model of Human Occupation Clearinghouse, Department of Occupational Therapy, College of Applied Health Sciences, University of Illinois at Chicago.

Kielhofner, G., Mallinson, T., Forsyth, K., & Lai, J-S. (2001). Psychometric properties of the second version of the Occupational Performance History Interview. *American Journal of Occupational Therapy 55*, 230–207.

Lai, J-S., Haglund, L., & Kielhofner, G. (1999). The Occupational Case Analysis Interview and Rating Scale: Construct validity and directions for future development. *Scandinavian Journal of Caring Sciences, 13*, 267–273.

Lynch, K., & Bridle, M. (1993). Construct validity of the Occupational Performance History Interview. *Occupational Therapy Journal of Research, 13*, 231–240.

Mallinson, T., Kielhofner, G., & Mattingly, C. (1996). Metaphor and meaning in a clinical interview. *American Journal of Occupational Therapy, 50,* 338–346.

Mallinson, T., Mahaffey, L., & Kielhofner, G. (1998). The Occupational Performance History Interview: Evidence for three underlying constructs of occupational adaptation. *Canadian Journal of Occupational Therapy, 65* (4), 219–228.

Moore-Corner, R., Kielhofner, G., & Olson, L. (1998). *Work Environment Impact Scale (WEIS) (Version 2.0).* Chicago: Model of Human Occupation Clearinghouse, Department of Occupational Therapy, College of Applied Health Sciences, University of Illinois at Chicago.

Prellwitz, M., & Tham, M. (2000). How children with restricted mobility perceive their school environment. *Scandinavian Journal of Occupational Therapy, 7,* 165–173.

Velozo, C., Kielhofner, G., & Fisher, G. (1998). *A user's guide to the Worker Role Interview (WRI) (version 9.0).* Chicago: Model of Human Occupation Clearinghouse, Department of Occupational Therapy, College of Applied Health Sciences, University of Illinois at Chicago.

Velozo, C., Kielhofner, G., Gern, A., Lin, F., Azhar, F., Lai, J., & Fisher, G. (1999). Worker Role Interview: Toward validation of a psychosocial work-related measure. *Journal of Occupational Rehabilitation, 9* (3), 153–168.

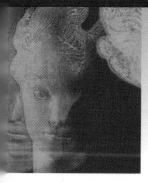

16

Assessments Combining Methods of Information Gathering

- **Kirsty Forsyth**
- **Gary Kielhofner**
- **Melinda Blondis**
- **Renee Hinson-Smith**
- **Sue Parkinson**

This chapter discusses three assessments that combine different methods of gathering information. They are:

- The Assessment of Occupational Functioning-Collaborative Version (AOF-CV)
- The Model of Human Occupation Screening Tool (MOHOST)
- The Occupational Therapy Psychosocial Assessment of Learning (OT PAL).

These assessments each represent distinct formats and purposes. The AOF-CV was originally designed as an interview to gather information on persons living in institutional settings and was later expanded for a broader audience. It has been revised so that it can be administered as a self-report or an interview. The MOHOST was initiated by a group of practitioners as a flexible means of gathering information on clients in a relatively short-term setting. Finally, the OT PAL incorporates observation along with brief teacher, student, and parent interviews to gather information on students.

The Assessment of Occupational Functioning-Collaborative Version

The original Assessment of Occupational Functioning (AOF) was developed for use in long-term institutional settings (Watts, Kielhofner, Bauer, Gregory, & Valentine, 1986). Later revision of the assessment resulted in

a more generic version suitable for a variety of contexts (Watts, Brollier, Bauer, & Schmidt, 1989). The current Assessment of Occupational Functioning-Collaborative Version (AOF-CV) is a semi-structured assessment that gives clients an opportunity to report about their occupational participation (Watts, Hinson, Madigan, McGuigan, & Newman, 1999). It is unique in that it may be administered as either an interview or as a self-report with therapist follow-up.

The AOF-CV is designed to yield a general overview of a person's occupational participation. It provides both qualitative information and a rating profile that reflect clients' views of their own strengths and limitations in personal causation, values, roles, habits, and skills. The assessment aims to efficiently generate a picture of numerous complex and interrelated factors that influence engaging in those things persons need and want to do.

Whereas the AOF-CV has been predominantly researched with psychiatric clients, the authors also recommend the instrument for use in physical disability settings. As a screening instrument, it identifies those areas of a client's occupational functioning that require more in-depth evaluation. Therapists have reported that the AOF-CV is useful for assisting treatment and discharge planning within a range of settings. The AOF-CV is particularly useful for occupational therapists in acute care settings in which there is pressure to develop specific, focused assessment protocols for each client.

Assessment of Occupational Functioning-Collaborative version (AOF-CV)	*Provides information on the client's view of his or her own strengths and limitations in personal causation, values, roles, habits, and skills. Yields qualitative information and a quantitative profile of factors affecting occupational participation*	*Copies of the AOF-CV are available from the Virginia Commonwealth University Department of Occupational Therapy web site: http://views.vcu.edu/sahp/occu/*

Administration

As noted above, the AOF-CV may be administered as either an interview or as a self-administered questionnaire with therapist follow-up. The interview/questionnaire consists of 22 questions. When administered as a self-report, the client responds to the questions in writing. After reviewing the client's responses, the therapist briefly discusses them with the client to clarify and gather additional information necessary for completing the rating scale. When conducted as an interview, the therapist treats the questions as a semi-structured interview, probing and asking additional questions as necessary. The questions (whether used as an interview or self-report) are designed to elicit the client's perception of his or her occupational functioning. The AOF-CV requires about 20–30 minutes when administered as an interview and about 12 minutes when self-administered with therapist follow-up.

After the interview or self-report with follow-up are finished, the therapist completes a rating scale. The rating scale is in the form of questions about the client's functioning (e.g., "Does this person demonstrate personal values through the selection of well-defined, meaningful activities?") which are scored using a five-point rating scale. When completed, the rating scale provides a profile of strengths and weaknesses that is useful to guide treatment and/or discharge planning.

Dependability

A number of studies (Brollier, Watts, Bauer, & Schmidt, 1988; Watts et al., 1986; Watts, Brollier, Bauer, & Schmidt, 1988; Viik, Watts, Madigan, & Bauer, 1990) provided evidence of test-retest and interrater reliability and content and concurrent validity of the AOF-CV rating scale. More recent research on the AOF-CV examined its content validity and the appropriateness of its terminology across cultures (Elliott & Newman, 1993; McGuigan, 1993). Content validity was examined by surveying experts from several English-speaking countries. Findings indicated that while the language of the instrument seemed to pose no problems, there was a need to interpret items relative to cultural values. A study by Elliott and Newman (1993) also explored the value of the AOF-CV as a self-administered evaluation. This study provided evidence that the AOF-CV can effectively be used as a self-assessment with therapist follow-up. Overall, clients were able to answer 89% of the questions as a self-report, requiring only limited follow-up by therapists. The study stated that those who were more able to complete the AOF-CV in the self-report format had achieved a higher level of education and had greater verbal ability.

Phil

Using the AOF-CV to Gain Insight

Phil was 36 years old. He was diagnosed with multiple sclerosis (MS) 4 years previously. Since then, he had been progressively debilitated with no remission. He was hospitalized during an exacerbation of MS and subsequently transferred to an intensive rehabilitation unit. Although he received outpatient occupational therapy and physical therapy in the past, this was his first inpatient rehabilitation admission. At the time he transferred to the rehabilitation unit, his physical limitations required that he use a powered wheelchair for mobility. During hospitalization, he had attempted ambulation and stand/pivot transfers with very limited success, even with maximal assistance.

The therapist administered the AOF-CV as an interview with Phil. She used the AOF-CV in this rehabilitation setting as a means of gaining insight into clients' views of their own situations and as a guide to make therapy more responsive to clients' needs. What the interview revealed is discussed below, and Phil's ratings on the AOF-CV rating scale are shown in *Figure 16-1*.

Phil was divorced 2 years after his diagnosis was made. He was estranged from his youngest child, a daughter who lived in another state with her mother. Phil lived in a house with his two sons, aged 14 and 10. This house was not wheelchair-accessible. Phil was previously employed full time as a roofer but could no longer work.

Phil reported that his two most important sources of meaning are his family and his work. However, both have been disrupted in the past 4 years. Phil's future goals were to walk again and to participate in the things he did before the onset of MS. He avoided any suggestion that his illness will likely progress and require accommodations. Consequently, he had no plans to adapt his home and had not considered the possible impact on his children.

Phil deeply wanted to be in control of his life. He reluctantly admitted that he is greatly reliant on other people. He noted, "Other people make suggestions of what I should do in every aspect of my life, but I reserve the right to say `yes' or `no,' even though they are probably right." Phil refused to discuss what was likely to be the future course of his illness. He had almost no knowledge about MS and rejected the idea of receiving education about the disease and its prognosis. Ironically, his lack of being informed greatly decreased his sense of control. He admitted that family members and friends often had to make medical and physical decisions on his behalf since he would not become involved in anything that pertains to his illness and disability. Phil also reported feeling that his sons were getting out of hand, since

he could no longer watch or discipline them. His authority had been greatly eroded by the fact that he had to rely on them to perform all of the household tasks as well as help him with aspects of his self-care.

Phil's previous interests all had involved physical activity. He enjoyed playing golf and basketball, playing sports with his sons, helping neighbors with odd jobs, and working as a roofer. Participating in these interests was no longer possible or has been radically altered. He continued to watch sports on television and to attend sporting events. He tried to spend time with his sons, but couldn't do things with them as before. Phil indicated that he has not attempted to find new things to do and insisted that he didn't want to explore things he might do from a wheelchair. Nonetheless, he reported feeling quite depressed at not having enjoyable things to do.

Prior to the onset of his illness, Phil had many roles including being a parent, husband, worker, friend, sports participant, church member, and club member. His remaining role was being a parent, and it had been radically altered as he had become so dependent on his sons and had no contact with his daughter. He indicated being very depressed over the loss of these roles. Up until 4 months before his hospitalization, he independently performed his morning self-care, completed simple home management tasks such as cleaning and meal preparation, and cared for his children. During the most recent exacerbation, Phil had remained in bed when his children were not home because he needed assistance to move around the home. For the past 3 years, he had a homebound routine, except for occasional trips to sporting events and movies. He wanted to expand his routine to include more community activities when he felt better.

Phil's view of skills was fraught with conflict. His mounting impairments and swift decline in performance conflicted with his need to believe his condition would markedly improve. Consequently, he tended to deny his limitations, which further restricted his performance. He was able to communicate on a superficial level. However, he admitted having difficulty discussing personal issues. He reported trouble discussing his illness with his sons. Phil admitted that his anger and poor communication had made his sons somewhat fearful and distant from him.

FIGURE 16-1   Phil's Ratings on the Assessment of Occupational Functioning.

Volition					
Values	5	4	3	2	1
Does this person demonstrate his/her values throughout the selection of well-defined, meaningful roles?				▩	
Does this person demonstrate his/her values through the selection of personal goals?				▩	
Does this person demonstrate socially appropriate values through the selection of personal standards for the conduct of daily activities?		▩			
Does this person demonstrate temporal orientation through expressed awareness of past, present, and future events and beliefs about how time should be used?	▩				
Personal Causation	5	4	3	2	1
Does this person demonstrate personal causation through an expressed belief in internal control?				▩	
Does this person demonstrate personal causation by expressing confidence that he/she has a range of skills?		▩			
Does this person demonstrate personal causation by expressing confidence in his/her skill competence at personally relevant tasks?					▩
Does this person demonstrate personal causation by expressing hopeful anticipation for success in the future endeavors?			▩		
Interests	5	4	3	2	1
Does this person clearly discriminate degrees of interests?		▩			
Does this person clearly identify a range of interests?			▩		
Does this person routinely pursue his/her interests?					▩
Habituation					
Roles	5	4	3	2	1
Does this person demonstrate an adequate array of life roles (family member, student, worker, hobbyist, friend, etc.)?				▩	
Does this person have a realistic concept of the demands and social obligations of his/her life roles?			▩		
Does this person express comfort or security in his/her major life roles?				▩	
Habits	5	4	3	2	1
Does this person demonstrate habit patterns through well-organized use of time?			▩		
Does this person report that his/her habits are socially acceptable?				▩	
Does this person demonstrate adequate flexibility in his/her habits?			▩		
Occupational Performance Skills					
	5	4	3	2	1
Does this person have adequate motor skills neccessary to move himself/herself or manipulate objects?					▩
Does this person have adequate skills for managing events, processes, and situations of various types?				▩	
Does this person have communications and interpersonal skills necessary for interfacing with people?				▩	

Key: **5** = Very highly; **4** = Highly; **3** = Moderately; **2** = Little; **1** = Very little

Therapy Implications

The AOF-CV results made it clear that any successful rehabilitation had to begin with addressing Phil's view of his situation. Phil's unwillingness to address his physical limitations, combined with his poor prognosis, was his greatest liability. Before he could benefit from rehabilitation efforts addressed at functional skills, his perspective on his disability and his future had to be addressed. Once Phil was able cognitively and emotionally to perform an accurate self-evaluation, he would be able to better plan for the future, communicate his needs, and participate in rehabilitation. From the evaluation, it was apparent that Phil's difficulty in facing his limitations and prognosis was exacerbated by his loss of participation in positive, meaningful activities. Therefore, the most likely point of intervention was to acknowledge these losses and to work with him to identify how he could reclaim some of his occupational participation without the necessity of regaining all his physical abilities. Since Phil had lost meaning, self-confidence, and felt most out of control in his parent role, this role was a possible beginning point. This was also a place to begin because his sons had expressed a willingness to help their father with his physical limitations and they were at critical ages when his parenting was important for their futures. Once Phil began to feel a greater sense of control and possibility for his future, interventions such as environmental adaptation, energy conservation, and alternative activity exploration were undertaken. *Figure 16-2* illustrates the specific strategies for intervention derived from the AOF-CV that correspond to the areas assessed.

During the rehabilitation stay, the therapist had a degree of success in implementing her plans with Phil. The team was very supportive of the therapist's aims to address Phil's personal causation. The team as a whole worked to provide realistic information to Phil about his condition and prognosis. Additionally, because Phil was very involved in a local church, his pastor worked with the team to provide Phil emotional support and spiritual guidance in coming to grips with his situation and its meaning for him. Phil was able to make some progress in facing the implications of MS and in collaborating to make changes to improve his function. Phil accepted and learned to use a number of adaptive aids to support toileting and bathing. Phil was given

FIGURE 16-2 Areas and Strategies for Intervention With Phil.

Area	Strategies for Intervention
Values	• Identify with Phil his highest priorities for occupational participation • Assist Phil to develop realistic goals for occupational performance within areas of highest priorities • Begin process of long-term goal-setting strategies to accommodate for his prognosis of declining functional status, as he is able to cope with the prognosis and its implications
Personal causation	• Identify an area of great importance (e.g., parenting) and work with Phil to participate in this occupational area despite his impairments • As he can accept the information, increase Phil's knowledge of MS and functional implications • Work with Phil to plan for and adapt the home environment to enhance his performance and control
Interests	• Introduce modifications to past interests and explore their satisfaction with Phil • Provide opportunities for Phil to explore new areas of interest based on factors that provided him satisfaction in the past • Work with Phil to plan current and future increased participation in interests to reduce feelings of loss and depression
Roles	• Explore modifications of roles to allow Phil to retain as many roles as possible • Work with Phil to identify and plan for the self-care management role (see discussion in Chapter 5) and its implications for his ability to participate in other roles
Habits	• Educate Phil on energy conservation and adaptations to increase activity level • Work with Phil to plan and implement present routines and plan future routines

continued

FIGURE 16-2 *(Continued)*

Area	Strategies for Intervention
Skills	• Identify in collaboration with Phil physical impairments and abilities with an aim to adapt the environment to minimize the impact of his limitations and to enhance his performance
	• Provide support and training to enhance Phil's interpersonal communication skills and ability to emotionally cope with his disability through better planning and communication

a narrow manual wheelchair so that he could transfer from his powered chair to it in order to maneuver in his narrow hallways and bedroom. He was reluctant to accept further adaptations at the time.

Phil returned to rehabilitation about 1 year later, severely impaired. The therapist revisited some key questions from the AOF-CV with Phil. At this point, he had come to grips with the reality of his MS and expressed fears about what it would mean. Phil noted that at home his older son was taking care of him. Phil would lie in bed all day, since he had become too weak to transfer into or use his manual chair, until his sons came home and then the sons would cook meals, assist Phil with his activities of daily living, and help him do some activities out of bed. Phil acknowledged that this was not a satisfying way to live, and he was willing to try a variety of strategies to improve it.

Phil still very much wanted to attempt walking, and the team decided to validate his values by letting him try. He was fitted with braces but was unable to ambulate with them due to limited arm strength. On the other hand, he did make some modest physical gains in rehabilitation that improved his performance capacity. However, the most important changes were based on adapting his environment to enhance his occupational participation.

The local Rotary Club adapted Phil's home, providing ramps, a new walk-in shower, a better bed, and widened hallways. They arranged to adapt the family vehicle so that it could accommodate Phil and his powered wheelchair. Phil also made plans in therapy for the kinds of things he wanted to do, and problem-solved with his therapist to remove any ob-

stacles. This whole process of environmental adaptation, planning for greater control, and focusing on how Phil could realize some of his values and interests in his everyday life gave him new hope. Phil returned home, and the next period of time was very good for him. His acceptance and increased knowledge of MS, as well as new-found freedom in mobility within and outside his home and increased ability to manage his own self-care, gave him a measure of control over his life and allowed him less dependence on and greater involvement with his children. Phil's improved quality of life also affected his sons' lives after Phil died some months later.

After Phil's death, his older son lived independently and his younger son went to live with his mother and sister. The sons were grateful for the improved final months with their father. The therapist's use of the AOF-CV with Phil and others like him served as the basis for the occupational therapy department in this rehabilitation setting to garner team support for and to develop new programs addressing the psychosocial aspects of physical disability, which had previously not been systematically addressed. Clients on the rehabilitation unit have received the new programs positively.

As this case illustrates, the AOF-CV provides an efficient means of identifying the client's status and making apparent issues that need to be addressed in therapy. It also points to areas that may need further evaluation. This case, in particular, illustrates how issues that often go unattended and unresolved in physical rehabilitation can be approached. The AOF-CV is equally useful in identifying salient psychosocial issues in clients with a wide range of impairments in a variety of service contexts. The AOF-CV itself begins a process of collaborative dialogue with clients that can help the therapist design therapy that addresses the clients' greatest concerns and fears.

Model of Human Occupation Screening Tool (MOHOST)

The MOHOST (Parkinson & Forsyth, 2001) was developed to provide an assessment that covered the majority of MOHO concepts, allowing the therapist to gain

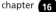

an overview of the clients' occupational functioning. The information gathered helps the therapist to complete discharge and treatment planning and to identify areas that require further assessment or intervention. It is also considered useful to screen referrals to occupational therapy to determine their appropriateness. The MOHOST seeks to objectify the kinds of information a therapist using MOHO would gather as part of regular practice. It is the most flexible of the MOHO-based assessment tools in terms of data collection methods and has been designed so that it can be used with a wide range of clients with psychosocial and/or physical impairments.

The MOHOST grew out of the efforts of a group of occupational therapists in Great Britain who were concerned that their clients' low levels of functioning and/or short lengths of stay were such that more lengthy and complicated initial assessments were not feasible. Therefore, it is designed to be flexible in use and is quicker and more straightforward to complete. It aims to capture the clients' relative strengths, highlighting the impact of volition, habituation, and skills on occupational performance. It is useful for treatment and discharge planning and for documenting change.

The MOHOST consists of a 20-item rating scale with items representing volition, habituation, and skills. Each item is rated with a four-point scale. *Figure 16-3* illustrates the rating scale and some items from the MOHOST. As the items show, criteria for making the ratings are built into each item, thereby making the rating process more straightforward for therapists. Most of the information for completing the ratings can ordinarily be gained from informal observation of the client, but the MOHOST is designed so that the therapist can gather data through whatever means are most practical. There is a short form for recording the information gathered in the MOHOST, and this is illustrated in the case that follows.

Administration

The data collection method has been designed to be flexible to meet multiple needs. The criteria for completing the scale are that the therapist must have basic information about the client's occupational life and performance and that the client's performance has been consistent throughout the assessment period. This information is usually gained primarily through observation; however, it may be supplemented or achieved through talking to the client, ward/residential staff, and/or relatives. The assessment enables clinicians to flexibly gather information about the client from as many sources as are available and practical. If necessary, therapists can build up an understanding of their clients' occupational participation over a period of time to complete the assessment. When therapists have enough information, they complete the rating form. Ratings can be recorded onto the simpler summary sheet that also has a place for a brief qualitative report. The MOHOST can be used at regular intervals to document the client's initial status and general progress thereafter.

Dependability

The MOHOST was initiated by a group of practitioners. Since it has been used in various formats for some time, it has been extensively pilot-tested. Consequently, the current version of the MOHOST reflects a great deal of practical experience. It has been revised from earlier for-

| Model of Human Occupation Screening Tool (MOHOST) | *Captures clients' relative strengths, highlighting the impact of volition, habituation, and skills on occupational performance* | *Information on ordering can be found at the Model of Human Occupation Clearinghouse web site at:* *http://www.uic.edu/hsc/acad/cahp/OT/MOHOC Or go to: http://www.uic.edu Link to:* *1) Academic Departments* *2) Applied Health Sciences* *3) Occupational Therapy* *4) MOHO* |

FIGURE 16-3   Sample Items From MOHOST.

Self-Belief • Self-confidence • Belief in skills • Belief in effectiveness	4	Anticipates success, recognizes strengths, aware of limitations
	3	Demonstrates questionable ability to remain hopeful of success
	2	Difficulty sustaining confidence about overcoming limitations/failures or overly confident
	1	Pessimistic, feels hopeless about influencing outcomes or highly overconfident
		Other:...
Routine • Balance • Structure • Productivity	4	Has a routine that supports responsibilities and goals, can change routine when needed
	3	OT questions appropriateness of current routine
	2	Difficulty organizing routines to meet occupational responsibilities
	1	Chaotic routine, routine unable to support responsibilities and goals
		Other:...
Problem-solving • Judgement • Adaptation • Decision-making • Responsiveness	4	Shows good judgement around anticipating adapting difficulties that arise
	3	Demonstrates questionable ability to make decisions based on difficulties that arise
	2	Difficulty anticipating and adapting to difficulties that arise
	1	Unable to anticipate and adapt to difficulties that arise and make inappropriate decisions
		Other:...
Cooperation • Relationships • Collaboration • Rapport • Respect	4	Sociable, supportive, aware of others, sustains engagement, friendly
	3	Demonstrates questionable social skills
	2	Difficulty with cooperation (shy/inappropriate/distracted)
	1	Unable to cooperate with others to complete occupation
		Other:...

Key: **4** = Competent; **3** = Questionable; **2** = Ineffective; **1** = Deficient

mats into a format that reflects lessons learned from development and psychometric testing of other MOHO assessments (e.g., the format of the rating scale and criteria attached to items). Currently, several phases of pilot testing have been completed and the MOHOST is about to enter the empirical test of its psychometric properties.

Andrew

Using the MOHOST to Gain a New Perspective

Andrew was in his late 30s and was diagnosed with schizophrenia 10 years ago. He completed an art degree but has never had a job or formed any major relationships. It was likely that he had impairments related to his mental illness for some considerable time before he came to the attention of psychiatric services. He had been able to remain living in the community due to the substantial help that he received from his parents.

Andrew had multiple psychiatric hospitalizations in his history. He was generally admitted to the hospital in an extremely distressed and agitated state, voicing paranoid delusions of a religious nature. He had never responded very well to medical treatment, and once, when the occupational therapist attempted to interview him during a previous hospitalization, Andrew answered most of the questions with "I don't know" or "I've never thought about it." Over the years, his symptoms had become more florid, and he attempted to commit suicide on several occasions. He had also assaulted staff when they have questioned him regarding his symptoms or when they have simply been in his way. Given that Andrew heard voices telling him to kill himself and that he had identified himself as living inside other people, he was thought to present a considerable risk both to himself and to the general public.

For much of his last inpatient admission he was uncommunicative and hostile. He neglected both his hygiene and his diet but would spend long periods writing furiously (and for the most part illegibly). Eventually, he made some improvement and started to attend the Open Art session on the ward for up to 10 minutes at a time. The artwork that he produced began to include some recognizable images in addition to apparently random scribbles. He expressed an interest in attending further occupational therapy, and after much deliberation, the team agreed that he could be accompanied to groups in the main day therapy area. His initial program was based on simple occupational forms that Andrew valued, where social interaction would not be the primary focus. These included art, yoga stretches, gardening, and table tennis.

The occupational therapist decided to use the MOHOST at this point to evaluate his progress and gain insight as to how to continue with him. The therapist completed the MOHOST based on her knowledge of Andrew from observing him in the groups and on the ward. Using the MOHOST as a structure, the therapist created the following account of Andrew's occupational performance. The MOHOST report she completed is shown in *Figure 16-4.*

Andrew appeared to be unaware of his limitations. He did not voice any difficulties in performance despite his overt impairments. He made no spontaneous reference to his future. He was able to make choices within structured situations (e.g., choosing art materials or making a drink when thirsty). However, he still needed prompting to manage personal activities of daily living. Moreover, he occasionally engaged in activities that appeared to be the product of delusional impulse (e.g., shaving off all his body hair).

Andrew's long-held interest in art had recently resurfaced. He could be readily engaged in selected activities related to art and express satisfaction in these activities. He also enjoyed physical exercise and pursued activities independently, but he continued to express no clear interest in his general surroundings. Likewise, he clearly valued the intervention of the occupational therapist, but the value that he placed on wider relationships was unclear. He still regularly asked his parents to leave when they came to visit him.

Andrew's sleep pattern had recently improved, and his ability to follow a routine was much better. He was aware of times and appointments and could cope with a certain amount of imposed structure. His responses had become much less unpredictable, and he had proved able to tolerate new situations. However, his interactions with the staff and his parents continued to center on his immediate needs rather than any long-term social or productive focus.

There were several indications that Andrew's sense of responsibility had recently improved. He had accepted feedback and had made appropriate requests (e.g., for permission to take some art materials to the ward). He also regularly thanked the occupational therapy staff for their support.

Whereas Andrew had not previously made eye contact, he began to do so readily but his gaze still tended to be fixed and his facial expressions and use of gestures continued to be limited. His progress was more evident in his improved ability in initiating and sustaining conversation, in responding to greetings and disclosing information appropriately, and in demonstrating basic listening skills. His speech was also much clearer and of a more normal rate and flow, although his intonation was unvaried and he interacted only when approached, continuing to isolate himself on the ward.

Andrew remained dependent on others to anticipate difficulties and make appropriate decisions. He continued to be anti-social at times. Therefore, his occupational therapy program had been designed to reduce risk by minimizing any pressure to make complex decisions.

Andrew had retained information given to him and showed some evidence of previous experience using art materials and practicing yoga. He initiated tasks but was unable to sustain concentration for any length of time when undirected. With encouragement, he would return to tasks to complete

FIGURE 16-4   Andrew's Ratings and Analysis of Strengths and Limitations on the MOHOST.

Andrew does not express his feelings but has clear interests. He has also proved able to tolerate new situations and to demonstrates a degree of responsibility. His interactions remain limited but improve when there is a practical focus, and he is able to plan and organize activities with support. He continues to be restless and distractible, and has difficulty coping with a marked hand tremor.

SUMMARY OF RATINGS

| Motivation for Occupation | | | | Pattern of Occupation | | | | Communication and Interaction | | | | Process Skills | | | | Motor Skills | | | |
Self-belief	Goals	Interest	Values	Routine	Flexibility	Responsibilities	Role behavior	Body language	Conversation	Expression	Cooperation	Knowledge	Planning	Organization	Problem-solving	Posture and mobility	Coordination	Strength and effort	Energy
4	4	4	4	4	4	4	4	4	4	4	4	4	4	4	4	4	4	**4**	4
3	**3**	3	3	3	**3**	3	3	3	3	3	3	**3**	3	3	3	**3**	3	3	3
2	2	2	**2**	2	2	**2**	2	2	**2**	**2**	**2**	2	**2**	**2**	2	2	**2**	2	2
1	1	1	1	1	1	1	**1**	**1**	1	1	1	1	1	1	**1**	1	1	1	**1**

Key: Competent [4]; Questionable [3]; Ineffective [2]; Deficient [1]

them, and he had been able to cope with a 30-minute yoga session. He was able to follow verbal instructions adequately, but his work was disorganized. He required prompts to tidy up.

Andrew's balance was reasonable and he was capable of running at speed but there was a certain rigidity in his gait and posture. His movements lacked fluidity and appeared awkward and clumsy at times. Most noticeably, his hands shook uncontrollably when he was not engaged in activities requiring hand-eye coordination. He had no evident problems with strength and effort, however, and was able to calibrate force sufficiently well to play table tennis. Overall, Andrew remained restless, and he still had periods of overactivity when he would dance or perform press-ups. He also continued to write or draw at a furious pace before losing focus and ending activities abruptly.

Impact of Using the MOHOST

Completing the MOHOST helped not only the occupational therapist but also the multidisciplinary team to look at Andrew's skills afresh. If the tool had been used just a few weeks previously, it would have reflected primarily major deficits. Now the MOHOST highlighted some strengths, providing a clear indication of Andrew's improvement.

The MOHOST also highlighted the importance of employing the following strategies in occupational therapy:

- Encouraging Andrew's interests and values
- Discussing Andrew's progress with him at regular reviews to help him to build on his success
- Supporting Andrew to rebuild a satisfying routine
- Introducing consideration of some occupational goals.

As the therapist implemented these strategies, Andrew responded as follows. He expressed that he wanted to use the gym and computing facilities. Later, he also wanted to join a baking group. The therapist recognized that these would provide opportunities to develop his motor, process, and communication/interaction skills and thus encouraged and supported his involvement.

His motivation to participate in these occupations was strong enough to allow the therapist and other staff to begin to negotiate with Andrew to make a number of positive changes. First, while Andrew had previously refused medication that could help to reduce his tremor, he agreed to take it when it was pointed out that it would probably enhance his performance. Moreover, the ward staff was also able to broach the sensitive issue of hygiene with Andrew and to work with him toward improving this. Andrew's hands were always heavily nicotine stained, and he took up his parents' suggestion to try nicotine gum, which helped him to smoke less. The occupational therapist shared with Andrew that she had observed him having difficulty seeing objects up close when engaged in therapy. Andrew consequently agreed to wear his spectacles more, which undoubtedly helped him to be more aware of his surroundings and may have contributed to his handwriting becoming more legible.

Occupational therapy had led the way in achieving a rapport with Andrew that began to extend to other staff members. The MOHOST also gave a tangible way of measuring Andrew's progress and helped to boost everyone's hopes that Andrew was making some improvement. In particular, it provided growing evidence that Andrew was capable of responsibility, cooperation, and flexibility, which was crucial to the difficult decisions that the team had to make regarding risk assessment.

At the time that this case study was written, Andrew's recovery was far from assured. The therapist planned to continue using the MOHOST in documenting his progress and ensuring a systematic,

ongoing assessment of his occupational needs. In Andrew's case the MOHOST proved to be an effective assessment for guiding intervention and documenting his progress.

As this case illustrated, the MOHOST can provide a systematic framework for pulling together and documenting a client's occupational status. For clients who are problematic and low functioning, it can highlight strengths on which therapy can build. Also, in cases in which progress is slow and uncertain, it can provide a concrete means of documenting change for the therapist, the client, and the team. Finally, when a new client's baseline level of functioning is unknown, the MOHOST can provide a valuable tool for gaining an overview of occupational competence.

Occupational Therapy Psychosocial Assessment of Learning

The OT PAL (Townsend et al., 2001) is designed for use within a school-based setting with children ages 6–12 years. It is designed to assess students who are experiencing difficulty fulfilling expectations and roles in the classroom. The OT PAL is designed to capture information on psychosocial factors (beyond performance capacity) that influence a child's learning.

The OT PAL includes a quantitative rating scale consisting of 23 items that reflect a student's volition (ability to make choices) and habituation (roles and habits). This scale provides a profile of the student's volitional and habituation strengths and weaknesses. Because the OT PAL does not gather information on per-

Occupational Therapy Psychosocial Assessment of Learning (OT PAL)	*Assesses students by capturing information on psychosocial and environmental factors that impact on a child's learning. Focuses on volition (ability to make choices) and habituation (roles and habits)*	*Information on ordering can be found on the Model of Human Occupation Clearinghouse web site at:* http://www.uic.edu/hsc/acad/cahp/OT/MOHOC *Or go to:* http://www.uic.edu *Link to:* **1) Academic Departments 2) Applied Health Sciences 3) Occupational Therapy 4) MOHO**

formance capacity or skills, other assessments must be selected to provide this information.

The therapist collects information for completing the scale through observation supplemented with semi-structured interviews with the teacher, student, and parents. The interviews are designed to have the teacher, student, and parents offer different perspectives about the student's performance, behaviors, beliefs, and interests related to school. In addition to the rating scale, the OT PAL also provides the structure to gather and report qualitative information on:

- The student's classroom
- The behavioral expectations in the classroom
- The teacher's style of teaching and managing the classroom
- The student's ability to meet these expectations
- The student's beliefs about his or her abilities as a learner within the school environment.

This information allows the occupational therapist to determine the quality of fit between the student and the classroom environment and how the latter affects the student's performance.

Administration

The OT PAL is designed so that it can be flexibly adapted to each child and school setting. The OT PAL involves completing the following forms:

- A pre-observation and environmental description worksheet that gathers information about basic characteristics of the student and the classroom
- The rating scale
- Brief teacher, student, and parent narratives that summarize the three interviews
- A summary form that summarizes student-environment fit, lists students' strengths and weaknesses, and describes any intervention plan.

Ordinarily, the therapist begins by preparing for the administration of the OT PAL (e.g., scheduling observation and interviews) and completing the preobservation and environmental description forms. Next, the therapist observes the student in the classroom and other school settings as indicated and feasible. An observation of at least 40 minutes is generally necessary to gather sufficient information for completion of the rating scale. The teacher, student, and parent interviews are administered after the observation because part of their purpose is to gather information that sup-

plements and confirms/corrects the observation. Each interview takes approximately 15 minutes. The parent interview may be conducted as a written questionnaire or via telephone. After the therapist finishes the information-gathering process, he or she completes the rating scale and forms. This process leads naturally to development of intervention plans and recommendations to others in the school setting. Because of the comprehensive nature of the OT PAL, it is a useful assessment for giving input to the school team for planning how to best meet a child's educational needs.

Dependability

The OT PAL was originally developed in Utica, New York. Two years of pilot testing involved a national group of school-based occupational therapists who provided feedback on the assessment's clarity, ease, and usefulness to occupational therapists and teachers. Content validity was examined by reviews of two rounds of experts. With each round the assessment was further refined. After this, a first version of the OT PAL was turned over to a research team in Illinois. The instrument was further piloted and revised. Case studies were performed to assess and demonstrate the practical utility of the assessment. At the time of this writing, data are being collected to further examine the psychometric properties of the OT PAL rating scale.

Gerald

The Use the OT PAL to Evaluate Adjustment to First Grade

Gerald was 7 years and 11 months old and was in first grade. He was diagnosed at age 5 with acute lymphocytic leukemia and received chemotherapy for 2 years. Gerald was no longer receiving leukemia treatment but still experienced fatigue and weakness. He had also been identified as having sensory integrative dysfunction, which affected his attention span, arousal levels, spatial orientation, postural control, visual motor skills, visual perceptual skills, and bilateral integration. Gerald had several adaptations in his classroom environment to improve his organization and attention span. He also had a classroom aide during half the school day to provide extra needed assistance.

Because Gerald faced numerous challenges in the classroom, the therapist decided to administer the OT PAL as a means of gathering information on his overall adjustment to first grade in anticipation of a school team review. The assessment illuminated both strengths and concerns for Gerald in the areas of making choices, habits/routines, and roles. Below is a discussion of the information that was discovered through the OT PAL and its implications.

Volition

Gerald displayed a positive sense of personal causation with reference to his academic ability in certain aspects of classroom performance. His behaviors in the classroom clearly showed that he was highly motivated to demonstrate his competence. For instance, he actively participated in classroom discussion by consistently raising his hand in response to the teacher's questions. When observed, he volunteered to go up in front of the room during a classroom activity to write his answer to one of the questions on the board. The teacher reported that he took pride in his work and routinely drew attention to himself whenever he did well on a classroom task.

Although Gerald appropriately seized opportunities to display his competence in certain areas of academic performance, other actions indicated a challenge or threat to his personal causation. For example, because he had difficulties focusing, organizing his school materials, and maintaining the pace of his individual work, he tended to rely heavily on his aide to scaffold his performance. Moreover, he had trouble when he needed to make self-directed choices and relied on his aide for guidance. In these situations, the more self-assured attitude he displayed when answering or performing publicly was replaced with a sense of insecurity.

He also did things that indicated that he either overestimated what he could do or attempted to hide his limitations. For example, Gerald offered to help another student carry the basket of lunches to the lunchroom (a job that the students do in each classroom), but he was unable to do his part because of decreased strength and endurance. In addition, Gerald's teacher reported that students often rejected him during recess because of his limited motor capacities. For example, he wanted to play kickball, but the students did not want him on their team because he was not very good. Overall, Gerald appeared to be working very hard to maintain a public image of competency.

Sometimes he managed competent performance. On other occasions he failed publicly or lapsed into an insecure, dependent mode. While variation in belief in skill is typical of his age, Gerald fluctuated to extremes. This, combined with the negative social feedback he received because of his motor limitations, indicated that his personal causation was at risk.

Gerald strongly valued being able to perform in the classroom. For example, it was clear that he cared about receiving the symbolic star or smiley-face on his assignments. It was also very important for Gerald to be looked upon and treated as normal. He went out of his way to be involved in classroom activities and discussions just as other children. However, he had substantial difficulty maintaining normal involvement in some classroom activities and during recess. He got clearly upset and frustrated when he could not do what other children did or was not invited to join in. Gerald also placed a high premium on his teacher's and parents' opinions about him as a student. The teacher and his parents saw him as working extra hard to earn their positive image of him as a student. For example, he was especially careful to follow classroom rules in order to be seen as a good student.

Gerald named his favorite subjects without hesitation during the student interview. His reason for liking these subjects was that they were easy for him and he performed them well. While interests often coincide with what one does well, his stated reasons for interests in school highlight how the need to feel and be recognized as competent dominates Gerald's volition.

Habits and Routines

Figure 16-5 illustrates the habituation portion of the OT PAL rating scale as it was completed for Gerald. He readily described the routine of the school day. He showed a good understanding of what to do throughout the day, such as hanging up his coat and book bag when he arrived in the morning, going to his desk, and listening to the teacher's directions. He even explained that the daily schedule varies depending on the day (i.e., music lessons on Tuesdays and Thursdays).

However, according to Gerald's teacher, most of the time he struggled to keep up with his classmates in relation to school routines even with help from the part-time aide. Both his level of energy and difficulties with focusing, attending, and organizing hampered keeping up with routines. For example, he was generally slower than peers in writing and had difficulty arranging classroom materials to complete assignments. He was provided with a number of classroom adaptations to improve his organization and to help him find materials more efficiently, which only partly compensated for his difficulties. Gerald's teacher reported that he was not able to organize his assignments in keeping with classroom routines without the help of his part-time aide. The teacher reported that he also needed assistance making sure he was bringing home the necessary books or worksheets to do his homework. Another factor that contributed to Gerald's difficulty completing classroom activities within allotted time was his periodic removal from the classroom for occupational therapy, physical therapy, and social work. As a consequence of all these things, Gerald was often catching up on assignments during free time. This tended to mark Gerald as different from the other students, thus undermining his attempts to appear normal.

Roles

Gerald strongly identified with and attempted to meet expectations of the student role in the classroom. He accepted the teacher's authority, asked for help appropriately, tried hard as a student, and participated in activities and class discussions. Gerald had difficulty transitioning between group roles, particularly from leader to follower. He wanted to be in a leader role, apparently because it gave him a feeling of competence.

Gerald's teacher noted that his opportunities for interaction with peers, which are also part of the student role, were more challenging for him. His classmates generally accepted and interacted with him as a member of the classroom. However, he was sometimes teased and others did not defend him when this happened. Moreover, he had only a couple of classmates who would actually do things regularly with him outside of structured classroom activities. He was not invited to interact with others, and as noted above, was not welcomed as a participant in sport activities.

His teacher reported that, aside from rare occasions of aggressive behaviors, Gerald managed to work adequately with his classmates. However, at the beginning of the year, he had much more difficulty. He used to touch students inappropriately and display aggressiveness. His touching inappropriately had stopped and his aggressiveness had decreased. His interactions with classmates had gradually improved as Gerald had become familiar with his classmates and they with him. Because of his trouble working with students in the beginning of the year, his teacher had some concerns about Gerald meeting and interacting with new students in second grade. She reported that if there was a problem between Gerald and another student, it was usually with a student who was not in Gerald's classroom.

Student/Environment Fit

Overall, Gerald's school environment supported his participation in school and learning. Gerald sat in the back of the room and at times had difficulty attending to the tasks at hand. However, this problem appeared more related to Gerald's need to move around at times and his short attention span rather than particular features of the classroom. Gerald was provided with and utilized a move-and-sit cushion (a pad he sits on to meet his need for movement and help increase his attention span). The pad had improved his distractibility. In addition, Gerald used a desk that opens and closes, a basket, and a part-time aide. The desk and basket enabled him to find supplies more easily and to be more organized. Gerald's part-time aide greatly supported his performance in the classroom. The classroom milieu was also highly structured, which helped Gerald to stay focused. Finally, the classroom provided some avenues for Gerald to feel a positive sense of personal causation related to his academic ability.

The desks in the classroom were arranged in groups of four (with assigned seating), facilitating Gerald's positive interactions with other students. Generally, Gerald could work with other students, although they tended to marginalize and sometimes tease him during open activities and recess.

Gerald was able to interact well with his teacher, readily asking for help and offering answers during group discussions. Gerald's teacher was a good match for him, as she has high expecta-

FIGURE 16-5 Gerald's Ratings and Comments on the Habits/Routines and Roles Section of the OT PAL Rating Scale.

II. Habits and Routines—The student	N/O	4	3	2	1
A. Demonstrates school routines comparable to peers. Comments: *Gerald occasionally demonstrates the ability to keep up with his classmates in relation to the school routines, but often he struggles and needs assistance*				▨	
B. Adheres to routines within the school day. Comments: *Gerald is aware of routines within a school day. He periodically needs verbal cues to assist him with his routine.*			▨		
C. Completes activities within time guidelines (e.g., finishes assignments/ tasks in a timely manner). Comments: *Does not always complete task within time guidelines because he is often slower than his peers in writing tasks.*				▨	
D. Maintains desk in a manner in keeping with classroom routines. Comments: *Even with adaptations, he still has trouble finding certain materials. It took him a longer time to find a book as compared to peers.*				▨	
E. Maintains personal belongings in keeping with classroom routines. Comments: *Knows where his belongings should be kept, but his book bag and jacket were on the floor (not the appropriate place) during the observation.*				▨	
F. Organize assignments and projects in keeping with classroom routines. Comments: *Tends to fall behind*	▨				
G. Completes smooth transitions between routine activities (i.e., efficiently ends and begins another). Comments: *Gerald is often the last one in the class to complete a transition and often needs verbal cues regarding the new activity in which he just transitioned.*				▨	
III. Roles—The student	N/O	4	3	2	1
A. Demonstrates a well-established student role (i.e., accepts teacher's authority, asks for help appropriately). Comments: *Demonstrates many behaviors attached to the student role; however, he needs to be more self directed.*			▨		
B. Demonstrates smooth transition between roles (i.e., switches smoothly from leader to follower). Comments:	▨				
C. Responds acceptably to diverse roles adopted by others. Comments:	▨				
D. Assumes roles consistent with classroom/school expectations. Comments:	▨				
Key: **4** = Competent performance; **3** = Questionable performance; **2** = Ineffective performance; **1** = Deficient performance; **N/O** = Not observed					

tions for all the students but considers each student's circumstances. She considered each student individually, identifying their academic and emotional needs, and worked hard to meet those needs.

Implications of the OT PAL Assessment

The OT PAL identified Gerald's strengths and weaknesses in the areas of volition and habituation. *Figure 16-6* summarizes Gerald's rating scale scores. Equally important to the profile of strengths and weaknesses is the qualitative information gathered about Gerald. His greatest strength was his volitional desire to be a good student and the sense of efficacy he had concerning some aspects of his classroom performance. Gerald's volitional strengths were particularly important given his substantial habituation and performance capacity weaknesses. However, aspects of Gerald's volition were at risk and needed to be supported and developed.

Supporting Gerald's volition meant paying attention to the strong values he held about being a student and bolstering his sense of personal causation. It was important to Gerald to be seen as a good and normal student, and this needed to be supported as much as possible. His limited motor performance barred him from a number of classroom and other activities, frustrating his attempts to be competent and to fit in. Additionally, a number of factors in the classroom tended to make Gerald stand out, and these needed to be considered and minimized.

First, consideration was given to minimizing how Gerald's limited strength and endurance affect his performance and what can be done about it. Fatigue, in particular, is a common problem following chemotherapy, and its extent and duration is a matter of great variation. Since the pace at which Gerald would regain these capacities was unknown, it was important to adapt circumstances in the interim to allow Gerald to participate more inside and outside the classroom. For example, carrying the lunch to the cafeteria was modified to involve pushing a cart.

Gerald at times relied heavily on his aide. Although this support was useful for him, it increasingly made him stand out from the other students. Moreover, growing independent of his aide in the future would further enhance his feelings of efficacy. The main function that Gerald's aide served for him was to help him organize his materials and focus on his schoolwork. Even though Gerald was provided with desk and basket adaptations to help him organize and find needed materials efficiently, he had not learned to use these resources optimally. The therapist and the aide worked together to develop an organization process that worked best for Gerald. Importantly, Gerald was involved in helping to plan this process. The therapist consulted with the aide concerning the importance of Gerald's growing more independent of her help and assisted her in planning how to gradually allow Gerald more responsibility and autonomy as he could handle it. This strategy enabled Gerald to develop habits to support his own competence in school.

Another area of concern was that Gerald needed to catch up on missed assignments during

FIGURE 16-6   Summary of Gerald's Ratings on the OT PAL Scale.

Volition — Student chooses to:										Habits and Routines — The student:						Roles — The student:			
Begin activity with direction	Begin self-directed activity	Stay engaged	Continue/transition with direction	Discontinue activity with direction	Discontinue self-directed activity	Engage with peers given direction	Engage with peers self-directed	Follow social rules	Show preferences	Demonstrates routines	Adheres to routines	Completes activities	Maintains desk	Maintains belongings	Completes transitions	Demonstrates student role	Transitions smoothly between roles	Responds to diverse roles	Assumes school-related roles
N/O	N/O	N/O	N/O	N/O	N/O	N/O	N/O	N/O	N/O	N/O	N/O	N/O	N/O	N/O	N/O	N/O	**N/O**	**N/O**	**N/O**
4	4	4	**4**	**4**	4	4	**4**	**4**	**4**	4	4	4	4	4	4	4	4	4	4
3	3	**3**	3	3	3	**3**	3	3	3	3	**3**	3	3	3	3	**3**	3	3	3
2	2	2	2	2	**2**	2	2	2	3	**2**	2	**2**	**2**	**2**	**2**	2	2	2	2
1	**1**	1	1	1	1	1	1	1	2	1	1	1	1	1	1	1	1	1	1

Key: **4** = Competent; **3** = Questionable; **2** = Ineffective; **1** = Deficient; **N/O** = Not observed free time. It was important for Gerald to get free time to let off steam, which helped him focus throughout the rest of the school day. Moreover, having to work on schoolwork when other students were engaged in free activities set Gerald apart from the other students. Thus, an alternative schedule for Gerald to receive therapies that minimized interference with classroom work was developed.

▄▄▄▄▄▄▄▄▄▄▄▄▄▄▄▄

As this case illustrated, the OT PAL can be very useful in the school context for identifying the status of volition and habituation and their contribution to how a child is adapting to school. The assessment also highlights factors in the school environment that support or constrain the student. Because of its focus, this instrument is well suited to complement capacity or perfor-

mance-oriented assessments used in the school context.

Conclusion

This chapter presented three diverse assessments that have in common the combination of flexibility in the use of more than a single method of data collection. Each method of data collection has its strengths and weaknesses, and assessments that use a single method (interview, self-report, or observation) are designed to make the most use of the methodology they employ. These assessments, by combining or allowing alternative approaches to collecting information, are designed to maximize the use of mixed methods.

References

Brollier, C., Watts, J. H., Bauer, D., & Schmidt, W. (1988). A content validity study of the Assessment of Occupational Functioning. *Occupational Therapy in Mental Health, 8* (4), 29–47.

Elliott, K. R., & Newman, S. M. (1993). *A concurrent validity study of the 1991 research version of the Assessment of Occupational Functioning.* Unpublished master's degree research project. Department of Occupational Therapy. Virginia Commonwealth University, Richmond, VA.

McGuigan, P. M. (1993). *Content validity of the 1991 research version of the Assessment of Occupational Functioning.* Unpublished master's degree research project. Department of Occupational Therapy. Virginia Commonwealth University, Richmond, VA.

Parkinson, S., & Forsyth, K. (2001). *A user's manual for the Model of Human Occupation Screening Tool (MOHOST) (Version 1.0).* Unpublished manuscript. UK MOHO.CORE, University of London.

Townsend, S. C., Carey, P. D., Hollins, N. L., Helfrich, C., Blondis, M., Hoffman, A., Collins, L., Knudson, J., & Blackwell, A. (2001). *The Occupational Therapy Psychosocial Assessment of Learning (OT PAL). (Version 1.0)* Chicago: Model of Human Occupation Clearing-

house. Department of Occupational Therapy. University of Illinois, Chicago.

Watts, J. H., Brollier, C., Bauer, D., & Schmidt, W. (1988). A comparison of two evaluation instruments used with psychiatric patients in occupational therapy. *Occupational Therapy in Mental Health, 8* (4), 7–27.

Watts, J. H., Brollier, C., Bauer, D., & Schmidt, W. (1989). The Assessment of Occupational Functioning: The second revision. *Occupational Therapy in Mental Health, 8* (4), 61–87.

Watts, J. H., Hinson, R., Madigan, M. J., McGuigan, P. M., & Newman, S. M. (1999). The Assessment of Occupational Functioning—Collaborative version. In B. J. Hempill-Pearson (Ed.), *Assessments in occupational therapy in mental health.* Thorofare, NJ: Slack.

Watts, J. H., Kielhofner, G., Bauer, D., Gregory, M., & Valentine, D. (1986). The Assessment of Occupational Functioning: A screening tool for use in long-term care. *American Journal of Occupational Therapy, 40,* 231–240.

Viik, M. K., Watts, J. H., Madigan, M. J., & Bauer, D. (1990). Preliminary validation of the Assessment of Occupational Functioning with an alcoholic population. *Occupational Therapy in Mental Health, 10* (2), 19–33.

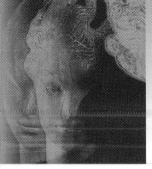

17

How to Know the Client Best: Choosing and Using Structured Assessments and Unstructured Means of Gathering Information

- **Gary Kielhofner**

- **Kirsty Forsyth**

The previous five chapters presented and discussed MOHO-based approaches to gathering information on clients. This chapter focuses on how to appropriately choose and use assessments in practice. The idea for this chapter came out of many discussions with therapists about their considerations and dilemmas in assessment.

These conversations have underscored the practical factors that influence how therapists go about assessment. They also revealed a number of fallacies that can lead to unfavorable decisions regarding assessment. Our perspective in this chapter considers how to be realistic while also doing what is in the best interest of the client. Because the issues addressed herein have arisen from therapists' questions about assessment, the chapter is presented as responses to their most common questions.

How Much Information Do I Need to Gather When Evaluating a Client?

As noted in Chapters 11 and 12, therapists gather information to create a conceptualization of the client's situation that will guide therapy decisions. Consequently, therapists should gather enough information to avoid harm and maximize benefit to the client. From the perspective of MOHO theory, this means that a therapist will minimally raise and seek answers to questions pertaining to the client's occupational adaptation, volition, habituation, performance capacity, and

environment as occasioned by the client's circumstances. The questions that the therapist raises will indicate the kind of information that needs to be gathered to generate an adequate understanding of the client's situation. The following case illustrates the importance of this point.

Henrietta

Henrietta is 75 years old and has osteoarthritis. The second author on this chapter received a referral to see Henrietta for occupational therapy. The referral further stated that Henrietta had recently been hospitalized after sustaining a fractured femur. At their first meeting, Henrietta indicated that she was familiar with occupational therapy. Several months ago, she first received occupational therapy as an inpatient following a mild stroke. She remembered that the therapist had asked her about her physical limitations and then recommended that Henrietta receive bathing equipment. Henrietta recalled that initially she was extremely excited at the prospect of being able to bathe again.

Henrietta then came to the occupational therapy department, where the therapist demonstrated how to use the bathing equipment. She then asked Henrietta to try using the equipment to get in and out of the bath. Henrietta remembered that she managed this simulation well and she never saw the occupational therapist again. In fact, the therapist had documented in Henrietta's file that she was able to "transfer in and out of the bath using the bath board and seat." After Henrietta was discharged, another community-based occupational therapist had visited her home once to install the equipment.

When asked where the bathing equipment was now, Henrietta answered, "in the closet . . . I never use it." Instead, Henrietta had been washing herself at the bathroom sink. The following is why Henrietta had abandoned the bathroom equipment and begun washing at the sink. First, Henrietta's bathroom at home was much smaller than the one in the hospital. Consequently, she had difficulty maneuvering into position while using her walker. Second, she could not gather and organize all the needed bathing objects within reach, which frustrated her. Third, Henrietta had attempted to bathe in the morning, as had always been her habit. However, because this was before her pain medication had begun to have an effect, she was in pain. Fourth, Henrietta found it very anxiety-provoking to do the routine she had simulated in the hospital with the bath full of hot water and steam.

Despite these factors and because bathing was so important to her, Henrietta chose to continue with the bath. As she proceeded, she realized that she had forgotten some of the therapist's instructions for how to use the bath board and seat. Consequently, she was only able to maneuver part way onto the bath equipment. After several attempts, her skin became sore and she decided she could not manage and gave up.

Henrietta was so flustered by this negative experience and so unsure of her capacity to use the bathing equipment that she resolved never to try bathing with the equipment again. So, she asked a neighbor to remove the bathing equipment. Then she put it permanently in the closet.

Following this, Henrietta chose to bathe in the best way she could: washing at the bathroom sink. However, her endurance was severely taxed by this bathing process. It was during this morning wash at the bathroom sink that Henrietta, exhausted, slipped and fractured the neck of her femur. The two occupational therapists' failure to do adequate assessment had contributed to Henrietta's fall and fracture.

Clearly, the therapists needed more information about Henrietta than they gathered. They might have recognized the need to gather more information had they generated the following MOHO-based questions:

- Did Henrietta have adequate motor and process skills to manage bathing at home with the prescribed equipment?
- What was Henrietta's daily habit of bathing? How would this habit influence her success in bathing?
- When the new equipment (objects) are put into the physical space of Henrietta's bathroom along with other objects (her walker, soap, shampoo, towels, robe, etc.), how will the overall bathroom space and objects collectively impact her performance?
- How will Henrietta experience her first attempt to bathe at home?
- Will she feel an adequate sense of efficacy to continue using the equipment?

Gathering adequate information to answer these questions would have pointed to the utility of:

- Helping Henrietta find a way to transport/arrange her bathing objects in reach of the bathing seat
- Solving problems of dealing with limited maneuvering space
- Providing further training and practice in the use of the adaptive equipment under real life conditions
- Giving her verbal encouragement and reassurance to reduce her anxiety
- Altering daily habits so that she could bathe in the afternoon or evening when she had less pain.

Even if Henrietta had not been able to bathe with these interventions, the therapist could have worked with her to establish a different, safe way of getting washed. Had the original occupational therapist taken a bit more time to gather information or had the community therapist gathered information while installing the equipment and followed up later, Henrietta might well have been able to bathe safely. Certainly, the additional time and cost of doing adequate assessment would have been substantially less than the expense of Henrietta's hospitalization for the hip fracture. As this case illustrates, taking time to do adequate assessment can be very cost-effective. Failing to gather adequate information can have high human and economic costs.

Why Can't Assessments Be Simpler, Quicker, and Easier to Use?

Assessments that are simple, quick, and easy to use have intuitive appeal. Those that require training or study can be intimidating. Those that require adherence to a protocol, reflective thought, and use of standardized forms and rating scales can seem unnecessarily burdensome. Not surprisingly, then, therapists often relate that they are not using structured assessments because they take too much effort, preferring instead an approach with ease and simplicity.

Simple and easy assessments might be adequate if our clients' occupational problems were simple and easy to manage, but this is hardly ever the case. Most persons come into occupational therapy with significant impairments and major disruptions to their lives. Others struggle with declining function or recurring exacerbations of their diseases. A large proportion of clients face the task of rebuilding all or part of their lives. In short, their occupational problems tend to be complex and challenging. Such problems hardly suggest that the criteria for assessing them should be ease and simplicity.

Easy and simple assessment methods risk misunderstanding and oversimplifying a client's situation. This can readily lead to therapy that fails to meet clients' needs and, in the worst case, does harm. In thinking about assessment, therapists should recall Trombly's (1993, p. 256) warning that "we cannot ethically treat what we do not measure." Using simple and easy assessments that fail our clients is not only bad practice but also ethically questionable.

The MOHO-based assessments discussed in the previous chapters are designed to provide therapists with the best possible means of gathering relevant, sound, and thorough information. Most reflect years of development and have been studied and refined to enhance their de-

pendability and practical value. Importantly, they were created with the aim of making them effective means of gathering information. The amount of effort each assessment takes is proportional to the kind of information it gathers. One should always consider not only how much effort an assessment takes, but also the value of the information it yields. For example, a life history interview takes the most effort, but sometimes this information is also most critical to providing good therapy.

What Do I Do About Time Constraints in Selecting Assessments?

The following is a good exercise. Examine every aspect of the information gathered on clients and ask, "How does this information influence what I do with a client?" A surprising number of therapists who try this exercise realize they are collecting information that does not consistently influence what they do. This insight allows them to cease gathering information that does not impact therapy and focus on what really makes a difference.

Another strategy to achieve more efficiency in assessment is to overlap assessment and intervention. It is possible to do some assessment while engaging in therapy. It is also the case that one can accomplish therapeutic aims during assessment. The following are examples of doing assessment during therapy:

- An interview can be done while making a splint or helping a client practice a skill
- Observation of volition or skill can be done during a therapy session in which the client is performing
- Self-administered assessments can be incorporated into group interventions aimed at helping clients solve problems or set goals related to their occupational adaptation.

The following are examples of how therapists accomplish therapeutic aims during assessment:

- During an interview, the therapist builds rapport with a client
- As part of assessment, the therapist provides feedback to a client or shares information about the client's situation
- Engaging in an assessment helps a client clarify values

> *Simple and easy assessments might be adequate if our clients' occupational problems were simple and easy to manage.*

- Participating in an assessment process gives a client a more realistic view of personal capacity.

As these examples illustrate, the line between assessment and intervention need not be starkly drawn. In the best therapy, assessment and intervention are interwoven. The therapist's use of both structured assessments and informal methods of information gathering can be readily woven into the process of therapy. Therapists who are creative in how they integrate assessment and intervention make time for more comprehensive assessment.

A final, important strategy is to make the case to appropriate persons that the assessment is worth the time it takes. No one would trust a physician who saved time by going straight into surgery without lab tests and other information about the patient's condition. Therapists who can justify the importance of the information they wish to gather are often able to negotiate for the time. Even when assessment means using time that would ordinarily be spent in intervention, it may be justified as a means to assure that the intervention is optimal for the client.

If I Have to Choose Between Different Kinds of Information to Gather, Shouldn't I Focus on Performance Capacity?

A common misconception is that when priorities must be set for assessment, the best strategy is to focus on performance capacity since it seems most relevant to function. To the contrary, we argue that the most indispensable part of assessment is to gain an understanding of a client's volition and habituation. Recall that in Henrietta's case habituation contributed to her difficulties and volition determined the decision to use her bathing equipment. Both directly impacted how she functioned.

> *Failing to take time to do adequate assessment can result in wasted time in therapy.*

The following is another example of why volition and habituation information is so important. Chuck Close, an acclaimed American painter who had a spinal blood clot that left him paralyzed from the neck down, eventually returned to painting. When interviewed on the U.S. National Public Radio show, *Fresh Air*, he had the following to say about occupational therapy:

> I remember rolling down the hall one day and seeing the name on the door that said "Occupational Therapy." I said, "Oh great, they'll help me get back to my occupation." But in fact it was much more about stacking spools and making things out of pipe cleaners.

Consequently, Close's wife intervened to tell the therapists about her husband's volition. She pointed out to the therapists that it was most important to him to find a way to return to painting. As he notes,

> She convinced the therapists to stop trying to convince me to do things that I didn't need to do, and to get back to what really mattered, and they found me a space in the basement of the building and I equipped it as a studio and managed to start painting while I was still in rehabilitation. (Gross & Miller, 1998)

The occupational therapist would have gotten much more directly to the business of helping Close do what he valued and what constituted his most important life role by using such assessments as the Occupational Performance History Interview (OPHI-II) (Kielhofner et al., 1998) or the Occupational Self Assessment (OSA) (Baron, Kielhofner, Iyenger, Goldhammer, & Wolenski, 2002).

Close's remarks also underscore another important issue. Sometimes therapy can take up time doing things that do not really benefit the client. Failing to take time to do adequate assessment can result in wasted time in therapy. Taking enough time to do adequate assessment of volition and habituation is often the most efficient thing to do.

Failing to adequately assess volition and habituation of clients can also result in therapist and client working at cross-purposes. Take for example the client, Tom, described by Helfrich and Kielhofner (1994). Tom's therapist found him uncooperative and disruptive in therapy. He appeared unmotivated to engage in occupational therapy groups and often challenged the therapist, disrupting the group. In fact, Tom was a highly motivated client with a strong desire to move beyond his psychiatric hospitalization and get back to living and working in the community.

While the therapist shared this same goal, her lack of information about Tom's occupational narrative resulted in a missed opportunity to make therapy more meaningful and engaging for him. Tom saw his hospitalizations for exacerbations of his bipolar condition as detours from his real life as a newspaper professional. He saw much of his occupational therapy experiences as putting him in the role of a patient rather than helping him re-enter the worker role. In Tom's case, the OPHI-II and the Role Checklist (Oakley, Kielhofner, Barris, & Reichler, 1986) would have been ideal assessments. They would have provided critical information for making his therapy more meaningful and relevant.

As these two case examples illustrate, failure to gather adequate information on a client's volition or habituation can readily result in therapy that is not meaningful for the client. When this is the case, time can be wasted and clients can feel frustrated that their needs are not met. Another way of framing this is that assessment must be client-centered (Law, 1998). From the perspective of MOHO, client-centered assessment means gathering information on the client's values, interests, personal causation, roles, and habits.

How Can I Assess the Volition of Clients Who Are Too Low Functioning to Relate Their Desires and Perspective?

We have often heard therapists indicate that they cannot apply the concepts of volition to their clients whose level of functioning is too low. This has always perplexed us because clients, who are least able to self-describe and self-advocate, most deserve careful assessment of their volition. A very touching and telling lesson in this regard is contained in the book, *A World Without Words*, by Goode (1994). The book's author, a sociologist, engaged in a longitudinal study of two young women who were blind, deaf, and had severe cognitive

impairments. They had no language and, therefore, could not tell anyone what they thought and felt or what their actions meant. Nonetheless, those responsible for their care went about doing all kinds of things that changed their actions, modified their experiences, and controlled their context. As Goode documents, a substantial amount of what was done in the name of service to these young women did not make their lives better and frequently made them substantially worse.

Elsewhere, Goode (1983) discusses Bobby, a man with Down's syndrome and severely limited cognitive and linguistic capacity. For many years, Bobby had been a resident in a state hospital. Goode (1983, p. 241) observes that in Bobby's medical record from the state hospital, the occupational therapist had written:

> "Time and effort . . . are not suggested as prognosis for improvement is poor . . . maintain client in a protected environment as he can never function independently."

Ironically, at the time Goode met Bobby, he was living in a residential facility in the community, pretty much relying on his own devices to get along. Goode makes the point that none of Bobby's professional caregivers, including the occupational therapist, had taken adequate time to assess Bobby.

As it turns out, and as Goode meticulously demonstrates, Bobby had well-formulated ideas about what he liked and what was important in his life. Given adequate opportunity, Bobby was able to make these things known. Goode acknowledges that, while Bobby had very severe cognitive and linguistic deficits:

> " . . . it was equally valid and far more beneficial for Bobby and us to see him as a man with an unusual countenance, different ways of thinking and evaluating, trying to explore and master his everyday world." (Goode, 1983, p. 254)

Goode's argument makes the point that people who are extremely limited in their ability to tell about themselves nonetheless have their own perspectives on their own lives. They have thoughts and feelings pertaining to what they care about (value), things they enjoy (interests), and ideas about how they can best accomplish what they want (personal causation).

There are ways that a therapist can readily gain insight into the volition of lower functioning clients. The

Volitional Questionnaire (VQ) (de las Heras, Geist, Kiel-hofner, & Li, 2002), the Pediatric Volitional Question-naire (PVQ) (Geist, Kielhofner, Basu, & Kafkes, 2002), and the Model of Human Occupation Screening Tool (MOHOST) (Parkinson & Forsyth, 2001) work well with such clients. Additionally, therapists can make good use of unstructured means of assessment for such clients.

If My Practice is Based on MOHO, Is It Okay to Use Assessments Other Than Those Derived From MOHO?

The answer is, of course, yes. There are several reasons for this. Therapists often use MOHO in combination with other practice models or with theories borrowed from other disciplines or professions. When this is the case, assessments that correspond to those models and theories may be used.

In other circumstances, the occupational therapist may use assessments other than those derived from MOHO because they are part of an interdisciplinary ap-proach or because administration or regulatory bodies requires their use. When this is the case, therapists may use MOHO-based assessments to complement such data collection. Additionally, such assessments should be examined carefully for whether the information they provide is useful to consider as part of a thera-peutic approach guided by MOHO.

A third reason for using assessments with different origins is that there are no MOHO-based assessments available for a given client group or situation. We will discuss this more later, but in such circumstances, ther-apists should be careful to consider how the informa-tion gathered by such assessments relates to the con-cepts for which they are seeking information on the client.

For a variety of reasons, then, therapists basing practice on MOHO will use assessments other than those presented in the previous chapters. When this is the case, it is important to consider why one is using the assessment, what kinds of information it provides, and how it can best be used in relationship to the model and the MOHO-based assessments that are be-ing used.

Do I Consider the Client's Diagnosis in Selecting Assessments and, If So, How?

None of the MOHO-based assessments are designed for use with clients from a specific diagnostic group. MOHO focuses on understanding the impact of a dis-ease or impairment on the person's occupational life, not on the disease or impairment itself. Therefore, most of the assessments will work with clients who have a wide range of diagnoses.

This is not to say that the therapist should ignore the diagnosis or impairment in selecting assessments. Two important considerations in selecting assessments that do emanate from the client's diagnosis or impair-ments are:

- Whether the diagnosis or nature of the impairment has implications that are better addressed by certain assessments
- Whether the client's impairment limits the client's ability to do what is necessary to participate in the assessment.

Some MOHO-based assessments are particularly rele-vant to a given population. For example, the NIH Ac-tivity Record (ACTRE) (Furst, Gerber, Smith, Fisher, & Shulman, 1987; Gerber & Furst, 1992) gathers informa-tion on pain and fatigue. Therefore, for clients who are likely to experience pain and fatigue that impacts their occupational performance, the ACTRE would be the better choice.

When a diagnosis is known to routinely produce certain kinds of occupational consequences, it may war-rant use of particular assessments. For example, chronic, severe depression typically results in severe volitional problems. For this reason, the Volitional Questionnaire is frequently an assessment of choice for these types of clients. Another example is that traumatic injuries or catastrophic illnesses that significantly alter a person's life (e.g., persons with spinal cord injury or persons with AIDS) often produce changes in interests and participa-tion in interests, changes in roles, and changes in occu-pational identity and occupational competence. For this reason, such clients would be good candidates for use of the Modified Interest Checklist, the Role Checklist, and the OPHI-II, since all three assessments provide in-formation on changes that occur as the result of dis-eases or impairments that change a person's life.

Knowing what implications for assessment emanate from a client's diagnosis or impairment requires that the therapist have two kinds of information. First, the therapist must have some knowledge of how the diagnosis or impairment is likely to impact the client occupationally. Second, the therapist must know the content and organization of the MOHO-based assessments. When these two factors are known, the therapist can make intelligent matches.

What Should I Do When Clients' Impairments Limit Their Ability to Participate in the Assessment?

Most of the assessments discussed in previous chapters require at least minimal abilities as illustrated in *Table 17-1*. These client requirements are based on the ordinary protocol for administration of the assessment. For example, interviews require verbal abilities, whereas self-reports require the ability to read and write.

In a number of instances, the administration can be altered to accommodate client limitations. For example, a client whose motor abilities impair speech could respond to an interview using augmented communication, or a client with motor limitations that prevent writing can respond to self-reports verbally. Most manuals for MOHO-based assessments provide guidelines for whether and how the administration can be accommodated and still maintain the psychometric properties of the assessment.

Whenever client limitations are of the kind that such an accommodation of the assessment cannot be made, there are often still alternatives. For instance, therapists have often found it useful to ask family members to respond to the Role Checklist or the

TABLE 17-1 Client Requirements for Participation in MOHO Assessments

Assessment	Client Requirements to Participate
Assessment of Communication and Interaction Skills	Engage in some social interaction
Assessment of Motor and Process Skills	Perform an occupational form (simple to complex)
Assessment of Occupational Functioning	Answer interview questions (interview format) Read and write (self-report format)
Child Occupational Self Assessment	Concentrate, read, and write
Interest Checklist	Read and write
Model of Human Occupational Screening Tool	Minimally interact with the environment
NIH Activity Record	Concentrate, read, and write
Occupational Circumstances Assessment-Interview and Rating Scale	Answer questions
Occupational Performance History Interview-II	Answer questions
Occupational Questionnaire	Concentrate, read, and write
Occupational Self Assessment	Concentrate, read, and write
Occupational Therapy Psychosocial Assessment of Learning	Participate in school and answer questions
Pediatric Interest Profiles	Look at pictures or read, use a crayon or write (depending on which profile is used)
Pediatric Volitional Questionnaire	Minimally interact with the environment
Role Checklist	Concentrate, read, and write
School Setting Interview	Answer questions
Volitional Questionnaire	Minimally interact with the environment
Worker Role Interview	Answer interview questions
Work Environment Impact Scale	Answer interview questions

OPHI-II on behalf of a client. However, when someone is asked to be a proxy for a client who cannot respond, it is best to think of it as an informal assessment.

How Do I Consider The Client's Age In Selecting Assessments?

Some MOHO-based assessments are designed for clients within a specific age range. Other assessments are designed to span adolescence and adulthood. A few assessments, by virtue of their content, will be most appropriate for persons of certain ages. For example, the Worker Role Interview (WRI) (Velozo, Kielhofner, & Fisher, 1998) and the Work Environment Impact Scale (WEIS) (Moore-Corner, Kielhofner, & Olson, 1998) will be appropriate for persons of working age, whereas the Occupational Therapy Psychosocial Assessment of Learning (OT PAL) (Townsend et al., 2001) and the School System Interview (SSI) (Hoffman, Hemmingsson, & Kielhofner, 2000) are both designed for children who are students.

Table 17-2 lists all the MOHO-based assessments, indicating the age groups with which the assessments are used. More specific information on age-appropriateness of each assessment will ordinarily be covered in the manuals or texts that present the assessments. In the end, appropriate use of the assessments in terms of age will depend on a therapist's judgment. For example, the appropriateness of some assessments that require more abstract thought and self-reflection will depend less on chronological age and more on intellectual development and personal maturity of the client. Therapists should always be vigilant to consider a client's developmental readiness and ability to participate in any assessment process.

Do Cultural Differences Affect The Use Of MOHO-Based Assessments?

Most early assessments developed for use with MOHO were first developed in the United States. As they were increasingly used with persons from different cultures elsewhere in the world, it became apparent that subtle cultural biases were built into some of the assessments. To overcome this, a concerted effort has been made to modify early assessments and to develop new assessments in ways that are not culturally biased. For instance, most of the newer assessments have been developed in collaboration with persons representing multiple cultures and languages.

Moreover, research indicates that many of the MOHO-based assessments do not reflect cultural biases. For example, studies of the Assessment of Motor and Process Skills (AMPS) (Fisher, 1999) have indicated that it is free of cultural bias (Fisher, Liu, Velozo, & Pan, 1992; Goto, Fisher, & Mayberry, 1996). Studies of the WRI (Haglund, Karlsson, Kielhofner, & Lai, 1997), the WEIS (Kielhofner, Lai, Olson, Haglund, Ekbladh, & Hedlund, 1999), the OPHI-II (Kielhofner, Mallinson, Forsyth, & Lai, 2001), the ACIS (Haglund, Kjellberg, Forsyth, & Kielhofner, 2001), and the OSA (Kielhofner & Forsyth, 2001) indicate that these assessments are valid cross-culturally and when administered in different languages.

Assuring that assessments are relevant and valid with persons from diverse cultural backgrounds requires ongoing development and research. Such work is being undertaken across the MOHO-based assessments. Nonetheless, therapists should always be vigilant to consider whether an assessment is valid for clients based on their cultural background.

A further point needs to be made about MOHO-based assessments in relation to culture. Because the theory of this model incorporates culture into its concepts (e.g., volition and social environment), many of the assessments are specifically designed to capture a client's unique cultural perspective. For example, the OPHI-II elicits and considers culturally influenced values, interests, roles, and occupational narratives. For this reason, such assessments are particularly useful when therapists desire to gather information about the client's culturally influenced thoughts, feelings, and actions.

Can MOHO-Based Assessments Be Used To Show Client Change And The Outcomes Of Therapy?

A number of MOHO-based assessments can be used to document change in clients and to evaluate the impact or outcomes of therapy. *Table 17-3* lists the assessments

TABLE 17-2 MOHO-Based Assessments, Concepts on Which They Provide Data, Methods They Use, and Populations for Which They Are Designed

Assessment	Occupational Adaptation		Volition			Habituation		Skills			Performance	Participation	Environment Impact		Method of Data Gathering			Population			
	Identity	Competence	Personal Causation	Values	Interests	Roles	Habits	Motor	Process	Communication/ Interaction			Physical	Social	Observation	Self-report	Interview	Children	Adolescents	Adults	Elderly
Assessment of Communication and Interaction Skills		X								X	X	X		X	X				X	X	X
Assessment of Motor and Process Skills								X	X		X	X			X			X	X	X	X
Assessment of Occupational Functioning		X	X	X	X	X	X									X	X			X	X
Child Occupational Self Assessment	X	X	X	X	X	X	X					X	X	X		X		X	X		
Interest Checklist					X											X			X	X	X
Model of Human Occupation Screening Tool	X	X	X	X	X	X	X	X	X	X	X	X	X	X	X				X	X	X
NIH Activity Record					X	X	X					X				X				X	X
Occupational Circumstances Assessment-Interview and Rating Scale	X	X	X	X	X	X	X					X	X	X			X		X	X	X
Occupational Performance History Interview-II	X	X	X	X	X	X	X	X	X	X	X	X	X	X			X		X	X	X
Occupational Questionnaire			X	X	X		X									X			X	X	X
Occupational Self Assessment	X	X	X	X	X	X	X					X	X	X		X			X	X	X
Occupational Therapy Psychosocial Assessment of Learning			X	X	X	X	X	X	X	X		X	X	X	X			X	X		
Pediatric Interest Profiles					X											X		X	X		
Pediatric Volitional Questionnaire		X	X	X	X							X	X	X	X			X	X		
Role Checklist				X		X										X			X	X	X
School Setting Interview												X	X				X	X	X		
Volitional Questionnaire		X	X	X	X							X	X	X	X			X	X	X	X
Worker Role Interview		X	X	X	X	X	X						X	X			X		X	X	X
Work Environment Impact Scale												X	X	X			X		X	X	X

> *A number of MOHO-based assessments can be used to document change in clients and to evaluate the impact or outcomes of therapy.*

whose formats would gather quantitative data for evaluating client change and demonstrating impact. It also indicates the type of change that the assessment would capture.

Most of the assessments are being developed with careful attention to the measurement properties that are essential to being able to capture change and thus document outcomes.

Creating a sound measure is a long process that involves a series of studies. Some MOHO-based assessments have very clearly demonstrated measurement properties, while others need further investigation. In selecting an outcome measure, therapists should become familiar with the research documenting each as-

sessment's psychometric properties. Currently, for several of the assessments, true measures can only be derived from computer analyses. Ongoing and planned research will result in paper-and-pencil methods of scoring the assessments that yield true measures. As these are available, they will facilitate the everyday use of the assessments to determine client change.

Which assessment one chooses for capturing change or demonstrating program outcomes depends on what changes services are designed to achieve. Outcome measures must be targeted to those aspects of clients that the services aim to achieve.

How Do I Go About Choosing Which Assessment(s) To Use?

Choosing which assessments to use routinely is one of the most important decisions therapists make about their practice. As we have stressed throughout this chapter, assessment has a direct effect on the quality of therapeutic reasoning as well as the relevance and im-

TABLE 17-3 MOHO Assessments Suitable for Indicating Client Change and Program Outcomes

Assessment	Type of Change Captured by Assessment
Assessment of Communication and Interaction Skills	Change in skill
Assessment of Motor and Process Skills	Change in skill
Child Occupational Self Assessment	Change in values and competence
Model of Human Occupational Screening Tool	Change in volition, habituation, skill, and environmental impact
NIH Activity Record	Change in participation and in fatigue, pain, perceived competence, interest, and value in what one routinely does
Occupational Questionnaire	Change in participation and in competence, interest, and value in what one routinely does
Occupational Self Assessment	Change in values and competence as well as in environmental impact
Occupational Therapy Psychosocial Assessment of Learning	Change in student's adaptation to the student role and its demands
Pediatric Interest Profiles	Change in interests, perceived competence, and participation
Pediatric Volitional Questionnaire	Change in volition (motivation to do things)
Role Checklist	Change in roles and value assigned to roles
Volitional Questionnaire	Change in volition (motivation to do things)
Worker Role Interview	Change in psychosocial readiness for work

pact of therapy. Consequently, one should carefully choose which assessment or assessments to incorporate into practice. We recommend the following steps in making an informed decision:

- Becoming familiar with all potentially relevant MOHO assessments and identify those that appear most suitable for use
- Piloting these assessments in practice to evaluate their utility
- Developing an assessment strategy that allows flexibility to meet individual client needs.

Identifying and Examining Potentially Relevant Assessments

This first step involves simply becoming familiar with the range of assessments developed for use with MOHO. Table 17-2 provides an overview of the assessments. It allows you to identify those that are potentially most suitable. Another resource for identifying potentially relevant assessments is *Figure 17-1*. The figure categorizes MOHO-based assessments according to whether they are general (providing data on many MOHO concepts and designed for use across practice settings) or specific (focused on one or a few concepts and/or designed for specific practice settings). By examining this figure, you can further focus your initial selection of assessments. For an initial evaluation, you may want to choose an assessment that covers the majority of the MOHO concepts. This will give you a global picture of this person's occupational life. These assessments are noted at the top of Figure 17-1. Secondly, if the types of clients you see tend to have specific weaknesses or challenges, you may choose an assessment that focuses on that specific area. These are noted in the middle of Figure 17-1. If you are working in a specialized setting, such as a school or a work rehabilitation program, you should consider the assessments listed at the bottom of Figure 17-1.

Once you have selected potentially relevant assessments, the next step is to become familiar with them. The previous chapters provide overviews and case examples for each assessment. This information should be sufficient to determine whether a given assessment has potential relevance. Finally, you should examine copies of the assessments in order to study them more carefully. It is also useful to read articles

that discuss the assessment's development and/or use in practice. The bibliography at the end of this text is a source for identifying such publications. They often offer suggestions and information that can help a therapist think further about the relevance and utility of an assessment.

Piloting Assessments in Practice to Evaluate Their Utility

After having selected those assessments that appear to be most relevant, you should spend some time trying each one out in your setting. This will allow you to determine whether one assessment works well across your clients, or whether you need alternative assessments. For example, if you would like to do interviews with your clients, but have clients with a range of personal characteristics, you might want to have available more than one interview. Then, when you encounter a new client, you can decide which interview to do with that particular client.

You should also try out specific assessments to see how useful the information provided on the assessment is for clients. Once again, you may find that a specific assessment almost always provides useful information on clients, and you may decide to use it with all clients. On the other hand, you may find that it is more suited to one subgroup of clients and decide to use it regularly only with that subgroup.

Piloting the assessments also gives you an opportunity to test out which assessments best meet your own working style and the overall needs for information in your setting. It also allows you to find out which assessments are best suited to your clients. In short, it provides the practical experience with the assessment that helps you further refine choices.

Developing an Assessment Strategy

You may find a single assessment that meets all your needs. However, you will more likely find it helpful to create an information gathering strategy with optional assessments and a means to decide which to use for specific clients. What we mean by this is best illustrated through an example. Let us consider an occupational therapist working in a psychiatric rehabilitation setting. The assessment strategy shown in *Figure 17-2* is viable for such a setting. Because most of the clients com-

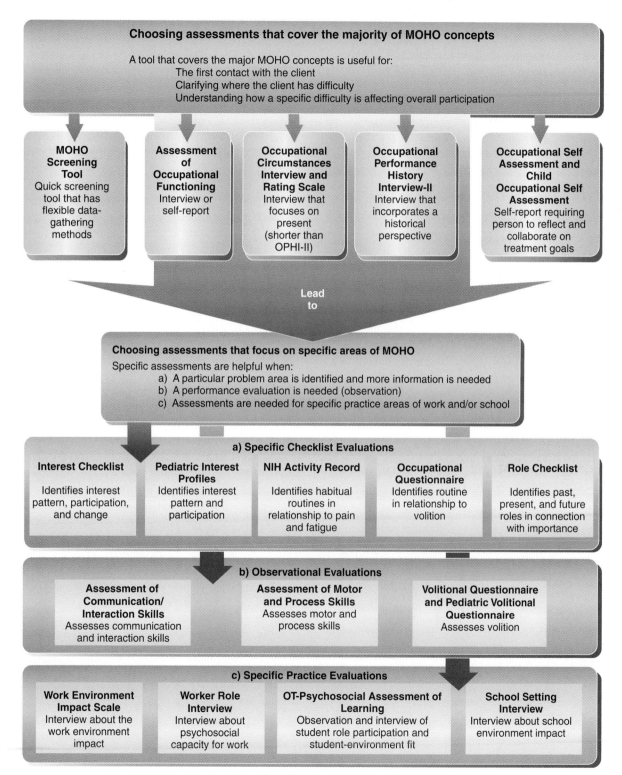

FIGURE 17-1 A Decision Tree for Selecting MOHO Assessments.

You may find a single assessment that meets all your needs. However, you will more likely find it helpful to create an information gathering strategy with optional assessments and a means to decide which to use for specific clients.

ing into the setting are initially functioning at too low a level for an interview, the therapist has chosen to begin the MOHOST as the overall assessment to be used with all clients. In cases in which a client does initially have the ability to engage in an interview, the therapist has identified the OCAIRS (Version 2.0) (Haglund, Henriksson, Crisp, Freidhiem, & Kielhofner, 2001) as the primary interview to be done. This interview may be done on only a small number of clients as an initial assessment. It may be done later with some clients when they progress to the point of being able to participate. Other clients who progress and identify the goal of returning to work or achieving employment may be interviewed with the WRI or the WEIS. Since the WEIS is designed to interview clients concerning a specific job setting or type of job setting, only those clients with

previous employment will ordinarily be candidates for this assessment.

The assessment strategy shown in Figure 17-2 also indicates that when the MOHOST identifies problems in skills, the AMPS or the ACIS (Forsyth, Salami, Simon, & Kielhofner, 1998) may be done. Finally, when clients show more extreme problems in motivation, the VQ may be used. Since these are all observational assessments, they can be done on clients who are at a lower level of functioning than is required for the interviews.

Such a strategy allows for many different configurations of assessments to be done according to client needs and characteristics. One client may be assessed only through repeated applications of the MOHOST to monitor progress and identify intervention needs. Another client, who showed clear problems in communication/interaction, may be assessed with the ACIS following the MOHOST. Repeated use of the ACIS may be used to monitor the client's needs and response to social skills training. Still another client who shows some cognitive impairment that affects occupational performance but wants to live in the community may be assessed (following the MOHOST) with the OCAIRS and the AMPS to gather critical information for intervention and discharge planning.

As this example illustrates, having a strategy of assessment allows the therapist to be:

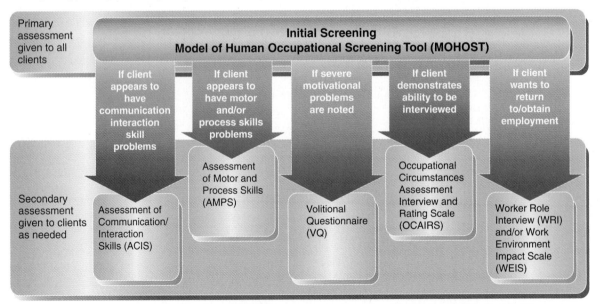

FIGURE 17-2   Example of an Assessment Strategy for a Psychiatric Rehabilitation Setting.

- Efficient by avoiding assessments unnecessary or unsuitable for clients
- Client-centered by choosing assessments that reflect client needs and characteristics
- Comprehensive by getting information that is needed to understand the client's specific occupational problems/challenges in order to design the best intervention.

Developing an assessment strategy will take some time and experimentation, but it is the surest means of doing optimal assessment for clients.

What Should I Do If There Is No Assessment To Meet My Client's Needs?

The number of MOHO-based assessments has grown over the years. However, there may not be an assessment appropriate to meet your circumstance or client. When you have exhaustively examined and tried the assessments discussed in the previous chapters and found nothing suitable, the following are options:

- Consider an unstructured method of data gathering
- Look for assessments not developed under MOHO theory but compatible with it
- Collaborate with researchers to develop a new assessment.

When formal assessments are not available, one option is to use unstructured or informal methods of data collection. These methods are most suitable when they supplement or build on some formal assessment. Their value and the guidelines for use that help to assure that one gathers dependable information are discussed in Chapter 12.

The use of assessments not specifically developed for use with, but that are compatible with, MOHO has always been part of the practice of therapists who use

MOHO. When using such assessments, therapists should review the content of such assessments to establish their relevance to MOHO concepts. This means carefully examining the kind of information the instrument gathers and asking about its relevance to each MOHO concept. One way of doing this is to take the questions posed in Chapter 11 and determine the extent to which an assessment gives answers to those questions.

Although we do not advise the use of "home-grown" assessments without study of them, it is possible for therapists to work in collaboration with researchers to develop a new assessment to meet their needs. Many of the assessments in the previous chapters came from such efforts. This is, of course, a long-term solution, but one which may benefit others who have similar assessment needs.

Therapists who believe they have been through a rigorous process of exploration of the current MOHO assessments and have identified an assessment need that is not addressed by a MOHO-based assessment, are encouraged to contact the MOHO Clearinghouse (mohoc@uic.edu) or post a message on the MOHO listserv. The listserv can be joined by visiting the MOHO Clearinghouse web site (http://www.uic.edu/ahp/OT/MOHOC).

Conclusion

This chapter addressed a number of questions that practitioners routinely ask in reference to selecting and using assessments. In answering them, we tried to offer a perspective that addresses both the standards of assessments our clients deserve and the logistics faced by practitioners. This chapter provided a number of guidelines and resources that we hope will guide therapists through the process of selecting and using the best possible assessment strategies for their practice.

References

Baron, K., Kielhofner, G., Iyenger, A., Goldhammer, V., & Wolenski, J. (2002). *The Occupational Self Assessment (OSA) (Version 2.0).* Chicago: Model of Human Occupation Clearinghouse, Department of Occupational Therapy, College of Applied Health Sciences, University of Illinois at Chicago.

de las Heras, C. G., Geist, R., Kielhofner, G., & Li, Y. (2002). *The Volitional Questionnaire. (VQ) (Version 4.0).* Chicago: Model of Human Occupation Clearinghouse, Department of Occupational Therapy, College of Applied Health Sciences, University of Illinois at Chicago.

Fisher, A. G. (1999). *Assessment of Motor and Process Skills 3rd Edition.* Ft. Collins, CO: Three Star Press.

Fisher, A. G., Liu, Y., Velozo, C. A., & Pan, A. W. (1992). Cross-cultural assessment of process skills. *American Journal of Occupational Therapy, 46,* 876–885.

Forsyth, K., Salamy, M., Simon, S., & Kielhofner, G. (1998). *The Assessment of Communication and Interaction Skills. (Version 4.0).* Chicago: Model of Human Occupation Clearinghouse, Department of Occupational Therapy, College of Applied Health Sciences, University of Illinois at Chicago.

Furst, G., Gerber, L., Smith, C., Fisher, S., & Shulman, B. (1987). A program for improving energy conservation behaviors in adults with rheumatoid arthritis. *American Journal of Occupational Therapy, 41,* 102–111.

Geist, R., Kielhofner, G., Basu, S., & Kafkes, A. (2002). *The Pediatric Volitional Questionnaire (PVQ) (Version 2.0).* Chicago: Model of Human Occupation Clearinghouse, Department of Occupational Therapy, College of Applied Health Sciences, University of Illinois at Chicago.

Gerber, L., & Furst, G. (1992). Validation of the NIH Activity Record: A quantitative measure of life activities. *Arthritis Care and Research, 5,* 81–86.

Goode, D. (1983). Who is Bobby? Ideology and method in the discovery of a Downs syndrome person's competence. In G. Kielhofner (Ed.), *Health through occupation.* Philadelphia: FA Davis.

Goode, D. (1994). *A world without words: The social construction of children born deaf and blind.* Philadelphia: Temple University Press.

Goto, S., Fisher, A. G., & Mayberry, W. L. (1996). The assessment of motor and process skills applied cross-culturally to the Japanese. *American Journal of Occupational Therapy, 50,* 798–806.

Gross, T., & Miller, D. (Executive Producers). (1998, April 14). Interview with Chuck Close on *Fresh Air.* Philadelphia: National Public Radio.

Haglund, L., Henriksson, C., Crisp, M., Friedhiem, L., & Kielhofner, G. (2001). The *Occupational Circumstances Assessment-Interview and Rating Scale (OCAIRS) (Version 2.0).* Chicago: Model of Human Occupation Clearinghouse, Department of Occupational Therapy, College of Applied Health Sciences, University of Illinois at Chicago.

Haglund, L., Karlsson, G., Kielhofner, G., & Lai, J. S. (1997). Validity of the Swedish version of the Worker Role Interview. *Scandinavian Journal of Occupational Therapy, 4,* 23–29.

Haglund, L., Kjellberg, A., Forsyth, K., & Kielhofner, G.

(2001). *The measurement properties of the Swedish version of the Assessment of Communication and Interaction Skills (ACIS).* Unpublished manuscript, Queen Margaret University College, Edinburgh.

Helfrich, C., & Kielhofner, G. (1994). Volitional narratives and the meaning of therapy. *American Journal of Occupational Therapy, 48,* 319–326.

Hoffman, O, R., Hemmingsson, H., & Kielhofner, G. (2000) *A user's manual for the School Setting Interview (SSI) (Version 1.0).* Chicago: Model of Human Occupation Clearinghouse, Department of Occupational Therapy, College of Applied Health Sciences, University of Illinois at Chicago.

Kielhofner, G., & Forsyth, K. (2001). Development of a client self-report for treatment planning and documenting therapy outcomes. *Scandinavian Journal of Occupational Therapy, 8 (3),* 131–139.

Kielhofner, G., Lai, J. S., Olson, L., Haglund, L., Ekbadh, E., & Hedlund, M. (1999). Psychometric properties of the work environment impact scale: A cross-cultural study. *Work, 12,* 71–78.

Kielhofner, G., Mallinson, T., Crawford, C., Nowak, M., Rigby, M., Henry, A., & Walens, D. (1998). *The Occupational Performance History Interview (Version 2.0) OPHI-II.* Chicago: Model of Human Occupation Clearinghouse, Department of Occupational Therapy, College of Applied Health Sciences, University of Illinois at Chicago.

Kielhofner, G., Mallinson, T., Forsyth, K., & Lai, J. S. (2001). Psychometric properties of the second version of the occupational performance history interview (OPHI-II). *American Journal of Occupational Therapy, 55,* 260–267.

Law, M. (1998). *Client centered occupational therapy.* Thorofare, NJ: Slack.

Moore-Corner, R. A., Kielhofner, G., & Olson, L. (1998). *Work Environment Impact Scale (WEIS) (Version 2.0).* Chicago: Model of Human Occupation Clearinghouse, Department of Occupational Therapy, College of Applied Health Sciences, University of Illinois at Chicago.

Oakley, F., Kielhofner, G., Barris, R., & Reichler, R. K. (1986). The Role Checklist: Development and empirical assessment of reliability. *Occupational Therapy Journal of Research, 6,* 157–170.

Parkinson, S., & Forsyth, K. (2001). *A user's manual for the Model of Human Occupation Screening Tool (MO-HOST) (Version 1.0).* Unpublished Manuscript, UK MOHO CORE, University of London.

Townsend, S. C., Carey, P. D., Hollins, N. L., Helfrich, C., Blondis, M., Hoffman, A., Collins, L., Knudson, J., &

Blackwell, A. (2001). *The Occupational Therapy Psychosocial Assessment of Learning (OT PAL) (Version 1.0)*. Chicago: Model of Human Occupation Clearinghouse, Department of Occupational Therapy, College of Applied Health Sciences, University of Illinois at Chicago.

Trombly, C. (1993). The issue is—anticipating the future: Assessment of occupational functioning. *American Journal of Occupational Therapy, 47*, 253–257.

Velozo, C., Kielhofner, G., & Fisher, G. (1998). *Worker Role Interview (WRI) (Version 9.0)*. Chicago: Model of Human Occupation Clearinghouse, Department of Occupational Therapy, College of Applied Health Sciences, University of Illinois at Chicago.

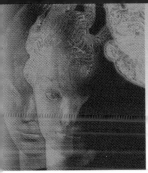

18

The Process of Change In Therapy

- **Gary Kielhofner**
- **Kirsty Forsyth**

ffective occupational therapy enables clients to change. This chapter addresses the following three questions pertaining to client change. What kinds of change takes place in therapy? How does this change take place? What is the client's role in change? Before addressing these questions, we will first examine why client change is the focus of therapy.

Client Change is the Focus of Therapy

Sometimes therapy is discussed in terms of whether the approach is remediative (i.e., aimed at producing a change in the client to reduce impairment) versus compensatory (i.e., aimed at producing a change in the environment to accommodate a permanent impairment). In the latter case, it is implied that the environment changes, but the client does not. However, claims that clients do not change when therapy is compensatory only make sense when one considers the intervention and the client narrowly. For example, when a client has motor or cognitive limitations, therapists must consider whether the clients can improve motor or cognitive capacities or whether the client must find ways to compensate for these impairments. However, the latter, compensatory strategy will still require the client to change. That is, the client may need to do some or all of the following:

- Incorporate new objects (e.g., adaptive aids) into performance
- Develop a new sense of capacity that enables choosing to do things within one's ability and seeking assistance with those that are not
- Alter habit patterns to accommodate limitations in capacity
- Find new interests to replace those that had to be relinquished.

Thus, compensatory strategies do not avoid client change. All occupational therapy targets some form of change.

Centrality of Clients' Doing in the Change Process

Only clients can accomplish their own change. As seen in Chapter 3, the development, continued existence, and transformation of people's characteristics depend on what they do. Volition, habituation, and performance capacity are fashioned, maintained, and changed by being put to use. What clients do and how they think and feel about their doing drives change.

We will use the term occupational engagement to refer to client doing, thinking, and feeling in the midst of therapy. The term engagement is used in the American Occupational Therapy Association Practice Framework to connote not only client doing, but also to im-

> **All occupational therapy targets some form of change.**

> **Only clients can accomplish their own change.**

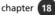

ply choice, motivation, and meaning (Commission on Practice, American Occupational Therapy Association). Consistent with the argument made here, the framework also views engagement as a key element of therapy.[a] Hence, **occupational engagement** is defined as clients' performance of one or more occupational forms and the attendant thoughts and feelings that occur as part of therapy. This definition underscores two points:

- For doing to be therapeutic it must involve an actual occupational form, not a contrived activity
- For the client to achieve change through doing, what is done must have relevance and meaning for the client.

It is a longstanding occupational therapy tenet that what the client does in therapy should have relevance and meaning. Nonetheless, reports of persons with disabilities suggest this is not always so. For example, Callahan, an accomplished cartoonist who incurred a traumatic spinal cord injury, recalls with appropriate sarcasm:

> When I was able to sit up in the chair long enough, I began two hours . . . of occupational therapy daily . . . I remember having my hands harnessed for long periods of time to a rolling-pin-like apparatus that sanded a piece of wood. A bright future as a finish sander stretched before me if I played my cards right. (Callahan, 1990, p. 74)

The anthropologist Robert Murphy in his memoir, *The Body Silent*, has a similar complaint about the meaningfulness of what he did in occupational therapy:

> . . . I thought some of the exercises ridiculous. Nonetheless, visitors to our house still scrape their feet on the doormat that I made in O.T. Yolanda is

the only person who knows its origins, a sign of the care I have taken to keep secret the indignities visited upon me . . . (Murphy, 1990, pp. 54–55)

Finally, Robert McCrum, a British novelist and literary editor, writing about his recovery from a stroke recalls:

> The part of convalescence that I found most profoundly humiliating and depressing was occupational therapy . . . I was reduced to playing with brightly colored plastic letters of the alphabet, like a three-year-old, and passing absurdly simple recognition tests. Sitting in my wheelchair with my day-glo letter-blocks I could not escape reflecting on the irony of the situation. (McCrum, 1998, p.139)

These three commentaries underscore the need for therapists to pay attention to the occupational forms in which clients' engage. For therapy to be successful, it must enable clients to feel competent and achieve satisfaction by doing things that matter to them. Since the client's occupational engagement is the central force in change, therapists must carefully consider what they are asking clients to do in therapy.

Kinds of Change That Occur Through Therapy

MOHO can be used as a framework for identifying kinds of change that take place in therapy. The Section II Master Table (see column 4, page 347) lists changes corresponding to MOHO concepts. These changes correspond to the kinds of client problems and challenges identified in the third column of the table. Importantly, the table is not intended to be exhaustive. Rather, it provides an indication of the kinds of change with which a therapist using MOHO would be concerned.

To appreciate fully each kind of change listed in the table, it is necessary to have the background provided in theoretical chapters of Section I of this book. For example, the table lists the following changes related to personal causation:

- Enhance understanding of performance capacities (strengths and weaknesses)
- Focus attention to more accurately understand how limitations and assets affect occupational performance

---

[a]The American Occupational Therapy Association's Occupational Therapy Practice Framework (Commission on Practice, AOTA) identifies the use of enabling activities and adjunctive methods as legitimate components of therapy. Enabling activities are designed to improve specific performance capacities and skills and can include contrived activities designed to exercise capacity. Adjunctive methods prepare the client for performance by affecting performance capacity; they include such things as exercise, physical modalities, and splinting. The rationale for enabling activities and adjunctive methods is provided by other models of practice. Their rationale derives from concepts other than those proposed by MOHO, which focuses specifically on the role of occupational engagement to facilitate change.

- Develop emotional acceptance of limitations and pride in occupational abilities
- Reduce unnecessary feelings of dependence, resentment, or guilt associated with reduced participation
- Increase facility in choosing to do occupational forms consistent with performance capacity
- Build up confidence to approach occupational forms within performance capacity
- Increase knowledge and acceptance of using adaptive aids and/or environmental modifications to augment capacity
- Increase willingness to ask for help when needed
- Reduce anxiety and fear of failure in occupational performance
- Build up confidence to face occupational performance demands
- Improve facility to sustain effort for attaining goals and/or completing performance
- Widen expectation of success in performance
- Extend readiness to take on occupational challenges and responsibilities
- Increase sense of control in occupational outcomes.

These changes reflect the concepts of self-efficacy and sense of personal capacity discussed in Chapter 4. Similarly, the section on performance capacity indicates changes in the lived body, a concept discussed in Chapter 6. They are as follows:

- Develop new ways of attending from and to the body
- Incorporate altered/estranged parts of the body and necessary new prosthetic/orthotic/adaptive devices into self and into occupational performance
- Increase feeling of how to do things with an altered body or bodily capacity
- Increase understanding and better management of such things as altered bodily sensations, hallucinations, pain, fatigue, and altered perception to minimize interference with occupational performance.

The full logic for the personal causation or lived body changes noted above and in the table is contained in the discussions in Chapters 4 and 6. Consequently, to appreciate and use the kinds of changes noted in the table, it will be helpful to refer back to the relevant theoretical discussions.

Equally important will be comparing the descriptions of change in the table to one's experiences with clients in practice. Going back and forth between the systematic way of thinking about change provided by the table and everyday practice situations will enrich one's understanding of the table's contents and of clients. Furthermore, it will inevitably reveal additional types of change pertinent to MOHO concepts not listed in the table.

A Taxonomy of Occupational Engagement

This section more specifically examines how a client's doing, thinking, and feeling propel the kinds of changes noted in the Section II Master Table. A first step is to consider more specifically what happens during occupational therapy. When clients engage in an occupational form in therapy or as a result of therapy, volitional, habituation, and performance capacity are all involved in some way. For example, in any moment of therapy a client may be:

- Drawing on performance capacity to exercise skill in occupational performance
- Evoking old habits that shape how the occupational performance is done
- Enacting or working toward a role
- Experiencing a level of satisfaction/enjoyment (or dissatisfaction/displeasure) with occupational performance
- Assigning meaning and significance to what is done (i.e., what this means for the client's life)
- Feeling able (or unable) in doing the occupational form.

All these complex dimensions of what the client does, thinks, and feels shape the change process.

As previously noted, the central component of change is the client's occupational performance. As defined in Chapter 8, to perform is to do an occupational form. How the client goes about doing an occupational form is critical to the type of change it may produce. Moreover, surrounding performance are processes that involve thinking and emotion that are also central to change. Recognizing this, we can begin to identify client actions that occur in therapy and that drive change. Below, we will offer a preliminary taxonomy of such client actions. The aim is to provide a more structured way for thinking about what clients do, think, and feel in therapy.

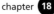

Choose/Decide

Client choices and decisions are central to effective therapy. As discussed in Chapter 2, activity choices shape what we do in the immediate future. Such choices and decisions are often the first step toward change. Such things as selecting what to do, how to do it, and what to aim for are also central to therapy as they represent the client's volitional involvement in the therapy process. Persons **choose** or **decide** when they anticipate and select from alternatives for action. A wide range of choices and decisions may take place in the therapy context. The following are examples:

- A child in therapy chooses to play with a new toy that previously seemed too challenging
- A client decides to focus on a particular short-term goal in therapy
- A client selects a particular piece of adaptive equipment to use for doing activities of daily living
- A client chooses to engage in a valued occupational form despite some anxiety and fear of failure
- A client chooses to indulge a particular interest by selecting what to do in a leisure group
- After being shown alternative ways of performing, a client decides on a particular technique
- A client chooses whether to have a personal care attendant for self-care to have more energy and time to devote to work.

By making such choices and decisions, clients can shape the nature of their own therapy and what that therapy aims to accomplish. The very process of making choices can help clients feel more in control of their lives. Often, when the client has limited performance capacity, making choices and decisions is one of the most empowering things the client can do. Finally, choices and decisions are critical since they influence what will change, what will remain the same, and how the change will unfold.

Commit

For long-term change to occur in therapy, clients must **commit** themselves to undertake a course of action for accomplishing a goal or personal project, fulfilling a role, or establishing a new habit. As discussed in Chapter 2, occupational choice always involves commitment because it requires one to sustain action over time. Committing to a course of action is also an act of hope

since the client's intention is to achieve some goal, occupy a place in the social world, or modify his or her lifestyle in anticipation of improving life. Some examples of committing in therapy are:

- After a period in a supported living facility, a client concludes it is time to work toward living independently in an apartment and commits to that goal
- A client in a rehabilitation program who has been out of work for years following onset of chronic disability resolves to work again
- After examining their daily routine, a group of clients agree together to develop long range plans for achieving more productive lifestyles. They all agree to set weekly goals and report their goal accomplishment to each other.

As the examples indicate, commitment ordinarily follows a process of information gathering and reflection, so that clients have an idea of the obligations they are assuming. The process of commitment is closely tied to development of occupational identity and competence since it involves decisions about how the occupational narrative will be continued or changed.

Explore

As discussed in Chapter 10, the first stage of change involves exploration. **Exploration** includes investigating new objects, spaces, and/or social groups and occupational forms; doing things with altered performance capacity; trying out new ways of doing things; and examining possibilities for occupational participation in one's context. The following are some examples of exploration:

- A client with hemiplegia explores different techniques for putting on clothes
- A client with a recently acquired cognitive disability tries to do a familiar occupational form, exploring how altered capacities impact performance
- A client recently discharged from an institutional setting to a community group home walks in the neighborhood to see what is in it and joins a leisure activity in the evening to see what the other residents are like
- A child tries out a new communication device to see how it works
- An older person, who gave up a hobby because of fading vision, tries using larger materials and tools

to see if doing it is still enjoyable with the modifications

- An adolescent in a work program tries out different occupational forms to see what kind of productive activity is most satisfying to do.

Exploring options, feelings, and experiences is central to making informed decisions in therapy. Successful exploration is especially important with individuals who have a newly acquired disability.

Identify

Identifying refers to locating novel information, alternatives for action, new attitudes, and new feelings that provide solutions for and/or give meaning to occupational performance and participation. Locating this information can result from such processes as discussion with therapists, self-reflection, examining alternatives, or hearing feedback. Some examples of identifying are:

- After hearing feedback on performance and discussing it with the therapist, a client identifies that the interpersonal difficulties he experiences are related to skill problems in the physical domain
- During the Occupational Performance History Interview (Kielhofner et al., 1998) a client identifies with therapist feedback that the occupational narrative underlying her life story is a tragedy, something she would like to change
- A client who is anxious identifies the specific occupational forms and performance contexts that cause the most anxiety
- Following a therapy session, a client reflects and recognizes that her fear of failure gets in the way of her finishing things.

As the examples indicate, identification involves insight into something of which the client previously lacked awareness. Such insight supports change because it gives the person critical information to know what to do or to guide decisions.

Negotiate

When possible, the client should be involved in a process of negotiation throughout therapy. The onset of disability often results in new situations and experiences that create a gap between disabled persons' and others' perspectives, desires, and expectations. More-

over, the client will sometimes differ with the opinion of the therapist concerning the nature of impairments and their consequences. **Negotiation** involves give and take with others that creates mutually agreed-upon perspectives and/or finds a middle ground between different expectations, plans, or desires. The following are examples:

- A client's therapist recommends that the client use a certain piece of bathing equipment. The client prefers not to depend on the equipment and agrees to try alternative methods of bathing first
- On advice from the therapist, a client negotiates with the supervisor at work for accommodations that could enhance work performance
- After attending an energy conservation program, a client negotiates with family members for how household chores can be fairly redistributed in the family
- Clients in a leisure-planning group have differing ideas about what to do in the next outing. They agree to plan for two outings so that both ideas can be accommodated.

Negotiation can be difficult for clients, given the power differential that often exists between health care providers and clients. By giving clients clear messages that they can negotiate, the therapist creates a more collaborative context. By creating a vision of therapy goals and procedures, negotiation can positively affect a client's willingness to cooperate in therapy. Moreover, negotiaton with others in one's environment is critical to filling roles effectively and otherwise participating in the social context.

Plan

Because impairments can impose new conditions that invalidate habitual ways of doing things, it is often critical for clients to think through how they will go about doing something before they attempt it. Moreover, when persons are attempting a new performance or a new pattern of participating in occupations, they are more likely to be successful when they have created an agenda for doing so. **Planning** refers to establishing an action agenda for performance and/or participation. The following are examples:

- A client, who wants to start exercising regularly by swimming, finds out where the nearest swimming pool is located, calls and ascertains the hours it is open, and locates a bus route for getting there

- Clients in a work program are getting ready to go on job interviews. With the guidance of the therapist they consider what to do if the interviewer asks about gaps in their employment history and whether and how to disclose the nature of their disabilities
- Clients in a cooking group plan the content of the meal, make up a grocery list, decide where to go for the groceries, and anticipate how much money they will need to make the purchase.

By focusing on the steps required for doing something, planning helps to assure success. Also, because planning makes the process of accomplishing something concrete, it can allay a client's anxiety about performance.

Practice

Clients **practice** in therapy when they repeat a certain performance or consistently participate in an occupation with the effect of increasing skill, ease, and effectiveness of performance. Practice aims to enhance effectiveness on doing an occupational form and/or participating in an area of occupation, such as self-care, work, school, or leisure. The following are some examples of practicing:

- A client participates in a daily leisure group, doing a variety of social occupational forms, and in the course uses and refines communication/interaction skills while building a sense of efficacy in being able to interact with others
- A student with problems in process skills practices doing his school tasks using a set of visual cues that help develop habits for better organizing and sequencing actions to meet the expectations of the student role. In the course of this process the client also identifies more strongly with the student role and more clearly internalizes its expectations
- A client in a vocational program twice role plays a job interview before actually going on the interview to internalize the attitudes and behaviors that are appropriate to someone applying for a job
- A client does her daily routine of hygiene using adaptive equipment, learning how to better handle and adjust the equipment and forming a habit of

going through the self-care routine and developing a sense of efficacy in doing it

- A child plays several times a day with an adapted toy, developing a sense of how it feels to do the action and experiencing a sense of pleasure in being able to manage it effectively.

The key element in practice is that a client has the opportunity to repeat something to consolidate the volition, habituation, performance capacity, and environmental factors shaping an effective and satisfying way to perform and/or participate.

Re-examine

Therapy is often a time when clients must leave behind perceptions, feelings, beliefs, and patterns of acting that are no longer valid or that have led to difficulties. **Re-examination,** then, involves critically appraising and considering alternatives to previous beliefs, attitudes, feelings, habits, or roles. The following are examples:

- A client, whose habits have contributed to dissatisfaction with everyday life, considers alternative ways of organizing the daily routine to include more enjoyable things
- A client, whose sense of capacity has always underestimated strengths, reflects with the therapist on successes achieved in therapy and what they said about the client's abilities
- A client, who has had the goal of returning to a particular job, considers the gap between the job demands and current capacity and begins to think about what other types of work might be possible.

Letting go of thoughts, habits, responsibilities, and ways of doing things is not always easy, but unless the client is able to recognize the problems associated with them and also see alternatives, change cannot occur.

Sustain

One of the challenging aspects of therapy is sustaining effort over time despite such things as difficult barriers, pain, failures, and slow progress. By its nature, therapy can be taxing for clients. However, as noted earlier in this chapter, change requires repeated action over time. **Sustain** refers, then, to persisting in occupational performance or participation despite uncertainty or difficulty. The following are examples:

- Despite feeling anxious, a client completes all the steps required of an occupational form. This reinforces for her that, despite her doubts, she did have adequate capacity
- A child, whose distractibility makes it difficult, manages to stay focused throughout a classroom exercise. Afterward, he has a sense of accomplishment
- A client, who has returned to work after an accident, goes to work each day despite experiencing mild pain and concerns over re-injury. With the therapist's reassurance that there is no serious risk, in time the client feels less pain and more secure
- After a long period of isolation, a client is trying to become more socially active. After joining a club that meets weekly the client persists in going, although feeling socially inadequate and tempted to stay home. Each time, however, the client enjoys it and experiences more confidence.

As the examples indicate, persistence takes effort but has its rewards in feelings of accomplishment, new learning, and development of a sense of efficacy.

Summary

This section identified a number of processes that characterize client thinking, feeling, and doing in therapy. As noted at the outset, these do not exhaust the possibilities for what clients do to achieve change. However, they do provide a detailed way of thinking about occupational engagement. In the Section II Master Table (see column 5, page 347), examples of these types of occupational engagement are given corresponding to types of client change to which we referred earlier. By examining the table, one can see what kinds of occupational engagement are proposed as contributing to different types of change. Together these two pieces of information are useful for establishing therapy goals and strategies, as discussed in Chapter 20.

The Process of Change in Therapy

We have just examined types of changes that can occur as a result of therapy, but we still need to consider the change process itself. Based on discussions of change, especially Chapters 3 and 10, the following two key elements of change in therapy can be identified:

- Change in therapy is dynamical. That is, it involves simultaneous and interacting alterations in the person, the environment, and the relationship of the person to the environment
- Change in therapy is part of a history of change in a person's life. Therapy enters a client's unfolding life and its impact is in terms of that life.

The following sections discuss each of these characteristics of change and their implications for how therapy can best enable client change.

Dynamical Changes

Change involves complex reorganization in which multiple, simultaneous alterations resonate with each other. As seen in Chapter 3, volition, habituation, performance capacity, and environmental conditions form a heterarchy interacting with and influencing each other. When one element changes, the total dynamics of this interacting heterarchy shift and result in the emergence of new thoughts, emotions, and actions. Over time this process takes on a life of its own, cascading forward as one event builds on another. Therapy serves to stimulate, support, nudge, and otherwise enable the change process. This dynamic process of change in therapy can best be illustrated through a case example. *Figure 18-1* illustrates some key features of the dynamic change processes that are discussed below.

Julie

Julie is 4 years old and lives with her mother, father, and 6-year-old brother in a small town. She has severe cerebral palsy resulting from anoxia at birth. She experiences fluctuations in tone (i.e., she is very "floppy" much of the time but also has a marked extensor thrust). She has limited head control and disconjugate eye movements. She cannot talk and has other oral-motor problems. Julie can make her pref-

---

Change involves complex reorganization in which multiple, simultaneous alterations resonate with each other.

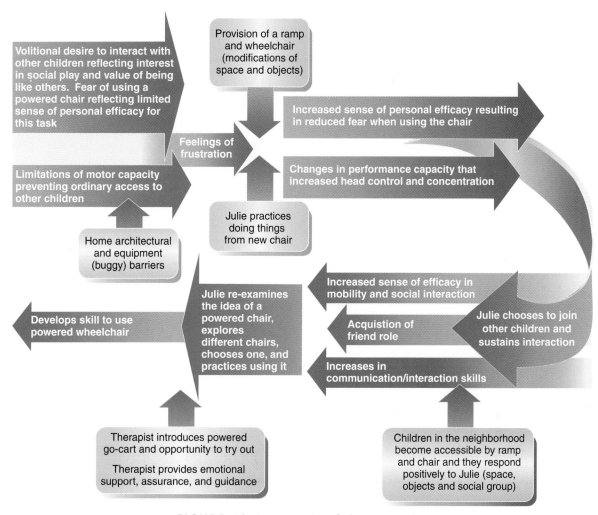

FIGURE 18-1 Dynamics of Change in Julie.

erences clear and she is generally cheerful and interested in things going on around her. For example, Julie is passionate about computer games and single-switch toys.

Despite her communication impairments, Julie very much values interacting with other children. Her mother notes it is important to her to wear clothes and have her hair done like other children, and Julie very much wants to do things that she sees other children do. Recently, her mother has observed that Julie becomes upset and irritable when her brother goes out to play in the street with other

children. Julie spends most of the day in an adapted chair or buggy, both of which are difficult to get out of the house. Therefore, she cannot readily go out and join the other children. Instead, she watches the children play in the street from the front windows of the house. Julie's sense of inefficacy in achieving something about which she cares deeply is clear in the frustration she shows while passively watching the other children. Consequently, the therapist and Julie's mother together decided it was essential to enable Julie to play with other children. As a first step the therapist recommended that a ramp be installed at the front door of the home.

Julie is unable to propel a chair herself and would benefit from a powered chair. However, Julie is quite fearful of being in a powered chair. The therapist previously gave Julie opportunities to try out such chairs. When she did so, Julie had difficulty controlling her body and the chair. She clearly felt out of control in the chair and was too anxious to be able to learn to use it. Julie instead used a buggy in which she felt safe, but which had to be propelled by others.

Now that Julie wanted to play with other children, the buggy posed a constraint because it did not allow her to be in a position in which she could play. Therefore, the therapist tried out a number of different seats and wheelchairs with Julie, finally settling on one with small wheels that needed to be pushed by another child or attendant, and from which Julie could safely play in the street.

To use the new chair Julie had to practice doing things in it. Consequently, she improved her head control and concentration, and increased her sense of efficacy to the point at which she could use the chair without fear. The neighborhood children welcomed Julie and willingly propelled her chair along as they engaged in play. Soon she was routinely part of the group of children, was confident in joining them, had developed a friend role, and was learning to communicate with them in simple ways. Bolstered by a growing success in joining and interacting with friends at play, Julie became ready to try out in occupational therapy a variety of self-powered go-carts. After some exploration she found one with which she was comfortable and selected it. She became very motivated to master navigation with the chair. After a period of practice she developed the necessary motor and process skills for effective maneuvering of the chair. When Julie went to school a year later, she was using her own motorized chair.

As the case illustrates and Figure 18-1 shows, the changes in Julie over time represent a complex resonating process. Certainly Julie went from being afraid and unable to use a powered chair to feeling effica-

cious and being skilled at using one, but the process of change underlying it involved interacting changes in her volition, habituation, performance capacity, and environment. Therapy impacted the process at key points as shown by the darker arrows in Figure 18-1. Other environmental factors, such as the children's acceptance of and willingness to play with Julie, are also important. Note also how the environmental impact of an object (the buggy) changed once Julie wanted to play. Whereas it previously supported Julie's functioning, her new volitional desire meant that its impact had become constraining. As pointed out in Chapter 7, the impact of any environmental feature will depend on the volitional and other characteristics of the person. When something changes in the person, the impact of existing features of the environment may change. This is an example of how elements of the person and environment resonate in change.

Julie's volition, habituation, and performance also changed together. She simultaneously increased confidence for interacting with children, assumed the player role, and developed new communication/interaction skills for socializing with the children in play. Julie's own thoughts, feelings, and actions were central to her change. Her choice to interact with the children was necessary to the change. By sustaining social play with the children she developed new skill and confidence. Finally, she reexamined whether she wanted a powered chair, explored different chairs and selected one, and then practiced with the selected chair. Therapy could only remove constraints and provide opportunities and resources that enabled Julie to undertake the change process herself.

A final aspect of the case worth noting is Julie's progression through stages of change relative to her feelings of efficacy in using new chairs. As noted in Chapter 10, the process of change ordinarily takes place in three stages: exploration, competence, and achievement. Moreover, the client must first be ready to embark on the change process. Julie was initially not volitionally ready for using a powered wheelchair. However, her volitional desire to engage in play with neighborhood children initiated her exploration of a new wheelchair and her positive experience in being able to engage in play, which further propelled her toward a readiness to explore, gain competence in using, and finally incorporate the powered chair into her life when she went to school. The case illustrates that it is important to appreciate when a client is ready to change and to anticipate that each client's sequence of change will have its own unique route.

Change in the Context of an Unfolding Life

Any change that therapy enables is alteration within the larger life of the client. Consequently, the role of occupational therapy is to enter into a life that has both a past and a future extending beyond the therapeutic process. Therapy is a unique and bounded event, the goal of which is to contribute positively to the course of the client's life. Successful therapy always proceeds with appreciation of the life the individual has lived and might live in the future (Helfrich, Kielhofner, & Mattingly, 1994).

The kind of change that should take place in therapy depends on the client. Impairments leading to disability may come as a condition in the beginning of life, as a traumatic event in the prime of life, as a progressive encroachment on life, as recurring interferences with life, or as a waning near the end of life. The impact of any disabling condition depends on the life it has entered into and of which it is now a part. Impairments precipitate disability not only because they reduce capacities, but also because they disrupt an unfolding life.

The following case illustrates how change in therapy can relate to a client's unfolding life.

Harold

Harold was 42 years old, married, and had one child. For a few months he had been training for work as a corrections officer for a federal prison. He was preparing to take a series of physical and mental exams that would certify him for the job. At the same

> *Therapy is a unique and bounded event, the goal of which is to contribute positively to the course of the client's occupational life.*

time, he rented and farmed several acres of land. During the spring wheat harvest he accidentally caught his right, dominant hand in a combine mechanism, resulting in a crush amputation of his thumb, index, middle, and ring fingers at the metacarpophalangeal level. Following surgery and a continuing course of therapy, he was able to develop only a marginally functional grasp using his thenar eminence and the remaining fifth digit, which was restricted in active flexion and extension.

While therapy needed to enhance Harold's performance capacity, it was equally important to consider and address how the impaired hand had impacted on Harold's life. From the beginning of his rehabilitation, Harold wished to continue his training and pursue his goal of permanent employment as a corrections officer. Because his ability to physically respond to prisoners in an emergency was affected, he negotiated a placement as the officer in charge of a main gate, which minimized direct contact with prisoners. This position, however, required that he do additional paperwork related to prisoners' coming and going.

Harold was initially provided a prosthesis, which would allow him to write with his dominant hand, but he identified that wearing it inside the prison made him appear vulnerable and disadvantaged him against a potential assailant. Thus, after discussing it with his therapist, he chose instead to change hand dominance, learning to write with his left hand. With practice his writing became legible but slow. Because prison reports must be error free and completed quickly, he could not afford to lose further time by having to redo reports. Therefore, the therapist and he decided to explore the effectiveness of altering how he did this occupational form. Eventually, he practiced and developed a new habit of composing reports in his head before writing them down.

Harold identified other adaptations necessary for his job and for preparation to take certification exams. For example, he required more time to take notes from books in preparation for exams. This meant that he must devote more time to studying. Consequently, he decided not to attempt to farm, giving up this second work role, at least temporarily.

Harold continued to negotiate role responsibilities. For example, he requested and secured permission to take written exams under altered conditions so as not to be penalized by his slow writing. To pass the performance component of the corrections certification exam he had to deliver a number of accurate shots to a target with both a shotgun and a .38 caliber revolver, accurately firing two rounds of ammunition during a timed test. He planned and practiced a new way of completing this occupational form of firing, unloading, reloading, and firing the guns with the dual challenges of changed handedness and an impaired right hand. He readily managed to develop a process for reloading the shotgun without trouble, but getting small bullets in and out of the six-shot revolver was harder. The test required delivering 10 accurate shots out of 12. After exploring with different solutions, he developed the following routine. He fired one round of six shots. Then, to save time, he loaded and fired only four additional bullets. By delivering ten well-placed shots within the time period, he passed the exam.

Harold encountered problems with the injured hand in a whole range of situations. He consistently chose to substitute process skills for impaired motor skills such as handling and gripping. Moreover, he modified many habits of performance to compensate for the lost function and still be able to carry out some important occupations. For example, Harold chose to retain his hobby of cutting firewood. He managed to do this by changing the chain saw he used. He sold his large saw and purchased a smaller one, which he could handle safely. Moreover, he learned to rely on good planning to avoid unsafe situations in which he might lose control of the saw.

The changes that Harold made in objects, occupational forms, skills, habits, and roles allowed him to pursue his occupational narrative despite clear decrements in his performance capacity. He successfully completed the entire certification process, passed probation, and secured a permanent job as a corrections officer.

Throughout therapy it was important that the therapist pay attention to the life that Harold was attempting to realize. The therapist had to consider with Harold how his impairment affected what he wanted and needed to perform and to work with him to achieve workable solutions. Harold's therapy was effective because it enabled him to make changes that continued his life in the direction he wanted it to go.

CHANGE AS CRAFTING AN OCCUPATIONAL NARRATIVE

The reader will recall from Chapter 9 that crafting one's occupational life involves organizing the components of one's occupational identity into a narrative and operationalizing it in ongoing life. Harold exemplifies someone who had a clear occupational identity and knew what story he wanted to enact. Unlike Harold, many clients will have more difficulty identifying and constructing their occupational narratives. In such instances, change in therapy means enabling the client to recraft the occupational narrative.

When persons experience disability, they also experience a threat to or disintegration of their ongoing occupational narratives. Consequently, a core problem for many clients is to figure out where life will go next. As seen in Chapter 9, telling and living a story requires an appropriate plot and supporting metaphors to infuse the events of a life with coherence, wholeness, and direction.

Clients often face great challenges to finding a meaningful life plot. For example, when challenged with his own saga of life-threatening disease and disability, the novelist, poet, and lyricist Reynolds Price clearly outlined how he set about to narrate his experience:

> Now at last I must enter what was plainly a war, with life-or-death stakes, and assume the fight in the only way I knew to fight . . . I'd be myself to the outer limit of all I could be, resourceful as any hunted man in the bone-dry desert, licking dew

---

Living with a disability is consistent with living a fulfilling and joyful life. However, it has little to do with living a life that is normative or dictated by one particular set of values.

from cactus thorns. So, even that early, I'd cast my-self as the hero of an epic struggle, and I saw both the ludicrous melodrama of that role and the urgent need for it. (Price, 1994, p. 31)

A decade after his battle began, Price emerges clearly victorious:

I know that this new life is better for me, and for most of my friends and students as well . . . in the ten years since the tumor was found, I've completed thirteen books . . . I sense strongly that the illness itself either unleashed a creature within me that had been restrained or let him run at his own hungry will; or it planted a whole new creature in place of the old . . . (Price, 1994, pp. 189–193).

While few possess the eloquence of Reynolds Price, all clients must find stories compelling enough to carry them forward. Otherwise they languish.

Living with a disability is consistent with living a fulfilling and joyful life. However, it has little to do with living a life that is normative or dictated by one particular set of values. For example, Deegan (1991) notes that:

Too often we project traditional "American" values on disabled people, for example, rugged individualism, competition, personal achievement, and self-sufficiency . . . For some psychiatrically disabled people, especially those who relapse frequently, these traditional values of competition, individual achievement, independence, and self-sufficiency are oppressive. (Deegan, 1991, p. 52)

Each person with a disability must discover and enact an occupational identity and competence that incorporates the disability as part of the life to be lived. As Vash (1981) notes:

Acceptance of disability evolves gradually, for most people, over a span of years filled with instructive experience. It comes seldom, if ever, as a *coup de foudre* followed by getting on with life. Instead, the process of living teaches, little by little, that disablement needn't be viewed as an insurmountable tragedy . . . As the struggles to survive, work, live, and play show evidence of some success, individuals find awareness of disablement slipping longer and oftener into the background of consciousness. Eventually, for some, it may come to be seen as a positive contributor to life in

its totality—a catalyst to psychological growth. Since these changes take time, trial, error, and correction to unfold, forward movement does not always look like progress. (Vash, 1981, p. 124)

Living with a disability is a highly personal matter. Each person must construct his or her own story of what it means to be a person with a disability. All therapists have encountered persons who truly believe that their lives have been destroyed by disability and who go on to live lives much more constrained and unhappy than might have been otherwise. Then there are those who create positive occupational narratives for themselves. Consider, for example, John Callahan's reflection:

. . . I'm more surprised than anyone that I have adapted to this way of life. Sometimes I still wake in panic in the night when I discover I cannot move my legs, just as I did sixteen years ago on that night in L.A. And I panic again at the thought of having to spend the rest of my life in this condition. I wonder if I will survive it. It's true I've had to be a scrapper. I've had to work exceedingly hard to survive; before all else, it takes me three hours just to get ready in the morning. But deep inside I know I'm always right where I'm supposed to be at the time. (Callahan, 1990, p. 217)

As Callahan notes, adjustment to disability is ongoing, done in each moment of living. Moreover, as Vash (1981) notes, it also requires that one look forward through an unfolding narrative:

I have been disabled since I was sixteen, yet hardly a week goes by, nearly thirty years later, that I don't make some discovery or improvement that in one way or another makes my disability less handicapping. Since I hope that happy process never stops, I have to say that I hope I am never fully "rehabilitated." My physical abilities are still increasing. When, with age, they begin to decrease I fully expect to continue or accelerate in the psychological and spiritual discoveries that make my disability not only less handicapping, but a matter of trivia compared with the nonphysical realms of discovery and improvement I am experiencing. (Vash, 1981, pp. 2–3)

Change in therapy can play an important role in assisting persons to construct and live their occupational narratives. As DeLoach and Greer (1981) note, early in the process of living with a disability:

> Both the miracles we hope for and the miseries we fear are failures of the imagination, which tends to use the imagery supplied by daydreams and nightmares to fill what is at first a vacuum, virtually devoid of any experience, with relevant facts. (DeLoach & Greer, 1981, p. 251)

The occupational therapy process can facilitate movement back and forth between the telling and living of a life story, helping to achieve a synthesis between what is desired and the reality of what is possible. In therapy, clients' courage to imagine can be supported and they can test the reality of their imaginations. Through these means, the most challenging and important aspects of change may be accomplished.

Key Terms

Choose/decide: To anticipate and select from alternatives for action (e.g., choose an occupational form or select goals).

Commit: To obligate one's self to a course of action for accomplishing a goal or a personal project or fulfilling a role or establishing a new routine.

Explore: To investigate new objects, spaces, and/or social groups and occupational forms; do things with altered performance capacity; try out new ways of doing things; and examine possibilities for occupational participation in one's context.

Identify: To locate novel information, alternatives for action, and new attitudes and feelings that provide solutions for and/or give meaning to occupational performance and participation.

Negotiate: To engage in give-and-take with others that creates mutually agreed on perspectives and/or finds a middle ground between different expectations, plans, or desires.

Occupational engagement: Clients' performance of one or more occupational forms and the attendant thoughts and feelings that occur as part of therapy.

Plan: To establish an action agenda for performance and/or participation.

Practice: To repeat a certain performance or consistently participate in an occupation with the effect of increasing skill, ease, and effectiveness of performance.

Reexamine: To critically appraise and consider alternatives to previous beliefs, attitudes, feelings, habits, or roles.

Sustain: To persist in occupational performance or participation despite uncertainty or difficulty.

References

Callahan, J. (1990). *Don't worry, he won't get far on foot.* New York: Vintage Books.

Commission on Practice, American Occupational Therapy Association. (2001). *Occupational Therapy Practice Framework.* Unpublished Working Paper.

Deegan, P. E. (1991). Recovery: The lived experience of rehabilitation. In R. P. Marinelli & A. E. Dell Orto (Eds.), *The psychological and social impact of disability* (3rd ed.). New York: Springer-Verlag.

DeLoach, C., & Greer, B. G. (1981). *Adjustment to severe physical disability: A metamorphosis.* New York: McGraw-Hill.

Helfrich, C., Kielhofner, G., & Mattingly. C. (1994). Volition as narrative: Understanding motivation in chronic illness. *American Journal of Occupational Therapy, 48,* 311–317.

Kielhofner, G., Mallinson, T., Crawford, C., Nowak, M., Rigby, M., Henry, A., & Walens, D. (1997). *A user's guide to the Occupational Performance History Interview-II. (OPHI-II). (Version 2.0).* Chicago: Model of Human Occupation Clearinghouse, Department of Occupational Therapy, College of Applied Health Sciences, University of Illinois at Chicago.

McCrum, R. (1998). *My year off: Recovering life after a stroke.* New York: WW Norton.

Murphy, R. F. (1990). *The body silent.* New York: WW Norton.

Price, R. (1994). *A whole new life.* New York: Atheneum.

Vash, C. L. (1981). *The psychology of disability.* New York: Springer.

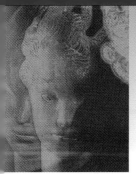

19

Therapeutic Strategies for Enabling Change

- **Gary Kielhofner**
- **Kirsty Forsyth**

hapter 18 examined client change in therapy. It examined the kinds of changes that take place and the process of change. Finally, it examined the role of the client's occupational engagement in driving change. This chapter builds on those discussions and answers the following question: How does an occupational therapist using MOHO interact with a client to support occupational engagement and facilitate desired change? In answering this question, the chapter begins with a broad discussion of the therapeutic use of self. Then, the chapter focuses on specific therapeutic strategies that follow from MOHO theory.

Therapeutic Use of Self

The relationship between therapist and client is always an important determinant of the success or failure of occupational therapy (Hopkins & Tiffany, 1983; Peloquin, 1990). Two elements are indispensable to the therapeutic relationship:

- Empathy
- Trust.

In what follows, these elements are discussed, with particular note as to how the use of MOHO concepts is related to these components of the therapeutic relationship.

Empathy

Empathy requires that therapists seek to understand the thoughts, feelings, and needs of clients and to actively communicate this understanding to the client (Burke &

Cassidy, 1991; Burke & DePoy, 1991; Peloquin, 1990, 1995). Achieving empathy requires careful listening to what clients have to say about their lives and about their ongoing experience of therapy. Empathy further involves a genuine effort to take on and appreciate the client's perspective (Peloquin, 1995; Tiffany, 1983). MOHO concepts focus specifically on the client's perspective and life. A therapist who uses the concepts from volition will take care to understand what a client values, how a client finds satisfaction and enjoyment in life, and what thoughts and feelings a client has about capacity and effectiveness. Moreover, the concepts of habituation lead a therapist to consider what the client's everyday life is like and what roles and responsibilities the client has. The concept of the lived body calls the therapist to attend to the nature of experiences the client has as a result of impairments. Environmental concepts require therapists to develop an appreciation of the physical and social context in which the client lives and participates. Finally, the concepts of occupational narrative (and the related concepts of identity and competence) orient the therapist to understanding the story that the client is living and with which the client makes sense of life. Taken together, MOHO concepts represent a comprehensive agenda for developing an empathic understanding of the client.

> *Taken together, MOHO concepts represent a comprehensive agenda for developing an empathic understanding of the client.*

Trust

Establishing trust between client and therapist is essential to collaboration and to maximizing clients' occupational engagement and investment in therapy (Peloquin, 1995; Tiffany, 1983). Therapists build trust through honesty and openness with the client. Developing a MOHO theory-based conceptualization of the client's situation facilitates honesty and openness for the following reasons. The therapist will have developed an understanding of the client that considers the client's thoughts and feelings and recognizes the client's strengths. Being able to communicate this understanding conveys to clients that the therapist is genuinely attempting to understand their viewpoints and concerns and views them with respect. At the same time, therapists' theoretically driven insights to clients' problems and challenges provide a basis for honest sharing of concerns about clients' lives and the difficulties they face. Clients who recognize that the therapist has taken time and effort to develop a thorough understanding of them will more readily trust what the therapist has to say.

Trust also requires therapists to recognize and respond to the client's needs and struggles. Therapists who use their conceptual understanding of the client to guide actions with the client will inevitably communicate their understanding and responsiveness. Indeed, the most powerful tool a therapist has for building trust is responding to clients in a way that reflects a deep understanding of them.

Therapeutic Relationship and Client Occupational Engagement

In the previous chapter, we argued that the central factor driving change was the client's acting, thinking, and feeling. What role, then, does the therapeutic re-

> *Clients who recognize that the therapist has taken time and effort to develop a thorough understanding of them will more readily trust what the therapist has to say.*

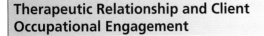

> *... the role of the therapist is to support and thereby enable clients to do what they need to do in order to change.*

lationship have in creating this change? This question is important because some perspectives suggest that it is the relationship between the therapist and the client that drives the change. However, this is not how MOHO theory explains client change.

From the perspective of MOHO, the therapeutic relationship is not the primary dynamic of change. Rather its usefulness is in supporting client occupational engagement as shown in *Figure 19-1*. This does not diminish the importance of the therapeutic relationship. Rather it recognizes that the role of the therapist is to support and thereby enable clients to do what they need to do in order to change. The therapist carries out this role by engaging in therapeutic strategies that follow logically from MOHO. These strategies, along with the therapeutic relationship, support and enable the client's occupational engagement as shown in Figure 19-1. We will consider them next.

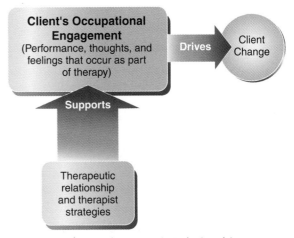

FIGURE 19-1 Therapeutic Relationship Supports Client Occupational Engagement, Indirectly Influencing Change.

Nature of Therapeutic Strategies

A **therapeutic strategy** is a therapist's action that influences a client's doing, feeling, and/or thinking to facilitate desired change. Many strategies identified below will also be used in association with theoretical approaches other than MOHO. What links these strategies to MOHO theory is the logic or rationale with which they are undertaken. That is, these strategies are undertaken with an aim of achieving types of changes articulated by MOHO concepts. Therefore, in discussing each strategy we will link it to MOHO concepts.

Although we can only generally link these strategies to theoretical concepts, the therapist using such strategies uses them in a very particular way. That is, as discussed in Chapter 11, the therapist creates from the MOHO concepts a conceptualization of the client's situation. This conceptualization points toward what changes need to take place. Furthermore, it provides a background against which the therapist decides:

- What kind of client occupational engagement is needed to achieve the desired changes
- What kinds of therapeutic strategies will support and enable the client's occupational engagement and change process.

Therefore, therapists should always have a conceptualization of the client that guides what therapeutic strategies are selected and used. Moreover, the strategies should be used reflectively so that the therapist can adjust their use in the course of therapy to meet client needs. The strategies we will discuss are validating, identifying, giving feedback, advising, negotiating, structuring, coaching, encouraging, and providing physical support. These are not meant to be an exhaustive list of therapeutic strategies. Rather, they represent the kinds of strategies that therapists undertake to support client occupational engagement.

Validating

To **validate** is to convey respect for the client's experience or perspective. Service providers often overlook or fail to take seriously the experience of people with disabilities (Toombs, 1992; Wendel, 1996). Therapists must carefully attend to and acknowledge the client's experience whether it is the lived body experience, the experiences associated with volition (enjoyment, painful

loss of capacity, anxiety), or experiences stemming from societal reaction to the disability. Negative experiences such as pain, anxiety, hallucinations, shame, and/or anger may interfere with the client's occupational engagement. Therefore, validation of experience sometimes requires the therapist to help the client manage the experience to do something positive.

Each moment of therapy is potentially charged with thoughts and feelings that accompany what a client does. Consequently, a client's experiences resonate outward to larger implications, intentions, worries, hopes, and disappointments. Validating these experiences is essential to effective therapy. Validation is also important for very low functioning clients with limited communication abilities. In these circumstances, validation may involve things as simple as acknowledging the presence and unique identity of a client. Such validation can serve to scaffold the volition of persons who lack sufficient internal volitional motives.

Some examples of validation are:

- A client diagnosed with schizophrenia is severely withdrawn. Each day the therapist visits the client briefly at the same two times. The therapist greets the person by name, reintroduces herself, and makes comments related to the client's past interests. After a week the client makes eye contact
- A child becomes very flustered in therapy. The therapist offers him the opportunity to take a break and she acknowledges that therapy is sometimes hard work
- A client with recent spinal cord injury is planning a first weekend home since being in rehabilitation. In the midst of the process the client becomes tearful and shares his fears about managing everything and facing neighbors and old friends from a wheelchair. The therapist acknowledges that this is a challenging situation and that most clients are very anxious on their first trip home
- A student who has been struggling to master use of a computer achieves something she has never done before. She lets out a shriek of pleasure. The therapist rushes over and gives her a round of applause and congratulations
- A client begins participating in the Occupational Circumstances Assessment-Interview and Rating Scale

(OCAIRS). As the client talks about her life she stops suddenly and indicates that she does not feel able to go on answering questions. The therapist acknowledges she was talking about an extremely difficult topic and that her life experiences must have been very hard to bear. The therapist also points out how useful the information was and how grateful the therapist was for the client's honesty and willingness to share her experiences. She offers to continue the interview at a later point, if the client prefers.

As the examples illustrate, therapists must first attend to clients' experiences before they can validate them. This means taking care to observe how the clients act and react in therapy, looking for signs of enjoyment, anxiety, boredom, investment, outrage, shame, excitement, and so forth. Finally, simply asking the client about and demonstrating an active interest in the client's thoughts and feelings are also important.

Identifying

Therapists need to be able to **identify** for clients a range of personal procedures and/or environmental factors that can facilitate occupational performance and participation. For example:

- A therapist becomes aware that a client is very anxious and flustered attempting to use public transportation. The therapist suggests a number of ways the client can manage the anxiety, including some ways she can ask for assistance if she is not sure what to do
- A client with AIDS has been out of work for 3 years due to complications of the illness. He now wants to return to work but is worried about how he can manage the medications he must take several times a day. The therapist uses her understanding of his legal rights for workplace accommodation to suggest the possible different kinds of reasonable accommodation that he can request
- The therapist shares a range of strategies a client with unilateral neglect can use to help notice things on the neglected side of her body
- Through observation, the therapist comes to understand and notes occupational forms a person with a stroke is able to do with and without assistance
- A client has stated that he wants to go to a day center. The therapist compiles a list of possible day centers for the client within a reasonable traveling distance.

In sum, the therapeutic strategy of identifying provides the client an understanding of the personal and environmental opportunities and resources. It can also provide the client information about options for enhancing occupational performance and participation in work, play/leisure, and activities of daily living that clients wish and need to do.

Giving Feedback

Therapists gather information to arrive at a conceptualization of a client's situation. For example, therapists using MOHO draw conclusions about a client's performance capacity, habituation, volition, and environmental impact to understand how these factors influence a client's skill, performance, and participation. Therapists also draw on this conceptualization to form an understanding of ongoing action of the client. When therapists share their overall conceptualization of the client's situation or their understandings of the client's ongoing action, they are **giving feedback.** Some examples of giving feedback are:

- A client has agreed to be observed with the Assessment of Motor and Process Skills. After completing the observations, the therapist shares the results of the assessment with the client and explains what it revealed
- A therapist has observed a client informally during therapy. These observations confirm what the therapist learned in the initial interview—that the client holds impossibly high standards that result in constant self-devaluation. The therapist reminds the client of this conceptualization since she previously shared it with the client. She now presents her observations of how the client has continued to devalue her own performance over the past two therapy sessions. The therapist also provides an alternative interpretation of the client's performance that emphasizes a number of strengths
- In a cooking group a client refuses to collaborate with other clients. Afterward, the therapist asks to speak with the client and notes that, while he has agreed that his non-cooperative behavior gets him into trouble, he still does it
- A client, who has difficulty performing self-care,

states that she is afraid she will end up in a nursing home. The therapist indicates that while she still has difficulty, she has made significant progress, which bodes well for her return to independent self-care

- An adolescent with mental retardation participates in an occupational form that he initially hesitated to do. After the session the therapist praised him for making a difficult choice and for completing the occupational form.

As the examples illustrate, giving feedback can serve a variety of purposes such as:

- Helping a client have a more accurate sense of capacity or understand a performance problem
- Letting a client know the value (positive or negative) of a behavior
- Reframing a client's interpretation of something
- Offering a different vision of the future than that held by the client.

Consequently, feedback can provide information that enhances skill and performance. Giving feedback that reframes something can address volition by influencing how clients interpret, experience, or anticipate the future.

Advising

Therapists **advise** clients when they recommend intervention goals and strategies. Thus, advising involves:

- Sharing what outcomes appear feasible and desirable
- Indicating possible options for achieving outcomes in therapy.

Advising should take place as part of a give-and-take process whereby the client and therapist mutually decide on therapy goals and strategies. However, because the therapist has collected information and used it in combination with MOHO concepts to create a conceptualization of the client's situation, the therapist is in a position to make recommendations for the client's consideration. These recommendations ordinarily contain information or insights beyond the client's thoughts and feelings. Therefore, sharing the advice with the client can serve to broaden or alter the client's perspective.

In the process of advising, a therapist may seek to persuade a client to make a particular informed choice or decision. For example, a therapist often provides the rationale for a given option with an eye to influence the client to agree to select that option or to make a particular commitment. Therapists most often seek to persuade a client when the client hesitates, has difficulty making a choice in therapy, or has problems committing to a particular long-term goal, project, role, or change in lifestyle. For example, a therapist may advise a client on such basic things as which occupational form to undertake in a work setting, school, or day center and such complex things as whether it makes sense for a client to commit to a goal of living independently. Sometimes advice seeks to persuade a client against a particular choice or commitment. This occurs when the therapist's conceptualization of the client indicates that certain choices may produce undesirable consequences or that certain desired goals are not feasible.

To advise a client effectively, the therapist must seek to understand the client's volition. For example, the therapist may consider what volitional factors are influencing a client's difficulty in making a choice. Alternatively, the therapist may consider what factors contribute to a client's strong preference or commitment to a choice that is not adaptive (e.g., feelings of inefficacy, not seeing the value of doing something). By doing so, the therapist can give honest advice with empathy for the client's perspective and desires.

Whereas advice and the persuasion that often goes with it can be a useful therapeutic strategy, therapists must be careful to advise without coercing the client. Persuasion occurs when the client, in response to information and suggestions, changes his or her own mind freely. Coercion occurs when the client gives in against his or her will. Coercion should never be a part of the process of advising a client.

Some further examples of advising are:

- A therapist recommends to a client who is nearing discharge from physical rehabilitation that he should complete a home visit to ascertain environmental changes needed to support performance after discharge
- A therapist advises a client with a mild cognitive problem about which occupational forms may pose safety risks. The therapist further recommends that the client should practice them in therapy to develop safe habits

- A therapist advises a client with brain injury that learning to drive is not currently feasible given the client's visual and perceptual deficits. The therapist also suggests that the client explore use of public transportation to achieve the client's goal of working
- A student is having difficulty beginning schoolwork. The therapist advises the student as to which steps to take first and how to approach the schoolwork.

Advising clients is important to client-centered practice because it allows the client to make informed decisions. It is important that the therapist take the time to explain to the client the rationale behind the advice, so the client can truly make informed decisions.

Negotiating

Therapists **negotiate** when they engage in give-and-take with the client to achieve a common perspective or agreement about something that the client will or should do in the future. Negotiation occurs when the client and therapist have differing information or viewpoints about some aspect of the client's occupational circumstances. Negotiation may be necessary to resolve disagreement between the therapist and client. Other times the therapist and client are simply comparing and reconciling their different perspectives.

Negotiation implies that the therapist must be careful to be aware of and elicit client views. Without such efforts the client's viewpoint can be obliterated by institutional routines or by the plans of service providers including the therapist. Thus, negotiation begins with a respectful elicitation of a client's thoughts and feelings throughout the therapy process. Some examples of negotiation are:

- A client states uncertainty over whether occupational therapy can do anything for him. The therapist presents a number of changes he could achieve and how they would be achieved in therapy. The therapist then asks for the client's perspective on this information and whether he thinks the changes seem valuable to him. After deliberation they agree on therapy goals that incorporate both the client's ideas and some of what the therapist envisioned
- A therapist notes that a client is unwilling to work toward a level of independence in self-care that is easily within his reach. The therapist discusses this

with the client, asking for the client's perspective. As a result, the therapist comes to understand that the client has different, culturally specific criteria for judging the situation. He views it as a matter of honor that his family should take care of him. After learning his perspective, the therapist acknowledges it, but points out how it can create difficulties for him and his family. While the client is not able to accept the therapist's viewpoint, he does agree that they can continue to discuss the topic as part of his therapy

- A student informs the therapist he plans to drop out of high school because he is so frustrated. The therapist talks with the student to ascertain his sources of frustration. She then offers to convene the school team to talk with the student about what things can be changed. The student agrees to attend the meeting to see if things can be improved enough to convince him to stay.

As the examples indicate, negotiation always requires respect for and understanding of the client. It often means that the therapist must be willing to compromise, to see things differently, or to depart from usual procedures.

The give-and-take of negotiation can be very important to empower clients. Successful negotiation requires the therapist to understand what the client is being asked to concede and to make sure to offer incentives that are worth it to the client. Furthermore, therapists must model the same openness and flexibility of thinking and acting that they are asking of clients.

Structuring

Therapists must often structure clients' occupational engagement. **Structuring** refers to establishing parameters for choice and performance by offering clients alternatives, setting limits, and establishing ground rules. Structuring can often serve to create reasonable demands for clients to make choices, perform, maintain habits, and fulfill roles. Some examples are:

- Stating the importance of mutual respect and collaboration in a goal setting group
- Offering a child the choice between two different toys in a therapy session

- Letting a client know that if he experiences too much pain or fatigue during a session practicing dressing, he can take a break
- Communicating to clients during a goal setting exercise that members of the group are expected to set goals, follow through on what they committed to do, and report back to the group
- Informing a client in a work program that she is expected to arrive on time and stay focused on work responsibilities
- Organizing a personal care session with a client who has a hip replacement to introduce and practice with a long-handled shoehorn, stocking aid, and elastic laces. Due to the client's lack of mobility the therapist places all the needed objects within the client's reach.

Structuring can give a client a sense of control and safely make opportunities and constraints in the environment clear. Structuring can be used to convey expectations and is useful for helping clients to internalize role scripts and to learn to be effective members of groups. Moreover, external expectations can be a support to volition (Jonsson, Josephsson, & Kielhofner, 2000). That is, persons can find it easier to be motivated to do things when others expect them to do so.

Coaching

Therapy involves clients in such things as exploring new ways to perform or practicing performance to increase skills. Therapists **coach** when they instruct, demonstrate, guide, verbally prompt, and/or physically prompt clients. Some examples of coaching are:

- During a role-playing exercise designed to help a client with a psychiatric condition learn and exhibit effective communication/interaction skills, the therapist demonstrates assertive behavior and then guides a client through how to assert himself in a simulated interaction
- While trying a new occupational form, a therapist helps a client with head injury problem-solve by cueing her to notice what is happening
- Serving as a job coach for a client with cognitive impairments in a supported employment program, a therapist demonstrates to the client how to greet fellow workers

- A therapist guides a pediatric client with perceptual-motor difficulties as she engages in gross-motor play. The therapist demonstrates how to do something, reminding the child to pay attention to bodily experience. Once the client begins, the therapist prompts her on how to move
- Working with an adolescent whose performance anxiety often gets in the way of enjoyment, the therapist redirects his attention to aspects of the performance that may be enjoyable or satisfying.

As the examples illustrate, coaching is often directed to enabling clients to develop performance capacity and enhance skill. However, coaching also influences a client's volition in that during a performance it can redirect the client's attention to aspects of the performance to affirm satisfaction and enjoyment. Coaching may also take place in the context of role performance and therefore support the client to engage in roles effectively.

Encouraging

Therapy often involves clients in such things as exploring new situations, choosing to take risks, and sustaining effort when it is difficult. Therapists enable clients to do these things by **encouraging** them. That is, they provide emotional support and reassurance to clients. The following are examples of encouraging:

- A therapist reassures a child who appears anxious that the purpose of a game in therapy is to have fun. She does this through her smile and exaggerated actions since it is not clear if the child understands language. The therapist confirms this when the child makes a mistake by laughing and hugging her
- A client is anxious about the transition to independent living. The therapist indicates to the client that he feels the transition will go well and uses phrases like "things are going to be OK" and "everything will work out"
- An elderly client is becoming discouraged while practicing a self-care routine. The therapist uses phrases like "you can do it," "you're nearly there," and "you're doing great" to keep her going within the occupational form.

As the examples show, encouraging is ordinarily necessitated because of clients' personal causation difficulties and/or because of gaps between their performance capacity and the things they are attempting to do. Encouragement scaffolds the client's volition, enabling them to feel greater confidence, to relax and enjoy themselves, and/or to recall why something is worth the effort. In short, it serves to elicit positive thoughts and feelings about performance.

Providing Physical Support

Lack of motor skills may require a therapist to provide physical support. **Physical support** is when the occupational therapist uses his or her body to provide support for a client to complete an occupational form or part of an occupational form when the client cannot or will not use his or her own motor skills. Occupational therapists who work with clients who have physical disability are likely to use this strategy frequently as this client group often has reduced motor skills. Therapists working in psychiatry may also need to use this strategy as there can be lack of motor skills associated with this client group (e.g., an older person with dementia, side effects of medication, physical deconditioning). Some examples are:

- A client is unable to open a jar while making a meal. The therapist loosens the top on the jar to make it easier for the client to use his weakened grip to open the jar
- The therapist uses her body to support a client who has had a stroke to get out of bed in the morning and transfer to a chair. The therapist then retrieves the client's clothes from the wardrobe and positions the clothing within reach because the client has an impaired transportation skill
- Within his morning routine, a client who has Parkinson's disease has difficulty bending to his feet. The therapist helps him to wash his feet, get socks over his toes, and put on his shoes
- An older client who walks with his walking frame to the kitchen to make breakfast loses his balance, requiring the therapist to gently put her hand on his back to provide stability until he regains his balance
- A person who has had schizophrenia for many years and has reduced physical flexibility due to side effects of medication requires the therapist to get some woodwork materials for him from a high shelf because he has an impaired reach skill
- A child who reaches for a toy requires the therapist to stabilize the child's base of support, which allows her to have a more effective reach skill.

This strategy focuses on the physical aspects of completing occupational forms and can be used with any client who is experiencing reduced motor skills.

Using Therapeutic Strategies to Support Client Change

The strategies just presented are used by therapists to influence and complement the occupational engagement of a client. They are ultimately aimed at enabling the client to achieve specific kinds of changes. The final column of the Section II Master Table (pages 346–355) indicates therapeutic strategies that support client occupational engagement to achieve changes related to MOHO concepts. For example, the following strategies are given related to supporting client occupational engagement for achieving changes in the client's sense of capacity:

- *Validate* how difficult it can be to have a damaged or altered body
- *Structure* the therapeutic environment to allow the client to experience using his or her body within meaningful occupational forms
- *Advise* the alteration of daily habits, using energy conservation techniques and written and verbal cues
- *Coach* the person in the use of new objects and adapted methods of completing occupational forms
- *Coach* the person by verbal cueing to overcome subjective experiences of the body
- *Provide* physical supports when needed to support lack of performance capacity
- *Encourage* the person when he or she is engaged in occupational forms. This encouragement should be highly empathic and attentive to understanding the lived body experience
- Encourage the client when using adaptive strategies.

As noted earlier, the logic for the strategies follows from the theory. Therefore, the strategies in the table take their logic from the corresponding discussions in the earlier theory chapters. The logic for these strategies and change that these strategies are meant to support are found in the Chapter 4 discussion of volition and more specifically of personal causation. Therefore, in considering these strategies, therapists should be mindful of the theoretical concepts behind them. As noted earlier, the strategies discussed in this chapter (that are presented in Section II Master Table) are not meant to be exhaustive. Rather, they provide a starting point for thinking about what a therapist can and should do to support clients' occupational engagement and change processes.

Therapists will employ a combination of these strategies in each encounter with a client. While these strategies should be used genuinely and naturally as situations arise, it is important that the therapist be reflective about using strategies. This means anticipating, when possible, the kinds of strategies that might benefit a client. It also means carefully monitoring a client's needs throughout therapy to select appropriate strategies. Having an awareness of the strategies discussed above is the first step in being reflective.

The previous chapter noted that therapeutic change is a dynamic unfolding process. To effectively use therapeutic strategies, the therapist must monitor the unfolding events that are part of the change process. Changes in personal causation, interests, values, roles, habits, performance capacity, skill, and performance will often occur together and influence each other in therapy. Moreover, the therapist will also need to consider how the environment affects the change process. Change cannot be fully preplanned. Rather, by monitoring how things are unfolding, therapists can implement useful therapeutic strategies that can be devised to support the unfolding reorganization of the client.

Putting It All Together: Two Case Examples

The following two case examples are given to illustrate how the therapeutic strategies and principles offered here can be implemented. The first client is from the first author's practice; the second client's therapist is the second author.

Jim

Jim was an adolescent client in a psychiatric setting. He had a history of depression, chronic school truancy, and substance abuse. A few months before, he ran away from home and had been living with friends and on the streets of Los Angeles. One of the aims of therapy was to improve Jim's very poor personal causation. During several successive occupational therapy sessions, Jim engaged in woodworking. His sense of capacity and personal efficacy was very low. Jim was initially very reluctant to try woodworking even though it was clear that he was very attracted to doing it when he saw other adolescent clients in the woodshop. The therapist had to carefully advise and encourage Jim to undertake a personal project (making a small table), assuring him that he would coach Jim in the necessary skills and help him through each step. Consequently, Jim made the occupational choice to undertake this project.

Despite increasing skill and success in each subsequent session, Jim persisted in downgrading his own capacities. Moreover, he needed encouragement to get started and to continue during each therapy session. Unsure of each new step, he required encouragement and coaching to keep him involved and help him know how to undertake the step. After each session Jim was quick to attribute positive outcomes to the therapist's assistance and difficulties to his own lack of skill. Each time this occurred, the therapist carefully gave Jim feedback to reframe how he was interpreting the session, guiding him to think about what he had accomplished during the session. The therapist also pointed out increases in his performance that had occurred across sessions and how much less support he had needed during each successive session.

These strategies seemed to help Jim the next session. However, over several sessions he seemed to become even more agitated and upset over minor failures, even though his overall skill in performance was increasing. At the end of one therapy session he disavowed interest in the woodworking and pronounced it "a stupid waste of time."

The therapist was able to recognize Jim's struggle with his growing interest in woodworking and his increasing valuation of being good at it. As these two volitional changes took place, they raised the stakes for Jim's personal causation, making any of his lingering thoughts and feelings about not being effective more painful.

The therapist used the following statement that reflected strategies of feedback, validation, and encouragement. "Jim, I don't believe that you think woodworking is stupid. In fact, I think that you really want to do it more than ever, which makes you more concerned over whether you can do it well. That makes you anxious. I know it doesn't feel good. But, if you avoid it, you're never going to see how good you can be at doing this. Even though it's hard for you, remember that I'll support you and I have confidence that that you can do it." Jim listened but did not say anything in response before leaving. Jim arrived at his next therapy session to announce that he had been working on a plan to make a piece of furniture and requested additional time in the woodshop to undertake this project.

Let us consider in even more detail what happened across these few therapy sessions. *Figure 19-2* illustrates the key processes involved. Jim entered therapy with a particular, stable volitional pattern: a sense that he could not succeed, accompanied by a tendency to disavow interest in things. It became clear in therapy that Jim did see working with the kind of equipment that was in the woodshop (e.g., table and band saws, electric drill press) as symbolizing a world of technology and competence—a world he dared not imagine entering despite his attraction to it. By avoiding it, he could avoid the pain of failure. The therapist had to begin by advising and encouraging Jim to try and choose a personal project. As Jim worked on this project, it was necessary to provide ongoing encouragement, coach-

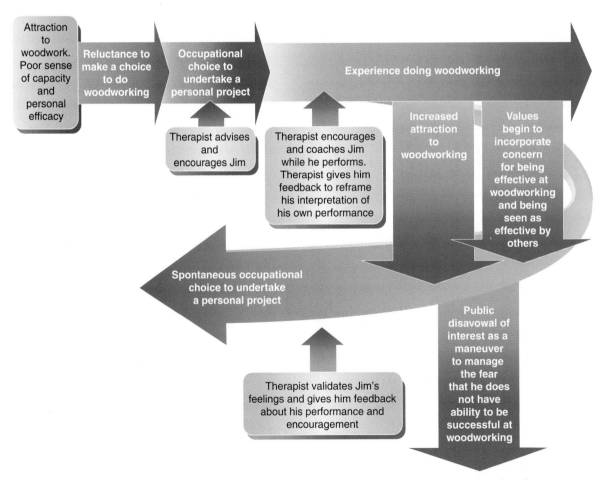

FIGURE 19-2 Therapist Strategies and Dynamics of Jim's Change During Woodworking.

ing, and feedback about what appeared to be going on. Jim was able to progress volitionally so that he enjoyed and increasingly valued woodworking. However, this raised the stakes for him, and given his limited sense of capacity, Jim became overwhelmed with fear of failing. His protestations of disinterest were maneuvers to avoid the possibility of painful failure. The therapist provided Jim further feedback about his improving performance along with validation and encouragement. This empowered Jim to understand his own situation and reconsider his own volitional self-understanding. This allowed him to imagine success and allowed his interests and values to energize him toward an independent occupational choice for a personal project.

Importantly, this choice proved to shift Jim into a new mode of action. He was soon proudly showing other clients and therapists the progress of his work and insisting that the therapist let him do every step of the project on his own. By the time he was discharged, he had negotiated access to a neighbor's workshop and had several woodworking projects planned to help furnish the semi-apartment in which he lived in the basement of his parent's home. Of course, the most important transformation in Jim was the development of his personal causation. He achieved and was able to generalize a growing sense of capacity and personal efficacy. He was beginning to see himself as a person effective in realizing values.

Betty

Betty was 71 years old. The therapist joined the inpatient rehabilitation ward when Betty had already been in the ward for 2 weeks. When the therapist first went to see Betty she was slumped in her chair. She had a right hemiplegia with no active range of motion in her right arm. She had some leg movement although it was restricted. Her mouth was slightly drooped and her speech slurred.

The therapist identified that Betty seemed discouraged and gave Betty feedback about this. Betty agreed, and indicated that she did not really see the point of therapy given her slow progress and acknowledged that she was overwhelmed by the uncertainty of her future. The therapist validated

Betty's feelings. Given Betty's despondence and reluctance for therapy, the therapist stopped by Betty's room at the end of each day to see her for a few minutes. This had the advantage of making a daily connection with Betty and gave her the sense she mattered to the therapist.

During one of these brief visits, the therapist advised Betty that the best way to feel more control over her situation was to identify some goals of her own for therapy. The therapist encouraged Betty to complete the Occupational Self Assessment (OSA), indicating that it would help her think about what was most important to her and what she would want to accomplish in therapy. With some coaching, Betty was able to complete the OSA in her next therapy session and she selected four OSA items as priorities for change:

- Taking care of myself
- Getting along with others
- Working toward my goals
- Having a satisfying routine.

The therapist asked Betty to discuss her choices. Explaining her first priority, Betty stated that she lived alone and prided herself on being able to take care of herself. She lived in a first floor rented flat in Edinburgh, Scotland, where she had lived for 51 years. She was very emotionally attached to her home. She had moved there when she married and had raised her child there.

She was also very particular about her self-care. She took a bath and put on make-up everyday. She set her hair in curlers every Saturday night so that she would look "presentable" for church on Sunday. She preferred to wear skirts, jumpers, and tights and was very particular about her clothes, as she did not want to be "mutton dressed as lamb."

Betty had an active and structured routine at home. She got up at 7:30 AM and would then take a bath and get dressed. She made her bed and opened the curtains. Then she prepared a light breakfast of cereal and toast. Most of her morning consisted of household duties of cooking, cleaning, and hand laundry. Betty stated she was very "house proud" and previously managed all her own housework. She had a light meal for lunch and a snack at teatime. Afternoons she shopped in her neighborhood, entertained or met friends, walked and sat in the park, or went into the city center using public transportation. She would go out everyday and walk to local shops. Weekends were different. On Saturday she prepared soup that she would eat during the week. She went to church on Sunday and visited with her daughter and friends both days. She enjoyed reading and watching a few favorite TV shows in the evening, going to bed by 10:00 PM. Betty described this routine as full, noting that there was always something to do at home and that she felt always "on the go." Her priority of being able to take care of herself meant getting back to this routine.

When asked about her second priority, getting along with others, Betty furnished the following information. Betty and her husband had managed a pub for most of their working lives. Betty served drinks and meals in the lounge bar for 24 years, until her husband's death 27 years earlier. She was very proud of this job and valued it very much. She regretted having to retire when her husband died, but she was not able to run the pub herself. When asked what she particularly enjoyed about this job, she quickly indicated it was the social aspect.

She considered herself an outgoing person who also led a very social life at home. For example, she has a friend across from her flat who joined her for a meal once a week. She met another friend in town for a coffee a couple times a week. Several neighbors and their daughters visited her routinely, so she ordinarily entertained one or more guests each day, often for tea. When the therapist asked her why she had asked for no visitors and had chosen a private room in the rehabilitation hospital since this isolated her, Betty stated that she felt very conscious of her drooping mouth and felt that she could not communicate anymore with others the way she was used to doing.

Betty's OSA priority 3 was "working toward my goals." To Betty this meant "getting home as quickly as possible." Her OSA priority 4 was "having a satisfying routine." Explaining this, Betty shared that she was extremely bored in rehabilitation. She felt that she could not do anything herself, which also made her feel helpless and frustrated. Her perception was that other clients, relatives, or nurses completed everything for her. She still wakes at

7.30, but now lies in bed thinking about how dependent she is until the nurses get to her around 8.30. She says starting her day this way makes her feel especially depressed and useless.

The therapist validated Betty's feelings by carefully listening to her and indicating that she realized Betty was in a very difficult emotional situation. She also advised Betty that there were things that could be done to help her achieve her goals and to make things more tolerable for her in the hospital. They negotiated that she should set therapy goals and discussed the possibilities. Betty indicated that for her, a very important goal was to return home to live alone. Betty and the therapist also agreed that two other, shorter term goals were that she would have a productive and satisfying routine within the hospital environment and would feel confident interacting with other clients in occupational therapy.

At the next therapy session the therapist suggested structuring the following schedule for Betty in the hospital. During weekdays there would be a specific personal care program that would happen between 7:30 and 8:30 AM. This would be carried out by a member of the occupational therapy team or a selected nurse. Breakfast would be at 9:00. Then, Betty would read the newspaper until the occupational therapy session at 10:00. The occupational therapy session lasted until noon. Lunch on the ward was between noon and 1 PM. Betty attended physical therapy for an hour after lunch. She then rested for an hour before receiving visitors. The therapist negotiated with Betty's family to arrange a rotation of visitors at this time. The therapist also arranged for a TV to be brought into Betty's room so that she had some entertainment at night. Weekends were also scheduled to allow for maximum use of time. Betty's daughter volunteered to support Betty with outdoor occupational forms on the weekends in the mornings. This required Betty to be issued an attendant propelled wheelchair. The therapist coached the daughter in its use, including car transfers, and gave the daughter and Betty an opportunity to practice these skills. A hairdresser was arranged for Betty for Saturday afternoons. Arrangements were also made for her minister to visit her on Sunday, until she felt able to go to church with her daughter.

This restructuring of Betty's routine was effective in allowing her to find her ongoing experience personally satisfying.

Betty was highly committed to achieving independence in the area of self-care due to her value of privacy and her pride in her appearance. The therapist structured self-care sessions so that Betty could develop skills in personal care without feeling overwhelmed and concluding that she could not do anything. The Assessment of Motor and Process Skills (AMPS) showed that Betty had deficits in walking, stabilizing, aligning, positioning, reaching, and coordinating. The therapist, therefore, coached Betty to get out of bed safely and obtain objects from the wardrobe by providing verbal instructions and prompts. Betty stated she felt physically unsure when bathing, which made her very anxious. Therefore, the therapist provided physical support and encouragement to reassure her. The OT also advised Betty to use a bath board and seat to get in and out of the bath. The OT structured the environment to include this equipment. Betty explored the new objects and practiced them with substantial coaching and encouragement from the therapist.

However, Betty became despondent over the procedure and an alternative was quickly identified. The OT advised that there was another piece of equipment that would provide more support and require less physical capacity from Betty. Betty explored using this equipment and was able to use it with encouragement from the therapist. Practice was arranged so that Betty could generate habits around the use of the equipment.

Betty was very particular about dressing. She insisted on using her clothes and did not wish to explore alternative clothing. The therapist validated this desire despite it posing greater functional challenges for Betty. Due to Betty's affected arm and her subsequent skill deficit with reaching, coordinating, manipulating, and gripping, the therapist coached Betty in one-handed techniques to put on clothes. Betty was very anxious while attempting dressing. Since being in hospital she had failed repeatedly to complete parts of her personal care routine. Consequently, she expected failure again. Betty struggled with positioning garments to allow

easier access. She would forget the technique and be unable to sustain performance. The therapist was careful to respond to Betty's anxiety and provide validation and encouragement that reassured her. She also provided physical support and coaching to ensure that Betty would be able to succeed and complete the occupational forms.

Therefore, despite difficulty, Betty sustained her performance. Based on this success, Betty began to practice putting on her jumper while in the ward during the day. Initially, Betty felt exhausted after personal care sessions and required therapist feedback to reframe her discouragement by stressing what she had accomplished. The therapist structured Betty's social environment by informing the nursing staff of Betty's routine and arranging for both nursing staff and the occupational therapy assistant to support Betty to practice dressing to create habits around these new ways of doing things.

Betty also attended an occupational therapy session in the department daily. The sessions were held in the morning with several other clients who attended at the same time. The therapist was careful to structure Betty's experience. In the early sessions Betty was more of an observer and completed an occupational form on her own with coaching from the therapist. Initially she was self-conscious because of her drooped mouth and did not want to socialize. Therefore, working within a parallel group situation without high demands for interaction was less threatening for her. Gradually she began to interact more. The therapist then paired her with others to complete occupational forms in a cooperative group situation. The therapist purposively paired Betty with a talkative client who would stimulate communication. Betty soon made friends and asked to be moved from the side room in the ward to be nearer her friends from occupational therapy in the main ward.

In this parallel group context, the therapist offered Betty increasingly challenging occupational forms. Since Betty had been a homemaker who routinely entertained people, she was keen to do things that contributed to that role. The therapist identified the kinds of occupational forms that were within Betty's performance capacity, advising Betty on what she might choose to do. First, Betty tried a ready mix sponge cake that only required stirring in a few ingredients and baking. This provided her with instant success, promoting her sense of capacity. Betty shared the cake with a few other clients. The therapist had previously coached these clients to encourage Betty with positive feedback. Similarly, the therapist told nursing staff about Betty's accomplishments and asked them to reinforce this achievement. Subsequently, Betty undertook a range of more challenging occupational forms including making sandwiches, cheesecakes (a favourite of her friend who used to visit), simple meals, and soup.

Betty was very particular about soup. When the therapist advised Betty to consider using canned soup because it would be more convenient, given that she was now effectively one handed, Betty refused and negotiated to try to make her own soup from raw ingredients. She had made soup every week of her married life and used to give it to her visitors when they called. She stated she was known for her soup all over Scotland, and it was a source of pride. In addition, she pointed out that canned soup simply did not have the same nutrients as homemade soup. As Betty and the therapist discussed soup, it became clear that making soup was an important form of leisure participation for Betty. It structured her day and provided enjoyment when shared with her visitors. Therefore, the therapist validated Betty's choice to attempt making soup from raw ingredients. She advised Betty about adaptive equipment she would require for vegetable preparation and coached Betty in their use. Although it was difficult and took Betty a whole morning to complete the soup, she sustained her performance because she found it meaningful and satisfying. The first session made it apparent that once Betty was set up to prepare the vegetables, she could spend all morning engaged in this occupational form with minimal support from occupational therapy staff. Next, the therapist arranged it so that on days Betty made soup it was taken to the ward for lunch. In this way Betty received glowing feedback from the other clients and ward staff.

The occupational forms were structured to provide the opportunity for Betty to develop and/or compensate for skill deficits. For example, Betty had difficulty with transporting objects. Initially, due to her lack of confidence and motor skills, the therapist organized the needed objects within reach to allow Betty to experience success and enjoyment. As Betty gained a better sense of her own capacities and efficacy, especially her recognition that she could succeed despite her impairments, the therapist decided to introduce more challenge. For example, Betty became responsible to collect needed objects. To help her, the therapist advised Betty to explore adaptive objects such as different trolleys and/or a pocketed apron. Betty chose to use an upright trolley and the therapist coached and encouraged her to practice so that it became more habitual. The therapist initially had to closely supervise and provide physical support to reduce the risk of falling. In addition, Betty was easily fatigued so that her endurance needed to be increased. Initially, she used a chair with supportive arms; with time, she was able to work from a tall stool that allowed her to maintain a semi-standing position and stand for short periods.

Betty's success inspired several other clients who wanted to be involved. Therefore, a "soup group" was created. Members worked toward their own occupational goals within this common occupational form. Betty's role was to organize everyone and welcome new members. At the end of 3 weeks, both the team and Betty's family could see major improvements in Betty's mood, social ability, and performance capacities. For example, one nurse who had been on holiday noted that Betty had become a "completely different person" who was chatty, motivated, and engaged in life again. Another nurse commented, "occupational therapy had given Betty back a sense of who she was." Betty continued to make improvements and was discharged to her home.

Figure 19-3 illustrates the key processes involved in Betty's therapy. Betty initially could not engage in therapy because she was anxious and discouraged by her lack

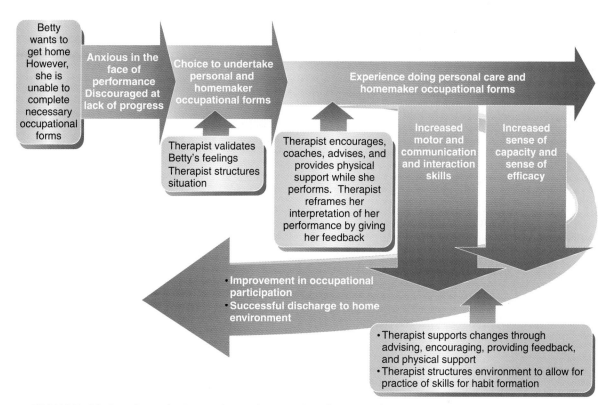

FIGURE 19-3 Therapist Strategies and Dynamics of Betty's Change During Occupational Therapy.

of progress. The therapist had to deal with Betty's anxiety and discouragement by first validating Betty's feelings. The therapist also structured her environment quickly to show Betty that she was committed to supporting Betty's recovery. As therapy unfolded, other strategies were used to facilitate improvement in communication and interaction skills and Betty's volitional status. These included encouraging, structuring, coaching, advising, giving feedback, and providing physical support.

Key Terms

Advise: Recommend intervention goals and strategies to the client.

Coach: Instruct, demonstrate, guide, verbally prompt, and/or physically prompt clients.

Encourage: Provide emotional support and reassurance.

Conclusion

This chapter presented and discussed a number of strategies that therapists use to facilitate and complement clients' occupational engagement. As noted at the outset, the discussion is not intended to be exhaustive. Rather, the purpose of this chapter is to begin to identify strategies that take their logic from or clearly contribute to changes conceptualized by MOHO.

Give feedback: Sharing an overall conceptualization of the client's situation or an understanding of the client's ongoing action.

Identify: Locating and sharing a range of personal, procedural, and/or environmental factors that can facilitate occupational performance and participation.

Negotiate: Engage in give-and-take with the client to achieve a common perspective or agreement about something that the client will or should do in the future.

Physically support: To use the physical body to support the completion of an occupational form or part of an occupational form when clients cannot or will not use their motor skills.

Structure: Establish parameters for choice and performance by offering clients alternatives, setting limits, and establishing ground rules.

Therapeutic strategy: A therapist's action that influences a client's doing, feeling, and/or thinking to facilitate desired change.

Validate: Convey respect for the client's experience or perspective.

References

Burke, J. P., & Cassidy, J. C. (1991). Disparity between reimbursement-driven practice and humanistic values of occupational therapy. *American Journal of Occupational Therapy, 45,* 173–176.

Burke, J. P., & DePoy, E. (1991). An emerging view of mastery, excellence, and leadership in occupational therapy practice. *American Journal of Occupational Therapy, 45,* 1027–1032.

Hopkins, H. L., & Tiffany, E. G. (1983). Occupational therapy: A problem solving process. In H. L. Hopkins & H. D. Smith (Eds.), *Willard and Spackman's occupational therapy* (6th ed., pp. 89–100). Philadelphia: JB Lippincott.

Jonsson, H., Josephsson, S., & Kielhofner, G. (2000). Evolving narratives in the course of retirement: A longitudinal study. *American Journal of Occupational Therapy, 54* (5), 463–470.

Peloquin, S. M. (1990). The patient-therapist relationship in occupational therapy: Understanding visions and images. *American Journal of Occupational Therapy, 44,* 13–21.

Peloquin, S. M. (1995). The fullness of empathy: reflections and illustrations. *American Journal of Occupational Therapy, 49,* 24–31.

Tiffany, E. G. (1983). Psychiatry and mental health. In H. L. Hopkins & H. D. Smith (Eds.), *Willard and Spackman's occupational therapy* (6th ed., pp. 267–229). Philadelphia: JB Lippincott.

Toombs, K. (1992). *The meaning of illness: A phenomenological account of the different perspectives of physician and patient.* Boston: Kluwer Academic Publishers.

Wendel, S. (1996). *The rejected body: Feminist philosophical reflections on disability.* New York: Routledge.

20

Putting Theory into Practice

- **Kirsty Forsyth**
- **Gary Kielhofner**

Therapists frequently consider theory more ornamental then instrumental because its relationship to practice has not been made sufficiently explicit. Even when therapists find that theory helps them understand clients, it is not always clear how to translate that understanding into a plan of action. Consequently, theory can often fail to impact how therapy is planned, implemented, and evaluated.

Therapists who do use occupational therapy theory are often unsure about how to communicate the underlying ideas to the client and others (e.g., family, caregivers, peer professionals) and how to document the goals, process, and outcomes of therapy. Reflecting the theory in the process of communication and documentation is also important because the client and others need to know what the therapist is thinking and why things are being done. Part of the responsibility of using theory is to let others know what you are doing.

Communication and documentation are also important means of establishing the credibility of a health profession. Occupational therapists often report that they find it challenging to articulate the theoretical basis for practice. More than ever before, it is important that occupational therapists clearly document the rationale, process, and outcomes of service.

This final chapter of Section II addresses these issues and focuses on the following questions. How does a therapist use MOHO theory to plan, implement, and evaluate therapy? How does one communicate MOHO concepts underlying practice to the client and others (e.g., family, caregivers, peer professionals)? How does one document MOHO-related goals, process, and outcomes of therapy?

Previous chapters have:

- Presented questions that can guide assessment (Chapter 11)

- Identified the kinds of client strengths and problems/challenges that such questions may help identify (Chapter 11)
- Described assessments that therapists can use to identify strengths and problems/challenges of clients, and discussed how to choose and use them (Chapters 12–17)
- Identified types of change that takes place in therapy and the kinds of client doing that contribute to such change (Chapter 18)
- Identified the role of the therapist and therapeutic strategies that enable the client to achieve changes (Chapter 19).

We will build on this information to discuss how it is integrated and used when the therapist is planning, implementing, and communicating about therapy. Throughout the chapter, the authors refer the reader to various resources in previous chapters and discuss how to use them as part of an integrated process.

Process of Therapy

According to the American Occupational Therapy Association's (AOTA) "Occupational Therapy Practice Framework" (Commission on Practice, AOTA), the therapy process is represented as involving three main processes:

- Evaluation
- Intervention
- Outcomes.

Evaluation involves creating an understanding of the client's perspectives, priorities, concerns, and problems. It also involves identifying the client and contextual factors that facilitate or interfere with performance.

Intervention involves planning, implementing, and reviewing therapy. Outcomes involve determining the extent to which targeted goals were achieved.

As shown in Figure 20-1, we conceptualize planning, implementing, and evaluating therapy as a six-step process that corresponds to the processes outlined in the AOTA practice framework. Throughout these steps, the therapist engages in therapeutic reasoning that involves the active use of theory. Theory should help the therapist to grasp the complexity of client problems and appreciate the factors supporting or hindering progress in therapy.

As shown in Figure 20-1, the first step is applying the questions given in Chapter 11 (or creating one's own set of questions derived from MOHO) as a framework for approaching information gathering. The second step involves using structured and unstructured means to collect information from and about the client. The third step involves arriving at a conceptualization of the client, as discussed in Chapter 11. This step includes identification of client strengths

and weakness and considering the overall dynamics of the client's situation. The conceptualization of the client's situation represents a synthesis of the general concepts of the theory with the particular information about the client. Together, steps 1–3 make up what the AOTA practice framework refers to as evaluation.

Based on the conceptualization that emerges from the first three steps, the therapist plans the therapy process in the fourth step. This fourth step involves:

- Creating therapy goals with the client
- Deciding what kinds of occupational engagement will enable the client to change
- Determining what kind of therapeutic strategies will be needed to support the client to change.

The fifth step involves implementing therapy and reviewing it by continually collecting new information to determine whether clients are progressing as planned. Steps 4 and 5 correspond to the practice framework intervention process. The sixth and final step, which corresponds to the practice framework outcomes process,

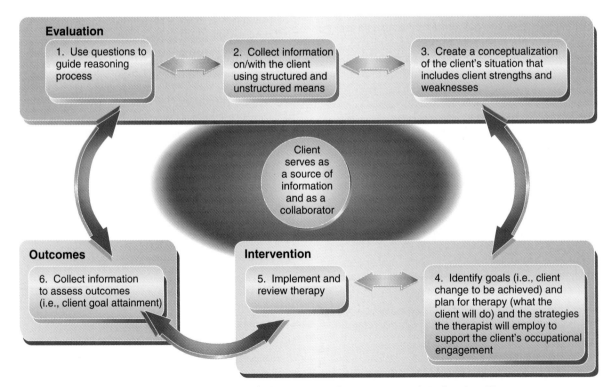

FIGURE 20-1   The Process of Planning, Implementing, and Evaluating Therapy.

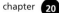

is to determine whether the client has attained therapy goals.

Although these are presented and discussed as a series of steps, it is important to realize that the process should be seamless. That is, one step flows into the next and the therapist moves back and forth between steps throughout the course of therapy.

Complimenting Figure 20-1 and the process it illustrates, the Section II Master Table (pages 346–355) includes the questions, strengths, problems/challenges, changes, client engagement, and therapeutic strategies identified in previous chapters. Throughout this chapter, as the therapy process is discussed, the authors will refer to the Section II Master Table, which brings together information from several previous chapters.

Client-Centeredness in Therapy

As indicated in Figure 20-1, the client must always be at the center of this process. The MOHO approach to client-centered therapy is to integrate a conceptual understanding of the client with attention to the client's experience and desires. Whenever possible, the process should be undertaken with the collaboration of the client. Throughout the process, the therapist must communicate with the client, seeking client input and validation, and engaging the client to collaborate in planning, implementing, and evaluating therapy.

Client-centeredness should extend to those clients who are unable to verbalize and/or be active in collaboration. There are two main strategies for doing this. First, the therapist can collaborate with family members or others who care about and can serve as advocates for the client. Second, the therapist works to understand the client's view of the world, what matters to the client, what the client enjoys, and how the client feels about his or her abilities. This can be achieved

> *The MOHO approach to client-centered therapy is to integrate a conceptual understanding of the client with attention to the client's experience and desires.*

through careful observation of the client's volitionally relevant actions as discussed in Chapter 13.

Terminology in Communication and Documentation

The words that are selected to describe therapy are very important. Deciding whether and how to use MOHO terminology in communication and documentation requires consideration of several factors. MOHO terms, like those of any other professional language, offer benefits and pose challenges.

Occupational therapists acquire the professional languages of several disciplines and theoretical perspectives. The terms resuscitation, repression, and reinforcement reflect medical model, object relations, and behavioral concepts, respectively. Complex conditions or procedures can be conveyed and immediately understood when such professional terminology is used.

A common example of how a professional term can efficiently convey complex information and facilitate communication between professionals is medical diagnosis. The term Alzheimer's dementia conveys the following, rather complicated meaning:

> . . . The development of multiple cognitive deficits manifested by both 1) memory impairment (impaired ability to learn new information or recall previously learned information), 2) one (or more) of the following cognitive disturbances: a. aphasia (language disturbance), b. apraxia (impaired ability to carry out motor activities despite intact motor function), c. agnosia (failure to recognize or identify objects despite intact sensory function), d. disturbance in executive functioning (i.e., planning, organizing, sequencing, abstracting). The cognitive deficits in Criteria 1 and 2 each cause a significant impairment in social or occupational functioning and represent a significant decline from a previous level of functioning. The course is characterized by gradual onset and continuing cognitive decline. The cognitive deficits in Criteria 1 and 2 are not due to any of the following: 1) other central nervous system conditions that cause progressive deficits in memory and cognition, 2) systemic conditions that are known to cause dementia, 3) substance-induced conditions. The

deficits do not occur exclusively during the course of a delirium. The disturbance is not better accounted for by another Axis I disorder (DSM-IV-TR, 2000).

As the definition illustrates, using diagnostic terms allows those who know the meaning of terminology to share common perspectives and to convey information succinctly.

Similarly, MOHO terminology can also be used to convey complex concepts to those who are familiar with the model. For example, the term volition denotes a complex idea about how persons are motivated toward their occupations. To those who know its meaning, volition will convey several concepts. When someone refers to a volitional problem, those who know the terminology can anticipate that the problem involves the client's values, personal causation, and interests. They can further expect that the problem is manifested in how clients anticipate, choose, experience, and interpret what they do. In this way, MOHO terminology can succinctly convey information.

The major disadvantage of all professional language is that everyone needs to have a common understanding of the terms. It is therefore ineffective to use MOHO terms with colleagues or clients/relatives who will not understand what the words mean. Some MOHO terms such as volition, personal causation, and roles have meanings not readily understood. Other terms, such as interests, values, and habits, contain meaning beyond but still consistent with ordinary usage. Still other terms, such as skill, have a meaning within the MOHO context (i.e., a quality of actual occupational performance) that may be quite different than everyday usage (i.e., underlying capacity). Therefore, therapists should carefully decide when and how they use MOHO terms in communicating to clients, lay persons, and other professionals.

Communication and MOHO Terminology

There are circumstances in which it is appropriate to use MOHO terms in communication. These include when:

- The primary or exclusive audience is other occupational therapists who are familiar with MOHO language

- Clients are empowered by learning the MOHO concepts as a means of increasing understanding and control over their own circumstances
- Other professionals are receptive to becoming familiar with occupational therapy terminology.

MOHO language is intended to facilitate communication of ideas between occupational therapists. It can be particularly helpful when therapists are discussing clients, plans for therapy, and so on. Whereas clients ordinarily require that we communicate to them in everyday language, there are occupational therapists who empower their clients to learn basic MOHO language and concepts. In one community occupational therapy program, Reencuentros, in Santiago, Chile, clients are educated on the basic language and views of MOHO as part of their therapy. An important lesson from this experience is that client-centered therapy includes not only respecting clients' perspectives, but also enriching clients' understanding of their own situations.

We have routinely used MOHO language both with clients and other professionals in practice contexts with positive results. Most clients are responsive to a therapist's attempts to explain the ideas they are using. Moreover, other professionals are often quite willing to acquire a basic understanding of one's professional terminology. Therapists have often noted to us that they have been surprised by how quickly teams pick up MOHO terms. Often, the therapist's lack of confidence in using the terminology, rather than resistance on the part of other professionals, prevents use of MOHO terminology in an interdisciplinary context. Nonetheless, therapists do need to be sensitive to the demands they put on other professionals for learning their terminology. It is important to decide which terms one would like interdisciplinary colleagues to understand and to take the time to explain them. Finally, a willingness to attend to the perspectives and language of others goes a long way in encouraging them to attend to our own.

Recently, a colleague shared the following experience about introducing MOHO terminology in a psychiatric setting. Initially, the psychiatrist and other team members were skeptical about such terms as volition and personal causation. The therapist asked that the team give him an opportunity to use these and other terms since it represented his professional language. The psychiatrist agreed as the leader of the team that he would entertain the idea of the therapist using the terms in team discussions, provided it became clear how these terms added to understanding of the client and planning interdisciplinary care. Within a few months, the psychiatrist had not only developed an understanding of the terms, but also habitually ventured his own observations of client volition and habituation, asking for the therapist's expert opinion.

Using MOHO language in a multidisciplinary context can convey that the occupational therapist has a specific domain of interest and expertise to contribute to the team. For example, a psychologist recently approached the first author, upset because she felt that occupational therapists were claiming motivation as their domain. She felt that motivation was a psychological term and area of expertise. The first author explained that occupational therapy's interest in motiva-

tion was based on the concept of volition and offered a brief explanation. Following this, the psychologist realized that her concerns with motivation and occupational therapy concerns were actually complementary rather than competitive or duplicative.

Moving Between MOHO Terms and Everyday Terms

Most therapists will find it necessary to develop facility in moving back and forth between using MOHO terminology and expressing MOHO concepts in ordinary language. All professionals who wish to be effective in interacting with those who do not share their expertise must know how to explain themselves in everyday language. *Table 20-1* lists some common MOHO terms and ways they can be expressed in everyday language. Therapists may wish to expand and modify this table

TABLE 20-1 MOHO Terms and Explanations in Everyday Language

Concepts from MOHO	Ways of Explaining the Theory/Concept to Clients
Person	
Volition	• Your motivation for the things you do in everyday life and for choices you make about what you do with your life. • Motivation is based on what we perceive to be interesting and valuable and what we believe ourselves capable of doing.
Personal Causation	How effective you feel in accomplishing the activities in your everyday life.
Values	What is important and meaningful to you and what your goals are.
Interests	What you enjoy or find satisfaction in doing.
Habituation	Your lifestyle and typical routine of daily activities.
Roles	The positions in life you hold and the responsibilities associated with them, such as being a spouse, parent, worker, student.
Habits	The routine way of doing activities, and your daily routine.
Performance Capacity	Physical and mental abilities. Subjective experience of symptoms of illness/impairment.
Environment	
Spaces	The physical places where you work, play/relax, study, take care of yourself, rest and sleep (e.g., classroom, kitchen, bedroom, office).
Objects	Tools, supplies, furniture, appliances, clothes, vehicles, and other things you use, interact with, wear, or otherwise make part of your everyday life.
Occupational Forms	The everyday activities you do.
Social Groups	The people you interact with in daily life (coworkers, classmates, family members, roommates, neighbors, etc).

for their own everyday use, particularly when talking with clients and their families.

Documentation and MOHO Terminology

Since written documentation is primarily intended for professional audiences and aims at accuracy and completeness, a strong case for using MOHO terminology can be made. Consider for example the following client note in ordinary language:

> Edna lacks confidence and is overly dependent.

Using MOHO language makes the definition of the problem more specific:

> Edna's personal causation is characterized by lacking a clear sense of her own capacity. As a result, she anticipates performance situations with anxiety and frequently chooses to avoid doing things for which she has adequate skills. She also habitually seeks advice and help from others which leads to her being unnecessarily dependent on others.

As the example illustrates, using the terminology of a theoretical model can result in documentation that is more precise and detailed. Moreover, while the first statement describes Edna's behavior, it does not explain it. The second statement offers an explanation that also provides a rationale for the following interventions:

- Advise Edna on a course of therapy that will be graded to be increasingly challenging to her sense of capacity
- Provide Edna with feedback about her occupational performance to enable a more accurate sense of her own capacities
- Encourage Edna to sustain performance in the face of anxiety

> *Precision in language, including the use of theoretical terms, can clarify what we understand clients' difficulties to be and how we plan to address them.*

> *Formulating therapy requires therapeutic reasoning beyond the guidelines presented here. Consequently, the process . . . and the information in the Section II Master Table should not be viewed as rigid or inflexible. Good therapy requires creative application of the concepts and tools provided by a conceptual model of practice.*

- Structure the environment to provide the opportunity for Edna to practice more autonomy.

Precision in language, including the use of theoretical terms, can clarify what we understand clients' difficulties to be and how we plan to address them. One of the best ways to explain occupational therapy is to demonstrate how its concepts frame problems and solutions.

Implementing the Process

The following sections examine each stage of the therapy process outlined earlier, discussing how it is undertaken. In so doing, we discuss not only the therapeutic reasoning involved, but also how the therapist communicates and documents each step. In each discussion, we refer to sharing information and collaborating with the client. However, it should be understood that when the client is not capable, therapists would share information and collaborate with others close to the client, such as a family member. Also, in many instances, the therapist will share information and collaborate with both the client and family member(s).

This process and the materials in the Section II Master Table, to which we will frequently refer, are not recipes for implementing MOHO interventions. Although they provide guidelines for formulating therapy, the actual process should always be infused with the specific information about clients, the circumstances, and the unfolding dynamics of therapy. Formulating therapy requires therapeutic reasoning beyond the guidelines presented here. Consequently, the process we will discuss below and the information in the Section II Master Table should not be viewed as rigid or inflexible. Good therapy requires creative application of the concepts and tools provided by a conceptual model of practice.

Steps 1 and 2: Using Questions and Selecting and Using Assessments to Collect Information

As discussed in Chapter 11, therapeutic reasoning begins with translating concepts from MOHO into questions that guide how one approaches gathering information about a client. In step 2, the therapist selects and uses the most appropriate structured assessments and unstructured means of information gathering. Chapters 12 through 17 provided detailed resources for MOHO-related information gathering.

The Section II Master Table lists the questions first discussed in Chapter 11 along with corresponding client strengths and problems/challenges that therapists may discover. Reviewing these columns of the table should provide helpful guidelines for the first two steps. That is, when thinking about use of assessments, it is helpful to reconsider the fundamental questions one is trying to answer with reference to the client. Similarly, it is useful to remind oneself of the kinds of client strengths and problems/challenges for which one should be looking. With time and experience, the process will become more tailored to one's own circumstances and more automatic.

We recommend that therapists develop their own tables with questions, strengths, and problems/challenges that are more specific and reflective of their clients. Such a table should continue to evolve over time as one develops a deeper appreciation of one's client group. Moreover, the process of creating and updating such a table helps one become more reflective in practice. Finally, it can be a useful tool in communicating one's perspective to others.

COMMUNICATING ONE'S THEORY AND QUESTIONS TO CLIENTS

Therapists should begin to communicate to clients the theory they are using from the beginning of therapy. Consider that, from the first encounter, most clients will begin forming impressions about the kind of help they might receive from the therapist. It is important to help the client have an understanding and expectations that are as accurate and realistic as possible.

How much one says and how to frame it depends on the client. Most of the time, however, therapists will use everyday language to explain their theoretical approaches. The following are examples of how therapists might orient a client to the theory and questions they will be using.

Sara

Sara was a college-educated, 44-year-old woman recently diagnosed with multiple sclerosis. Her therapist introduced MOHO as follows:

> As an occupational therapist, I work from a perspective that is concerned with how Multiple Sclerosis has affected your ability to participate in the things that are important to you—for example, your work, taking care of yourself, your leisure activities. I'll want to get to know what is important to you and how you feel your illness has affected your ability to do what you need to do and like to do. I will also want to know something about your major life responsibilities and your everyday routines.
>
> We'll work together to figure out ways we can minimize any problems in your everyday life and how you can best go on with life in a meaningful way. We can make changes in your environment or in how you go about doing things that allow you to be more effective in getting done what you need and want to do.

Melissa

Melissa was a 65-year-old woman who had limited cognitive capacities due to Alzheimer's disease. Her therapist used a much briefer explanation:

> My job is to help you manage things and be able to do what's most important and enjoyable to you.

Mike

For Mike, a 10-year-old with cerebral palsy, introduction to the school therapist's use of MOHO was as follows:

I'm here to make sure you are managing okay in school and liking it. I want to find out how you are doing with such things as getting to your classes, doing homework, dressing for gym, eating lunch, getting along with your classmates and your teacher. I'd also like you to tell me what you do well and what is harder for you. Lastly, I want to know what's most important for you and what you like in school.

As the examples illustrate, it is possible to give clients, in terms suited to their ability to understand, an indication of the therapist's concepts and approach. Even though terms like volition and personal causation were not used in these explanations, the therapists nevertheless conveyed to the clients that they were concerned with volitional issues.

Explanations of one's concepts may be expanded or reduced depending on the response of the client. The point is to meet clients where they are, respecting their emotional states, cognitive abilities, background, and other characteristics. When clients are nonverbal, communication may occur primarily through the therapist's actions. This means, for example, conveying one's intention to know what the client values and enjoys by responding to any indication of these things by the client. Similarly, one conveys concern for personal causation by respecting a client's need to feel some sense of personal control.

Clients who are uncooperative present some of the largest challenges. However, one of the best tools a therapist has for dealing with uncooperative clients is the concept of volition. What appears to be a lack of cooperation from the therapist's viewpoint is always a volitionally driven client decision. No single strategy will work, but respect for the client's viewpoint, however different from that of the therapist, is a constant principle. If therapists can understand the client's volitional perspective, they can often derive appropriate strategies. An excellent example is the case of Claudio in Chapter 21.

The process of communicating with the client only begins with the first encounters in therapy. As time goes on, therapists should reveal more and more to their clients about their perspectives. Once again, how this is done should be based on what the client is able to grasp and integrate.

COMMUNICATING ONE'S THEORY AND QUESTIONS TO OTHER PROFESSIONALS

It is useful and important to make known one's theory and approach to gathering information to others such as peer professionals. This can be done in a variety of ways. One might do so formally by giving a presentation at a team meeting or by providing in-service training. One can also do it informally by sharing anecdotal information about clients in which theoretical concepts are embedded. Discussing clients in team meetings or when consulting with another professional often provides an excellent opportunity to mention and explain the concept one is using.

In the end, it is important that other service providers and professionals have some understanding of one's theoretical perspective and its implications for what one does in therapy. Others' interests or abilities to understand MOHO concepts will, of course, vary. Therefore, one must judge when and how to communicate the information to others.

EXPLAINING ASSESSMENTS TO CLIENTS

It is extremely important to explain planned assessments to the client if at all possible. Clients often perceive a large power differential between themselves and the therapist. Assessment can seem mysterious and frightening to a client. Clients may have no idea why the therapist is asking questions or gathering information. They may fear that the therapist will discover something negative about them. Clients may be concerned that the therapist will gain information that affects them (e.g., where they can live, how much freedom they have, how much help they receive).

Consequently, the therapist should explain to the client (and/or family member) in terms that can be understood:

- Why the assessment would be done
- What is entailed in doing the assessment
- What the assessment is likely to reveal
- How the information will be used.

Additionally, the therapist should assure the client (and/or family member) that the information learned in the assessment process will be shared with the client. Most MOHO assessments gather information on the client's viewpoint, concerns, and desires. Therefore, it is appropriate to inform the client that one of the main aims of the assessment process is to clarify and assure that the client's desires and needs will be addressed seriously in therapy.

The following are examples of how the therapist might explain the use of assessments to a client.

The Occupational Self Assessment (OSA)

> It would be very helpful for me if you would complete a short form called the Occupational Self Assessment. It will take you about 10 to 15 minutes. The form asks you to look at a number of statements about how you do things in your everyday life. You will indicate on the form how well you do the things listed and how important they are to you. I'm asking you to fill out this form because I want to know what's important to you. I also want to know where you think things are going okay and where you might feel you have some problems. When you have finished this part of the form, we will look at it together and then you and I will use it to decide what things you would most like to change about your life.

The Occupational Performance History Interview-Second Version (OPHI-II)

> As we begin therapy, I'd like to get to know you better. I'm interested in how (name the injury or disability) has affected your life. I would also like to know how you see your future and what we can do in therapy to make things better for you. In order to do this, it would be very helpful for me to sit down with you for a while and talk about your life. After we have done so, I will fill out some forms and share them with you. This might not only help me understand you better, but it might give you some new ways to think about your life.

The Assessment of Communication and Interaction Skills (ACIS)

> You and I have agreed that sometimes it is not so easy for you to talk and get along with others. It would be really helpful for me to see you in different social situations to gain a better understanding of what actually happens. After I've spent some time with you in these situations, I will fill out some forms. We will look at these forms together to see what things you do well and what things you might want to work on in therapy so you can feel more confident about getting along with others.

These examples only illustrate how one may introduce an assessment. Therapists should develop their own styles of doing so and modify what they say according to each client's unique characteristics. A client who is anxious may need to be reassured. A client who is cognitively disabled or confused will need a simplified explanation. Of course, it is not always possible to explain the intended assessment to the client. Sometimes clients are too cognitively or emotionally constrained to understand or accept the information. On other occasions, clients may be uncooperative. In these situations, therapists must make careful decisions about how to proceed with assessment. For example, a therapist may decide to discreetly observe a client with the aim of gaining information helpful to intervention or to achieving a more collaborative relationship with the client.

EXPLAINING ASSESSMENTS TO OTHER PROFESSIONALS

Explaining the use of assessments to other professionals should also be aimed at elucidating the purpose, process, and content of assessments. Additionally, some professionals will be interested to know whether the assessments that the therapist is using are valid and reliable. MOHO assessments have been or are in the process of careful development and study. This can and should be emphasized when explaining them to other professionals. Having an awareness of the kinds of research that has been done to assure the dependability of an assessment is useful for being able to speak to its value. This does not mean that a therapist should be prepared to recount all the research, but to know something about how an assessment has been studied is a good idea.

When a therapist decides to use an assessment regularly, it is a good idea to become familiar with the kinds of studies that have led to the development of the assessment. The kinds of information provided in Chapters 13 through 16 will be a useful beginning. Also, most MOHO-based assessments have manuals that discuss the research behind the assessment in ways that therapists and other professionals can readily understand.

Documentation provides an excellent opportunity to explain assessments to other team members. In documentation, the value of the assessment in identifying client problems can be readily demonstrated. The following is an example of a summary report of an ACIS evaluation with Rachel who, before a psychotic episode, was actively involved in community activities. She was having difficulty effectively engaging in socially based activities.

Rachel

Rachel wanted to be able to return to her community-based activities that were largely socially based. Rachel was observed in social activities using the Assessment of Communication and Interaction Skills. It revealed the following strengths and weaknesses. Rachel's nonverbal interactions were appropriate (i.e., eye contact, gesturing, touching others). She maintained interactions even when she felt disoriented. She was able to engage others and readily initiated conversation with others. She had trouble focusing in conversation (i.e., jumped from one topic to another). When distressed, she increased the pace and volume of her speaking to the effect that others became uncomfortable. She had difficulty picking up others' cues and respecting their needs or desires in social interaction. Her skill difficulties significantly impacted her ability to engage in socially based activities.

As the example illustrates, sharing what an assessment reveals about a client demonstrates its utility.

Step 3: Creating a Conceptualization of the Client's Situation

In this step, the therapist synthesizes information collected with MOHO concepts to create a unique explanation or understanding of each client (see Chapter 11 for a detailed discussion of this process). The therapist will go back and forth between the theoretical concepts and what is learned about the client. The strengths and problems/challenges listed in the Section II Master Table (pages 346–355) will be helpful. However, the therapist must go beyond listing client characteristics to consider how various characteristics are dynamically interrelated. This means using concepts from Chapter 3.

This step is best illustrated through a detailed example. Therefore, the following is an account of how the first author engaged in this step of conceptualizing a client's occupational circumstances.

Ruth

Ruth was 70 years old and had sustained a stroke that resulted in a left-sided hemiplegia. When the therapist joined the team and took over Ruth's therapy, Ruth was 4 weeks into a rehabilitation program. Nursing staff described Ruth as initially very motivated for therapy. However, she had become withdrawn, noncompliant, and depressed. The physician was considering antidepressive medication. Nursing staff also considered Ruth a safety risk, as she would try to do things for which she had questionable capacity. Consequently, nursing staff indicated that they "had to keep a constant eye on her." They also noted that Ruth had stated her intention to discharge herself from the hospital against medical advice.

Given Ruth's mood and apparent disinterest in rehabilitation, the therapist decided to assess her using selected portions of the OPHI-II and informal observation. The therapist felt that asking Ruth to do anything more would not be successful, given her withdrawal and apparent intention to discharge herself.

During the interview, which was conducted as an informal conversation, the therapist emphasized to Ruth the importance of her being able to say how she really felt about her situation. This was reinforced through active listening and an attitude of empathy to Ruth's experience and viewpoints.

Ruth characterized her mood as being "fed up." When asked to explain what this meant, Ruth described herself as previously being a very independent person who now was "useless." She had lived alone without family and always made her own decisions and looked after herself. She also valued her privacy and felt that her most private self-care routines were now exposed to "strangers."

Moreover, she complained that staff kept telling her she could not do things for herself, which made her feel even worse. She stated she had been a "doer" all her life and was now reduced to a "watcher." Even at 70, she kept her own apartment, went out every day on public transportation, assisted two friends with domestic chores, was actively involved in her church, and had a busy social life.

She felt that being in the hospital was a waste of time, since all she was doing was sitting around feeling bored. She questioned the value of the rehabilitation hospital when she could feel more comfortable at home and could, at least, try to do things on her own there. Ruth stated that she had no interest in occupational therapy since being in therapy would only reinforce what she could not do. She also admitted to fears that the therapist might discover something that would prevent her from being allowed to go home.

From informal observation, it was apparent that Ruth's motor skills were so limited that she could not perform even her basic personal care. When attempting transfers and walking, she was clearly at risk for falling.

With this information, the therapist was able to construct the following conceptualization of Ruth's situation. Ruth's personal causation was extremely limited because she felt incapable and unable to effect outcomes she desired. Because this was so emotionally painful for her, she was unable to fully think about the extent of her limitations. She also experienced her environment on the ward as constraining her choices to do things. Her social environment (nurses) was reinforcing this on a regular basis. Moreover, her previous experience in occupational therapy had led to her focus on her limitations, reinforcing her lowered personal causation. Added to this, Ruth's value system made the loss of capacity, privacy, and independence particularly painful for her.

Ruth's former active routine and roles such as a home maintainer, religious participant, caretaker, and friend had all been eliminated by her stroke and the subsequent rehabilitation hospital routine. Her loss of a familiar and stimulating routine and her loss of occupational roles had left her with a sense of boredom and alienation. Moreover, her current routine was passive and without meaning or satisfaction, so that it further eroded her already compromised volition.

Ruth's rehabilitation experience was extremely demoralizing for her since it assaulted rather than supported her volition. She was forced into losing choices and being passive. She was confronted with her limitations. Ruth's lack of role-related responsibilities and routine contrasted with the high level of activity from which she previously achieved satisfaction. Being forced to sit and watch when her volition was organized around actively doing things was intolerable for her.

If she returned home, she would be extremely limited. Given that Ruth had only recently sustained the stroke and had started to regain movement, the best way forward was to have Ruth engage in a rigorous therapy program. Going home at this point would not only compromise possible gains in her performance capacity, but would likely result in further deterioration of her volition and habituation. Ruth would, therefore, be very unlikely to be able to live independently, requiring institutional placement.

This conceptualization of Ruth's circumstances made it apparent that unless things were radically altered, she would discharge herself with the likelihood that she would be permanently reduced to a passive and dependent state. In this case, with only the limited information that could be gathered on Ruth given her depressed mood and disinterest in therapy, the therapist was able to construct a conceptualization of Ruth's circumstances. We will see later how the therapist used this information.

Communicating Step 3 to the Client

Sharing the therapist's conceptualization with the client is particularly important for any client who is able to understand and emotionally deal with the information. In addition to letting the client know how the therapist understands the client, sharing this information allows the therapist to validate with the client whether it is accurate. Sharing the conceptualization is also an example of the therapeutic strategy of feedback discussed in Chapter 19.

Negotiating with the client at this stage to arrive at a common understanding of the client's situation is often critical to support the next steps in therapy. Of course it is not always possible to share all details of the therapist's conceptualization. Therapists have to carefully couch explanations in terms clients can understand. One exception to this is that therapists sometimes teach elements of the theory to clients as a way to empower them to better understand their own circumstances.

Client-centered practice requires that therapists share their views of the client's situation. Sharing such information gives the client critical information for engaging in the collaborative process. The optimal goal of a client-centered relationship is to allow clients to determine their own vision of the future under the professional guidance of the therapist.

One of the biggest challenges to client-centered practice is a disparity in the therapist's and the client's perspectives (McGavin, 1998; Missiuna & Pollack, 2000; Sumsion & Smyth, 2000). In the event of such a disagreement, it becomes necessary to negotiate with the client. Arriving at a common perspective is important because it helps to ensure that both the therapist and the client are committed to a shared vision of therapy.

While the client is viewed as an equal and active member in the collaboration process, it is the therapist's responsibility to initiate this step and to facilitate action on the part of the client. Occupational therapists have full responsibility for contributing ideas, suggestions, and cautions as well as defining boundaries beyond which therapists cannot go, regardless of a client's wishes (E. Townsend, personal communication, November 4, 1997). The therapist must provide clients with reasonable visions of the likely outcomes of certain decisions and gently challenge the client's perspective if it appears to be unreasonable. The process of communicating this step will be illustrated by returning to the example of Ruth.

Ruth: Part 2

Communicating the therapist's conceptualization to Ruth was particularly challenging since Ruth had already "lost faith" in rehabilitation. The therapist realized it would be necessary to reframe the experience of being in the hospital and re-engage Ruth in a therapeutic process that would be meaningful enough for her to want to stay in the hospital and work to improve her abilities.

The therapist began by validating Ruth's experience and her concerns about staying in the hospital. The therapist explained how she appreciated Ruth's experience of therapy as only making her feel more ineffective, her feeling that she had no control over her privacy and choices, and her boredom with the hospital routine. The therapist also advised Ruth of the difficult challenges Ruth would face if she discharged herself home without further therapy.

The therapist negotiated that she would arrange to change Ruth's routine to be more satisfying and would support her to make choices consistent with her abilities. The therapist gave Ruth a vision of how her experience of therapy could be different and the kinds of meaningful occupations in which she could engage as part of therapy. Finally, she shared information about improvements she believed Ruth could realize in therapy and how they would impact on her ability to live at home and regain important parts of her life.

Reluctantly, Ruth initially committed to stay 2 more weeks after negotiating with the therapist to determine specific goals that focused on improving her ability to return to live at home. The therapist acted swiftly to put in place what had been negotiated. Ruth ended up staying 4 weeks and making gains that significantly improved her performance of self-care and domestic occupational forms before being successfully discharged home.

While the therapist was successful in sharing her conceptualization with Ruth, other clients may either accept or reject the therapist's opinion at this stage. Additionally, there may be times when either the therapist or the client chooses to terminate the therapeutic relationship when they cannot agree. Other times, negotiation may mean that the therapist will support the client with a decision that the therapist perceives as less than optimal, but which is more desirable than terminating therapy.

For example, Ruth was competent to make her own decisions. Therefore, if Ruth had made an informed decision to discharge herself, the therapist would have supported her to make the transition home with the least risk. The therapist would also have documented the areas of concern along with the strategies and environmental supports that were put in place to facilitate Ruth's discharge.

DOCUMENTING STEP 3

Documentation of the therapist's conceptualization of the client is important because it provides the rationale for the goals and therapeutic strategies. The following is the note that was written for the chart concerning Ruth. MOHO language was not used because other occupational therapists in the department were not familiar with MOHO language.

Ruth: Part 3

On initial contact, Ruth stated that she didn't want to be involved in therapy and planned to discharge herself home. Prior to the cerebrovascular accident, Ruth lived alone independently. Her very active lifestyle included daily use of public transportation, active involvement in a church group, supporting two friends with household chores, and regular socialization. Now, she felt she had lost control over her life and access to the things she valued and enjoyed doing. It was also important for Ruth to be able to complete her personal care routine herself as she strongly valued privacy and independence. Ruth's experience in rehabilitation was that she could not enact her most important values and she did not feel that rehabilitation had helped her progress toward achieving them.

Two separate observations of her personal care routine revealed that she was extremely limited in her ability to complete self-care activities due to motor skill deficits. She was unsafe transferring from one surface to another, and was unable to walk independently due to lack of balance. The risk was greater when she was walking as part of some larger activity (e.g., collecting clothes from the closet when it was twice as necessary to prevent Ruth from falling). She required physical support to transfer to a commode. Her walking deficit also limited her ability to move objects around her environment while doing activities. She could not bend and reach for objects from a standing position. She was unable to use her affected arm within activities. This reduced her ability to complete parts of activities in her usual manner (e.g., buttoning shirts, stabilizing her body while she reaches for an object). She became quickly fatigued. On the other hand, Ruth's process skills were effective. Notably, she could think through how to complete some aspects of the activities by adapting to her motor skills deficits.

Ruth overestimated her abilities (or ignored risk), which led her to make decisions to do things beyond her current abilities, threatening her safety. Ruth justified her choices by saying she will never get better if she doesn't try things. Ruth found it extremely painful to face her limitations and felt that therapy underscored her limitations. She also felt that staff members were overprotective and interfered with her choices and privacy. Ruth was demoralized by the loss of her previous routine and the roles she had as a friend, caretaker, home maintainer, and religious participant.

Given Ruth's limited motor skills and a lack of social support, it would be difficult to facilitate a successful discharge at this stage. She had no family for support. Home health services would not be sufficient to support Ruth with personal care and homemaking activities. Further, the extreme alteration in Ruth's lifestyle would place her emotionally at risk. A likely outcome of discharge against medical advice would be that Ruth would need readmission.

Ruth was a good candidate to continue in rehabilitation for the following reasons: a) her stroke was recent and she was beginning to show motor gains, b) she had strong process skills and could readily learn to problem solve how to perform safely, and c) she was very motivated to return to and remain in her home and had a successful history of independent living.

I shared my reasoning with Ruth and discussed in depth her concerns about staying in the hospital. After much negotiation, Ruth has agreed to an occupational therapy program of 2 weeks with specific goals aimed at a successful discharge home.

As the note illustrates, documentation of the therapist's conceptualization of the client's situation serves to communicate critical information to others and to illustrate the therapist's rationale for action. It is also an excellent way to demonstrate the utility of MOHO concepts to other team members.

Step 4: Identifying Goals and Plans for Client Engagement and Therapeutic Strategies

Goals indicate the kinds of client changes that therapy will aim to achieve. The types of client change identified in Chapter 18 and listed in the Section II Master Table (pages 346–355) will be useful guides for generating therapy goals. Nonetheless, it should be remembered that the types of change listed in the table are not meant to be exhaustive. Therapists may identify other types of change that are indicated by the client's strengths and problems/challenges and the therapist's conceptualization of the client's situation.

Setting goals (and thereby identifying the types of client change that will be targeted in therapy) links directly to the next part of this step, which is to plan what will happen in therapy to achieve the goals. This consists of a description of:

- The client occupational engagement that will take place in therapy to enable change
- The strategies the therapist will use to support the client's change.

As discussed in Chapter 18, the central factor driving client change will be the occupational forms in which the client engages. Therefore, therapy always involves consideration of the occupational engagement that will occur during therapy and/or how therapy will guide the client to engage in occupational forms outside the context of therapy.

As discussed in Chapter 19, therapists can employ a variety of strategies that support client engagement and the kinds of changes therapy is intended to achieve. Both of these aspects of the therapy plan will need to be monitored and modified in step 5 as therapy unfolds. Nonetheless, it is important that the therapist begin with a plan for what will occur in therapy to support goal attainment.

Identifying the types of client engagement and therapist strategies that will help achieve the planned

changes can be facilitated by referring to Client Occupational Engagements and Therapist Strategies columns of the Section II Master Table (pages 346–355). These contain guidelines for these two elements of therapy that correspond to types of change listed in the table. Once again, these should be taken only as general guidelines, and the therapist should be thoughtful and creative in undertaking this step.

COMMUNICATING AND COLLABORATING WITH CLIENTS TO GENERATE THERAPY GOALS AND PLANS

Successful therapy depends on a client's willingness to accept the goals and plans of therapy. Therefore, the therapist must communicate and collaborate with the client to identify the intended goals and therapy plan. How this is done will depend on the client and must be built around the client's perceptions and desires.

Studies have shown that clients do not know about or agree with the therapist's goals. For example, one survey found that therapists routinely developed goals without involvement of the client (Neistadt, 1995). Another study indicated that goals tend to be formulated by health professionals and not owned by the client. (Playford et al., 2000). Consequently, therapists need to be vigilant to assure that goal setting is accomplished, to the extent possible, in collaboration with clients.

Enabling the client to see the relevance of goal setting is a common challenge. Not all clients will understand or appreciate what goals are and why they are important (Playford et al., 2000). When a client is not familiar with goal setting and why it can be helpful, the therapist should discuss with the client the importance and utility of therapy goals. The following are some reasons that can be shared with clients:

- Selecting goals will give you something to aim for
- Goals can allow you to focus on the positive state you want, not the problem state you are in
- Goals can help you monitor your own progress and achievement
- Clearly stated goals provide focus for therapy and an avenue for communicating between client and therapist during the therapy process.

Once the client has an understanding of why goals might be helpful, the therapist can facilitate the client's participation in goal setting.

Clients who understand the value of goals should be encouraged to generate their own goals. Clients often set different goals than their therapist or guardians (McGavin, 1998; Missiuna & Pollack, 2000). By allowing clients to initiate ideas for goals, the therapist ensures that goals will be relevant to the client's perspective. Moreover, goals that result from a collaboration with clients result in better outcomes (Linton, Jannert, & Overmeer, 1999). Of course, for many clients, negotiating goals will require a substantial help and support from therapists. Some clients will require the therapist to lead the process. The following example illustrates a collaborative approach to establishing goals and therapy plans in a way that respects and responds to the client.

Elsie

Elsie was a 45-year-old client in a mental health setting. When she discussed what she saw as her major problem with the therapist, she referred to it as lacking the "ommpphh" to do what she wanted and needed to do. The client's concept of "ommpphh" was clearly how she thought about her problem. In fact, she even expressed it in a poem, entitled "my get-up-and-go has got up and gone." Because this is how she saw the problem, she saw therapy as a way to get her "ommpphh" back.

Elsie's occupational therapist collaborated with her in setting goals for therapy, one of which they agreed would be: Improve Elsie's "ommpphh"! What the therapist appreciated was the necessity of validating and reflecting in the goal how her client perceived her own difficulty. Moreover, because Elsie's perspectives were validated, she was much more motivated to engage in therapy.

Making sure that goals reflect client perspectives becomes even more important for clients who are unable to advocate and negotiate for themselves. For example, when working with nonverbal clients, it is still possible and important to consider the client's perspective and desires. This can best be accomplished through careful assessment of the client's volition. Previous chapters have discussed methods for gathering information on the client's volition. An understanding of a client's volition enables therapists to create goals that will have meaning for their clients even when those clients have difficulty letting others know about their occupational needs and wants.

The Need to Set and Document Measurable Goals

One of the keys to being able to evaluate therapy outcomes (step 6) is to assure that, in step 4, one has created and documented measurable goals. Therapists often omit writing goals in documentation (Neistadt, 1995), which hampers identification of the outcomes of therapy. One common reason put forward for not documenting goals is that all the client's goals are the same and writing them down is duplicative. However, client-centered practice requires individualized goals. Another reason put forward is the lack of time. However, without documentation of occupational therapy goals and outcomes, there is no evidence of the value of service. Routinely creating and documenting measurable goals is a fundamental obligation of every therapist.

There are many ways to structure measurable goals for therapeutic interventions. Unfortunately, when therapists do set goals, they are often vague (Neistadt, 1995). In what follows, we suggest how to set goals with necessary specificity.

Goals can be long or short term. Long-term goals should be specific about the overall outcome of occupational therapy and are most useful for determining therapy outcomes. Because they project a greater distance into the future, they may need to be adjusted as the therapy unfolds.

Long-term goals are accomplished through a series of short-term goals. Typically, short-term goals imply a sense of sequencing and priority (Trombly, 1995). Short-term goals can mean setting daily goals in an acute care setting. Short-term goals enable the therapist to better review therapy (part of step 5) and de-

> *Routinely creating and documenting measurable goals is a fundamental obligation of every therapist.*

termine that appropriate progress is being made. Creating both long-term and short-term goals is helpful because it provides an understanding of what is being worked on immediately and what overall outcome is desired.

To be measurable, a goal should contain:

- Action: What the client will do to demonstrate that the occupational goal has been achieved
- Setting: The specific setting where the client will do it (e.g., within the ward or within the client's home environment)
- Degree: The circumstances under which the client will do it (e.g., independently, with physical support, with verbal cueing, using adaptive equipment, using compensatory techniques)
- Timeframe: The timeframe within which the client will be able to do it.

A goal with all these elements clearly indicates what therapy aims to accomplish and provides a way of determining if clients are achieving their goals. *Table 20-2* provides examples of possible measurable goals. The table is not exhaustive, and the goals are not meant to be exemplars of possible goals but may be used as a starting point for developing your own measurable goals.

As an example, we will use this framework to create measurable goals for Elsie, who was discussed earlier. The therapist discussed with Elsie how she defined "ommpphh." Potentially, many issues affecting Elsie's "ommpphh" could be identified (e.g., it could be a motivational problem or a problem with the skill of endurance). On discussion, Elsie identified that she had difficulty completing her occupations because of reduced physical endurance. Therefore Elsie's long-term goal of increasing her "ommpphh" yielded the following short-term, measurable goal that was entered into her chart:

> Within 4 weeks, Elsie will exhibit enough endurance skill to complete her personal care and homemaker routine within her home environment independently.

Below are two additional examples of client scenarios and goals related to MOHO concepts. Each goal presented contains elements associated with a measurable goal.

Beatrice and Jack

Personal Causation Goal

Following a stroke, a client, Beatrice, stated that she was anxious about her occupational performance. Having assessed Beatrice's motor and process skills, the occupational therapist noted from other informal observations that Beatrice's personal causation was leading her to avoid choosing to do things that were well within her performance capacity. Consequently, the therapist identified the following goal:

> Within 7 days, Beatrice will improve her personal causation as evidenced by independently choosing to engage in personal and domestic occupational forms in line with her performance capacities in the ward setting.

Role-Related Goal

Jack, a 42-year-old client in a community-based work rehabilitation program for persons with psychiatric impairments, reported that he received negative feedback from the supervisor in a business in which he was placed for work training. Discussion with Jack and with the supervisor indicated that Jack was unaware of many of the subtle role-related expectations in the work setting. The therapist concluded that for Jack to competently meet worker role performance demands, he had to identify and internalize appropriate expectations for the worker role in this setting. The following goal was established:

> Following three on-the-job coaching sessions, Jack will independently demonstrate consistent compliance with the expectations of the worker role at his work placement as judged by his supervisor.

Step 5: Implementing and Reviewing Therapy

Implementing therapy involves not only following the plan of action set out in the previous step, but also being vigilant to monitor how therapy is unfolding. As noted above, reviewing short-term goals is an essential part of this step. When the therapist reviews therapy,

TABLE 20-2 Examples of Measurable Goals Corresponding to MOHO Concepts

Volition	• Within [timeframe], [client] will be *able to identify* [number] of occupational form(s) that are significant to his/her occupational life [or role as a xxx] and which are commensurate with his/her current skills and abilities within [setting] independently [degree]
	• Within [timeframe], [client] will be *able to perform* in [name occupational form] in line with his/her performance capacity without a verbal report/observation of low confidence within [setting] independently [degree]
	• Within [timeframe], [client] will *make the choice* to engage in [name occupational form] having *identified* this as significant to his/her [successful performance of/or as a step in the progress towards] his/her performance as a [name role] within [setting] with [degree] support
	• Within [timeframe], [client] will be able to demonstrate *an ability to perform* in [occupational form] in line with his/her performance capacity within [setting] independently [degree]
	• Within [timeframe], [client] will be able to demonstrate *an ability to choose* to ask for help and use equipment where necessary within [setting] independently [degree]
	• Within [timeframe], [client] will state he/she feels like he/she *is in control* of the occupational outcome while successfully *performing* in [name the occupational forms], within [setting] with [degree] support
	• Within [timeframe], [client], will be able to *perform in valuable* occupational forms using adaptive equipment, within [setting] with [degree] support.
	• Within [timeframe], [client] will be able to *identify* [number] occupational goals, with [degree] support within [setting]
	• Within [timeframe], [OT] will be able to *identify* [number], occupational goals, that are based on the OT's understanding [through observation/proxy reports] of the client's occupational needs and wants within [setting]. (Useful with non-verbal clients).
	• Within [timeframe], [client], will be able to *identify* and *choose* to engage in the needed occupational performance for goal achievement [or state goals], with [degree] support within [setting]
	• Within [timeframe], [client], will be able to *sustain performance* in [name occupational action] involved in reaching their goal, with [degree] support within [setting].
	• Within [timeframe], [client], will be able to *identify* [number] interest to pursue, this will be achieved with [degree] support within [setting]
	• Within [timeframe], [client], will be able to *perform in* [number] interests, with [degree] support within [setting]
Habituation	• Within [timeframe], [client] will be able to *identify* the responsibilities for roles that are valuable and meaningful to the person, this will be achieved with [degree] support within [setting]
	• Within [timeframe], [client] will be able to *plan & meet* the responsibilities for roles that are valuable and meaningful to the person, this will be achieved with [degree] support within [setting]

(continued)

TABLE 20-2 (continued)

	• Within [timeframe], [client] will be able to *identify* roles that have the potential to be valuable and meaningful to the person, this will be achieved with [degree] sup-port within [setting]
	• Within [timeframe], [client] will be able to *practice* & develop a habit pattern that will support achievement of a single occupational form, this will be achieved with [degree] support within [setting]
	• Within [timeframe], [client] will be able to *practice* & develop a habit pattern that will incorporate a new object and/or new way of completing an occupational form, this will be achieved with [degree] support within [setting]
	• Within [timeframe], [client] will be able to *practice* & develop a habit pattern that will support achievement role performance, this will be achieved with [degree] support within [setting]
Skill	• Within [timeframe], [client] will be able to perform within [name the occupational form] using [name skills] within [setting], independently [degree]
	• Within [timeframe], [client] will be able to perform in [name the occupational form] using adapted techniques to support lack of skill within [setting], independently [degree]
Performance Capacity	• Within [timeframe], [client] will be able to incorporate damaged/estranged parts of the body into completion of occupational forms, within [setting] independently [degree]
	• Within [timeframe], [client] will be able to manage symptoms while engaged in [name the occupational forms] within [setting] independently [degree]
Environment	• Within [timeframe], [client] will be able to *perform* in the occupational forms they need and/or want to be able to do within [state the physical space] [setting], independently [degree]
	• Within [timeframe], [client] will be able to *perform* in the occupational form using adapted objects or new objects within [setting], independently [degree]
	• Within [timeframe], [relative] will be able to demonstrate an appropriate level of skill in supporting the client within their [setting] environment, independently [degree]
	• Within [timeframe], [relative] will be able to understand the client's abilities and limitations within their [setting] environment, independently [degree]
	• Within [timeframe], [client] will be able to *perform* in [name the occupational form] within their physical and social [setting] environment, independently [degree]
Key: The therapist should include the unique characteristics of the client within brackets.	

new information may emerge, which can result in one or more of the following:

• Confirmation of the therapist's conceptualization of the client's situation
• Changes in the therapist's conceptualization of the client's situation
• Confirmation of the utility of the planned client oc-cupational engagement and therapist strategies
• Modification of goals and/or planned client occupa-tional engagement and therapist strategies.

To the extent that therapy unfolds as anticipated, the therapist's conceptualization of the client's situa-tion was most likely accurate and the goals and plan of therapy were appropriate. However, therapists should always expect that at least part of what happens in therapy will be unexpected. When things do not turn out as expected, the therapist returns to earlier steps of generating questions, selecting methods to gather in-formation, conceptualizing the client's situation, set-ting goals, and establishing plans.

Once again, it is important to continue communication with the client as therapy unfolds. Feedback to the clients concerning their progress helps to solidify commitment to therapy. When clients have attained goals, it is important to recognize their accomplishment and to reinforce the efforts they have put forward to accomplish them. Honest discussion with the client about new problems or lack of progress is equally important to maintain trust in the therapeutic relationship. When clients fail to reach goals, the information should be shared in a supportive context that examines the reasons for failure and facilitates the problem-solving necessary to formulate attainable goals or to assure future goal attainment.

DOCUMENTING CLIENT PROGRESS IN THERAPY

As the therapist reviews therapy, it is important to maintain an ongoing record of therapeutic interventions and their outcomes. A central element of such documentation is reporting progress on short-term goal attainment. If the guidelines offered for measurable goals are followed, the therapist will already have decided what information to gather, when to gather it, and what criteria to apply to decide if the client has attained short-term goals.

For instance, consider the two examples offered above. In the case of Beatrice, the therapist would use informal observation 1 week from the time the goal was established to observe Beatrice's choices of personal care and domestic occupations on the ward. Her criteria for goal attainment is that Beatrice is able to independently make choices to do things in line with her skills.

In Jack's case, the therapist did not specify a given time but indicated that the evaluation is to follow three job-coaching sessions. According to the goal, the information to be collected is a report from Jack's supervisor and the criterion of success is that Jack shows consistent compliance with worker role expectations. As these two examples readily illustrate, careful work of creating measurable goals will make the process of collecting information to determine goal attainment relatively straightforward.

A variety of methods of reporting progress are used, but the most common is through progress notes in the client's chart or record. SOAP notes are commonly used. SOAP is an acronym for the four components of the note:

- Subjective information
- Objective information
- Assessment results
- Plan (Kettenbach, 1995).

For example, the following is a SOAP note for Beatrice.

S "I feel more confident to do things now."

O Beatrice was seen for 30 minutes for training in personal occupational forms at her bedside. Her performance capacities and how they matched to the demands of dressing were discussed with her. When coached to initiate dressing, Beatrice was observed to independently dress her upper extremities, which was in line with her performance capacity. Beatrice spontaneously asked for support with dressing (donning underwear, shoes, and pants) that could potentially threaten her safety if she attempted to complete them independently.

A Compared to previous sessions, Beatrice appeared more relaxed in both discussing and engaging in personal occupational forms. Her ability to recognize occupational forms that were within her capabilities has improved over the past week. This improves the likelihood that she can be safely discharged home.

P Continue Beatrice's engagement in personal occupational forms. Plan a home visit before setting the discharge date to assess Beatrice's ability within her home environment.

The following is a SOAP note for Jack:

S "I feel I am doing okay."

O Jack's time cards show that he has completed a full work timetable. Jack's work supervisor stated that Jack has improved and has shown several behaviors consistent with his worker role. However, Jack has been late four out of five days and has been frequently observed interrupting the work of colleagues with stories unrelated to the job.

A Jack appeared to be happy with his progress following the coaching sessions. He will benefit from a review of time management strategies to foster his ability to get to work on time and a discussion of how his tendency to interrupt coworkers impacts the team. A behavioral contract may be useful in changing Jack's behavior if his tendency to disturb coworkers persists after the problem has been addressed.

P Extend the goal timeframe and discuss supervisor's feedback with Jack.

Step 6: Determining and Documenting the Outcomes of Therapy

The final step in therapy is to assess client outcomes. By collecting information to determine whether clients have attained goals, therapists can determine and document the effectiveness of occupational therapy. Occupational therapy, in particular, needs documentation of service outcomes (Christiansen, 1996; Foto, 1996; Rogers & Holm, 1994). Although practitioners strive to make a unique contribution to important health and quality of life outcomes, there is little documentation of occupational therapy outcomes (Ellenberg, 1996; Gutman, 1998; Wood, 1998).

Outcomes can be determined by evaluating whether the client has achieved the stated short-term and long-term goals. When goals were not achieved, it is important to document the reason for the lack of success. The following is an example of this kind of documentation.

Beatrice: Part 2

Beatrice attained four of five of her short-term goals within the estimated timeframe. The fifth short-term goal, to evaluate Beatrice within her home environment, was being planned and would have provided the information needed to attain the long-term goals of successful discharge home. Beatrice, however, developed a chest infection and became ill. She will be reassessed when she is well enough for therapy, and goals will be reset.

Many MOHO evaluations (detailed in Chapters 13 through 16) are designed to be outcome measures and are appropriate to use before and after an intervention. In many cases, they provide clinical occupational profiles that can be compared to understand how a client has changed as a result of therapy. Outcomes of the client's progress can, therefore, be described in terms of change as measured by one of the assessments. Below is a note of the outcome of Rachel's therapy. Rachel had identified that she was having difficulty engaging in her community-based occupational forms. Her difficulties were due to deficits in her communication/interaction skills.

Rachel: Part 2

Rachel was involved in an occupational therapy program twice a week for 3 weeks that focused on engaging her in graded social occupational forms within her community. The therapist actively structured situations, coached Rachel, and provided feedback and advice. Rachel is now able to focus her conversations appropriately to the ongoing social action. Rachel effectively uses adaptive strategies to control the pace and volume of her speech when anxious or distressed. Rachel's ability to be attentive to the meaning of others' behavior and to respect their needs still requires coaching (minimal verbal cueing). The therapist recommended and helped Rachel arrange to attend community groups with a friend, who can provide her with these cues as needed. Rachel is now regularly attending these community groups with the support of her friend. Both Rachel and her friend report satisfaction with Rachel's ability to engage in social occupational forms.

Conclusion

This chapter discussed how a therapist can use MOHO theory to plan, implement, and evaluate therapy. Guidelines and examples of communicating MOHO concepts to clients and others (e.g., family, caregivers, peer professionals) were presented. Finally, how to go about documenting MOHO-related goals, processes, and outcomes of therapy was discussed.

As noted at the outset, this chapter builds on and directs the reader to use numerous resources, including the preceding chapters of this section and the Section II Master Table that follows this chapter. It should be apparent that this chapter is designed to be a resource to which therapists can turn. Because it attempts to synthesize much of the previously presented information and place it in a practical framework, the reader should find it a useful ongoing resource.

References

American Psychiatric Association. (2000). *Diagnostic and statistical manual of mental disorders* (4th ed., text revision). Washington, DC: Author.

Christiansen, C. (1996). Managed care: Opportunities and challenges for occupational therapy in the emerging systems of the 21st century. *American Journal of Occupational Therapy, 50* (6), 409–412.

Commission on Practice, American Occupational Therapy Association. (2001). *Occupational Therapy Practice Framework.* Unpublished Working Paper.

Ellenberg, D. B. (1996). Outcomes research: The history, debate and implications for the field of occupational therapy. *American Journal of Occupational Therapy, 50,* 435–441.

Foto, M. (1996). Outcome studies: The what, why, how, and when. *American Journal of Occupational Therapy, 50,* 87–88.

Gutman, S.A. (1998). The domain of function: Who's got it? Who's competing for it? *American Journal of Occupational Therapy, 52,* 684–689.

Kettenbach, G. (1995). *Writing SOAP notes* (2nd ed.). Philadelphia: FA Davis.

Linton, S., Jannert, M., & Overmeer, T. (1999). Whose goals should guide? A comparison of two forms of goal formation on operant activity training. *Journal of Occupational Rehabilitation, 9* (2), 97–105.

McGavin, H. (1998). Planning rehabilitation: A comparison of issues for parents and adolescents. *Physical and Occupational Therapy in Paediatrics, 18* (1), 69–82.

Missiuna, C., & Pollack, N. (2000). Perceived efficacy and goal setting in young children. *Canadian Journal of Occupational Therapy, 67* (2), 101–109.

Neistadt, M. (1995). Methods of assessing clients' priorities: A survey of adult physical dysfunction settings. *American Journal of Occupational Therapy, 49* (5), 428–436.

Playford, E., Dawson, L., Limbert, V., Smith, M., Ward, C., & Wells, R. (2000). Goal-setting in rehabilitation: Report of a workshop to explore professionals' perceptions of goal setting. *Clinical Rehabilitation, 14* (5), 491–496.

Rogers, J. C., & Holm, M. B. (1994). Accepting the challenge of outcomes research: Examining effectiveness of occupational therapy practice. *American Journal of Occupational Therapy, 48,* 871–876.

Sumsion T., & Smyth G. (2000). Barriers to client centeredness and their resolution. *Canadian Journal of Occupational Therapy, 67,* 15–21.

Trombly, C. A. (Ed.). (1995). *Occupational therapy for physical dysfunction* (4th ed.). Baltimore: Williams & Wilkins.

Wood, W. (1998). It is jump time for occupational therapy. *American Journal of Occupational Therapy, 52,* 403–411.

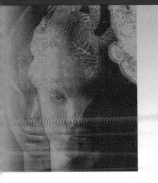

Section II Master Table

- **Kirsty Forsyth**
- **Gary Kielhofner**

The information in this master table is designed to stimulate thought. It is not exhaustive and it is not intended to be prescriptive. Further, it should be used in a flexible manner and should always be adapted to the unique characteristics of each client. Understanding this table requires that one read the rest of the text. Chapters 11, 18, 19, and 20 refer directly to this table.

Questions	Strengths	Problems/Challenges	Changes	Client Occupational Engagement	Therapist Strategies
PERSONAL CAUSATION					

Questions

- What is this person's view of personal capacity and effectiveness and how does it affect the choice, experience, interpretation, and anticipation of doing things
- What abilities or limitations stand out in this person's view of self
- Is the sense of capacity accurate
- Is this person aware of abilities and limitations
- Does this person feel in control of her or his own thoughts, feelings, and actions and the occupational consequences of these
- Does this person expect to achieve desired outcomes
- Does this person have confidence, anxiety, or other feelings in the face of change

Strengths

- Aware of capacity (strengths and limitations)
- Ability to choose occupational forms within capacity and take on appropriate challenges and responsibilities
- Adequate confidence to make decisions about engagement in occupational forms
- Seeks out appropriate occupational challenges based on an adequate knowledge of capacity
- Seeks assistance appropriately and makes use of environmental adaptations
- Feels in control of occupational performance
- Expects success within occupation
- Reasonable expectations of success in occupational performance situations
- Confident to face occupational performance demands
- Ability to sustain effort to attain occupational goals/complete occupational forms

Problems/Challenges

- Lack of awareness of capacity (strengths or limitations)
- Underestimation of abilities leading to:
  - Depending unnecessarily on others
  - Avoiding occupational forms commensurate with performance capacity, leading to reduced occupational performance
  - Failing to seek out occupational challenges that would promote learning/growth in skill
- Overestimation of abilities leading to:
  - Taking unnecessary risks by seeking challenges that are higher than performance capacity, resulting in poor occupational performance, danger, stress, damage, or injury
  - Failure to seek assistance appropriately or make use of needed environmental adaptations
- Feelings of lack of control over occupational performance leading to anxiety (fear of failure) within occupations
- Poor frustration tolerance leading to disengagement from occupational forms
- Poor concentration leading to difficulty in completing occupational forms
- Expectation of failure in occupational performance
- Avoidance of performance, failure to set occupational goals or lack of adequate effort to complete occupations, or lack of follow through on occupations/goals

Changes

- Enhance understanding of occupational capacities (strengths and limitations)
- Focus attention to more accurately note how limitations and assets affect occupational performance
- Develop emotional acceptance of limitations and pride in occupational abilities
- Reduce unnecessary feelings of dependence, resentment, or guilt associated with loss of participation
- Increase facility in choosing to do occupational forms consistent with capacity
- Build up confidence to approach occupational forms within capacity
- Increase knowledge and acceptance of using adaptive aids and/or environmental modifications to augment capacity
- Increase willingness to ask for help when needed within an occupational form
- Reduce anxiety and fear of failure in occupational performance
- Build up confidence to face occupational performance demands
- Improve facility to sustain effort for attaining goals and/or completing occupational performance
- Widen expectation of success in occupational performance
- Extend readiness to take on occupational challenges and responsibilities
- Increase sense of efficacy in occupational life circumstances

Client Occupational Engagement

- *Commit* to overcoming fear in occupational performance
- *Explore* alternative ways of doing an occupational form that compensate for performance capacity limitations
- *Re-examine* previously held beliefs about effectiveness in achieving occupational outcomes
- *Re-examine* anxieties and fears in the light of new performance experiences
- *Identify* occupational forms within/beyond performance capacity
- *Negotiate* an appropriate level of risk within occupational performance
- *Choose* to do relevant and meaningful things that are within performance capacity
- *Choose* to engage in occupational forms that challenge the person
- *Sustain* performance in occupational forms despite anxiety
- *Practice* asking for and using help appropriately
- *Practice* performance to reinforce sense of efficacy

Therapist Strategies

- *Structure* environment to allow clients to take risks safely
- *Validate* client's thoughts and feelings concerning performance capacities
- *Validate* how difficult it can be to do things that provoke anxiety
- *Identify* client's strengths and weaknesses in occupational performance
- *Give feedback* to client about match/mismatch between choice of occupational forms and performance capacity
- *Give feedback* to support a positive reinterpretation of their experience of engaging in an occupation
- *Advise* client to do relevant and meaningful things that match performance capacity
- *Advise* client to engage in occupational forms within performance capacity to assure high degree of success
- *Encourage* client to sustain effort in difficult occupational circumstances
- *Encourage* client to use performance capacities in the face of anxiety
- *Physically support* when necessary to ensure success
- *Coach* when appropriate, to ensure success

Questions	Strengths	Problems/Challenges	Changes	Client Occupational Engagement	Therapist Strategies
VALUES					

• What is the organizing theme in this person's sense of values
• What things are most important for this person to do
• What standards or other criteria does this person use to judge his or her performance
• Are the values to which this person ascribes really his or her own
• Can this person prioritize among what is important
• Is this person clear as to what his or her values are
• How do this person's values match or conflict with his or her performance capacity
• Does this person hold values that lead to adaptive occupational choices
• Does this person's values match or conflict with social and cultural norms
	• Identifies and engages in personally meaningful and valuable occupations
	• Readily sorts out what is most important in a situation
	• Employs realistic standards to evaluate self and others
	• Identifies values as own
	• Can readily identify and prioritize among goals
	• Can pursue and realize goals
	• Has values/standards consistent with capacity
	• Values lead to positive choices
	• Has values matched to context
		• Difficulty identifying and engaging in personally meaningful and valuable occupational forms
		• Difficulty sorting out what is most important in an occupational situation
		• Employs unrealistically high or low standards to evaluate self and others
		• Ascribes to values defined by others rather than self
		• Inability/difficulty identifying and prioritizing among occupational goals
		• Inability to pursue and realize occupational goals
		• Values/standards inconsistent with performance capacity
		• Values lead to negative occupational choices
		• Values conflict with context
			• Increase perception of self as realizing important values
			• Increase satisfaction from realizing occupational goals
			• Increase ease of identifying what is most important in an occupational situation
			• Develop more realistic values/standards for assessing self and others
			• Strengthen sense of what is most personally significant within occupational life
			• Increase ability to identity and prioritize among occupational goals
			• Increase ability to pursue and realize occupational goals
			• Increase tendency to sustain efforts to realize occupational goals
			• Adjust values/standards to match performance capacity
			• Develop values that support positive occupational choices
			• Develop values consistent with context (or find context consistent with values)
				• *Explore* occupational forms/environments embodying different values/standards
				• *Re-examine* current values in light of:
				  • Current performance capacities
				  • Environmental context
				• *Identify:*
				  • Appropriate standards for self and others
				  • Values consistent with capacity
				  • Realistic long- and short-term goals
				• *Choose:*
				  • To engage in valued/meaningful occupational forms
				  • Among occupational goals and values
				• *Negotiate* selection/application of occupational goals/values/standards
				• *Commit* to:
				  • Realistic occupational goals
				  • Attainable standards
				  • Plan for occupational goal attainment
					• *Validate* client's value system as important driver of the therapeutic plan
					• *Identify* conflicts between values and:
					  • Performance capacity
					  • Environmental values
					• *Give feedback* on how client's value standards:
					  • Do not seem personally cogent
					  • Lead to self-devaluation
					  • Set up unattainable standards/occupational goals
					• *Identify* realistic long- and short-term occupational goals with/on behalf of the client
					• *Negotiate* with client concerning:
					  • Values and standards to be applied in therapy
					  • Priorities of occupational goals
					• *Advise* client to:
					  • Select occupational performance and participation that reflect personal meaning
					  • Seek out environments consistent with occupational goals
					  • Change standards to be more consistent with performance capacities
					• *Structure* therapeutic environment to:
					  • Facilitate setting, planning, and realizing occupational goals
					  • Allow exposure to appropriate reference groups and role models
					• *Give feedback* on how the client is moving toward occupational goals

Questions	Strengths	Problems/Challenges	Changes	Client Occupational Engagement	Therapist Strategies
INTERESTS					
• Can this person identify personal interests • What occupations does this person enjoy doing • What are the aspects of doing that this person enjoys most (e.g., physical challenge, intellectual stimulation, social contact, and aesthetic experience) • Does this person do the things he or she enjoys • Is anything interfering with this person's feeling of pleasure and satisfaction in performance	• Able to identify interests • Able to pursue interests	• Inability to identify interests • No/limited feeling of attraction • No/limited pleasure in doing things • Disengagement from occupational forms • Inability to pursue interests leading to feelings of boredom • Feelings of frustration at lack of engagement in interests	• Changes in attraction, participation, and enjoyment/satisfaction • Greater desire to do things • Increased willingness to chose to engage in interests • Increased participation in things of interest • Greater sense of enjoyment/satisfaction in doing things	• *Commit* to developing interests • *Explore* opportunities to identify interests • *Re-examine* past interests • *Identify* potential interests • *Choose* between potential interests • *Plan* strategies of how to pursue interests • *Perform* interests • *Sustain* performance in interests • *Practice* pursuing interests	• *Structure* the therapeutic environment to offer ongoing opportunities and resources to identify interests and to support engagement in interests • *Negotiate* which interests will be the focus of therapy • *Validate* person's attraction to occupational forms • *Give feedback* as required while the person is engaging in the occupational form • *Identify* the essence of the attraction to the old interests if the person no longer has the skill to engage in that particular occupational form • *Identify* resources in the person's social environment to support identified interest • *Encourage* continued engagement in interests when clients get discouraged • *Advise* clients to readapt previous interests, explore new interests • *Coach* person to attend to pleasure in action

Questions	Strengths	Problems/Challenges	Changes	Client Occupational Engagement	Therapist Strategies
ROLES					
• What is the overall pattern of role involvement of this person	• Aware of responsibilities associated with success in various roles	• Poor awareness of responsibilities associated with success in various roles (poor role scripts)	Changes in identification with roles:	• *Commit* to altering roles	• *Structure* therapeutic environment to provide opportunities to discuss roles and their related expectations
• Does this person have roles that impact positively on his or her identity, use of time, and involvement in social groups	• Able to meet multiple role expectations	• Difficulty meeting multiple role expectations (role conflict)	• Improved awareness of responsibilities associated with success in various roles (poor role scripts)	• *Commit* to behaviors required to make changes in role scripts or role repertoire	• *Structure* environment to provide opportunities to engage in the behavior required by the role to allow for internalizing the role script and developing a supportive routine
• Is the person over- or under-involved in roles?	• Able to structure day through role involvement	• Difficulty structuring the day due to lack of roles (role loss)	• Increased perception of self as involved with roles that are necessary, desirable, developmentally appropriate	• *Explore* potential strategies for altering responsibilities and structure of the day	
• How important is each role to the person	• Positively identifies with roles	• Does not identify with roles	• Increased identification with self-enhancing disability-related roles (e.g., self-care manager, disability advocate/activist)	• *Explore* role responsibilities for identified valued roles	• *Validate* the challenges around role change and assuming responsibilities
• Can this person meet the obligations of each role			Changes in enactment of roles:	• *Re-examine* role responsibilities	• *Give feedback* on appropriateness of their understanding of role responsibilities
• Are collective role requirements too few, too demanding, or make conflicting demands on this person			• Increased effectiveness in meeting multiple role expectations through negotiation of realistic role responsibilities	• *Identify* valued roles	• *Identify* appropriate role behaviors or role conflicts
			• Improved routine due to role change	• *Negotiate* range and content of roles	• *Advise* the client to make choices (volition) around reducing their responsibilities
			• Perception of self in a more manageable and fulfilling number of roles	• *Choose* to prioritize specific valued roles to allow for reduced role conflict	• *Advise* the person to identify other ways of meeting their responsibilities that do not require time from them; discuss/negotiate roles and their related expectations
			• Improved routine due to role acquisition	• *Perform* behaviors consistent with role responsibility	• *Advise* the client to leave roles behind or to enter into new roles
				• *Practice* behaviors required for enactment of role	• *Coach* person in role enactment
					• *Encourage* people to make choices to engage in new roles (or old roles in an adapted way, e.g., with configuration of new role responsibilities)

Questions	Strengths	Problems/Challenges	Changes	Client Occupational Engagement	Therapist Strategies
HABITS					
• Does this person have well-established habits • What kind of routine does this person have and is it effective • What is this person's characteristic style of performance and is it effective • What quality of life is provided by the habitual routine of this person	• Has a habitual routine that allows for the completion of specific occupational forms • Able to internalize the habitual use of a new object or a new way of completing an occupational form • Routines are organized and allow for the completion of needed collection of occupations	• Difficulty completing a specific occupation due to lack of habitual structure • Difficulty internalizing the habitual use of a new object or a new way of completing an occupation • Disorganized routines that makes it difficult for the person to complete required occupation	• Changes in habits to accommodate an acquired impairment and/or enhance occupational performance and occupational participation • Increased effectiveness in completing a specific occupation due to acquisition/change in habitual way of doing it • Acquisition of a new habit pattern that incorporates a new object and/or new way of completing an occupation (e.g., acquiring a habit for using adaptive equipment or acquiring the habit of energy conservation in completing typical daily tasks) • Increased organization of daily routines that improve effectiveness in managing role-related responsibilities	• *Commit* to changing habits • *Explore* ways of organizing self and environment to support habit formation • *Re-examine* usefulness of previous habits structure • *Identify* new habitual ways of completing occupational forms • *Negotiate* options of altering methods of completing occupational forms or organizing occupational forms into alternative routine • *Choose* between different ways of doing or routines of doing • *Perform* one or more occupational form in a consistent manner to support habit formation • *Practice* actions that make up the intended new habit	• *Structure* therapeutic environment to support habit training within an occupation and/or routine; offer repetitive opportunities to engage in the routine • *Structure* usual environment with structures to support habitual routine, e.g., have a person in the social environment reinforce habits • *Negotiate* options of altering methods of completing occupational forms or organizing occupational forms into alternative routine • *Validate* that it is hard to change habits • *Identify* new habitual ways of completing occupational forms • *Advise* new habits around a particular occupational form or routine • *Coach* by giving consistent verbal prompts to reinforce habit • *Encourage* sustained effort until the person is able to complete the occupational form and/or routine

Questions	Strengths	Problems/Challenges	Changes	Client Occupational Engagement	Therapist Strategies
PERFORMANCE CAPACITY					
• Are there underlying impairments of performance capacities • What is the experience of the impairment and its implications for function being remedied or compensated for • Do any experiences interfere with this person's occupational performance and how so • What are the consequences of sensory, motor, or other capacities for this person's experience of performing occupational forms • How do experiences (e.g., pain, fatigue, dizziness, confusion, or altered bodily perceptions) influence this person's occupational performance	• Able to incorporate damaged/estranged parts of the body into occupational forms • Able to manage altered bodily experiences	• Difficulty incorporating damaged/estranged parts of the body into occupational performance • Negative experiences engaging in occupational forms due to altered bodily experiences (e.g., sensations, hallucinations)	• Develop new ways of attending from and to the body • Incorporate altered/estranged parts of the body and necessary new prosthetic/orthotic/adaptive devices into self and into task performance • Increase feeling of how to do things with an altered body or bodily capacity • Increase understanding and better management of such things as altered bodily sensations, hallucinations, pain, fatigue, pain, and altered perception to minimize interference with occupational performance	• *Commit* to changing performance capacity and/or to adapting for loss of performance capacity • *Explore* new ways of incorporating damaged/estranged parts of body • *Identify* strategies of how to manage altered bodily experiences • *Choose* new methods to complete an occupational form • *Perform* successfully by engaging in occupations incorporating damaged/estranged parts of body • *Practice* to ensure successful ongoing completion of occupational forms incorporating damaged/estranged parts of body	• *Validate* how difficult it can be to have a damaged or altered body • *Structure* the therapeutic environment to allow the client to experience using the body within meaningful occupational forms • *Advise* the alteration of daily habits using energy conservation techniques and written and verbal cues • *Coach* the person in the use of new objects and adapted methods of completing occupational forms • *Coach* the person by verbal cueing to overcome subjective experiences of the body • *Provide* physical supports when needed to support lack of performance capacity • *Encourage* the client when he or she is engaging in occupational forms; this encouragement should be from a highly empathetic other who is attentive to understanding the lived body experience • *Encourage* when using adaptive strategies

Questions	Strengths	Problems/Challenges	Changes	Client Occupational Engagement	Therapist Strategies
SKILLS					
• Does this person have adequate motor/process/ communication and interaction skill ability	• Has adequate motor/process/ communication and interaction skills to allow the client to engage in occupational forms	• Difficulty with motor/process and/or communication and interaction skills while performing an occupation	• Increases in skill within occupational performance by: • Acquiring new information that enhances skill • Learning a strategy that results in increased skill • Learning to use more adaptive skills to compensate for weaker skills (e.g., using process skills to make up for lack of motor skills) • Compensation for immutable impairments of performance capacity through learning to capitalize on changes in the environment (space, objects, forms, and groups)	• *Commit* to improving or compensating for lack of skill • *Explore* possible solution to skill deficit • *Re-examine* previous skill ability • *Identify* new ways of using current skill or adapting for lack of skill effectively that are acceptable and maintain the meaning of the occupational form • *Negotiate* solutions to difficulties with therapist when possible • *Choose* to use alternative methods of supporting skill deficit • *Perform* occupational forms that challenge the person's current skill level • *Practice* using the skill through repeated engagement in occupational forms that challenge the person to use the skill in a graded way • *Practice* substitution of certain skills for others (e.g., using process skills to organize occupation to adapt for the lack of motor skill)	• *Structure* environment to challenge skill ability • *Negotiate* with client around treatment strategies of improving skills or adapting for lack of skill • *Validate* how difficult it can be to have skill deficit • *Advise* the client to: • perform particular occupational forms that will build skill • Introduce new objects to compensate for lack of skill • Change the demands of the occupational form to accommodate the skill deficit; and/or • Change the social environment to support skill deficit (e.g., teach the spouse how to best support the client) • *Coach* by demonstrating, guiding and/or verbally instructing clients to enable them to show skill or effectively adapt for skill deficit and achieve effective performance • Provide physical support due to lack of motor skills • *Encourage* clients to sustain performance when they are showing signs of frustration or difficulty when trying to use their skills or learning how to adapt to skill deficit

Questions	Strengths	Problems/Challenges	Changes	Client Occupational Engagement	Therapist Strategies
PHYSICAL ENVIRONMENT					
• Do the spaces in which the person performs his or her occupations represent physical barriers or supports that impact on performance • Do the objects this person uses support performance • Do the spaces and objects constitute a physical environment with adequate resources for doing things this person needs and wishes to do	• Physical spaces supportive of occupational performance • Objects adequate to support reduced capacity	• Physical space cluttered, unsafe, or otherwise not supporting occupational performance • Naturally occurring objects not supportive of reduced performance capacity	• Change in physical space and objects to facilitate occupational performance and occupational participation through improving ease of access and use, including: • Adaptations to naturally occurring objects or new object	• *Commit* to habit training around altered space and new objects • *Explore* new ways of altering physical space and objects • *Re-examine* physical layout of environment • *Negotiate* possibilities for changing space and objects • *Negotiate* solutions to difficulties with therapist when possible • *Choose* appropriate physical environmental strategies	• *Validate* with the client how difficult and emotional it can be to alter physical spaces and use new objects • *Negotiate* possibilities for changing space and objects • *Advise* about the physical modification of home, school, and/or work space (e.g., moving furniture around to create more physical space) • *Identify* the learned habits that are attached to how the physical space has been set up within the person's environment • *Identify* the physical space required for the successful completion of occupational forms and the consequence of reduction of physical space for any new objects that are placed within the person's environment • *Encourage* person to make changes to physical environment

Questions	Strengths	Problems/Challenges	Changes	Client Occupational Engagement	Therapist Strategies
SOCIAL ENVIRONMENT					
• Does the environment provide appropriate occupational forms in which this person can engage • Do the occupational forms sufficiently challenge this person and provide a sense of worth • Do interactions with others support or inhibit this person's performance • Do the social groups of which this person is a member support the assumption of meaningful roles • What are the reactions of others in occupational behavior settings to this person's disability	• Family has the knowledge and skills that allows them to appropriately support their relative • Routine ways of completing occupational forms are in line with the person's capacities • Supportive social attitudes	• Family/family member do not have enough skill to support their relative's lack of ability • Family member does not have enough knowledge to support their relative's engagement in occupational forms • The usual way of completing an occupation is no longer supported by the ability of the client • Negative social attitudes, discrimination due to disability	• Immediate social group (family) is altered in ways to increase performance and/or participation: • Increase in information about client's needs and desires • Change in expectations for performance/participation • Increase ability of family member to provide support/assistance • Occupational forms performed in various contexts are altered, made available to allow better performance and greater participation: • Social attitudes and behaviors are more conducive to participation • Discrimination and other negative attitudes/practices are reduced • Laws and practices are made more conducive to participation	• *Commit* to altering social environment • *Explore* new social groups and occupational forms • *Re-examine* old social groups and occupational forms • *Identify* altered ways of completing occupational forms • *Identify* people in social environment who can support occupational performance • *Negotiate* with relatives about social environmental needs • *Choose* to complete occupational forms in new ways and/or enter into new social groups • *Practice* altered way of completing occupational form	• *Structure* environment to allow for repeated experience (habit training) until the relative has a high sense of personal causation about helping their relative • *Negotiate* with relatives about social environmental needs • *Validate* difficulties of changing social environment • *Identify* altered ways of having the social environment support the client to engage in occupational forms • *Identify* the relative's volitional process while he or she is helping the client • *Advise* relatives about the occupational forms the client requires support with and the client's abilities and limitations • *Advise* client and relative about available support networks • *Advise* about changing the demands of the occupational form and subsequent practice required for habit training • *Coach* family members in how to support their relative; this may require the family to be involved in the client's treatment sessions

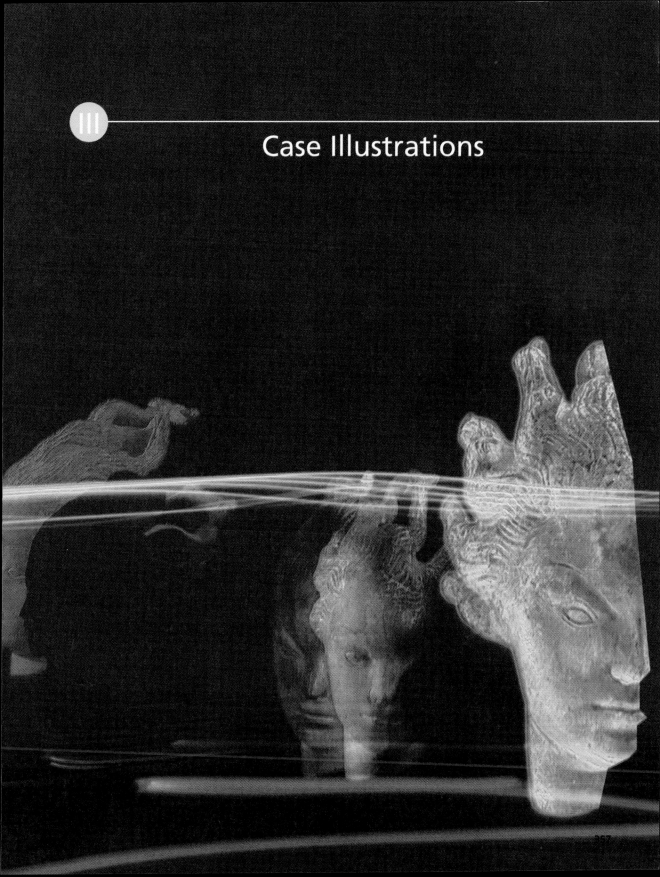

III

Case Illustrations

Introduction to Section III

Section III contains 5 chapters presenting 20 cases that illustrate the application of MOHO. Table STI-1 lists all the cases indicating the client's age, sex, diagnosis or impairment, the context in which therapy took place, and the chapter in which the case occurs. No single case employs every MOHO concept. Indeed, good use of MOHO involves recognizing those concepts that are most useful for a particular client and for deciding a course of intervention. Therefore, the cases should be viewed collectively as illustrations of a range of approaches to applying the model. Each case highlights an aspect of the process of therapy and change that occurs in therapy. For example, one case may have a stronger emphasis on volition, while another stresses performance skills. One case may emphasize the therapeutic reasoning process, while another emphasizes the client's occupational engagement and the strategies the therapist used.

It should be noted that the cases in this section have been partly fictionalized. We have changed some things about each client to preserve the person's confidentiality. Some of the cases are from the previous edition of this book. We still have included them because they are excellent examples. These cases were updated to reflect current concepts, terminology, and assessments. While not all details of each case are literal, each case faithfully presents the nature of the therapist's reasoning, the actual course of intervention, and the client's outcomes.

Case	Age	Sex	Diagnosis/Impairment	Context	Chapter
Alex	30	M	Spinal Cord Injury	Rehabilitation Setting	24
Barbara	33	F	Multiple Sclerosis	Rehabilitation Setting	21
Carl	32	M	Schizophrenia	Inpatient Unit	22
Claudio	47	M	Bipolar Disorder	Day Program	21
Dan	37	M	AIDS	Work Rehabilitation Program	23
David	8	M	Sensory Integrative Dysfunction	Private Practice	25
Esther	79	F	Cerebro-Vascular Accident	Skilled Nursing Facility	25
Fabrecio	40	M	Complex Regional Pain Syndrome	Outpatient Program	25
Fredrick	23	M	Depression	Rehabilitation Unit	24
Haydée	50	F	Cerebro-Vascular Accident	Residential Setting	21
Jesse	22	F	Head Injury	Rehabilitation Setting	24
Joan	79	F	Congestive Heart Failure	Home Care	23
Kim	16	F	Depression, Alcoholism	Inpatient Setting	24
Lars	88	M	Alzheimer's Dementia	Nursing Home	23
Marc	27	M	Paranoid Schizophrenia	Psychiatric Setting	23
Margaret	22	F	Profound Intellectual Impairment	Residential Setting	23
Nathan	7	M	Sensory Integrative Dysfunction	Private Practice	24
Paula	45	F	Learning Disability, Hemiparesis	Home Care	24
Robert	28	M	Autism, Intellectual Disability	Residential Setting	23
Sally	37	F	Arthritis	Outpatient Rehabilitation	25

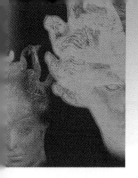

21

Recrafting Occupational Narratives

- Ana Laura Auzmendia
- Carmen Gloria de las Heras
- Gary Kielhofner
- Claudia Miranda

This chapter contains three cases. They each illustrate the process of rebuilding occupational adaptation in the face of significant life challenges. In each case, the client's occupational identity has been significantly eroded. Consequently, the course of therapy involved helping clients recraft occupational narratives for themselves and finding ways to put these narratives into action. The cases provide insight into the process of rebuilding occupational narratives as well as the complexities and challenges involved.

Transcending Adversity to Recraft a Narrative

This first case tells the story of a woman with physical impairments who has faced many major life challenges, only to face yet another. This case spans a 4.5-year period, illustrating that the recrafting of an occupational narrative can take a long time.

Haydée

Haydée was the widowed mother of three grown children and grandmother of seven. She led an active and independent life in Mar del Plata, Argentina, working as a school principal. Five days after her 50th birthday she suffered a cerebral vascular accident resulting in left hemiplegia. She received acute services at a local hospital and was transferred to a rehabilitation institute where she

made limited progress. The physician in charge of Haydée's rehabilitation wrote in her chart that she would "be confined in a wheelchair for the rest of her life."

Haydée was transferred to a nearby public geriatric residence. She was unable to get out of bed. Her impairments were significant. For example, she had lateral rotation and deviation of her neck due to contractures and she drooled uncontrollably. Finally, Haydée was severely depressed and withdrawn.

Initial Information Collection and Therapeutic Reasoning

Considering Haydée's physical impairments and her emotional status, the therapist decided to first establish a relationship with her through a series of brief unstructured interviews in which she could learn about, validate, and encourage her. In these conversations, Haydée sometimes talked of suicide. At other times she wanted to overcome her despair but did not know where to begin. Haydée's thoughts and feelings reflected her severely compromised volition. She felt totally robbed of control over her life. She had no interest in anything around her. She felt all her life plans as well as the lifestyle she valued had been destroyed.

Engaging Haydée

Because of her compromised volition, the only goal Haydée could see as possibly improving her life was to walk again. Therefore, her therapist decided not to negotiate a goal more in line with her current physical status. Rather, she met Haydée where she was and validated her one desire at the time, agreeing to see what could be done. Gait training services were not available in the nursing home. Consequently, the therapist attempted to refer Haydée to physical therapy, which was available through the rehabilitation facility. However, Haydée did not meet criteria for outpatient services because of the prognosis she had been given. Moreover, Haydée did not have the resources to purchase private physical therapy in the residence. Therefore, the therapist found an occupational therapy colleague who had the background to work with Haydée on ambulation and who agreed to see Haydée for a reduced fee that she could afford.

Because the therapist had demonstrated to Haydée a willingness to attend to her desires, she had gained Haydée's trust. She was able to use this as a foundation for advising Haydée to engage in other aspects of occupational therapy. The therapist worked with Haydée to enhance her occupational performance, through engaging her in doing things she enjoyed that also improved her scapular and neck mobility and sitting posture. The therapist also felt it was important to address the fact that Haydée had isolated herself from others due to her depression. Thus, she advised Haydée of the importance of reinvolving herself with others and persuaded her to join a creative activity group.

Haydée rapidly improved over the next few months. As she began to experience the return of her motor function, her volition improved as well. She felt more in control, enjoyed things she did, and saw herself as achieving things that mattered to her. Haydée showed such gains that she was readmitted to rehabilitation services on an outpatient basis while still living in the geriatric home.

Through concentrated rehabilitation efforts, Haydée continued to improve her upper extremity motor skills and occupational performance. In everyday activities such as eating she was beginning to use her left arm as an assist. She also began to walk with a tripod cane and the assistance of another person. Haydée became more socially active and regularly attended occupational therapy groups at the geriatric residence.

Dealing With a Devastating Setback

During an X-ray procedure to monitor her osteoarthritis and osteoporosis (conditions she had before her stroke), the technician fell with Haydée while assisting her to transfer from her wheelchair to a gurney. In the fall, Haydée fractured her affected left wrist. Six weeks later, when the cast was removed, Haydée had lost many of the fine motor abilities she had previously gained in her hand. Realizing her loss in function, Haydée became depressed and withdrawn again. Haydée's still vulnerable volition was clearly impacted by the turn of events over which she had no control and which had such negative consequences for the functional gains she had worked so hard to achieve. At this point, Haydée was not able to identify any goal for herself because she did not see how working toward something would really help her.

The therapist decided that Haydée needed an exploratory level intervention (as discussed in Chapters 10 and 18) that would allow her to regenerate some sense of control, regenerate some feelings of satisfaction in doing things, and experience realizing something of value. Because Haydée had such disrupted volition, it was clear that she would need a highly supportive environment that could scaffold her volition by providing external sources of confidence, interest, expectation, and value. The therapist also reasoned that this environmental support could best be achieved in a group context. Therefore, she began to encourage and persuade Haydée to join a group project.

Turning the Corner Through Engagement in a Group Project

At first Haydée was reluctant. However, with constant encouragement and statements of expectations that Haydée could and should do this for herself from the therapist, she agreed to join a project called, "The Puppet Workshop." A number of residents of the facility had planned, with the leadership of an occupational therapist, to implement a musical puppet show. For this project, they would make the puppets and stage, adapt the script of the musical for puppets, rehearse, and perform the show.

Becoming involved in this project provided the necessary momentum for Haydée. Moreover, she became an essential part of the group so that the group members began to provide the expectation for Haydée to participate that the therapist previously provided. Over time she improved her sense of efficacy and gained a feeling of satisfaction in doing things. Since she had more education than most residents, Haydée was recruited to write the adaptation of the play's script. At first she hesitated, but with some coaching and encouragement from the therapist, Haydée soon found that she was quite good at writing. Bolstered by her success in this task, she also showed interest in performing with puppets. However, when she first tried, it was difficult because of the functional restrictions of her left arm. However, with environmental adaptations and coaching, she was able to manipulate a puppet. Thus, she became a puppeteer.

The first puppet show was held at the geriatric residence for other residents and for family members. It was a great success. The puppet group was subsequently invited to perform seven more shows hosted by different community settings. One of the settings was the school where Haydée had formerly been principal. Haydée had suggested this setting. Performing there meant that she had to face the emotionally difficult challenge of reencountering her former colleagues and students. The experience of going to the school and seeing the children and teachers enjoy the puppet show was a great boost for Haydée. Once again, she began to feel that she could do something worthwhile.

Going back to her old school was only one of many social and physical challenges Haydée faced because of the puppet performances. For example, she also had to cope with a variety of architectural barriers that made it difficult to get onto the stages. With all these challenges and successes, the puppet project was an important achievement for Haydée. Involvement in working on the script and doing the performance stimulated Haydée's feeling of efficacy and enjoyment in writing. She began writing poetry and essays in occupational therapy. Moreover, her excursions into the community provided her with the opportunity to know that many barriers, physical and social, could be faced and overcome.

During this period, as Haydée began to show regeneration of her volition, the therapist also worked with her to establish a routine and to enhance her performance of self-care. Haydée was able to make steady progress. After some time, she indicated a desire to begin thinking about her future and what she would do with the rest of her life.

Administering the Occupational Performance History Interview-2nd Version (OPHI-II)

Because of Haydée's progress, the therapist felt it was an ideal time to administer the OPHI-II. Haydée had shown enough progress to be able to reflect on her life history and look to the future. The therapist did not complete the occupational behavior settings part of the OPHI-II since Haydée already had indicated a desire to move to a new living environment. As the OPHI-II scores on *Figure 21-1* show, Haydée had begun to rebuild her occupational identity, but her competence was still limited.

The process of engaging in the interview was important for Haydée. It allowed her to put into perspective the experiences of her life and to be reminded of her own strengths. Furthermore, through the process of telling her life story, Haydée was able to identify goals she wanted to strive toward in the future. The following is the occupational narrative that Haydée told in the interview.

Haydée began her story with her family, expressing that she had a wonderful childhood. Her parents were poor and worked hard to support 10 children. Haydée was the only one of her siblings to finish high school. She went on to obtain a diploma in teaching through her own fierce determination. Soon thereafter, Haydée married and had her first child. She went to work in a car dealership, since it allowed more flexibility than teaching. In the years that followed, she had a warm and loving relationship with her husband and together they had two more children.

However, with the birth of Haydée's youngest child things began to change dramatically. Her son was born prematurely, became dehydrated, and had convulsions. Then, when her son was 13 months old, her husband was killed in a car accident. Simultaneously, after 10 years of working for the dealership, she was suddenly laid off along with 7 other persons.

FIGURE 21-1   Haydée's Strengths and Weaknesses on the OPHI-II Occupational Identity and Competence Scales.

Occupational Identity Scale	1	2	3	4
Has personal goals and projects			░	
Identifies a desired occupational lifestyle			░	
Expects success				░
Accepts responsibility				░
Appraises abilities and limitations				░
Has commitments and values			░	
Recognizes identity and obligations				░
Has interests				░
Felt effective (past)				░
Found meaning and satisfaction in lifestyle (past)				░
Made occupational choices (past)				░
Occupational Competence Scale	1	2	3	4
Maintains satisfying lifestyle			░	
Fulfills role expectations		░		
Works toward goals		░		
Meets personal performance standards			░	
Organize time for responsibilities			░	
Participates in interests			░	
Fulfilled roles (past)				░
Maintained habits (past)			░	
Achieved satisfaction (past)			░	

Key : **4** = Exceptionally competent occupational functioning; **3** = Appropriate, satisfactory occupational functioning; **2** = Some occupational dysfunction; **1** = Extremely occupationally dysfunctional

Haydée even had to fight to receive a pension to which she was entitled. As she notes, "I never had time to grieve as I should have. Two days after my husband's death, I took my bike and went to apply for my pension. I didn't have time to cry." This incident typifies Haydée's view of herself as both a fighter and positive person. She refers to herself as both optimistic and obstinate.

Mustering her strength, Haydée immediately found a job teaching. It was a difficult challenge to be both a full-time worker and a single mother of three small children. As she saw it, she had no time for herself and insufficient time for her children. Nonetheless, Haydée excelled as a teacher, advancing to a substitute principal position. Her successes during this period in managing her household and raising children, while doing well as a teacher, greatly increased her sense of efficacy. She was very proud of her ability to set and achieve goals. As her children were grown and left the home, she set two important goals for herself. First she wanted to become a school principal. Second, she wanted to begin taking courses at a local university.

Shortly after Haydée reached the first of these goals, she had the stroke. The life she worked so hard to build collapsed, leading her to a state of despair and forcing her to live in a geriatric residence at the age of 50. Haydée saw the past months in the residence, and especially her experiences in the puppet workshop, as allowing her to begin rebuilding her life once again. Her success was reflected in her current routine, which was organized and balanced with different leisure, self-care, and rehabilitation activities. She engaged in a variety of interests and had goals to:

- Improve her walking
- Manage herself in a house
- Obtain a disability pension
- Work part-time as a writer.

She acknowledged that she had difficulty staying focused on and sustaining energy toward achieving her goals, so talking about them helped her commit to them.

As illustrated in Haydée's narrative slope (*Fig. 21-2*) she had made significant progress in reversing the tragic consequences of her stroke. Once again, she was finding a way to rise above adversity in reconstructing a vision of a life she wanted. Also, in beginning to think about her future narrative, Haydée was able to reflect on her past, identifying what she would like to do differently. For example, she noted how she had been so focused on her career, explaining, "I often would get only four hours of sleep. I was obsessed with work." Now she wanted to live her life in a less extreme way. She saw her stroke as an opportunity to reflect on her life and think about how she would live in the future. The therapist advised Haydée of the picture of her occu-

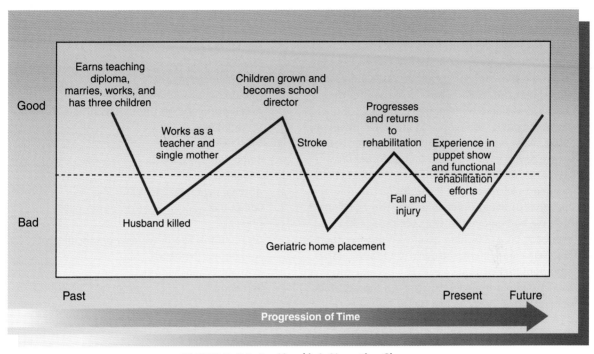

FIGURE 21-2 Haydée's Narrative Slope.

pational narrative, which came from the interview, and Haydée heartily agreed with it. She also concluded with the therapist's advice and encouragement that she would focus in the coming months on realizing the future she envisioned for herself.

Building a New Occupational Narrative

In the following months, Haydée worked hard to achieve the competence she envisioned in her narrative. She improved performance of her self-care activities, achieving independence in everything except bathing. She used her wheelchair to get around in the facility and walked around in her room with a tripod cane. Haydée undertook a 500-km trip on her own to complete the legal procedures to receive her pension.

During this time, Haydée continued to write. She completed a private book of essays and prose. To write effectively on the computer, she worked to improve her motor skills for typing in occupational therapy. Haydée continued to participate and often took on a leadership role in activities and outings organized by the geriatric residence. At the New

Year's party she danced for the first time. Haydée also began to go out alone to shop regularly, using a local taxi that accommodated her wheelchair.

Finally, Haydée achieved one of her most important dreams. She traveled by bus with her three children back to her hometown. There, she reencountered relatives and old friends that she had not seen for years. She also visited the cemetery where her parents and husband were buried. Haydée returned very enthusiastic with the plan to move to her native city in a short time.

The occupational therapist was concerned that it was not clear how the move would fit into the identity Haydée was constructing for herself. It seemed that Haydée was caught up in the emotion of the visit. Nonetheless, the therapist realized the importance of allowing Haydée to make her own decision and the need to support her to make a good decision. Consequently, she advised Haydée that she should make this decision very carefully since a move to a new environment could have many unanticipated impacts on her. She negotiated with Haydée that she should take time with this de-

cision. They agreed that Haydée would travel back
one more time to gather more information about
what her life could really be like there before making this important occupational choice. Haydée
made the trip with her daughter, traveling by bus.
During this visit, she was able to reinterpret the situation, realizing that her initial plan was not realistic. As she put it, "Everyone has his or her life set up,
what place would I occupy?" So she decided to
search for other alternatives for her future life.

After reflection, Haydée decided that she
needed to focus on her main productive role and
her goal of living independently. She recognized
that she had enjoyed writing and received positive
feedback on her writing abilities. With her therapist's encouragement, she decided to take a univer-
sity-sponsored writing course. She became the first
student with a disability to attend a literary workshop called, "Words Amidst Hands."

During this time she also continued in occupational therapy, practicing her skills in using the computer and focusing on her self-care. After a couple
of months she became totally independent in self-
care, including bathing. She began to practice other
activities of daily living such as sewing, washing, and
ironing.

All these efforts not only moved Haydée closer
to her objective, but also allowed her to realize her
long-standing values of independence, vitality, and
accomplishment in what she did. Haydée still had
some highs and lows. Nonetheless, despite occasional fears and uncertainties, Haydée continued to
strive to live her occupational narrative. In the
words of one of her poems:

Sometimes . . . .
I feel like:
Laughing or crying.
And I laugh or cry.
Sometimes . . .
I feel like:
Walking, running or dancing.
And I walk, run or dance.
Sometimes . . .
I feel like:
Going back to the classroom,
And seeing the eager gaze,
Of the children, waiting for their work.

And I go back to the classroom.
To enjoy those gazes.
Sometimes
I feel like:
Going back to my city.
And going through its streets.
And I return and go through its streets.
Sometimes . . .
I feel like:
Being with my parents,
In our home.
And I am with my parents.
Sometimes . . .
I feel like:
Going to the beach, with my grandchildren.
And I go to the beach,
With my grandchildren.
Sometimes . . .
I feel like:
Dreaming . . .
And . . . I dream awake.

Haydée in Perspective

The case of Haydée illustrates how the most effective
occupational therapy must be timed according to
client's needs and readiness for change. Haydée's therapist correctly reasoned that initial assessment was best
done though informal means and only later chose to
do OPHI-II at a point when she felt Haydée could emotionally face and benefit from reviewing her life. Haydée also illustrates that the course of therapy is not always linear. There are often times when a client will
regress or have difficulty moving forward due to complex combinations of personal and environmental factors. In particular, the process of rebuilding one's occupational narrative is extremely difficult when the onset
of a disability has completely altered it.

Transformation From Victim to Heroine

This case illustrates how recrafting of an occupational
narrative can take place in the context of physical rehabilitation. Therapists who concentrate their efforts

in rehabilitation on only the remediation motor and functional problems can miss what is most important to a client—to figure out what kind of life is possible. When devastating physical impairments invalidate an ongoing life story, their impact is much more far-reaching for the person than the functional limitations they impose. Attention to the disrupted life story and to how it can be rebuilt is the key to effective, client-centered therapy.

Barbara

Barbara was a 33-year-old single mother, diagnosed with multiple sclerosis 3 years earlier. For 5 years before her diagnosis she had intermittent symptoms such as weakness and pain in her back and lower extremities, blurred vision, and some slurring of her speech. Barbara was recently admitted to a rehabilitation center after several months of exacerbation. During the exacerbation she experienced dramatically decreased endurance and ascending muscle weakness that sometimes made it hard for her to breathe and swallow. During the worst of this period, she was unable either to walk on her own or to propel a wheelchair.

When the therapist first met Barbara she was depressed and anxious, but able to express her thoughts and feelings. She felt out of control, had lost her involvement in all her everyday activities, and was terrified about what the future had in store for her. Consequently, the occupational therapist was quite concerned not only about Barbara's physical condition, but also about her severely impacted volition.

Despite her depression and anxiety and even though she had no idea how to go about it, Barbara expressed a willingness to do all she could to get her life back in order. In large measure this was fueled by the fact that she was responsible for two children. The therapist reasoned that it would be useful to examine Barbara's occupational narrative along with her to help figure out where her life had been and might go in light of her disability. She first interviewed Barbara using the Occupational Performance History Interview-2nd Version (OPHI-II) and then collaborated with Barbara to complete the In-

terest Checklist and the Role Checklist. Because the impact of Barbara's environments could not be determined until her future performance capacity was better known, the therapist did not complete the occupational behavior settings portion of the OPHI-II. Her plan was first to get an overall picture of Barbara's life and how the multiple sclerosis had affected it, then to go on to assess Barbara's physical capacity and performance, gathering other information as needed.

Barbara's Occupational Narrative

During her interview, Barbara related the following narrative. During her senior year in high school she became pregnant. After graduation she married the father; her daughter was born soon thereafter. Barbara had only worked briefly as a waitress on weekends during school. Barbara did not enjoy this job. She disliked working with customers on a daily basis since she was a private person. For the next 2 years, Barbara's time was taken up with being a homemaker and mother. She had a second daughter 2 years after her first.

In the meantime, Barbara's relationship with her husband deteriorated badly. He was an alcoholic and physically abused Barbara. He also had been unable to hold a steady job because of multiple absences and a temper that got him into trouble with supervisors. Financial stress, combined with her husband's self-destructive drinking and his abuse of her, made life practically unbearable for Barbara. It became increasingly clear that her husband was not going to do anything about his drinking and abuse. Moreover, he had no prospects for work. Therefore, Barbara decided she would be better off alone with the children. Shortly after the birth of her second daughter, she divorced him.

Forced by the financial realities of being a single mother without the benefit of child support, Barbara returned to work. She found employment as a secretary in a construction firm, filing papers, typing, bookkeeping, and acting as a receptionist. With a great deal of effort, she managed to balance the demands of being a single mother of two children, working full-time, and maintaining a household. She did this for nearly a decade. During this time Barbara viewed herself as a fighter and a survivor who overcame a number of hurdles to be a good mother and provider.

Barbara was forced to resign her job 3 years earlier. Her multiple sclerosis had progressed to the point that she was unable, despite extreme effort and a supportive work environment, to fulfill her job responsibilities. In the 2 years before her resignation, Barbara frequently missed work due to fatigue and weakness.

In retrospect, Barbara felt that she had enjoyed her job. She liked the moderate contact with other people that her job demanded and felt that she did it well. She felt a sense of accomplishment in being able to hold the dual role of single parent and family breadwinner. Although it was hard, it was a source of great satisfaction to her that she had pulled her life together. However, Barbara had also felt guilty about not being with her children during the day. Barbara's values were organized around her view of her responsibility as a mother and her hard-won independence. Her children and the family which she and they constituted were of central importance. Fiercely independent, she wanted to be financially secure, and therefore not reliant on anyone else.

The advent of multiple sclerosis threatened all of Barbara's most basic values. She was plagued by the idea that she could neither be a good mother nor a source of income for her family. The entire life story she had constructed and lived had now come crumbling down. Her financial picture had become more and more negative as she lost her income and had to rely on social security income. She had grown dependent on her children and her parents. The independence and self-reliance she had worked so hard to achieve after leaving her husband had disappeared.

Just before her hospitalization, Barbara spent three-quarters of her waking day in bed watching television or talking to family members on the telephone. The other major portion of her day was spent talking with her children or directing them to get household chores completed. Barbara had no set schedule for meals or self-care activities. Household chores were completed sporadically by her children or her parents. When Barbara had more energy, she would get up and spend an hour or two folding clothes or straightening the house. As a consequence, she would be exhausted for the next 2 or 3 days.

Overall, her low energy level and tendency to fatigue easily meant that Barbara was unable to sustain even a resemblance of the active lifestyle she previously had when working as a single mother. Moreover, she no longer had access to the occupational forms that she enjoyed and valued and which gave her a sense of competence. Finally, the highly organized habits that had supported her earlier function had disintegrated to a haphazard and passive daily routine.

The impact of multiple sclerosis on Barbara's occupational identity and competence are illustrated in *Figure 21-3,* which shows the ratings the therapist gave her on the OPHI scales along with comments written by the therapist. At this point, Barbara felt her life was in a shambles. She was unable even to take care of herself. The future loomed ahead as a great blank. Despite the great strength Barbara had shown in the past, when confronted with the life change wrought by multiple sclerosis, she had no idea of where to begin in imagining a future for herself. This is illustrated in Barbara's narrative slope, which is shown in *Figure 21-4.*

Information From Other Assessments

Barbara identified family member as her only continuous role for the past, present, and future on the Role Checklist (*Fig. 21-5*). At this time, her daughters were 14 and 12 years old. She had been completely out of touch with her husband for 12 years and had depended only on the occasional support of her parents to assist in child rearing. Nonetheless, she did not indicate on the form that she was a caregiver to her children. When her therapist questioned why she did not consider herself currently in the role of caregiver to her children, she responded, "No, I'm inadequate. I can't handle those responsibilities. My parents are their caregivers."

Barbara identified the following roles as disrupted: worker, caregiver, home maintainer, and friend. She also felt that she had lost her friends. They had become uncomfortable as her disease progressed. Barbara very much missed social contact with others outside her family.

FIGURE 21-3 Therapist Rating of and Comments Concerning Barbara's Strengths and Weaknesses on the OPHI-II.

Occupational Identity Scale	1	2	3	4	Comments
Has personal goals and projects	X				Before MS had ongoing goals and projects, now has none since future is unclear
Identifies a desired occupational lifestyle		X			Desires previous lifestyle, but has no idea of what is possible now
Expects success	X				Feels hopeless about the future
Accepts responsibility			X		Has done her best in the face of disease process, does not know what to do now to be in control of life
Appraises abilities and limitations	X				Has no idea what they will be in future
Has commitments and values				X	Taking care of children, working
Recognizes identity and obligations				X	Strong sense of responsibility as a mother
Has interests			X		Mostly revolves around work and children
Felt effective (past)				X	Felt very effective in managing her substantial responsibilities
Found meaning and satisfaction in lifestyle (past)				X	Managed a challenging but satisfying and meaningful life as a working single mother
Made occupational choices (past)				X	Took control of her life with major choices
Occupational Competence Scale	**1**	**2**	**3**	**4**	
Maintains satisfying lifestyle	X				All areas affected by current limitations
Fulfills role expectations	X				"
Works toward goals	X				"
Meets personal performance standards	X				"
Organizes time for responsibilities	X				"
Participates in interests			X		"
Fulfilled roles (past)				X	Worker and single mother roles
Maintained habits (past)				X	Well-organized life despite multiple demands
Achieved satisfaction (past)				X	Satisfied with meeting challenges of her life

Key : 4 = Exceptionally competent occupational functioning; 3 = Appropriate, satisfactory occupational functioning; 2 = Some occupational dysfunction; 1 = Extremely occupationally dysfunctional

Barbara rated the roles of caregiver, home maintainer, and family member as very valuable. When the therapist pointed this out, Barbara agreed that if she could choose her future, these would be the roles she wanted to fulfill. Discussing the Role Checklist, the therapist pointed out that Barbara's biggest concern was being a burden to her children. They were just coming to an age when they needed more independence. Her concern about being a burden was even more acute, since she very much wanted for her daughters to have a better start in life than she had.

Together, the OPHI-II and the Role Checklist gave a detailed picture of how Barbara's life had been transformed by the steady progress of her multiple sclerosis. A previously self-reliant and determined woman, she had been transformed into someone who felt victimized and helpless. This transformation was also reflected in her change from a life filled with valued roles to one filled with losses.

Barbara identified 8 strong interests on the 80-item Modified Interest Checklist (*Fig. 21-6*). These interests mostly centered around family life, social-

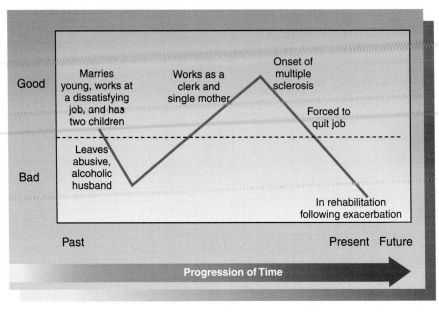

FIGURE 21-4   Barbara's Narrative Slope.

ization, and sports. Despite Barbara's regular involvement in these interests in the past, she had recently participated in only one interest, watching television. She agreed with her occupational therapist's advice that she needed to identify, develop, and pursue new interests. As suggested in her Interest Checklist responses, Barbara had seen a significant decline in the quality of her everyday occupational participation.

Barbara's Functional Decrements

Multiple sclerosis had imposed functional limitations that severely affected Barbara's occupational performance. At admission, Barbara could not completely dress herself or bathe; she reported that she had not been in a shower for well over a year and instead took sponge baths. She was unable to transfer from her wheelchair without assistance and could only propel it about 200 feet on a level sur-

FIGURE 21-5   Role Checklist.

Role	Past	Present	Future	Not at all Valuable	Somewhat Valuable	Very Valuable
Student						
Worker						
Volunteer						
Caregiver						
Home Maintainer						
Friend						
Family Member						
Religious Participant						
Hobbyist/Amateur						
Participant in Organizations						
Other						

FIGURE 21-6 Barbara's Responses on the Modified Interest Checklist (Only Those Items for Which There Was a Past or Present Interest Shown).

Activity	What has been your level of interest?						Do you currently participate in this activity?		Would you like to pursue this in the future?	
	In the past ten years			In the past year						
	Strong	Some	No	Strong	Some	No	Yes	No	Yes	No
Listening to popular music	▓			▓			▓		▓	
Holiday activities	▓			▓				▓		
Swimming	▓					▓				
Bowling	▓				▓					
Visiting	▓			▓						
Cycling	▓									
Child care	▓									
Cooking/baking	▓				▓					

face, requiring two or three rest stops to catch her breath.

Since Barbara's major life role at the time was as a homemaker, the occupational therapist continued an ongoing informal evaluation of Barbara's homemaking performance. Barbara reported that, for the past 5 months, she had managed to make only two or three meals for her family and had relied on her children or parents to do most homemaking tasks. She confessed that she was unsure of how to approach these tasks from a wheelchair. During an informal observation of her performance in the kitchen, Barbara was unable to maneuver her wheelchair to effectively transport items from the cabinets, stove, or refrigerator. It took her about 15 minutes to transport a single item from the refrigerator to a counter across the room.

Course of Therapy

Barbara came to occupational therapy twice a day. She came in a wheelchair or on a stretcher if she was too fatigued to sit. Her occupational therapist felt that the overall focus of her therapy would be to help her find a way out of her story of victimization and helplessness and to reinstate life roles. She realized that this would mean enabling Barbara to maximize her performance and participation despite her motor impairments. This would require adjustments in her environment.

Barbara's occupational therapy was developed to coordinate with physical therapy and nursing care. It was modified weekly according to Barbara's endurance level and strength. Her various therapies and self-care activities were scheduled hourly with half-hour rest periods between them. Barbara was unable to envision what was possible for herself or how her therapy should unfold. Consequently, the therapist collaborated with her by giving her routine feedback on her progress and its implications, advising her about new goals and approaches and then negotiating with Barbara to modify or refine them in ways that increasingly gave Barbara control over the course of her own therapy.

The occupational therapist began by advising Barbara about multiple sclerosis: the symptoms, possible precursors to exacerbations, and how she would need to have a flexible habit pattern in the future to accommodate fluctuations in her motor skills. In relating this information to Barbara, her therapist also began to portray ways in which she could retake control over her life and reinstate important parts of her former life. She began to encourage Barbara to reframe her occupational narrative by considering future scenarios. Throughout the hospitalization, Barbara's children and parents were also informed about multiple sclerosis and encouraged to support Barbara to envision her life in a more positive way.

Before relearning any self-care or homemaking skills, the therapist coached Barbara in how to integrate work simplification principles into what she did. Once she had the basic information, Barbara practiced work simplification within the hospital routine and occupational therapy sessions. Barbara also explored objects that would compensate for her limited motor skills (e.g., a reacher, a dressing stick, and a long-handled bath sponge).

During self-care and homemaking tasks, Barbara practiced planning her actions ahead of time, so that she could complete an occupational form with efficiency and minimal energy expenditure. With her therapist's advice, Barbara also identified when it was acceptable to ask for help from her children or parents to complete tasks. Before each weekend at home, Barbara developed a schedule with the advice of the occupational therapist. In doing this, Barbara learned the value of both planning ahead and of being flexible with her time according to her strength and endurance.

The occupational therapist worked with Barbara to gradually identify a future for herself. Together they explored what roles and activities were most important to her, using these as a basis to set goals. Barbara decided to set daily, weekly, and monthly goals and to identify which of these were of highest priority for her. In selecting occupational forms to use in the course of therapy, her therapist had two interrelated goals:

- Giving Barbara an opportunity to explore things that might become new interests
- Improving her strength, coordination, and endurance.

For example, Barbara chose to learn macramé. She learned the basic knots while sitting at a table and then was able to macramé with her arms up in the air, with the macramé secured to an overhead stationary object. As her strength and endurance improved, time spent doing macramé was increased and the wheelchair seat belt and armrests were removed. Later, she sat on the edge of a plinth while doing macramé to increase her stability.

As Barbara's motor skills improved, her occupational therapist began to advise her on ways that her environment could be modified to accommodate her limitations. Her therapist helped her to choose bathroom equipment that would enable her to be independent in self-care. The therapist fitted Barbara for an appropriate wheelchair and cushion, and she coached Barbara while she practiced wheelchair control and maintenance.

In preparation for her return home, Barbara also planned environmental adjustments to her house to improve accessibility. Finally, she began to participate in community excursions where she was able to put together all she had learned about energy conservation, work simplification, and use of adapted equipment. For example, she shopped in a local grocery store using a wheelchair grocery cart. In the final stage of her therapy, Barbara identified that she wanted to be independent in getting around in her community and needed to be able to drive a car. She received driving instruction and learned to drive with hand controls.

Barbara had to face the fact that the occupational narrative she had crafted and would have preferred to continue living was not going to be possible. The therapist validated Barbara's pain in coming to grips with this. At the same time, the therapist advised and encouraged Barbara to envision a new life story, which included probable further decrements in capacity and periods of exacerbation. Barbara commented that she had successfully faced adversity before when she became a single mother and that, by doing it again, she would continue to enact for her daughters a powerful example. Over time, Barbara was able to reframe her experiences in this way and increasingly saw herself as a heroine struggling against a mighty adversary. The transformation from victim back to heroine in her occupational narrative enabled Barbara to go on with her life.

Preparing for the Return Home

Approximately 2 weeks before her discharge, Barbara's occupational therapist accompanied her on a home visit. Barbara's parents met Barbara and the therapist to participate in the review of possible home modifications. Barbara lived in a one-floor ranch house. Neither of the two entrances to the home were wheelchair accessible, but a ramp and sidewalk could be constructed at the front entrance. The home was small and crowded with excess furniture. By rearranging the furniture, all the rooms were made wheelchair accessible except the utility room and the bathroom. Since neither of these rooms could be modified for improved accessibility, Barbara and the occupational therapist identified and practiced a system of transfers onto a chair and the commode. They were able to determine that the transfers were feasible so that Barbara could use the bathroom independently.

Barbara's father and mother were impressed with the improvement therapy had brought about in Barbara's ability for transfers and in her mobility throughout the house. They added suggestions for further possible home modifications. Both of Barbara's parents were extremely supportive. Her father planned to make the necessary home modifications with the help of Barbara's two brothers who lived nearby. Both of Barbara's daughters were accepting of their mother's illness and did extra household chores with few complaints. Her family admitted that in the past their willingness to help Barbara may at times have made her overly dependent and agreed to cooperate with her in the future to maintain the level of independence that she wanted to have in her life.

Constructing an Acceptable Life

As therapy proceeded, Barbara continued to recognize and accept her reduced capacities and other consequences of her disease. Importantly, she had begun to develop an image of how she could have a satisfying life that operationalized her value of independence. In part, this meant that she had a new definition of independence which allowed her to rely to some extent on her family while being on her own in every way that she reasonably could. Her occupational narrative and long-term goals were organized around being an independent homemaker and a caregiver to her children. She solidified the image of herself as an example to them of how to rise above adversity. She was able to enact this new narrative and to achieve her homemaker and mother roles, albeit in altered ways.

At discharge, Barbara was independent in self-care, homemaking, and wheelchair management. She could propel her wheelchair up and down ramps, on flat level surfaces, and over rough terrain. She was able to maneuver the chair around objects and through small hallways. She had completed adapted driving training, was able to drive using hand controls, and was able to put her own wheelchair in and out of her car. She identified this accomplishment as her "ticket to freedom." After discharge, Barbara was referred to a vocational counselor at the Department of Rehabilitation Services. Her goal of independent homemaking was recognized as a vocation. Therefore, it financed the recommended home modifications and the hand controls for the car.

Barbara no longer required her parents' assistance on weekends and she managed the cooking and cleaning and her own self-care independently with minimal help from her children. She began socializing again with some of her old friends and neighbors and joined a bimonthly bridge club. Barbara continued her new-found interest in macramé and gave away many of her projects as gifts.

Barbara in Perspective

Barbara recrafted her occupational narrative by identifying an acceptable lifestyle for herself and reinstating her most important roles. This required her to reframe what had happened to her. It also required that she redefine her roles and find new ways to enact values. In the end, her struggle with multiple sclerosis became another episode in which her fierce determination allowed her to prevail and create the kind of life she wanted.

The therapist enabled Barbara to envision a future life and to work toward achieving it. Improving motor skills, making environmental modifications, and learning energy conservation all became ways for Barbara to achieve occupational competence. However, without a narrative to enact, these practical approaches would have lacked the cogency they had for Barbara. As noted in Chapter 9, occupational identity is a prerequisite for occupational competence.

Reclaiming Life Roles

The following typifies the kind of disintegration of life that can occur for persons who have chronic mental illness. It also illustrates how persons who can seem very unmotivated and unlikely to benefit from therapy can become committed to the therapy process if the therapist carefully assesses and understands the past occupational identity of the client.

Claudio

Claudio was 47 years old when he became a client at Reencuentros, a community-based occupational therapy day program in Santiago, Chile. Referred by his psychiatrist, Claudio was still hospitalized and had begun taking medication that appeared to manage the symptoms of his bipolar disorder. Claudio had been legally detained in the psychiatric hospital, and the plan was that he would remain hospitalized but attend Reencuentros during part of the day.

Claudio had a long psychiatric history. He had been forcibly admitted to units of psychiatric hospitals several times in the past. Almost every time, Claudio managed very creative ways to escape. His aggressiveness had also led to him being incarcerated a number of times in the past. He had never managed to be compliant with taking his medication for long.

Claudio came from a large family of 10 brothers and sisters, all well educated, professional, and married, with three or four children each. Their father died when they were small, and their strongly religious mother raised them alone. Following his first bipolar crisis, the whole family supported Claudio and tried to help him. However, from the beginning Claudio refused their assistance. Over time he increasingly antagonized them, so that with the exception of his mother, he had no family contact. He was legally separated from his wife since divorce is not legal in Chile. Claudio had not seen his three children since they were quite small. Claudio, formerly a very successful engineer, had been unemployed for many years. In short, he had lost all his roles.

When he arrived at Reencuentros, Claudio appeared sad. However, he proudly and adamantly announced that he neither needed nor wanted occupational therapy. His previous experiences with occupational therapy during his hospitalizations were negative. He stated that he did not believe in occupational therapy, because he "was an engineer and he did not like to do crafts." He further asserted that occupational therapy was a "second class career," inferior to medicine, engineering, or law. It was, therefore, beneath him to receive services from an occupational therapist. Nonetheless, he said that would he evaluate the quality of the program and people in it, and based on his evaluation, would decide whether to participate.

The occupational therapist recognized that she had to validate Claudio's viewpoint. Therefore, she offered to talk to Claudio about Reencuentros and give him a tour to see if it would meet with his approval. After the tour, Claudio indicated that he was still skeptical but would come back to further evaluate the program.

Beginning Assessment

When Claudio returned the next day, the therapist decided to ask Claudio to complete the Role Checklist. She selected this assessment because it required little effort and it would allow Claudio to state his views of himself and be able to interpret his own responses. Thus he could maintain the control he clearly needed in the situation. After he completed it (see *Fig. 21-7* for his responses), she asked him if he would explain its meaning to her. Claudio noted that until the onset of his illness at age 32, he had participated in a full range of occupational roles. After his first manic-depressive episode, he soon lost every one of his roles.

He went on to say that he had been a very successful student at the University of Chile. He had held very important jobs in the private and public sector. In his last job, he was Director of Projects in a very large engineering firm, leading a team of 30 people. This role was the one he had valued most. He often worked long hours, finding pleasure and pride in his performance. Claudio indicated that he valued his family roles, especially the role of father, although his wife and children often felt he was too

FIGURE 21-7 Claudio's Scores on the Initial Role Checklist.

Role	Past	Present	Future	Not at all Valuable	Somewhat Valuable	Very Valuable
Student						
Worker						
Volunteer						
Caregiver						
Home Maintainer						
Friend						
Family Member						
Religious Participant						
Hobbyist/Amateur						
Participant in Organizations						
Other		Sick role				

absent. His view was that his work did not allow much time for his children. He also believed that rearing children was primarily a woman's responsibility.

He did spend time with his friends and volunteered for a political organization where he led social projects. He felt that he was well appreciated everywhere, except at home. He resented his wife's attitude toward his routine, and her demands that he be more involved with the children. Claudio admitted that during his manic episodes, he "got physical" with his children and wife. He also began to gamble and eventually lost all the family savings. He also admitted getting into conflicts that resulted in his being fired from his job. His wife legally separated from him, moved to an unknown address, and he received a court order taking away his visitation rights to his children.

The one role Claudio noted that he never lost was religious participant. However, he noted that instead of doing the usual things involved in participating in the Catholic Church, he participated in this role privately, reading scripture and praying for hours, days, and months on end. He mentioned a depressive period when he felt that his religion had saved his life.

After reflecting with the therapist on the meaning of his roles in the past and present, Claudio stated that his illness had driven away his wife, siblings, and friends and caused him to lose his job and his children. He recognized that in 20 years engineering had changed dramatically, and he did not have the current computer skills to do it. He stated passionately that the only thing he really wanted back was his role as a father. He said that the loss of his children had taken away the deepest source of meaning in his life. Claudio had not seen them since they were tiny children and now they were adolescents. He summed up saying, "If this program is any good, it will give me back my children."

In response, the therapist encouraged Claudio to participate in a self-help group in Reencuentros for parents that were in similar situations. The therapist explained that the group would provide him with support and realization that he was not alone in his estrangement from his children. She also noted that the group was a place where participants could plan how to achieve a healthy connection with their children. Claudio immediately agreed that this was a good idea.

The therapist also invited Claudio to be a volunteer at Reencuentros, suggesting that he could use his administrative expertise from the past to help other clients to learn administrative tasks. She offered this as a way of validating his past performance. Claudio stated that he was not ready to do this. It was clear that he did not feel he had the capacity to succeed. However, with encouragement from the therapist upon returning the next day, he did agree to try out this volunteer role as well.

Interviewing Claudio's Mother

The therapist decided to interview Claudio's mother to get more insight into his history. She used the OPHI-II as a guide to doing the interview. Claudio's mother validated what he had said in the discussion of the Role Checklist. She also gave important additional information. She noted that her sons had all followed their father's pattern, being proud, self-centered, and selfish. Claudio's interpersonal relationships and his social skills were a problem since his adolescence. He could not accept feedback or criticism. He was often in trouble with authorities and always in conflict with his wife and children as well as brothers and sisters. He had little tolerance for others' mistakes or problems.

After the onset of his mental illness, Claudio's basic interpersonal difficulties escalated to the point that his wife left him and barred him from his children. Similarly, Claudio's brothers and sisters had grown fearful of his aggressive behavior, choosing not to have contact with him. She confirmed that she was his only source of social support. While Claudio had no contact with his ex-wife and children, one of his sisters remained a very good friend of his ex-wife. Claudio was unaware of this.

Claudio's mother was worried that he would not stay on his medication and remain in the program. She noted that he had reached this same stage in treatment several times before (i.e., some stabilization of his symptoms). Then he would suddenly discontinue his medication and other treatment, diminishing its importance and saying "he was an intelligent man, who could manage by himself." Claudio had a brother with schizophrenia who still lived with her, but was functioning well.

Claudio's mother said his primary interests had been intellectual and social. He had liked to read, attend Catholic mass, and participate in social gatherings and organizations. At home, he preferred reading to spending time with his children or wife. Work had been Claudio's first priority, and succeeding was the thing he most valued. Claudio was always the best student in his school, excelled at the university, and had been considered a highly tal-ented industrial engineer. Claudio had always tried to maintain a public image as someone who was very accomplished. This had all been destroyed now. Although Claudio still tried to maintain a public front, his mother knew that deep inside he felt a terrible sense of failure.

When asked about the future, she indicated that when he was discharged, Claudio could live in her house where her other son with a mental illness also lived. However, she was concerned that these brothers did not get along. Claudio's mother planned that once he was settled there, she would move elsewhere, since the house was really too small for three people. Once she left, Claudio would have his own room, sharing a bathroom with his brother. She also had a little money that she would give him each month for food and transportation. She noted, apologetically, that the house was a mess and the room Claudio would occupy was used to store things since they had nowhere else to keep them.

Further Evaluating Claudio's Volition

The therapist reasoned that it was important to carefully evaluate Claudio's volition. She did this by using the Volitional Questionnaire (VQ) to observe him in Reencuentros' administrative area, where he had agreed to volunteer, and in the parental support group.

Observation in the Administrative Area

The administrative area is where the accounting, administrative, clerical, and communication tasks of the center take place. There, the center also operates a desktop publishing business that produces educational and advertising materials for businesses and health professionals as well as newsletters and fliers for family members and clients of the center. Clients with interest and skill participate in one or more of the roles in the setting while working on personal goals. The environment is very busy with many people at different functional levels working to do a wide range of things.

Claudio was familiar with the kinds of tasks that were being done and with the equipment used, although his knowledge of computers was based on much older computer systems. The therapist invited him to explore this environment and to identify tasks for which he could provide help. Claudio sat in the room, looking around at others and what they were doing for about 10 minutes. He got up to glance inside the separate computer room but came right back. When the therapist asked him what he thought, he told the therapist he did not know what to choose. She helped to structure things for him, reviewing alternatives with him and encouraging him to try some things with her. However, he was not willing to try doing anything.

The therapist validated his reluctance, telling him just to take his time and to consider further the various things he might do, with no pressure to get started. He stayed for the whole morning. His scores for session 1 on the VQ (*Fig. 21-8*) indicated that while his volition was severely compromised as indicated by many passive ratings, Claudio was able to show interest for the accounting area of the office, as he read the accounting books for half of the time he was there. Another task he attended to with curiosity was organizing materials for family education. Claudio was able to indicate preferences by commenting that these two areas seemed interesting to him.

The therapist gave feedback to Claudio, indicating that he did well during the morning since he had not been in a work environment for many years. She was impressed that he could concentrate on reading for so long. He told the therapist that he did not do well, that he was only pretending to read much of the time and that his concentration for reading was not good. The therapist coached Claudio to reframe his view. She explained that considering the long time he had spent inactive, he had done very well. Nonetheless, Claudio continued to make disparaging comments about himself. Later, after lunch, when the therapist encouraged him to consider participating in one of the two tasks for which he had shown interest, he refused, saying, "The tasks are too easy for me. They would only be boring." It was clear to the therapist that this was his way of saving face, when in fact he lacked the sense of capacity and efficacy to try them.

Observation in the Parents Self-Help Group

The Parents Self-Help Group met twice weekly. When Claudio joined the group, it had eight members including both women and men. The group had an agenda for each meeting, presenting what

FIGURE 21-8 Claudio's Scores on the Volitional Questionnaire Based on Two Observations 3½ Months Apart.

Environmental Context	Initial				3½ Months Later			
1. Shows curiosity	P	H	I	S	P	H	I	S
2. Initiates actions/tasks	P	H	I	S	P	H	I	S
3. Tries new things	P	H	I	S	P	H	I	S
4. Shows pride	P	H	I	S	P	H	I	S
5. Seeks challenges	P	H	I	S	P	H	I	S
6. Seeks additional responsibilities	N/A				P	H	I	S
7. Tries to correct mistakes	N/A				N/A			
8. Tries to solve problems	P	H	I	S	P	H	I	S
9. Shows preferences	P	H	I	S	P	H	I	S
10. Pursues activity to completion/accomplishment	N/A				P	H	I	S
11. Stays engaged	P	H	I	S	P	H	I	S
12. Invests additional energy/emotions/attention	P	H	I	S	P	H	I	S
13. Indicates goals	P	H	I	S	P	H	I	S
14. Shows that an activity is special or significant	P	H	I	S	P	H	I	S
Key : **P** = Passive; **H** = Hesitant; **I** = Involved; **S** = Spontaneous								

they had accomplished from the last week and helping members to find solutions to problems they encountered. Then, they discussed various topics and issues related to parenting. Group members also reported on their success in trying solutions and achieving goals that were generated at the previous meeting. The therapist who ran the group was also a parent and participated as a member and facilitator. It was an open and supportive group.

In the meeting Claudio appeared involved in the group. His attention and posture indicated an interest in others' experiences. When Claudio was asked to tell about his difficulties as a parent, he became very upset. With a great deal of support from other members, he was able to answer only a few general questions about his children. Claudio kept his head down when talking about his children, blushing and unable to answer when asked what he used to do with them. Members of the group reassured Claudio, telling him not to feel embarrassed because all of them had made mistakes with their children. Nonetheless, he was unable to say anything more and kept his head down. At the end of the meeting, he apologized, telling the others that he would try to come to the next meeting. The members told him that he had participated a lot for a first meeting and that he should feel good about himself. He responded that he felt he did not do so well.

Constructing an Understanding of Claudio's Volition

Claudio was a person with a broken occupational life who had lost his most valued roles. He had no hope to be able to rebuild his life again. Previously a person with a strong personal causation, he lacked a sense of capacity and efficacy, needing intensive support from his social environment to be able to participate. Despite this, Claudio did appear to want to reconnect with his children and he was able to show some interest in work-related occupational forms. The initial assessment gave the necessary information to begin the process of remotivation (a structured approach to reinstating volition developed at Reencuentros and documented in a manual) (de las Heras, Llerena, & Kielhofner, 2002). This approach is built around the exploration, compe-

tency, and achievement levels of change discussed in Chapter 10. Claudio needed to begin at the exploratory level. The therapist's aim was to facilitate his ability to make decisions to engage in occupational forms and to feel a sense of pleasure and efficacy in performance. In fact, the evaluation had already begun this process.

Facilitating Claudio's Decision-Making and Sense of Pleasure and Efficacy in Action

Claudio began regular participation in the administrative area and in the family group. In the former context, Claudio at first kept to himself working in the office area. He would not engage in anything that required him to work with others. Since Claudio was working on accounting tasks, an arrangement was made that the accountant who kept the books could supervise him. Together, they could talk in terms that Claudio knew from his management experience. The connection with the accountant was important for Claudio as it provided him validation. The therapist introduced the accountant to Claudio, and supervised his efforts to facilitate Claudio's occupational engagement. He first gave Claudio an overview of accounting practices at Reencuentros. Then he noted to Claudio that the system for registering data about income and expenditures needed improvement and he invited Claudio to think about the possibility of working with him to improve it. With constant encouragement, Claudio began to participate as the accountant's assistant for the first 2 months, working on this project.

At the end of the second month, he was still sometimes unsure of himself but was participating spontaneously and consistently. He was also beginning to show pride as he smiled each time he turned in work he had done. Up until this point he always worked under the direct supervision of the accountant who was only part-time in Reencuentros. Because of the progress in his volition, the therapist persuaded Claudio to also work when the accountant was not present. Claudio agreed, and was able to do this, asking for support if he needed it. As Claudio's sense of efficacy improved further, the therapist asked him to take on other responsibilities such as teaching basic accounting tasks to other members and taking payments from new members and creating receipts for them or their families. These responsibilities were important to him as they validated that he was trusted by the administration of the center. Increasingly, Claudio showed pride and satisfaction when he met with the accountant, helped others, and did his job well.

After another month and a half, Claudio began to come in late and to appear distracted as he worked. The therapist decided to observe him once again using the VQ (see Fig. 21-8). The observations suggested Claudio needed more challenge despite his refusal to accept more responsibility. This issue was taken up in the next phase of his intervention, which will be discussed later.

Beginning to Reapproach the Parental Role

Parallel with his accounting work, Claudio participated in the Parents Self Help Group. Other members of the group accepted and supported him. He continued to insist that the most important thing to him was to be with his kids, expressing immense pain at being away from his children coupled with anger toward his wife. He also felt very hopeless about any real possibility of seeing his children again. At first he would not accept responsibility for his own past mistakes. Led by the therapist, the female members of the group gave Claudio feedback on what had happened, helping him see the side of his wife and children. While he struggled with his own situation, Claudio took pride in helping others in the group, taking an interest in their struggles and outcomes. He was recognized in the group as being especially helpful to others. For the first couple of months, the main influence of the group was to validate his pain and give him feedback on his behavior and its effects on his family. With time, Claudio began to feel more comfortable admitting that he had not been a perfect parent. Other members of the group told their own stories, offering Claudio insight into how patience was required if he wanted to reconnect with his children. These stories also helped Claudio begin to fashion in his own occupational narrative a future in which he might be, once again, a father.

As Claudio's identification as a member of the group grew, he was increasingly able to reflect on himself and what he had done to contribute to the loss of his children. After 3 months he was ready to begin exploring what actions he needed to take to see his children again. Another important function of the group was that Claudio began to spend time in the role of a friend with individual members of the group, outside the formal group meeting time.

Building Claudio's Competency

Claudio's progress in his accounting assistant role and in his membership in the Parents Self Help Group indicated he was ready for the competency level of change. Additionally, the therapist felt that Claudio would benefit from individualized sessions with the therapist, which would help to establish goals for him. The therapist met with Claudio. After negotiating they agreed that Claudio's three main long-term goals should be:

- Being responsible for himself in the community (which would mean being discharged from the hospital)
- Taking on more responsibility in his work so that he felt more satisfaction in being productive
- Beginning to work to get closer to his kids.

The therapist met with Claudio and the psychiatrist to review his progress. The psychiatrist agreed that Claudio could be discharged under the condition that his medications were managed by someone other than himself, given his poor history of compliance. Claudio agreed that his mother (who was willing) could do it.

Being discharged meant that he had to live with his brother whom he did not like. It also meant that Claudio would eventually have to be responsible for cooking and organizing the house once his mother left. He did not like the prospect of doing this since he viewed it as women's work. He reluctantly committed to work toward these responsibilities to be free from the hospital.

The therapist began meeting weekly with Claudio to set concrete weekly goals aimed at moving toward his long-term goals and to identify strategies for accomplishing these short-term goals. Claudio expressed misgivings at starting this process, but the therapist indicated to Claudio that he was ready for this challenge and that she expected him to face it.

In their first session, the therapist shared with him the results of her most recent VQ observation of him in the volunteer work setting. She advised Claudio of her conclusion that his unwillingness to take on challenges more consistent with his skills was leading him to be bored in his work and not to derive the same satisfaction that he initially felt. She explained to him how his still weak sense of his capacities interfered with his ability to choose more challenging things to do, offering to coach him in this process.

Claudio rejected this explanation, indicating that the real problem was that he was tired because of his medications. The therapist validated his viewpoint by suggesting in response that they would set goals to increase his energy level. She then negotiated with Claudio to see what other things beyond his medication might be affecting his energy level. Their discussion led Claudio to recognize that his involvement in work painfully reminded him of his lost roles as an effective worker.

Suddenly, he asked to see the Role Checklist that he had filled out at the beginning of the program. When they completed another one, Claudio recognized that he had added the roles of volunteer and friend (*Fig. 21-9*). On reflection, he was able to reframe his experience as giving him hope that he could begin to reinstate his life again. The therapist also helped Claudio recognize that the volunteer role was meaningful to him and had value for others in the setting. Still, he recognized that he did not feel the same satisfaction in the volunteer role that he had felt at work. He saw it as hopeless that he would ever be able to work again as an engineer. The therapist validated his feelings, acknowledging that 15 years was a large gap in his career and he had a right to feel sad. At that, Claudio began to cry. The therapist responded with warmth and support. The whole interchange underscored Claudio's volitional struggle and the reasons for his ambivalence about his involvement in the volunteer accounting work.

After he recovered, the therapist advised Claudio that it was not clear what he might be able to do in the future related to work. She suggested that she would help him to assess his own skills and desires to identify and explore alternatives for work in the future. He agreed that this was a good plan and liked the idea that he would be responsible for evaluating himself.

The therapist then asked Claudio if he would like to help her to develop an economic forecast for Reencuentros in order to plan for the future. Claudio thanked the therapist for asking him to do this since it was an important task. He agreed to take on this project. Claudio worked on this plan for nearly a month. He needed ongoing support, as he would tend to view new challenges as insurmountable. For example, it became apparent that to do the economic planning, a certain software package was important. At first Claudio protested that he could not learn it, but with encouragement and coaching from the therapist he mastered it.

FIGURE 21-9 Claudio's Scores on the Follow-Up Role Checklist.

Role	Past	Present	Future	Not at all Valuable	Somewhat Valuable	Very Valuable
Student						
Worker						
Volunteer						
Caregiver						
Home Maintainer						
Friend						
Family Member						
Religious Participant						
Hobbyist/Amateur						
Participant in Organizations						
Other		Member of society	Member of society			

When the time came for him to present his recommendations, a meeting was set with the accountant and administrators of Reencuentros. Claudio was nervous but presented a well-done economic analysis of the center with recommendations for changes in the financial procedures. As he began to present his analysis and recommendations, he became quite animated and clearly felt proud about what he had accomplished. These recommendations included a proposal that the center should increase its charges for services. When the therapists questioned whether people would be willing to pay, Claudio responded, "The services here are very valuable to clients, they will be happy to pay for them." The therapists in charge of the program implemented most of Claudio's recommendations, which also served to validate for him the value of what he had accomplished.

Taking Responsibility for His Home

Claudio's next challenge was to take over responsibility for managing his home environment. While his brother kept the room in which he lived clean and organized, the rest of the house, including a combined living and dining room and Claudio's room, were ill kept. Claudio's room was so full of boxes that he barely had room to move about. When the issue of Claudio needing to manage his home came up in a community-living group, Claudio protested that he did not see why he had to do the cleaning, as it was women's work. Some female members of the group and the therapist gave him feedback and advised him that if he wanted to live there, he was responsible. They also pointed out that if he wanted to reconnect with his children, he would have to have a decent home in which to receive them.

Members of the group offered to help Claudio clean up his house and show him what to do to keep it clean and organized. Claudio reluctantly agreed. They planned to hold the next meeting of the group at Claudio's home to help him clean up and to teach him basic household cleaning tasks. After a long afternoon, his house became presentable. Claudio was able to recognize the transformation that had taken place and committed to continue cleaning the house.

Working in the Community

At this point, Claudio proposed to the therapist that he felt ready to begin the transition away from Reencuentros. With the therapist's help he was able to identify a business where he could begin working part time at a very basic job. The company involved computers. Claudio, at first, enjoyed the job very much, learning new computer skills and diligently discharging his responsibilities.

After a few months, in his monthly meetings with the therapist, Claudio began to complain that the work was not challenging enough for him. He also complained that he had lost so many years of working that he could not return to his engineering career. Over time the therapist helped Claudio realize that it was his own volition, not a lack of skills, that kept him from doing more. Claudio came to identify that his current values were such that he really did not want to take on more responsibility in work and that he needed to leave behind some of his other values of achievement. Eventually, he came to a point where he was satisfied with his job and planned to stay in it.

Reconnecting With His Children

As Claudio became stabilized in his home and job, he was ready to take on the biggest challenge of all, contacting his children. Claudio's mother had decided to tell him that his sister still maintained contact with his ex-wife and children. When Claudio learned this he wanted his sister to arrange a meeting with his children. However, she felt this was too drastic a step and suggested instead that he get a message to his former wife that he wanted to see his children. Claudio was afraid to make this contact himself and asked his therapist to do so.

When she realized how difficult this was for Claudio, she agreed. The wife explained to the therapist that she had remarried when the children were still young and that they now consider her new husband to be their father. Nevertheless, she agreed to let them know that their biological father wanted to contact them. At first, the children indicated they were not interested in seeing him. The oldest child remembered his father as a very frightening person, as he had seen him at his worst.

This news was devastating to Claudio, but in the parenting group other members told stories of permanent estrangement from their children and encouraged Claudio to be patient and persistent if he wanted to make contact. The therapist advised Claudio to focus on reconnecting with his siblings and their families. She noted that, perhaps, with time things would work out with his children. Claudio agreed to attend a family reunion that his mother arranged. This was an emotional gathering and it was followed by regular visits between Claudio and a number of his siblings' families. With time he was able to rebuild relationships with his brothers and sisters and their families.

At this point, seeing his progress, Claudio's sister, who maintained the connection with his former wife and children, agreed to plead his case. She spoke to the wife and children and explained how hard he had worked and the progress he had made. Subsequently, the children accepted an invitation to meet Claudio at his sister's house. This meeting was awkward, and Claudio was disappointed that there was no connection between them.

At the next meeting of the parenting group Claudio shared his experience and the group once again helped him see the progress he had made in meeting his children. They also helped him to come up with a plan for staying in touch with his children by phone and e-mail. Over the following months, Claudio continued to contact his children and they increasingly responded to his e-mails and phone calls, eventually coming to visit him at his house.

After a year had passed, Claudio's children, two of whom were in university, were seeing him regularly and even calling occasionally to ask for advice. Claudio maintained his job and kept his house in reasonable shape. Occasionally Claudio would call the therapist at Reencuentros to complain about some problem, to seek advice, or to report a new connection with his children. All in all, Claudio had put together and enacted a new occupational narrative for himself.

Claudio in Perspective

Claudio was a challenging client because of the chronic nature of his disability and his tendency to reject services. The therapist's approach that carefully met Claudio where he was represents the best of client-centered therapy. Importantly, the Role Checklist was the ideal way to begin assessment, since it gave him some validation for past performance and allowed him to open up in the informal interview that followed. At one point in his therapy, Claudio took the checklist in his hands and said, "This is what made me trust occupational therapy." Indeed, a central element in the success of his therapy was inspiring confidence in him that therapy could help him. The therapist was able to do this in part because she respected Claudio, despite his being difficult and demeaning to the therapist. In part, she was able to do this because she had a strong theoretical orientation and was able to explain her perspectives in professional terms that Claudio respected.

Discussion

Each of the cases in this chapter illustrate the human potential that exists even in the face of extreme adversity and personal failure. Life stories can be retold and rebuilt. However, the extent of the devastation of life faced by each of the clients in this chapter required substantial and long-term efforts on the part of therapists. It may be tempting to suggest that such intervention is not realistic because of restrictions on lengths of stay, reimbursement, and so on. However, what the cases cry out for is the advocacy of occupational therapists to secure services for their clients, whether on an individual level (as Haydée's therapist did), through the development of an independent program (as Claudio's therapist did), or through collective efforts of occupational therapists to achieve support for the kinds of service clients truly need.

Reference

de las Heras, C. G., Llerena, V., & Kielhofner, G. (2002). *Remotivation process: Progressive intervention for individuals with severe volitional challenges (Version 1.0).* Chicago: Model of Human Occupation Clearinghouse, Department of Occupational Therapy, College of Applied Health Sciences, University of Illinois at Chicago.

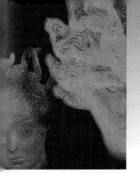

22

Applying MOHO to Clients Who Are Cognitively Impaired

- Gary Kielhofner
- Marianne Masako Ankersjö
- Frances Oakley
- Marian K. Scheinholtz
- Susan Anderson
- Luc Vercruysse

Clients who have cognitive impairments can pose significant challenges because of their functional limitations and/or problematic behaviors. Because of such challenges, these clients are not always recognized and treated as individuals with desires and preferences who need something meaningful to do. Since persons with cognitive limitations can lack the personal resources to advocate for their own perspectives and desires, therapists must advocate on their behalf and seek to empower them. This means putting in the time and effort to learn about their volition, habituation, performance capacity, and environmental context.

As the cases in this chapter illustrate, there are a number of formal and informal ways of gathering information on such clients that can help reveal their identities, desires, fears, and so on. These cases will also illustrate how gathering this information can lead to an understanding of clients that informs effective intervention.

Finding Peace

The case description that follows illustrates how therapists can use MOHO as an approach for both direct care and consultation with clients who have dementia in an institutional context. The case illustrates the impor-

tance of understanding how the environment impacts such clients and of appreciating their volition, habituation, and performance capacity. Lars, the man discussed in the following case, died approximately 1 year after the intervention described was completed. This case is dedicated to his memory.

Lars

Two years previously, at age 86, Lars was diagnosed with Alzheimer's disease and multi-infarct dementia. A year later, at age 87, Lars was no longer able to live alone at home and was admitted to a nursing home. During the first 6 months, he adjusted to the routine of the nursing home, performing his self-care with assistance.

The occupational therapist at this nursing home in central Stockholm runs therapy groups and provides individual intervention when residents require it. The therapist also works with nursing staff regarding self-care issues of residents. Finally, she provides consultation to nursing staff on managing special resident problems.

The Precipitating Problem
Six months before, Lars became agitated and was no longer able to follow the daily routine. He frequently refused to get out of bed in the morning.

He resisted getting cleaned and cared for by staff. Interactions with him often became tense and confrontational. Increasingly, Lars had become physically aggressive.

Lars also began to disrupt the ward in two unique ways. Ever since Lars came to the ward, he occasionally made some kind of noise, best described as a high-pitched vibrato singing. His singing became frequent and more intense. For as much as 4 hours at a time, Lars would sing while lying in his bed. Additionally, Lars often became restless, wandering into other residents' rooms. He sometimes did this at night, frightening others from their sleep. During the daytime he would enter other residents' rooms, lie down in their beds, eat their food and candy, and throw their belongings into their wastebaskets. When the staff tried to get Lars out of the other residents' rooms, he would become combative. He also threatened other residents who approached him.

At this point, the interdisciplinary team met to discuss Lars. At this meeting the occupational therapist agreed to assess Lars and to consult with the ward staff on ways to reduce Lars' disruptive actions and help him readjust his routine.

Information Gathering

The therapist decided to gather information through both structured and unstructured means. Her primary question was: Why had Lars' routine behavior changed so dramatically? Although it could be due to the progression of the dementia, the therapist decided to explore whether the causes might be related to Lars' volition, habituation, performance capacity, or his relationship to the environment of the nursing home.

The therapist conducted a semi-structured interview adopted from the Occupational Performance History Interview (OPHI-II) with Lars' son and daughter-in-law. The therapist gathered information on Lars' occupational history in hopes that his previous occupational life and characteristics might shed light on his present actions. She also did a series of brief informal observations of Lars and of the ward setting. Finally, she administered the Volitional Questionnaire (VQ) and the Assessment of Communication and Interaction Skills (ACIS).

Lars' Occupational History

For most of his adult life, Lars had owned and managed a small trucking company. He had one son. His wife had been ill for a long period and died when Lars was 75. Ten years before, at age 78, Lars was still running the trucking company and living alone in his house. At that time his son began to notice that his father had trouble calculating his workers' wages and other cognitive tasks. His father, who was always very private, became increasingly withdrawn. He would only talk if someone else first spoke to him.

Two years later, at the age of 80, he retired and sold his company because he could no longer manage it. This was difficult for Lars because his work was so central to his life. Four years later he had to stop driving, as he could no longer find his way around and sometimes forgot where he had parked his car.

According to his son, Lars was always fiercely independent and somewhat of a loner. For example, when he came home late in the evenings after being on the road all day, he read the mail and reviewed business papers over dinner. When the business had hard times or the mail contained bad news, Lars would read it and then silently leave the house and walk, sometimes for several hours. He always had a habit of taking long walks to cope with stress.

Lars was a handyman who could repair anything around the house, and when he was not working he kept himself busy with repairs and upkeep. When involved in a project, he would be singularly focused on getting it done, ignoring, for example, his wife's invitation to meals. He generally preferred solitary activities and limited his interactions with others to a few people with whom he was familiar and comfortable.

Lars' son noted that although Lars did not talk much, he had strong opinions about most things. When in a disagreement, Lars often lost his temper, shouted, and then walked away. According to Lars' daughter-in-law, Lars was a very shy man. She believed that he felt uncomfortable and self-conscious around others, especially around women. She also noted that he had a temper and strong opinions about almost everything. Nevertheless, he seldom expressed his views unless someone else said something that disagreed with them.

Despite his tendency to keep to himself, Lars was a neighborhood handyman who always could be called on to fix things. He obviously enjoyed being valued by others. He would willingly spend hours fixing a problem around their house. Other than home repair, Lars had no interest in other domestic activities such as gardening or home decorating. He also paid little attention to how he dressed.

Lars had been an outdoorsman who liked to hunt. He was very athletic and engaged in windsurfing and water-skiing when he was younger. He also liked motorbikes and owned one for a time. At home his leisure included reading trucking magazines and automobile magazines. While most of Lars' leisure interests were predominantly solitary and male-oriented, he did like music and dancing and would go to dances with his wife.

Lars was proud of his roles as husband and father. He saw himself as head of the house, taking seriously all the associated responsibilities. He was not particularly close to his son, but the son felt that his father had always provided well for him and cared for him. Lars also stoically provided and cared for his wife during her long illness. His whole pattern of doing things reflected his fierce independence and need to be in control of things. Although he helped others, he preferred going alone in his own life.

When Lars became a widower, he met Maggie who lived in a nearby neighborhood. He spent a great deal of time at her home under the auspices of doing home repair and chores for her. In time, she became his main concern, so he was routinely looking after her home. At one point they were engaged to be married. However, as Lars' dementia became apparent, they did not pursue it. Nonetheless, Maggie continued to present herself as Lars fiancé and remained a loyal and close friend who still visited Lars daily in the nursing home.

The Physical Environment
The ward was locked to prevent residents from leaving the ward unattended. It contained both single and double rooms, housing up to 40 residents. Each room had a washbasin, but showers and toilets were in a common space. The rooms were organized and decorated identically with the exception that residents could personalize their own space by displaying their own belongings. Aside from a few pictures

of his family, Lars did not have any decorations of his own in his room.

Ten residents shared one day room. There was one bigger room for events and meetings that could accommodate all the residents of the ward. Outside a small kitchen there was a large table, where residents could eat snacks. Architecturally, the large ward was not optimal. It was hard to find one's way to and from all the different areas. However, the environment was airy and lighted and there was an inner garden court with flowers and bushes.

The Social Environment
Lars' closest caregivers were a team of five staff members, four females and one male who worked the day shift. The male caregiver, Bengt, was primarily responsible for Lars' care and for communicating with Lars' relatives and other team members. Bengt was also responsible for buying things Lars needed, taking care of his clothes, and cleaning his room. When Bengt was at work he was always responsible for giving Lars a shower and helping him with other hygiene and dressing. Lars was much more comfortable around Bengt than other staff. When Bengt was off, the other four members of the team were usually responsible for helping Lars with his daily routines. However, the staffing patterns did not allow continuity of staff members who interacted with Lars. Additional personnel working weekends and nights and covering vacations also had occasional contact with and responsibility for Lars. In the course of a typical week, Lars interacted with as many as 15 different staff members. Generally, Lars was more comfortable with male staff and he became particularly upset when female staff members worked with him regarding personal hygiene.

Maggie came to visit Lars daily. His son and daughter-in-law visited him once or twice a month. Lars shared his room with another resident. However, Lars did not interact with him or any of the other ward residents, except in a structured group or when he was threatening them. He seldom engaged in group activities such as music and exercise sessions.

Lars' Volition
Nygård, Borell, and Gustavsson (1995) document how the progression of dementia represents a con-

stant assault on one's occupational self-image. In particular, the sense of self as effective in managing daily life becomes progressively eroded. This was certainly true for Lars.

As noted in his history, Lars had always been very skilled in fixing things and prided himself on his own independence and usefulness to others. With the progression of his disease, he had lost most of his abilities and with them his sense of efficacy and control. For example, he was unable to operate his electrical razor and thought that it was broken. Therefore, he took it apart and tried to fix it. He became befuddled and upset and destroyed the razor. Whenever he became confused or had difficulty doing something, he grew extremely anxious. Little in Lars' daily routine provided him with either a sense of being in control or pleasure. Finally, he was not able to do any of the things that formerly made him feel valued.

Observations With the Volitional Questionnaire

Lars' therapist observed him with the VQ during three different activities to determine how his motivation varied with environmental circumstances. The first observation was during a ball tossing game. The second was during an exercise group. These activities are routinely offered on the ward, although as noted above, Lars seldom participated in them. The third observation occurred by chance when Lars joined the therapist in a spontaneous activity. Ratings from these three observations are shown in *Figure 22-1*.

The ball tossing activity occurred in a secluded area on the ward. Ten participants sat in a circle, passing, tossing, or kicking different kinds of balls.

FIGURE 22-1   Lars' Scores on the VQ.

	Facility: Nursing Home											
Client: Lars **Diagnosis:** Alzheimer's dementia												
Area of Evaluate	**Ratings**											
	Session 1 Ballgame				**Session 2** Exercise				**Session 3** Scooter			
1. Shows curiosity	P	H	**I**	S	**P**	H	I	S	P	H	I	**S**
2. Initiates actions/tasks	P	H	**I**	S	**P**	H	I	S	P	H	I	**S**
3. Tries new things	P	**H**	I	S	**P**	H	I	S	P	H	I	**S**
4. Shows pride	**P**	H	I	S	**P**	H	I	S	P	H	**I**	S
5. Attempts challenges	**P**	H	I	S	**P**	H	I	S	P	H	I	**S**
6. Seeks additional responsibilities	**P**	H	I	S	**P**	H	I	S	**P**	H	I	S
7. Tries to correct mistakes	P	**H**	I	S	**P**	H	I	S	P	H	**I**	S
8. Tries to solve problems	P	**H**	I	S	**P**	H	I	S	P	H	**I**	S
9. Shows preferences	P	**H**	I	S	**P**	H	I	S	P	H	I	**S**
10. Pursues activity to completion/ accomplishment	**P**	H	I	S	**P**	H	I	S	P	H	I	**S**
11. Stays engaged	P	**H**	I	S	**P**	H	I	S	P	H	I	**S**
12. Invests additional energy/emotion attention	P	**H**	I	S	**P**	H	I	S	P	H	I	**S**
13. Indicates goals	**P**	H	I	S	**P**	H	I	S	P	H	**I**	S
14. Shows that an activity is special or significant	P	**H**	I	S	**P**	H	I	S	P	H	I	**S**
Key : **P** = Passive; **H** = Hesistant; **I** = Involved; **S** = Spontaneous												

A group leader directed and encouraged the members in this activity.

At first, Lars stood outside the group but watched with curiosity. When asked if he wanted to join in the game, he willingly sat in an empty chair offered to him. He was able to participate in the game with support from the therapist who was leading the game. With prompting, he made efforts to correct mistakes he made in following instructions of the group leader. When encouraged, he tried to solve a problem (i.e., the ball got stuck between chairs and he freed it). He did not interact with other participants except as was necessitated to pass or receive the ball. He stayed with the activity for the duration of the group, but was easily distracted from the game. Overall, he participated without enthusiasm, except that he occasionally smiled. The positive aspect of this activity for Lars was that it was a kind of sport.

The exercise activity also involved residents sitting in a circle. A staff member led the participants in a series of upper body and leg exercises. Lars sat during the entire activity with his arms in his lap, looking down at the floor. He did not react when his name was called and turned away when tapped on the shoulder. Lars appeared not to enjoy this activity since it involved everyone doing the same thing at the same time as they followed instructions from the leader.

As noted above, the third activity happened fortuitously. Staff used a three-wheeled cycle (which is propelled by kicking) to travel in the large corridors that connected parts of the facility. Lars was intently watching the therapist when she arrived on the cycle, and she offered him a ride. Lars cautiously stepped on the cycle and with encouragement from the therapist began to steer it while the therapist pushed him. Lars visibly enjoyed this activity. He smiled throughout and when asked if it is fun he answered an enthusiastic "yes." He maneuvered the bicycle very skillfully around the ward while it moved at a walking speed. He carefully avoided furniture and other residents. He was able to maneuver correctly even when going in reverse. He chose increasingly complex routes to take as the ride progressed, but declined to propel himself. This activity seemed especially enjoyable to Lars as it had some connection his past leisure activities and driving for a living.

The three observations highlighted that:

- Lars had the ability to become motivated if the activity fit with his interests and was not too demanding
- Lars liked activities that allowed him some measure of independence and safety
- Lars liked activities that connected in some way with his past leisure
- Lars' motivation was highly dependent on environmental circumstances.

Habituation

The ward had very strict routines. For example, breakfast was routinely served in bed. After breakfast, a staff member helped Lars to get groomed and dressed for the day. Lunch and dinner were taken outside the kitchen every day at the same time. With the exception of the groups that Lars only occasionally attended, his daily visit with Maggie, and personal grooming with the help of a staff member, he spent the rest of his time alone.

During the first 6 months of his stay at the nursing home, Lars had been able to follow the ward routine, cooperate with self-care, and attend some groups. He also had engaged in quiet activities such as reading automotive magazines. His daily visit from his friend, Maggie, had been and remained the highlight of his day.

Within the past 6 months his routine had become quite disrupted. Lars did have some good days in which he could participate in elements of the routine, but this was largely not the case. On rare, good days, Lars would cooperate with staff on personal hygiene, but most days he was uncooperative.

Lars had two kinds of days, walking days and lying-in-bed-and-singing days. During the former he was agitated and wandered around the ward, looking out of windows, lying down on couches. On days when he was particularly agitated, he wandered into other residents' rooms, sometimes lying on their beds, eating their food, and throwing their belongings in the trash. He also would push other residents around in their wheelchairs whether they wanted it or not, sometimes at a frightening, near-running speed. On his singing days, he stayed in bed, making his singing noise. During these days he was generally unwilling to get out of bed except for meals and to visit Maggie.

After lunch he returned to his walking or singing procedure until his friend, Maggie came for a visit. When she arrived he attended to her and appeared to calm down. They sat on a sofa in the open staircase area or in the inner garden during summertime. Maggie always brought candies; they sat together, holding hands, and Lars ate the candies. When Maggie left Lars generally went back to the procedure of the day, either singing or walking.

On days when Lars was doing better, he might join a group activity. He did attempt to help the staff by pushing or pulling a cart. On bad days, he became quite agitated, disrupted other residents, and could be combative when staff members tried to manage him. On several occasions when he was very agitated, he managed to escape and was found each time by the police, confused and upset, wandering in the neighborhood.

Performance Capacity

Lars had neither obvious sensory impairments nor musculoskeletal problems. He was fully ambulatory, although he walked with his back and head bent forward, taking small steps without swinging his arms. He had obvious cognitive problems associated with dementia.

While Lars could not report his lived experience, his therapist inferred the following from observation. Lars appeared to have difficulty organizing and making sense of much of what happened around him. When situations were unfamiliar or too complex, Lars became confused, apparently feeling out of control and frightened. He tended to get particularly upset when he felt cornered with no escape path. This occurred, for example, if a staff member happened to approach Lars when the wall was to his back and furniture to his side, blocking his movement.

When Lars was particularly agitated he stiffened and hissed like a cornered wild animal. When in this state, he would hit anyone who approached him. He apparently became aggressive in an attempt to maintain a sense of personal control and safety.

The following episode exemplifies how Lars' confusion and fear could escalate into a major confrontation on the ward. Lars enjoyed eating small candies. One day he found a nutshell of approximately the same size and put it into his mouth. He chewed the shell compulsively although it had punctured his gums and caused his mouth to bleed. When he realized his mouth was bleeding he became very upset. Staff members' attempts to help him spit out the shell only served to further agitate and frighten him. When their urging became stronger and they attempted to approach him, he became more frightened, started hissing, and tried to hit anyone in reach. Eventually, it took four people to hold Lars down while a fifth worked on removing the shell from his mouth. During the battle that ensued, Lars bit the staff member who was attempting to remove the shell.

Lars' sense of insecurity and fear that came from confusing or threatening situations appeared to be at the base of many of the difficulties the staff had managing him. His reactions, extreme as they could be, tended to provoke staff to action and their action, in turn, further upset Lars.

Occupational Performance Skills

Informal observation indicated that Lars' motor skills were basically intact and that he had major deficits in process skills associated with his dementia. Since his performance was limited and closely supervised, most of his performance problems were effectively managed when he was cooperative. When Lars was motivated (particularly when he was free from feeling threatened), he was able to cooperate with the supervision and assistance to complete basic activities of daily living. As the VQ observation demonstrated, he was also able to participate in simple leisure activities when he was positively motivated.

Lars' communication/interaction was clearly impaired. He only responded verbally to his son, Maggie, Bengt, his primary caregiver, and occasionally to ward staff with whom he was more familiar. Lars answered their questions by saying "yes," "no," "I don't know," or "I don't remember." He sometimes said the name of his friend, Maggie.

Because of Lars' difficult interactions, the therapist observed him with the ACIS. She completed the ACIS based on observation of Lars on the ward. Since his overall skill level did not vary much in different situations, the ACIS was scored only once from several observations. The therapist paid particular attention to environmental factors that affected whether he would use his existing skills. *Figure 22-2* shows the results of the ACIS observation. Observations of environmental factors that affected skills are noted in the comments section.

Overall, the ACIS observation revealed that Lars exhibited some very basic communication/interaction skills in the areas of physicality and relations when he trusted the person with whom he was interacting and when the occupational form was not too complex. The area of information exchange was

much more restricted. His communication was largely through body language, since his skill at speaking was restricted to a few words or phrases.

Formulation of Lars' Occupational Status

Based on this initial evaluation, the therapist developed the following formulation of Lars' occupational situation. Lars' occupational participation was limited to the area of activities of daily living and simple leisure pursuits that were available in the ward. Within these two areas his performance was restricted due to deficits in process and communication/interaction skills.

FIGURE 22-2   Lars' Scores on the ACIS.

Client: Lars					Observation Situation Nursing home ward	Comments
PHYSICALITY *Skills in this area basically adequate toward demands*						
Contacts	4	3	2	1	Holds hands with someone close to him	
Gazes	4	3	2	1	Looks at people only when interested in them	
Gestures	4	3	2	1	Gestures only when frightened/angry to threaten hitting	
Maneuvers	4	3	2	1	Able to maneuver in ADL and leisure when motivated	
Orients	4	3	2	1	Fine when he wants to interact; otherwise turns or walks away	
Postures	4	3	2	1	(Same as above)	
INFORMATION EXCHANGE						
Articulates	4	3	2	1	Articulation adequate but limited to a few words	
Asserts	4	3	2	1	Aggressive in asserting his desires	
Asks	4	3	2	1	Never	
Engages	4	3	2	1	Unable to initiate	
Expresses	4	3	2	1	Only in highly structured situation through body language	
Modulates	4	3	2	1		
Shares	4	3	2	1	Only through smiling	
Speaks	4	3	2	1	Only a few words	
Sustains	4	3	2	1	Cannot sustain interaction	
RELATIONS						
Collaborates	4	3	2	1	Variable, depends on motivation and whether person is familiar	
Conforms	4	3	2	1	Can follow basic rules in structured situation	
Focuses	4	3	2	1	Variable, depends on interest and relationship to person	
Relates	4	3	2	1	Relates only to a few close people	
Respects	4	3	2	1	Mostly unaware of others' wishes & reactions	

Comments: *Overall C/I is very restricted and dependent on either a clear structure or comfort/familiarity with person involved. When approaching him, staff should be aware of how their degree of familiarity affects his skill in interacting and adjust their behavior/expectations accordingly.*

Key : **4** = Competent; **3** = Questionable; **2** = Ineffective; **1** = Deficit

A number of Lars' past volitional traits still influenced his motivation. He still tended to be someone who would strongly protest his view of things. He continued to be a loner who only trusted a few people and who needed space when he was upset. When he felt contradicted or cornered he tended to react strongly. This tendency was exacerbated by the fact that his personal causation was severely eroded. He did not feel a sense of efficacy or control over his circumstances much of the time. When he felt out of control he became extremely anxious. When he was in such a state, he was not cooperative and was at risk to become aggressive or combative as a way to maintain some control over his situation and to feel safe.

Most of his past routines had been completely eroded. Since the spring when his disruptive behavior began, he had not been able to maintain even a basic self-care routine. The lack of familiarity in his routine also contributed to his anxiety and fear. When he became upset he wandered through the ward in the same way that he previously coped with stress through long solitary walks. When wandering, he sometimes entered other residents' rooms and became disoriented. He apparently threw their things into the wastebasket to make the room more like his own, which had few objects.

The emergence of Lars' uncooperative and combative behavior coincided with the beginning of summer vacations. Staff members with whom he had been most comfortable had been away on vacation and Lars was confronted with new faces, including less experienced personnel who had more difficulty understanding Lars and how to support his functioning. Also, with new staff the rhythm of the routine on the ward had changed. This change in the environment was the event precipitating Lars' negative behavior. Since that time, he had been unable to reestablish a routine and had been chronically anxious and out of control. The lack of continuity in staff members who dealt with Lars maintained this state of affairs.

Intervention

The therapist first developed the following recommendations that staff implemented:

- A structured daily schedule was developed for Lars so that all staff members knew exactly what things Lars did and could maintain the same routine. This helped Lars feel safe. The familiar routine also helped prevent Lars from becoming disoriented and confused
- Only male staff did personal hygiene with Lars, given his discomfort with women helping him
- When Bengt was not at work, persons who were familiar to Lars worked with him. Inconsistency of staff across the week was recognized as a general problem affecting other residents as well. Therefore, a work schedule and vacation rotation that allowed better continuity of staff familiar to residents was developed
- Lars was allowed to eat breakfast sitting at a table, dressed or in a morning robe, as he was used to doing at home. This facilitated getting him out of bed since he would always get out of bed to eat
- Lars' regular attendance at the more motivating groups was encouraged so that it became part of his habit structure
- When Lars was having a good day, staff offered him opportunities to be useful by helping with simple tasks or chores.

In her direct care role, the therapist's aim was to discover effective strategies for interacting with Lars. She planned to use this information to develop guidelines for nursing staff. As a first step, the therapist had to gain Lars' confidence. Given his suspicion of unknown faces and discomfort with unfamiliar women, the therapist's strategy was to become familiar to Lars.

She made a point of validating him by greeting him several times a day. She later began trying to encourage interaction by offering to shake hands with Lars whenever she encountered him on the ward. At first, he was very frightened and quickly walked away when the therapist approached him. After a while he stood still with an angry face, hissing and whistling and lifting up his right hand as if to strike the therapist. When she first offered a handshake, he would only hit her hand. Eventually, when she became familiar to him, he began to shake her hand when she greeted him.

After this basic level of interaction was established, the therapist was able to find moments in which Lars would accept her arm and they would walk around the corridors together. She knew that he felt an urge to walk to calm himself, but that the walks tended to result in his getting lost and wandering into residents' rooms. Consequently, her goal was to get him to walk with a companion.

During these walks the therapist talked slowly and calmly to him, sometimes singing quietly or humming. Through body language she identified for him that he could choose the way they would walk. As their walks became more regular, Lars began to answer simple questions. He sometimes allowed the therapist to choose the way in the walks and his willingness to do so was subtly communicated through his body language (i.e., it could be felt when walking with him). He also began to smile at the therapist during these walks.

In this way the therapist was able to identify a strategy for other staff to follow when establishing a relationship with Lars, including how to approach him in a stepwise fashion as the relationship with him was built. As these walks with staff became regular, Lars' wandering behavior became much less frequent. Moreover, if he did get lost, he was usually able to take redirection from a staff member who simply joined him and led the way back.

The therapist also worked directly with Lars to facilitate his participation in the music session and ball game on the ward. At the time the therapist terminated her direct intervention, Lars was able to attend groups sporadically and generally participated in and enjoyed them. The goal was still to make his attendance routine.

Lars' disruptive singing also decreased significantly. He became more cooperative with staff and was much less likely to become aggressive. He still exhibited some fear and anxiety, but staff members now knew how to avoid escalating his fears. He was able to establish a routine of activities of daily living that was comfortable for him.

Lars in Perspective

This case illustrates how negative or disruptive action can be related to the client's volition and habituation. Lars exemplified the fact that what a client with de-

mentia does is not simply a function of the cognitive impairment. It can sometimes be explained in terms of a person's previous occupational characteristics and experiences (Nygård et al., 1995). This case also illustrates the key importance of environmental factors in institutional settings. Environmental characteristics have an important and sometimes overlooked impact on the performance of persons with dementia (Borell, Gustavsson, Sandman, & Kielhofner, 1994; Borell, Sandman, & Kielhofner, 1991; Josephsson, 1994).

The therapist's approach in this case underscores the value of careful assessment in managing difficult behavior. As in this case, an occupational history is commonly done with a relative when the client is unable to respond to the interview (Oakley, 1987). Performing this kind of family interview followed by observations with the VQ is an effective approach with clients who are unable to articulate their own volition. The therapist's combination of direct services and consultation with nursing staff was an effective way to meet Lars' needs. In the end, occupational therapy greatly reduced Lars' problematic behavior and increased his ability to participate in self-care and basic ward routines. It terminated a cycle of negative affect and conflict that had emerged between Lars and ward staff. Most importantly, it increased the quality of Lars' last year of life.

Discovering and Supporting Volition

The following case documents intervention with Robert, who lived in an institutional setting. The interdisciplinary team referred him to occupational therapy because he was difficult to manage on the ward. In this and other similar institutional settings, behavior techniques (which in effect are punishments) are often used to manage aggressive behavior.

The occupational therapist in this setting had gained the respect of interdisciplinary staff by using an alternative approach, based on understanding the residents' volition. That is, the therapist had shown how withdrawn or aggressive behavior could be understood as being motivated by how residents saw their world through their own volition. When she gained an understanding of the resident's volition, she could recommend a plan of therapy that was most often more effective than behavioral techniques.

Robert

Robert was 28 years old. He had lived in an institutional environment in New England since the age of 4, when he was diagnosed as being both autistic and mentally retarded. Robert also had a seizure disorder for which he received anticonvulsive medication. He had been in several facilities during his childhood. When he was 12 he came to the state facility where he still resided at the time. Robert lived on a unit for residents with behavior disorders.

A physically unremarkable man of slight-to-medium build, Robert had no speech. He occasionally smiled or laughed to express happiness and usually did not respond at all when another person spoke to him. With few exceptions, such as eating, Robert did not spontaneously engage in what ordinary members of society would recognize as an occupational form.

Robert had difficulty performing and cooperating with personal hygiene. He sometimes took all his clothes off in front of others. He was physically aggressive to staff or residents when they came close to or touched him. Occasionally, he got so out of control that he damaged his own belongings and institutional property. These were the types of problems for which the interdisciplinary staff wanted assistance from the occupational therapist.

Assessment: In Search of Robert's Volition

The occupational therapist began with the following broad question: How did Robert make sense of himself and his environment? She wanted to know if Robert had identifiable interests and values and how these were expressed in his behavior, including his asocial actions. The therapist also wanted to know what kinds of feelings Robert might have related to control of his circumstances. Withdrawal and aggression are often closely related to anxiety and perceived threat. Consequently, the occupational therapist anticipated that Robert's personal causation might involve feelings about being unable to control his circumstances and that these feelings were related to his withdrawal and aggression.

Because Robert was incapable of any self-report or formal testing, the occupational therapist decided to conduct the evaluation mainly through informal observation. The therapist expected that she might infer from Robert's reactions to the environment what interested him and mattered to him and when he felt threatened or out of control. Moreover, the therapist expected the observation to provide cues about how the environment could be altered to support more positive behavior from Robert.

The therapist's first observation confirmed that Robert was extremely withdrawn. He would sit or stand in one position for long periods during which he did nothing but warily watch others. Robert occasionally exhibited stereotyped behaviors, such as rocking his body as he sat with his knees tucked under his chin. He resisted initial attempts of the occupational therapist to initiate interaction with him by turning away or gesturing aggressively.

The therapist decided that she would continue to observe Robert in a variety of settings and situations. She reasoned that by examining Robert in these different contexts, she might get additional information about Robert's volitional status. Since Robert was generally so withdrawn and inactive, she also decided it would be more informative to observe him briefly in a number of different contexts than to conduct a single more lengthy or formal observation. The occupational therapist did not formally use the VQ as a rating scale because she planned this series of very brief observations. Instead, she used the items on the scale as a general guide for her observations of Robert.

The therapist made the informal observations of Robert's behavior throughout the day in the various environments he occupied within the hospital. She also supplemented the information by interviewing staff concerning their perceptions of and interactions with Robert.

The therapist learned from observation and staff reports that Robert was able to feed himself using a spoon and to drink from a cup. He ate very fast without concern that he sometimes dropped food on the floor. He apparently had little understanding of or concern about personal hygiene. Robert would cooperate or resist a staff member's efforts at completing grooming according to whether he found the sensory stimulation enjoyable. For example, Robert, who liked the feeling of water, cooperated while being bathed by staff, although he made no attempts to wash himself. On the other hand, he resisted having his teeth brushed by staff, apparently because he did not like the feeling of the toothbrush or taste of the toothpaste.

Robert occasionally had toilet accidents during the day, although he could lower his pants and sit on the toilet without help. Consequently, the accidents appeared to be related to the fact that Robert did not always perceive the rationale for relieving himself on a toilet, especially if there was no ready access to one.

Robert could often be observed curled up asleep on the floor of the large room in which residents were kept during most of the day. Occasionally, Robert walked around the day area of the unit with no apparent aim. At other times, he sat with his knees drawn up to his chest, distancing himself as far away from other residents as possible. He frequently slapped, spat at, or threw spit at any staff or residents who came within a foot or two of him.

Robert was able to recognize from environmental cues when it was time for meals. He also performed some routine behavior at mealtime, such as waiting in the cafeteria line to be served. These observations of Robert's behavior suggested that he was clearly aware of his environment. He would conform to social norms, such as standing in line for food, when he was motivated.

At first, Robert appeared to prefer being alone. In particular, he liked to have some distance between himself and other residents. The occupational therapist wondered if this may have been a reflection of the potential of being attacked by other residents or having one's belongings or food taken. She reasoned that Robert's antisocial behavior might be a response to the chaotic environment of the ward. She resolved to continue to attempt to make social contact with Robert.

Despite Robert's consistent antisocial behavior, he showed that he actually wanted to have interactions with others. After the therapist had made clear to Robert through her behavior that she was not a threat, he made eye contact and sometimes

smiled in response to being lightly touched or softly spoken to. He even occasionally reached out to touch the therapist or hold her hand.

The occupational therapist observed that ward staff did not frequently approach Robert, except to stop his aggressive behavior. Robert had apparently come to know ward staff mainly as persons who forced him to do things that he did not want to do. They, in turn, saw him as a resistive and aggressive resident who needed occasional coercion to comply with unit procedures. Robert and the staff were clearly locked in an ongoing struggle.

Robert appeared to have some interests. He liked going out of doors, walking about, touching the grass, and feeling sunshine on his face. He liked playing in water and taking showers. His therapist could tell when Robert was interested in something by noting the frequency with which he tried to do things and by his affective responses, such as smiling or laughing.

Robert did not appear to care about his own clothing except as it affected his comfort or discomfort. He was unaware of when clothes were torn, backward, or inside-out. He could remove his shoes, socks, and shirts and did this when it pleased him, apparently unaware of others' responses.

An Explanation of Robert's Volition

Robert's occupational therapist constructed the following explanation of his volition. He had extremely limited comprehension of the social and cultural world around him. Moreover, his caretakers saw him primarily as a severely limited person with behavior problems. They sought to control Robert's problematic behavior but failed to invite him to participate with them in a positive way. Consequently, Robert did not internalize social values and therefore did not react like or understand the reactions of others to a variety of situations. For example, he did not experience shame at public nakedness. He did not show shame or disgust in response to his toileting accidents. He had no apparent regard for his appearance that suggested he did not have a view of himself as perceived by others.

While Robert did not share many of the culturally provided commonsense views of the world that ordinarily constitute volition, he did, nonetheless, possess an active volition. He clearly enjoyed certain activities that gave him basic sensory pleasure, including self-stimulation. He was attracted to other people and enjoyed simple interaction such as touching. Robert's values were:

- To do what he wanted
- To avoid being forced to do things
- To avoid aggression or loss at the hands of others.

His withdrawal and his aggression appeared clearly linked to these concerns.

Given Robert's level of cognitive functioning, he could not be expected to have a complex idea of his capacities or a very good grasp of how his behaviors were related to consequences. However, it was clear that he sensed threat and that he felt more in control of his circumstances when he was able to withdraw to a safe distance or when he aggressively drove others away. Through these behaviors, he managed to be somewhat in control.

Robert did not readily discriminate others' intentions toward him. Rather, he appeared to react on the basis of a feeling of threat or being unable to control his situation. Thus, his aggressive and withdrawn behaviors were overgeneralized, inconsistent, and not always related in the same way to others' actions. For this reason, Robert was a puzzle to those around him. Moreover, he did not appear to behave from a consistent set of inner desires or concerns.

Since this explanation of Robert's volition was composed from observation, and since Robert was incapable of verifying or refuting it, the occupational therapist could not know for certain how accurate it was. However, by using it to devise an intervention plan for Robert, she was able to test this explanation. If the intervention worked, she could have much greater confidence that her understanding of Robert's volition was accurate.

Robert's Environment

The occupational therapist's observations also revealed that Robert's volition was very much influenced by the environment of the state hospital. Further, it was clear that any intervention strategy would have to make use of that environment. Thus, the next step in information gathering was to examine the environment. The therapist wanted to gather information on the objects, spaces, occupational forms, and social groups and their impact on Robert. In addition, she also wanted to identify any factors in the environment that might help account for his withdrawn or aggressive behavior.

The environment that Robert occupied day-to-day consisted of five areas within and adjacent to the Behavior Disorders building: a day area consisting of two rooms where residents spent most waking hours, a small recreation room, a living area with bedrooms and bathrooms, a dining room, and an outside area immediately next to the building. The recreation room was not used for any particular purpose or for any regularly scheduled activities. Its main purpose, like the day room, was to contain residents where they could be more easily observed and managed.

The four areas inside the building were stark. Because of the residents' aggressive and destructive behavior, only objects that could be secured to the floor or wall were present. In the day rooms there were only plastic chairs and a few tables. Two benches were the only equipment in the area outside the building. Thus, there were very few objects present with which it was possible to do something. Not surprisingly, residents treated themselves and others as objects for use.

Staff occasionally brought objects, such as pegboards, bingo games, or other fine motor activities, into the living area when there were enough staff to supervise and when residents were generally calm. The only occupational forms routinely available in the environment were related to eating and hygiene. Residents were left to invent their own means of creating stimulation or activity. This is what many, including Robert, apparently did when they engaged in repetitive, self-stimulating behaviors.

The living area, with bedrooms and bathrooms, was the larger and more interesting area. However, resident access to this area was ordinarily restricted to times for sleeping and hygiene. Although there were two day areas on the wing, residents were usually confined to only one area where they could be more readily watched. Consequently, the day room was crowded. With residents forced to be in close proximity to each other, personal space was a commodity. It was not uncommon that residents appeared to react to someone else invading their personal space. Altercations over territory occurred regularly. The social environment was marked by periodic physical outbursts and assaults. It tended to be a threatening social environment where most interactions included some kind of altercation as residents got out of control or coercion as staff sought to manage behavior. It was not hard to see how such an environment would demand the kind of distancing and self-protective behaviors that Robert exhibited.

The only persons regularly in the environment were ward staff. The vast majority of their time and effort was directed to getting necessary routines of hygiene and eating completed and to avoiding or stopping problem behavior. There was minimal staff–resident contact, except for these routines and order-keeping purposes. Most of the time, the staff's interaction with residents was at least mildly coercive as they tried to move residents along the various routines of hygiene and meals with varying degrees of resident cooperation. Because staff members were constantly dealing with behavioral problems, passive withdrawn behavior was not seen as a problem. Indeed, a passive and withdrawn resident meant less work for staff.

Intervention

The occupational therapist reasoned that if Robert was to be encouraged to be less aggressive, he would also need to learn to be more comfortable in his environment. Also, if Robert could be enticed into positive interactions with his environment, he might learn not always to expect problems and to be more able to discriminate what was going on in the environment. To accomplish this, Robert initially needed to feel some degree of safety in the therapy environment and eventually in his living environment. The therapist validated Robert's need to feel safe by slowly initiating interaction, allowing him to become accustomed to her presence during each interaction and slowing letting him become more comfortable with her being around him.

Because Robert did not appear to have tolerance for long periods of interaction, the occupational therapist began with 15-minute sessions, scheduled 3 times per week. She began by observing Robert for approximately 5 minutes before treat-

ment. This observation period had several purposes. First, it enabled the therapist to determine Robert's emotional state before beginning treatment. Sometimes he was actually asleep, other times he was lethargic or passive, and sometimes he was very agitated. Second, the therapist could observe the climate of the immediate environment, such as whether it was crowded, whether nearby residents were agitated or noisy, or whether housekeeping or maintenance staff members were working on the unit. This information was used to determine whether therapy could be done on the ward or if Robert needed to be taken to a quieter or less crowded environment. Further, over time, it led to a better understanding of the relation of the environment to Robert's actions. Finally, it gave Robert time to be aware of the therapist and become accustomed to her presence.

Once the observation was over and the intervention was about to begin, the occupational therapist started by presenting, one at a time, various types of objects that she hoped would stimulate Robert's curiosity and elicit exploratory behaviors. She selected objects that provided sensory information and that could be easily manipulated. For example, she introduced to Robert a fuzzy animal that squeaked when he squeezed it. She showed him a mirror, which revolved within a plastic ring. She brought a bright-colored hard rubber ball with short flexible spines and a rhythm instrument that clanged when shaken. She always carried these objects to the unit in a bag or box. As Robert came to recognize the routine, he began to explore the bag or box to see what was inside.

Initially, the occupational therapist encouraged Robert by touching his hands, arms, face, and other body parts with some of the objects. His reaction ranged from accepting and noticing the stimulation to reaching for the object and poking, shaking, or pounding it against himself. When he was finished, Robert tossed the object several feet away from himself.

After approximately eight sessions, Robert demonstrated a preference for a spiny ball. The therapist attempted to gradually shape this interest into an occupational form—a simple game of catch. The therapist would retrieve the ball and roll it along the floor back to Robert. He would hold it a while and then throw it again. Often Robert purposely threw the ball away from the therapist and laughed mischievously. The therapist returned the ball to Robert and would gradually roll it to a point slightly further away from where he was sitting, so that he would have to retrieve it. Importantly, this game gave Robert a unique opportunity to influence the behavior of another in a socially appropriate and accepted manner.

There were still times when Robert slapped or spat at the therapist. To give Robert clear feedback, the therapist consistently stopped the interaction, firmly stated "No, Robert," moved approximately 8 to 10 feet away from him, and remained there until the negative behaviors ceased. Then she would walk back to him and reinitiate the interaction. In this way, Robert began to pay attention to others' reactions to his behavior. In one session, the occupational therapist moved away from Robert because he started to slap her. When he saw her reaction, he ceased the behavior, made eye contact with her, then rose and walked toward her reaching out for the object she held. Robert's ability to recognize how his actions influenced others was likely abetted by the fact he had seen how his behavior influenced the therapist's response in the game they played with the spiny ball.

Several specific objects and activities were further identified as ones Robert liked. One of his favorite activities was the game described above. He also demonstrated that he liked it when the therapist would bring the fuzzy animal close to and then lightly touch various parts of his face. In addition to the spiny ball, he developed a strong attraction to terry cloth and soft objects, and to rhythm instruments that made soft noises.

While the therapist made a great deal of progress in reducing Robert's aggressive and withdrawn behavior, she understood that the rest of his daily environment remained as before. Therefore, any positive experiences she and Robert had together could be erased by Robert's other experiences in the course of the day. Now that she had discovered some effective ways of interacting with Robert and mitigating his aggression, she could share them with other ward staff members.

During interdisciplinary meetings, the occupational therapist shared with unit staff the information she had gained about Robert's volition and about her success in interacting with him. At these meetings she encouraged and helped staff to view Robert as having values and interests and as being capable of behaving in a more positive fashion.

The occupational therapist modeled how to interact with Robert for other direct care staff on the unit. The following incident is an example. At the beginning of one session, the therapist wished to move Robert to a less crowded location. A direct care aide grasped Robert's arm to coerce him to follow her. Robert began to get upset and resist. The therapist intervened holding out one of Robert's favorite objects. He then voluntarily followed the therapist to the other area. Such incidents helped change staff views about Robert and about how they should interact with him.

More and more staff began to employ the approach suggested by the occupational therapist and began to see Robert in a different light (i.e., as a person who had feelings, who liked some things, feared others, and cared about what happened to him and about what he did). They used less and less coercion and instead coaxed Robert through his interests. Some staff even occasionally interacted with Robert in a playful way. With these environmental changes, Robert's behavior also began to change.

Staff members observed a significant decrease in Robert's aggression on the unit. They also reported that Robert had begun to approach staff to initiate interactions with them. Bolstered by their success with Robert, they continued to interact with him in this more positive manner. Staff members began to take it upon themselves to figure out new interests for Robert and prided themselves on getting him involved in simple activities. As the relationship between staff and Robert improved, they became more successful in getting Robert to go along with some self-care activities. For example, they introduced the toothbrush to Robert in a new way. Instead of forcing it on him for brushing his teeth, they let him explore it. As he became accustomed to it, he became cooperative while brushing his teeth.

Robert in Perspective

Learning about volition in such low-functioning persons as Robert is challenging. Nonetheless, the difficulty of learning about volition was clearly outweighed by the advantage of gaining an understanding of why Robert behaved as he did. As the case illustrates, this information is key to designing effective intervention.

Although it is true to say that Robert changed as a result of the intervention, the biggest change was in the dynamic relationship between Robert and the ward staff. They were no longer in an ongoing struggle. Robert came to see the staff as sources of enjoyment and not simply as sources of coercion. Moreover, as he developed some positive social connection with them, he was more able to respond to their desires and expectations for behavior. Staff members came to see Robert as a person with desires and needs and as capable of cooperation.

Finding a Life Role

Many persons with cognitive impairments related to chronic psychiatric illness live marginalized and unhappy lives because they cannot access meaningful roles. This case illustrates a straightforward intervention that aims to enhance quality of life for a person with limited cognitive resources and environmental supports.

Carl

Carl was 32 years old and had a diagnosis of chronic schizophrenia. He was admitted to a psychiatric hospital as his behavior deteriorated since stopping his medications approximately 6 weeks earlier. Carl had a long history of psychiatric hospitalizations dating back to when he was 16 years old.

Carl had an eighth-grade education. He lived with his parents and older brother in a two-bedroom apartment in a low-income neighborhood of Washington, DC. None of his family members were employed. Both of Carl's parents also had histories of mental illness.

When Carl was referred to occupational therapy, he was disoriented and reported hearing voices. He was extremely withdrawn and did not respond to verbal approaches. Carl required staff assistance for personal hygiene, grooming, and eating. He was unable to share any information about himself and preferred to stay in his room in the dark. However, he did venture out into other patients' rooms, gathering their plants and flowers into his own room.

The primary purpose of the hospitalization was to stabilize Carl on medication and quickly return him to the community. Thus, the occupational therapist had to decide how to accomplish the most within limited time. Specifically, the occupational therapist considered how she could:

- Achieve a small but significant improvement in Carl's life
- Attempt to break the revolving door syndrome.

The therapist knew from experience that medication would likely decrease Carl's symptoms. However, she also expected that upon discharge Carl would go back to watching television and in several months would likely be psychotic and back in the hospital. She decided to see if Carl could identify an occupational role around which he could organize his daily life.

Therefore, in gathering information the occupational therapist was guided by three theoretically based questions:

- Did Carl have any previous interests and experience that would suggest an appropriate life role for him
- How could Carl meaningfully fill his time with behaviors related to roles
- How could he find identity and satisfaction in his life.

Since Carl was initially too disorganized to participate in any formal data gathering, the therapist began by interviewing Carl's parents. They related that Carl had never worked and had no friends. He spent almost all his time watching television. They also noted that when his illness was in remission, he was able to attend to his self-care and to help a bit around the house. Finally, they mentioned that occasionally Carl would ride the bus to the local park where he would pick flowers and bring them home. This final bit of information stood out in the therapist's mind since it corresponded with his gathering flowers and plants from others' rooms. She decided to use it as the entry point for therapy.

Wooing Carl

At this point, Carl was so withdrawn that the first step was to attempt to woo him back into interacting with the environment. From observation and discussion with Carl's parents, the occupational therapist knew that plants and flowers were the one thing that attracted Carl. Since there were several plants in the occupational therapy room, Carl's therapist invited him to care for them. This strategy worked. Carl perked up and agreed to come into the occupational therapy room. Almost immediately he was repotting plants, planting seeds, and watering and pruning the existing plants. He did all of these things very well despite his previously regressed state.

Carl immensely enjoyed this activity with plants and stayed totally absorbed in it. Since Carl was still dysfunctional in his self-care, the occupational therapist decided to use his motivation for horticulture to influence his performance in this area. She set the expectation for Carl come to therapy appropriately dressed and groomed. The next day he started performing personal hygiene and dressing without staff intervention. It was clear that when motivated, Carl could function at a much higher level than when he had nothing to motivate him and organize his behavior.

The occupational therapist also observed that Carl preferred to work alone, remaining on the fringes of the group. He rarely interacted with others. The therapist decided that this aspect of Carl's behavior likely reflected a lifelong pattern and was not nearly as problematical for him as his inactivity. Therefore, she decided to support his continued engagement in mainly solitary activities.

As Carl became more verbal, the therapist encouraged and coached him to complete the Modified Interest Checklist and the Role Checklist. Her rationale in selecting these assessments was as follows. First, she wanted to determine whether Carl had any other strong interests, which could be capitalized on to motivate him. Second, because she hoped to find an organizing role for Carl, she wanted to identify his pattern of role identification. Carl's behavior in the hospital and his parents' reports affirmed that his skills were adequate for self-care and other basic activities.

So as not to overwhelm Carl, the therapist administered the Modified Interest Checklist verbally and only asked Carl to indicate his level of interest in each item and whether he had done it in the past. He reported a strong interest in gardening/yard work, in macramé that he had never performed, and in listening to the radio. He indicated some interest in woodworking that he had done during past hospitalizations, in television, and in ceramics that he had never done, in housecleaning, laundry, and in home repairs. He indicated that no other activities from the checklist were of interest to him. From the assessment it was apparent that Carl had few interests and limited experience doing things. It was also confirmed that Carl's dominant interest and the one in which he had the most experience was horticulture.

With the occupational therapist's coaching, Carl was also able to understand and complete the Role Checklist. Carl's responses on the Role Checklist are presented in *Figure 22-3*. He had no continuous roles but indicated that he saw himself in the past and future in the roles of home maintainer and hobbyist—both of which he checked as very valuable roles. When asked to clarify what kind of hobby he saw himself pursuing, Carl readily responded that it was involvement with plants and flowers.

Because of Carl's functional level, his living situation, and the short-term nature of his hospitalization, his therapist identified a single goal of engaging Carl in an occupational role that was meaningful to him, that matched his observed skills, and that would serve to organize his daily life. She encouraged Carl to pursue the role of hobbyist, built around his interest in plants and flowers. The therapist advised Carl of her goal and the reasons for it, and he readily agreed that it was a good idea. They negotiated that Carl would spend as much time as possible on his own in occupational therapy during the remaining days of his hospitalization.

In occupational therapy, Carl continued to work with plants. He even learned to make simple wooden hangers for his plants, incorporating his in-

FIGURE 22-3 Carl's Responses on the Role Checklist.

Role	Past	Present	Future	Not at all Valuable	Somewhat Valuable	Very Valuable
Student						
Worker						
Volunteer						
Caregiver						
Home Maintainer						
Friend						
Family Member						
Religious Participant						
Hobbyist/Amateur						
Participant in Organizations						
Other						

terest in woodworking. He learned to macramé simple plant hangers. Carl was very pleased with his accomplishments and indicated that he wished to incorporate these two occupational forms into his hobbyist role.

In preparation for his discharge, the occupational therapist worked with Carl to identify and plan for environmental supports for his new role. The plan was shared with his family and they agreed to support Carl by providing him basic supplies when needed and by expanding Carl's responsibilities in the home to include care of plants in the house and some yard work.

When he was discharged, Carl began to attend a psychiatric day treatment center 5 days a week. The therapist shared information about Carl's progress in the hobbyist role with the staff at the center. She recommended the kinds of supports that would help sustain this new role for Carl. These included providing opportunities for Carl to engage in the occupational forms he had begun in acute care. She also recommended social recognition of Carl's hobbyist role and integration of it into his activities at the center when possible.

The center staff agreed to continue Carl's hobbyist role in outpatient therapy at the center. After discharge, Carl was regularly attending the day treatment center on weekdays where he continued to work in horticulture. On weekends, he went to the park with a friend from the center to collect flowers that he often brought to the center on Monday morning. Carl was soon being recognized as the official "florist" for the center.

Carl in Perspective

In psychiatric acute care, the press of time along with the predominance of client symptoms often leads therapists to focus more on client functional deficits than on what clients can do with their lives. However, a major factor contributing to chronicity and especially the need for rehospitalization is that clients lack something meaningful to do with their lives. To the extent that if therapy addresses such needs, even in a limited way, it can contribute to the client's long-term occupational adaptation.

Recapturing Freedom

The following case tells the story of Marc, a 27-year-old Belgian man diagnosed with paranoid schizophrenia. According to the institutional records, Marc was the youngest of a family with two children. As a child, he had difficulty making friends. He felt inferior and was often teased, in response to which he became physically aggressive. As a teenager Marc had problems at school, was taking drugs, and got into trouble with authorities.

Marc had a very difficult relationship with his father, who had schizophrenia and who had been hospitalized multiple times. His father died suddenly when Marc was 19 years old. His mother, a teacher, found it very hard to manage the family after the death of her husband. Marc's psychiatric history and occupational therapy is described below.

Marc

At age 22, Marc was first hospitalized, complaining of constantly hearing voices that dominated his life. While hospitalized he began a relationship with another patient and following discharge lived mostly in her apartment in Brussels. During this time, he began training in carpentry, but stopped because of paranoid suspicions that he developed toward fellow trainees.

Shortly thereafter, Marc had to be readmitted to the hospital because he could not handle growing tensions between himself and his girlfriend. After a period of hospitalization he was discharged to a Psychosocial Center that provided partial residential care. While living there he began regularly using marijuana with two fellow residents and stopped taking his medication. His symptoms soon became so severe he was admitted to long-term psychiatric care. Marc spent the next 3 years in a psychiatric ward. During that period, he was socially isolated, sometimes even refusing to see his mother and girlfriend when they visited the hospital. Marc only rarely left the hospital, and his ability to do anything beyond minimal self-care was extremely restricted. Even the slightest demands for performance exacerbated his symptomatology. Over time his symptoms, especially the auditory hallucinations, worsened.

Just before being transferred to a ward designed for the most therapy-resistant clients, he had deteriorated even further. The overall focus of this new ward and its therapy services was to help clients find some comfort in life despite intractable, severe psychiatric disability. When he came to the ward, Marc suffered from more or less constant auditory hallucinations. The voices he heard accused and gave orders to him. Marc also suffered from ongoing paranoid delusions. Despite taking medications, Marc remained very psychotic and frightened.

Marc had lost all interest in doing things. His only activity was pacing or wandering about agitated. He rarely allowed any social contact with others. Most of the time he isolated himself, fretting over the voices he heard. After a few weeks, a medication change had a modest impact on Marc's psychosis so that he became somewhat more approachable. At this point the therapist began to invite Marc into the therapy workshop but Marc always declined.

The therapist consistently greeted Marc and had short conversations with him in an attempt to validate him and develop some rapport and trust. As Marc became more comfortable having short talks with the therapist, he decided to administer the Occupational Performance History Interview-Second Version (OPHI-II) to Marc in the hope of finding a way to better reach him. Although Marc had some difficulty attending and giving a detailed life history, some very useful information was revealed in the interview.

Marc told the therapist that there had been a period between when his father died and his first hospitalization that he had been able to function. This was the best period of his adult life. During that time he had first worked for a while as a truck driver. He had experienced his job as stressful, but it gave him a feeling of freedom that he very much appreciated. After the trucking job, he had also worked for a while on a farm which he liked because of the feeling of freedom he got from working outdoors. He also spoke about feeling free during a short period when he lived on his own in a room he could decorate himself.

However, this "freedom period" had not lasted long. His psychiatric symptoms became worse and he began to isolate himself in the room, listening to records. When he was not doing that, he wandered around in the city and frequented pubs. The people he met in the pubs reintroduced him to drugs, which contributed to his getting worse and ending up hospitalized.

One of the highlights of the interview was Marc's revelation that he had strong interest in photography. Marc had taken a class in photography.

He had even arranged a darkroom at home. He recalled that he had greatly enjoyed the development of black and white pictures that he made himself. His hobby had been interrupted by an exacerbation of his illness.

As shown on *Figure 22-4*, Marc's ratings on the occupational identity and competence scales reflect his severe impairment. The only present area in which he did not have a major problem was interests, and this was due to his identified interest in photography. Collaborating together, Marc and his therapist created his narrative slope (*Fig. 22-5*) that showed that Marc's one clearly positive life period

FIGURE 22-4   Marc's Ratings on the OPHI-II.

Occupational Identity Scale	1	2	3	4
Has personal goals and projects	■			
Identifies a desired occupational lifestyle	■			
Expects success	■			
Accepts responsibility	■			
Appraises abilities and limitations	■			
Has commitments and values	■			
Recognizes identity and obligations	■			
Has interests		■		
Felt effective (past)		■		
Found meaning and satisfaction in lifestyle (past)		■		
Made occupational choices (past)	■			
Occupational Competence Scale	**1**	**2**	**3**	**4**
Maintains satisfying lifestyle	■			
Fulfills role expectations	■			
Works toward goals	■			
Meets personal performance standards	■			
Organizes time for responsibilities	■			
Participates in interests	■			
Fulfilled roles (past)	■			
Maintained habits (past)	■			
Achieved satisfaction (past)		■		

Key : **4** = Exceptionally competent occupational functioning; **3** = Appropriate, satisfactory occupational functioning; **2** = Some occupational dysfunction; **1** = Extremely occupationally dysfunctional

was his "freedom period" when he lived in a room of his own, worked, and took up his photography hobby.

Based on Marc's history, the therapist reasoned that photography might be a way to engage Marc in doing something. The therapist explained to Marc that by taking pictures he would be able to walk about freely and capture some impressions that he could later develop in the darkroom. The idea the therapist explained was to see if he could recapture some of his old feeling of freedom from the good period of his life. When presented with this idea, Marc agreed to explore his old interest of photography. This was the first time he chose to undertake something in years.

With coaching from his therapist, Marc went to the library in the nearby village and found some books on photography. He checked out these books and began coming to therapy, during which time he read the books. Next, his therapist and he planned for Marc to go home for a weekend to find his old photography equipment. They located a small room in the occupational therapy building that they outfitted as a darkroom.

The therapist and Marc together decided to begin with developing some pictures from old negatives he still had from his schooldays. This turned out to be difficult for Marc because it brought back painful memories. After validating Marc's reaction, the therapist negotiated that he would find another source of negatives for Marc to develop. Consequently, some of the occupational therapy staff members brought negatives in with the request that Marc develop them and enlarge them. Marc did this for a couple days, but then indicated that he was not thrilled with the routine of developing old negatives.

He indicated that he would much rather develop pictures he took himself. The therapist then negotiated with Marc that he could go outside the hospital to take pictures, provided he was willing to join the organized excursions with other patients. Marc agreed. He began going on outings with other patients, taking pictures and even engaging in some social interaction with the others.

Up to this point the therapist had accompanied Marc into the darkroom, but as Marc had improved,

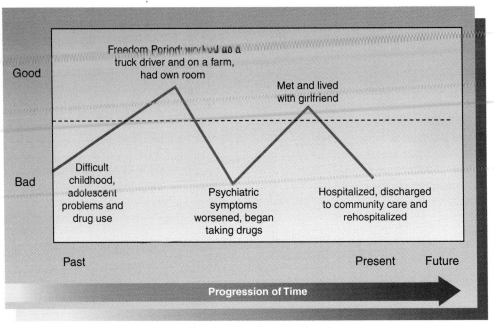

FIGURE 22-5   Marc's Narrative Slope.

the therapist suggested to Marc that he could begin developing the pictures on his own. Marc began to do this, but soon found that his auditory hallucinations became very upsetting to him when he was alone in the darkroom. The therapist supported and coached Marc to think about possible solutions to this problem. Marc identified the idea of taking a small portable radio with him into the darkroom. He tried this and found that it made him much more comfortable.

Soon, the therapist asked Marc if he would be willing to take pictures of other patients on these excursions. These pictures would be used in a newsletter that was regularly published by the patients in the hospital. Marc chose to do this and felt a sense of pride that he was asked to take on this role. During this time Marc began to improve in other areas. He became more social and more attentive to his own self-care. He began to take regular walks in the nearby village to shoot pictures.

Over time, Marc showed that he had a unique talent for photography. He made wonderfully expressive pictures and received praise for them from staff and patients alike. Bolstered by all this feed-

back Marc decided, with encouragement from the occupational therapist, to organize an exhibition of his pictures. He put together a beautifully designed exhibition in the hospital, which also served as his farewell. Shortly thereafter he was discharged to a psychosocial center in the village, Elsene. As a going away present, Marc gave his occupational therapist some framed pictures he had taken and developed.

Marc in Perspective

Marc was a particularly challenging case since his occupational identity and competence were so completely impaired. At the time he began therapy, Marc had no volitional desire to do anything. The value of learning about a client's past is underscored since it was a past interest from the one good period in Marc's life and the idea of recapturing some of the feeling of freedom from that period that re-engendered his desire for action. When clients cannot narrate for themselves a vision of a future, the therapist can sometimes find such a vision from the client's past, as Marc's therapist was able to do. While the severity of Marc's psychiatric disability was such that he will likely always need a supportive environment, he has, at the time of this writing, functioned well for 4 years in the community center. There, he has recaptured some sense of freedom.

Learning to Reach Out

Margaret was a friendly, sociable 22-year-old with short, curly red hair and a big smile. She was diagnosed with profound mental retardation and encephalopathy following a choking incident when she was a toddler. Margaret was unable to stand or walk and needed maximum assistance for mat or bed mobility. She had a custom manual wheelchair that she was unable to propel herself. Margaret had very little active movement in her legs and moved her arms with great difficulty due to abnormally high muscle tone and the persistence of primitive reflexes. She tended to keep both hands fisted, compromising her ability to grasp and release. She tended to keep her head rotated to the left with her neck hyperextended. She had difficulty bringing her

head to midline during grooming or looking down during tabletop activities. Although Margaret had very little expressive speech, she could understand some of what was being said to her and she did produce vocalizations to communicate.

Margaret lived in a facility for individuals with profound physical and mental disabilities and attended a developmental training program during the day. In this setting the occupational therapist mainly evaluated clients and consulted to direct care staff. Margaret also received services from an occupational therapy assistant in a small group setting every 2 weeks. This case discusses the therapist's use of MOHO in an annual evaluation and consultation process.

Margaret

Although Margaret's physical and cognitive limitations were very evident, these were not the only problems that had to be addressed to allow her to more actively participate. She also demonstrated low volition, as evidenced by her initial score on the VQ

FIGURE 22-6 Margaret's VQ Ratings Initially and 1 Year Later.

Client: *Margaret* Diagnosis:								
Area to Evaluate	**Initial Observation**				**Observation 1 year later**			
1. Shows curiosity	P	H	I	**S**	P	H	I	**S**
2. Initiates actions/tasks	P	**H**	I	S	P	H	**I**	S
3. Tries new things	P	**H**	I	S	P	**H**	I	S
4. Shows pride	P	**H**	I	S	P	H	**I**	S
5. Attempts challenges	**P**	H	I	S	P	**H**	I	S
6. Seeks additional responsibilities	**P**	H	I	S	**P**	H	I	S
7. Tries to correct mistakes	**P**	H	I	S	**P**	H	I	S
8. Tries to solve problems	P	**H**	I	S	P	H	I	S
9. Shows preferences	P	H	**I**	S	P	H	**I**	S
10. Pursues activity to completion/accomplishment	**P**	H	I	S	**P**	H	I	S
11. Stays engaged	P	**H**	I	S	P	**H**	I	S
12. Invests additional energy/emotion/attention	P	**H**	I	S	P	**H**	I	S
13. Indicates goals	**P**	H	I	S	P	H	**I**	S
14. Shows that an activity is special or significant	P	**H**	I	S	P	H	I	**S**
Rating Key: **P** = Passive; **H** = Hesitant; **I** = Involved; **S** = Spontaneous								

(*Fig. 22-6*). When the therapist observed Margaret during grooming and other activities, it was clear she did not have confidence in her ability to do them, even with assistance. Nor did she appear to have any desire to take an active role in doing these things.

Instead, her satisfaction came from interactions with and reactions of the direct care staff. For instance, she would laugh when a staff member encouraged her to try to move her arms to press a switch or to perform hand-over-hand assisted fine motor activities. She did not even attempt to look at what she was doing. Instead, she watched the reaction on her caregiver's face.

Margaret would indicate pride in her accomplishments (by smiling or laughing) only with much staff encouragement and rarely expressed a desire to try something again. She would rarely initiate any action, except with a great deal of staff encouragement. She rarely indicated goals such as how she wanted to do something or what she wanted to do. Despite her low personal causation, it was clear that Margaret had some interests and values. The most obvious was her interest in her personal appearance and her value of social interaction.

Because of her extreme physical limitations, the staff members tended not to expect or require much participation on her part. Also, because it was hard to know which activities were really enjoyable to Margaret, they did not readily try to elicit choices from her.

Recommending Goals and Intervention

The therapist recognized that Margaret needed an approach that would tap into her volitional strengths while providing physical support to facilitate her movement. Thus, the therapist devised goals and strategies for the staff to implement, based on using her strong interest in personal appearance and value of social interaction to encourage. The focus of these goals was to allow Margaret to more actively participate in self-care. For example, the therapist recommended the goal that Margaret would keep her hands open during the application of nail polish. The combination of physical facilitation techniques (e.g., hand massage) and Margaret's interest in getting a manicure proved successful. She not only reached this goal but also

began to demonstrate increased ability to grasp and release, particularly in her dominant, right side.

The therapist also recommended the goal that Margaret brush her hair with a long-handled hairbrush with assistance while looking in a mirror. Again, the combination of physical facilitation to relax her muscle tone with Margaret's pride in her beautiful curly red hair enabled Margaret to achieve success with this goal. She also demonstrated improved ability to bring her head to midline to look in the mirror during this activity.

Because of Margaret's value of social contact, the therapist also recommended the goal that Margaret would reach at least to midline with her right hand to shake hands with staff who approached her. To facilitate this goal, Margaret received physical facilitation, such as stretching on a therapy ball and passive range of motion in diagonal patterns. Margaret enjoyed this interaction with staff immensely and eventually attempted to shake hands as staff approached, without any verbal cueing. With practice she increased her skill in timing the opening of her hand with reaching for a staff member's hand.

Margaret was clearly pleased with her success and began to demonstrate active attempts to reach, grasp, and release in other activities. She was also beginning to make choices and to assert her need for physical assistance to do things she wanted to do. This, in turn, made staff more inclined to ask her to try new things.

A year later, Margaret had shown enough volitional desire and progress in occupational performance that she was moved from her developmental training classroom to a more vocationally oriented day program for higher-functioning clients. This new environment placed more emphasis on productive activities and put Margaret in contact with higher-functioning peers. For example, a number of clients had augmentative communication devices and/or power wheelchairs. Some clients were even able to talk. Instead of being in a classroom of 12 clients, Margaret joined nearly 30 clients in this new environment. This required her to further develop the skill of asserting herself to get her needs met.

Margaret began to thrive in this new environment. Her vocalizations increased and she used these vocalizations to gain staff attention. She also showed an increase in visual motor attention. Her ability to use her hands continued to improve with practice. With coaching, she could pick up an object, bring her arm across her body, and drop it in the appropriate container. This allowed her to do new occupational forms, such as sorting clips or filling potpourri sachets. Margaret showed her new volitional strength by becoming very vocal if she was not given an opportunity to participate when other clients were doing these kinds of things.

Finally, Margaret showed her increased volition by deciding on her own goal. She was able to communicate that she wanted to learn to do assisted tooth brushing. This occupational form was especially difficult for Margaret because she could not easily relax her right arm to flex her elbow in order to get the toothbrush to her mouth. Nevertheless, Margaret insisted that this be one of her new goals and was eventually able to achieve it.

During her last annual evaluation, Margaret's volition was again assessed using the VQ. As shown in Figure 22-6 her volitional ratings were significantly higher. She required less assistance to initiate actions and spontaneously showed that activities were significant to her. She showed pride and indicated goals with less cueing. She even sought challenges on occasion, when given encouragement. Margaret also indicated her preferences more consistently.

Direct care staff members noted the changes in Margaret. They saw that she was much more insistent on getting her needs met or in voicing her opinion by giving a "yes" or "no" response in a group setting. She insisted on being allowed to participate and derived pleasure from her accomplishments. Margaret also became popular with other clients, particularly one of her male classmates. She began independently reaching out to hold hands with him.

Margaret in Perspective

Margaret illustrates the extent to which volition can be an asset in achieving basic gains in motor capacity. She also illustrates how clients in long-term settings can settle into patterns of unnecessary passivity. Such patterns are often locked into place by the clients' lack of a sense of efficacy and by staff members' low expectations of clients.

Conclusion

When clients have significant functional limitations and/or problematic behavior, it can be difficult to discern the thoughts and feelings behind them. When this is the case, occupational therapists have a mandate to work toward comprehending the client's volition. It may be found in a person's past. It may be found in the subtle ways a client responds to circumstances in the environment. It is, however, always discoverable. No matter how impaired persons are, their volition exists. In their own ways, they experience and express it.

The cases in this chapter illustrate that therapists can find ways to understand and reach the client. With effort, therapists can discover things about their lower-functioning clients that not only make their volitional thoughts and feelings evident, but also provide essential information for designing effective therapy. When we do not understand the thoughts and feelings behind what lower-functioning clients do, we may miss the point of their communications and intentions and risk making their lives worse. When we are able to gain insight into their volition, we open up possibilities for truly client-centered practices that empower clients to more fully participate in occupational life.

References

Borell, L., Gustavsson, A., Sandman, P., & Kielhofner, G. (1994). Occupational programming in a day hospital for patients with dementia. *Occupational Therapy Journal of Research, 14*, 219–238.

Borell, L., Sandman, P., & Kielhofner, G. (1991). Clinical decision making in Alzheimer's disease. *Occupational Therapy in Mental Health, 11*, 111–124.

Josephsson, S. (1994). *Everyday activities as meeting-places in dementia*. Stockholm: Nordsteds Tryckeri AB.

Nygård, L., Borell, L., & Gustavsson, A. (1995). Managing images of occupational self in early stage dementia. *Scandinavian Journal of Occupational Therapy, 2*, 129–137.

Oakley, F. (1987). Clinical application of the model of human occupation in dementia of the Alzheimer's type. *Occupational Therapy in Mental Health, 7*, 37–50.

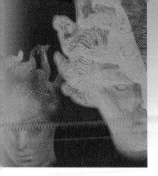

23

Facilitating Participation Through Community-Based Interventions

- **Gary Kielhofner**
- **Kim Bryze**
- **Lauren Goldbaum**
- **Dalleen Last**
- **Dommie Rey**
- **Laurie Rockwell-Dylla**

This chapter presents four cases in which therapists provided services to clients in community contexts. What most links the cases together is the extent to which therapy capitalizes on and enables the clients to participate more fully within settings of home, family, neighborhood, and workplace. The cases span childhood to old age and represent a range of cognitive, emotional, and physical problems and challenges.

The course of therapy for each of these clients takes place over several weeks or months. It naturally proceeds within the unfolding lives of the clients. Each of the cases illustrates in a different way how therapy can facilitate clients' occupational participation in a community context.

Recreating the Meaning of Home

Joan was a 79-year-old woman with myxedema (an extreme and disabling edema due to a thyroid abnormality) and a history of congestive heart failure. A couple weeks earlier, Joan's condition had worsened to the point that she was hospitalized and treated with medications aimed at eliminating some of the edema. She was given the choice to receive rehabilitation in the hospital or at home. Joan opted to return home to receive physical and occupational therapy services. The following case describes the course of Joan's home-

based intervention. It interweaves the themes of occupational identity and the meaning of home. Moreover, it demonstrates how therapy can enable persons to reclaim their lives and their environments.

Joan

The therapist arrived at Joan's home in a middle-class suburb of Chicago. There, she first encountered Joan's two adult daughters, Anne and Debbie, and Joan's 87-year-old husband, Art. Debbie led the therapist into the living room where the shades were down and curtains closed. Joan was sitting in a recliner and wearing a nightgown and robe. She sat with her shoulders hunched, clearly having trouble breathing. A fan in the corner of the room was blowing. Debbie explained that the fan helped reduce the moisture in the air, easing her mother's breathing.

The centerpiece of the former living room was a queen size bed with a comforter and embroidered pillows. While attractive, the bed evidenced that the living room had been transformed into a sickroom. Other objects completing the transformation were a bedside commode next to the television and a table that held pills, a cup of water, and a bell for summoning help.

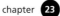

Joan's History and Current Performance

The therapist decided to conduct the Occupational Performance History Interview-Second Version (OPHI-II) as a group interview. She began the interview during the first visit and continued it over time as she continued to talk with Joan and her daughters. Since home health services extended over several visits, the ongoing interview allowed the therapist to build rapport and increasingly learn about Joan.

The following narrative emerged out of the interview. Many years ago, Joan developed a thyroid condition that Joan's physician thought had been cured with a newly approved medication. For several years, she had no symptoms and engaged in her normal routine of taking care of her family and her house, which had always been the focus of Joan's life. She had a satisfying life filled with cooking, cleaning, pursuing her hobby of crochet, and socializing with her family and friends.

Joan's illness re-emerged a year ago. The swift decline that followed led to the transformation of the living room into a sickroom and to a dramatic alteration of all their lives. Debbie recalled how her mother's eyes began to look "buggy," and how she began to retain so much fluid that her legs had become four times their previous size. As the edema progressed, Joan had increasing difficulty breathing and became increasingly fatigued with each passing day. Her symptoms progressed to the point that she was unable to cook or do heavy housework. From then on, she relied on help from her daughters.

Debbie and Anne both decided to restructure their lives, moving back home to become full-time caretakers. Debbie was single, had her own condominium, and worked as a freelance artist. She was spending increasing amounts of time at her family home rather than her own residence, so she decided it was best just to move back home. Anne was divorced and did not have children. She relinquished her apartment to return home and help her sister take care of their increasingly frail parents. They shared responsibility for meeting the medical, physical, and emotional needs of their mother and father as well as the responsibilities of maintaining the household.

As the year unfolded, Joan came to need help not only with homemaking, but also with her own personal care. She found it increasingly difficult to climb up and down the 14 steps to her bedroom and bathroom, so the family decided to move the bed down to the living room.

Joan's world slowly shrunk to her former living room. She ate her meals there. She was sponge bathed in the adjacent partial bathroom. She watched television from her recliner chair most of the day. She spent restless nights in her queen-size bed. Nearly immobilized, she had not been to other parts of the house for some time. Joan's occupational narrative was one of loss and retreat. As Joan and her family saw it, she had lost both life and her home as she retreated into her sick room.

After hearing this story of Joan's decline and observing Joan's fragile physical condition, the therapist explained her role and asked the family what they hoped to gain from therapy. The daughters told the therapist that it would help if their mother could become less reliant on them for her personal daily tasks. They all agreed together that this would be the primary goal of therapy.

The therapist next evaluated Joan's performance by asking her to demonstrate how she did her daily tasks. The observation revealed that Joan's edema, combined with her severely limited strength and endurance, made performing even her basic self-care routines nearly impossible. The therapist knew that achieving the overall goal of more self-reliance would require engaging Joan in occupational forms she valued, but was faced with the problem that Joan had such limited performance capacity that she could not effectively do them.

Course of Therapy

The therapist explained to Joan that to become more able to do things for herself, she would need to increase her strength and endurance. However, Joan was not convinced that she could do so and benefit from an exercise program on her own between therapy sessions. At the second visit, Joan admitted she was unable to follow through on the recommended exercises. She seemed very defeated when talking about her physical condition. In contrast, as they talked about Joan's lifestyle in her younger and healthier days, Joan enthusiastically reminisced about how she loved to cook and conjure up new recipes.

Since Joan did not have the physical capacity to get to the kitchen, much less participate in cooking, the therapist decided on the following strategy. She led Joan to participate in simple exercises for building strength and endurance while simultaneously enlisting Joan to share her store of expert knowledge about cooking. These conversations during exercise began Joan's return to the occupational form of cooking. The therapist did this by asking Joan for advice and suggestions about recipes and referring to Joan as her "cooking mentor." This process highlighted Joan's remaining capacity, her store of expert cooking knowledge. Consequently, Joan could experience culinary competence even though she did not have the motor capacity necessary to do the cooking itself. It also took her mind off the exercises and allowed her to put forth more effort.

As soon as Joan had enough capacity, the therapist encouraged Joan to try some cooking together with her. Joan agreed and referred to the process as getting her "kitchen coordination" back. Initially, Joan needed substantial assistance to do the cooking. Nonetheless, her position as the "cooking mentor" who supervised the therapist allowed Joan to feel satisfied with her performance.

Soon, Joan was regularly watching cooking shows and would share the latest recipes with the therapist when she came. One day, the therapist arrived to find Joan in the kitchen in the process of making chop suey. Joan had not independently made a sandwich—much less a whole meal—in well over a year! Joan enjoyed preparing the meal but found that it was overtaxing. Thereafter, she was content to assist her daughters with preparation of dinner, which was more in line with her physical abilities.

After the initial success with the occupational form of cooking, the therapist decided to find another occupational form from Joan's past for which she might have the physical ability. Joan had also shared with the therapist how she had loved to crochet and give her projects away as gifts. Her daughters showed the therapist beautiful and intricately designed afghans, curtains, towels, doilies, and pot holders that Joan had crocheted. Joan said that she had lost interest in crocheting because it was difficult due to her decreased eyesight.

Nonetheless, the therapist encouraged her to try crocheting again and advised Joan that if she started doing it, she might discover that she still enjoyed it and could do it. At the therapist's suggestion, Joan's daughters bought crochet yarn and set it on her table, just in case she wanted to try it. The presence of the crocheting objects in the environment gave Joan the opportunity and resources she needed. Eventually, she tried it. Joan found that she could still crochet by relying more on her sense of touch to compensate for her failing vision.

The therapist had learned over the sessions how important Joan's home had always been to her and the care with which she had decorated and maintained it. She advised Joan that it was possible for her now to reclaim her home. Joan enthusiastically responded to this idea as the next goal for therapy. As Joan's endurance and strength improved, the occupational therapist began to encourage and physically support Joan during each therapeutic session to walk to a different room of her home using her walker.

During these walks, Joan's husband offered encouraging comments, predicting, "Soon you'll be running around here." The walks also provided occasions for Joan to talk about the rooms and things that transpired in them, incorporating them once again as part of her life space. Next, the therapist persuaded Joan that since she was able to maneuver around her house, she should get back into the routine of having dinner in the dining room with her family. By incorporating the use of this space back into her daily routine, Joan was able to take a first step forward to restoring some of her previous lifestyle.

Soon, her walking had progressed to the point that her physical therapist thought she was ready to tackle the biggest physical barrier that faced her—the 14 steps leading to the upper level of her home. Joan not only had to overcome fatigue, but she had also experienced panic attacks with the physical therapist during sessions aimed at stair climbing. She clearly faced a personal causation hurdle related to walking up the stairs. She was afraid she would not make it up the stairs, needing to be carried down. She also had fears that she would not be able to make it back down the stairs and would be stuck upstairs. This prospect was upsetting to her since she had not been up the stairs in over a year and it had become foreign territory.

Given the fears that dominated Joan's personal causation with reference to climbing the stairs, she needed a great deal of encouragement from both the physical therapist and the occupational therapist. Joan eventually mastered three, then four, then five steps over a course of a few weeks. She gained not only strength, but also an increased sense of efficacy related to stair climbing. The occupational therapist and a physical therapist were both present when Joan finally made it all the way to the top.

The physical therapist felt that since Joan demonstrated the ability to climb all the steps, the physical therapy goals were accomplished. Thus, she decided to discharge Joan. At this point, the occupational therapist also had to consider whether to continue occupational therapy services. She consulted with Joan and the family and it became clear that Joan was not yet as self-sufficient as they all wished. With the goal that Joan continue to increase her functional mobility and independence, the occupational therapist was able to obtain approval from the insurance company to continue with therapy.

During the next phase of therapy, the therapist's goal was to help Joan be more independent once she was upstairs. To emphasize that Joan was moving from the sick role into her former home-maker role, the therapist framed the next phase of therapy as "shopping." Together, they shopped for appropriate adapted bathroom equipment, looking through pamphlets and catalogs. The therapist also arranged a demonstration of adapted equipment in her home. Together, the therapist and Joan collaborated to choose equipment that considered both Joan's physical needs and safety as well as her concerns that the equipment should complement the aesthetics of her home and not be institutional looking. With the addition of the equipment, Joan needed much less assistance from her daughters.

The therapist and Joan collaborated to identify her next goal, which Joan phrased as, "going outside to get a breath of fresh air and feel the sunshine." Joan was able to climb down the front steps with coaching from the therapist. She then transferred into her wheelchair that she used to visit the neighborhood. The therapist instructed the daughters on how to use the same procedure to assist Joan to get outside on a more regular basis. In some of her final sessions, Joan progressed to walking with her walker in the garden to look at flowers her husband had planted and in front of the house in order to reestablish friendships with neighbors she had not seen in months.

Conclusion of Services

Occupational therapy services were concluded when the therapist, in collaboration with Joan and her daughters, felt that their initial goal had been achieved. Joan's progress was evidenced by increased independence in self-care, assisting and supervising meal preparation, re-engaging in previous leisure pursuits, and getting around her home, yard, and neighborhood. Finally, Joan had started taking a more active role in household decisions.

Joan in Perspective

This case example has several features worth commentary. First of all, community contexts often provide opportunity for and call on the therapist to address not just the disabled person, but also family members and others as clients. The therapist effectively incorporated Joan's daughters and husband into assessment, goal setting, and intervention.

Second, the therapist was initially faced with a common dilemma. Joan did not have sufficient capacity to engage in the occupational forms that had meaning for her. The approach the therapist used (i.e., having Joan begin to re-engage in cooking by sharing her expertise verbally during exercises that prepared her occupational engagement) was a creative and effective way to resolve the dilemma. Moreover, while the therapist had to consider biomechanical factors throughout therapy, it was important that she framed the experience of therapy in response to Joan's occupational narrative as reclaiming Joan's life and her home. This kept the process motivating for Joan, as it allowed her to construct the competence to enact her identity.

Finally, the therapist had to decide and justify continuation of therapy after the physical therapist discontinued her intervention, based on Joan reaching the functional goal of climbing stairs. The occupational therapist's decision to continue therapy was based on an understanding that for Joan and her family, function meant reclaiming the competence to enact her identity. From this perspective, the therapist was able to justify and continue services to the point of achieving a better outcome for Joan and her family.

The Route to Full Participation in Family, Neighborhood, and School Contexts

Adam was 7.5 years old and attended second grade in a middle-class suburb of Chicago. Adam's therapy was precipitated by underlying sensory integrative problems that made it difficult for him to perform in play and school. As seen below, Adam first brought attention to the painful thoughts and feelings that surrounded his inability to fully participate in the occupations that make up the life of an ordinary second grader.

Adam

One day Adam came home from school with a troubled look on his face. When his mother asked him about his day, Adam had said, "Mom, something's wrong with me." She asked, "Does your stomach hurt? Do you have a headache?" Adam responded, "No, Mom, something is WRONG with me! I am not like the other kids. I'm afraid."

His mother encouraged Adam to tell her about his fear. In his own words, Adam explained that group activities and physical games at school were intimidating for him. He worried about these events before they happened. He felt terrified while he was involved in them. Afterward, he always felt like a failure. Over time, these cumulative experiences led him to conclude that there must be something very wrong with him. Added to this, Adam felt in-

creasingly isolated and different from the other children. He was lonely and pained by the idea that he did not belong with the others in school. Adam's mother offered the only help she could imagine in the form of advice to Adam. She suggested that he try harder and that he "be a friend to make a friend." Adam met these suggestions with tears and great frustration.

Consequently, Adam's mother decided to pursue the issue and requested a conference with his teacher. In conversation with the teacher, his mother learned that indeed, Adam was having difficulty in group situations such as in gym, recess, lunch, and during small group experiences in the classroom. His handwriting was less skilled than what would be expected in second grade. On the other hand, Adam was usually able to keep up with schoolwork that was to be completed individually.

Armed with both Adam's and the teacher's accounts, Adam's mother took it upon herself to learn more about the kind of problem he was experiencing and what kind of resources might be of help to him. She sought out information from friends who were also mothers of schoolchildren. One of these friends was an occupational therapist who recommended that Adam be evaluated by an experienced pediatric occupational therapist.

Adam's mother subsequently referred him to an outpatient pediatric occupational therapy clinic that specialized in interventions with children who had problems similar to Adam's. She voiced questions about his ability to keep up with other children his age in school and play. She emphasized that her primary concerns were Adam's lack of confidence and his view that something was wrong with him.

Adam's Assessment

Adam came to his first occupational therapy session accompanied by his mother. He was initially shy and quiet but was able to respond to the therapist's suggestion that he walk around and see the toys and equipment. As Adam explored, the therapist listened to the mother's thoughts and concerns about Adam. The information she shared led the therapist to suspect that Adam had sensory processing difficulties that contributed to his problems with physical and interactive situations in his daily life. Such problems are recognized and addressed from the perspective of sensory integration, another conceptual practice model (Kielhofner & Fisher, 1991). The therapist asked Adam's mother to complete a sensory integration-based developmental/sensory history form while she began to observe Adam directly. This form provided qualitative information regarding Adam's ability to perform developmental and sensory-based actions and supplemented what his therapist subsequently observed in the occupational therapy environment.

The therapist performed an observation that consisted of inviting and asking Adam to seek out sensory experiences and perform various motor tasks. She conducted this observation with two goals in mind:

- To informally assess Adam's responses to sensory information and his performance of motor tasks
- To formally assess his volition through use of the Pediatric Volitional Questionnaire (PVQ).

With regard to the latter, her volition questions centered on what he enjoyed and disliked, how he felt about his own abilities and performance, and what was important to him. She knew from the mother's report that Adam had a negative view of his capacities and she expected that the observation would

provide more information about the dynamics of how he acted and reacted in situations that called for motor skills.

Adam was quiet, passive, and compliant. He did not look directly at the therapist, except when she asked him to perform movements that involved his face and mouth. With encouragement, he attempted all tasks that the therapist presented to him, but his efforts were fleeting when he was asked to do something that he perceived as difficult. He was quick to say, "I can't" before he even attempted certain motor tasks. He was impulsive in his approach to doing visual-motor actions that the therapist requested, appearing to want to get them over with as quickly as possible. Nonetheless, he responded positively to encouragement and praise during the testing.

By the end of the evaluation session, Adam seemed more comfortable with the therapist and was more involved in his interactions with the therapist and with the physical environment. He appeared to enjoy the movement activities and play interactions with the suspended equipment once he became more comfortable and saw that no one was judging his performance. As shown in *Figure 23-1*, Adam's volitional ratings were mostly in the passive

FIGURE 23-1 Ratings and Comments on the PVQ from the First Observation of Adam.

Behavioral Indicators	Rating Scale				Comments
Explores novelty	P	H	I	S	*Looked around when encouraged*
Initiates actions	P	H	I	S	*Only when it was suggested what to do*
Task-directed	P	H	I	S	*Completed things he was asked to do with prompting/encouragement*
Shows preferences	P	H	I	S	*Liked suspended equipment*
Tries new things	P	H	I	S	*Tried out new equipment with encouragement/support*
Stays engaged	P	H	I	S	*Needed support to keep going*
Expresses mastery pleasure	P	H	I	S	*Seemed anxious through most of session; frequently said, "I can't"*
Tries to solve problems	P	H	I	S	*Did not attempt to problem-solve using equipment*
Tries to produce effects	P	H	I	S	
Practices skills	P	H	I	S	*Made no attempts to retry things*
Seeks challenges	P	H	I	S	
Organizes/modifies environment	P	H	I	S	
Pursues activity to completion	P	H	I	S	*Needed encouragement to keep going*
Uses imagination/symbolism	P	H	I	S	

Key : **P** = Passive; **H** = Hesitant; **I** = Involved; **S** = Spontaneous or hesitant range, indicating that in a context that required motor actions, his motivation was quite limited. As the therapist's comments suggest, Adam appeared anxious and fearful of being judged and had a negative view of his capacities. These characteristics interfered with his enjoyment and seemed to extinguish any desire to become really involved in the sensorimotor play the therapist had encouraged him to try.

Informal interviews with Adam and his mother also pointed out that his difficulties were affecting several parts of his life. Adam's problems had increased over the years as he was invited and expected to join other children in the neighborhood and school within various occupational forms that involved motor skills he had not developed. As a consequence, Adam's participation in childhood play had been negatively affected. The therapist learned from an interview with Adam's mother that Adam tended to play with children younger than his own chronological age and that he was unable to perform occupational forms done by other children his age (e.g., bike riding, in-line skating, street hockey, soccer). His play was limited to activities with minimal movement requirements, such as video games and reading.

Adam's participation in the family was also suffering. He clearly wanted to be helpful and useful in the family, but he was easily frustrated when his motor difficulties interfered with his helping. For example, he wanted to be able to help carry groceries for his mother, but he often dropped them, breaking items or making a mess.

Finally, Adam's problems affected his self-care. Adam was often frustrated and overly emotional when performing routine self-care. He had always been very particular with the textures of clothes he would tolerate and the foods he would eat. Adam had particular difficulty with those self-care activities performed infrequently, such as cutting his nails and cleaning his ears.

The Therapist's Conceptualization of Adam's Situation

Based on the initial observation, additional sensory integration evaluations, and informal interviews, the therapist arrived at the following conceptualization of Adam's situation. Adam was experiencing difficulty processing and interpreting tactile and movement information. His therapist noted that he had particular difficulties with hypersensitivity to tactile stimuli from the therapist's touch and in response to different objects (e.g., chalk, uncooked navy beans, sheepskin, etc.). His dyspraxia (inability to plan and execute motor skills) was particularly evident during fine motor, in-hand manipulation and during movements that required bilateral integration, sequencing, and anticipatory motor control (e.g., throwing and catching a ball and performing sequential jumping patterns).

Adam exhibited an inability to efficiently modulate or regulate incoming sensory information. Although this ability to modulate sensory information underwent a normal variation throughout the course of a day, Adam demonstrated an extreme variability in his ability to filter and regulate sensory/tactile information. He tended to underreact or overreact, or fluctuate between underresponding and overresponding, often without warning. This problem could have been very bewildering to those who interacted with Adam. Most importantly, it was highly frustrating and frightening to Adam. As he told the therapist in a later session, "I can't control how I react sometimes."

Adam's comment about his inability to control himself indicated the personal causation fear he had about his sensory processing problems. Moreover, the sensory integration problems likely contributed to and were exacerbated by his volition status. That is, it had become clear from Adam's behavior and self-report that he was plagued by a negative sense of personal causation that led him to expect failure and feel intimidated by sensory and motor-based actions. Consequently, Adam often rushed through or did his best to avoid such actions to circumvent the painful experience of seeing himself unable to tolerate or perform actions. Afterward, he felt an acute sense of failure.

With each new encounter, Adam repeated and reinforced his belief that he was incapable and his feeling of being out of control. Because of his feelings of incapacity and inefficacy, Adam's activity choices were not adaptive. He would not take moderate risks that would have given him opportunities for learning and success. He was also reluctant to join in the play activities in which his peers engaged (i.e., mildly competitive, skill-oriented games and sports). His negative personal causation and his modulation disorder together influenced his ability to interact effectively in social contexts, where touch and unexpected tactile stimuli were more unpredictable and where, as a consequence, he felt even more out of control.

Adam's volitional sense of threat and his anxiety also meant that he approached sensory and motor experiences in a suboptimal emotional state that exacerbated his performance problems and his reactions to sensation. Adam was clearly in the midst of an ongoing process that kept him in the grip of self-doubt and anxiety. This led him to avoid many learning and socializing experiences. Moreover, when he had to perform, he was so terrified that his emotional state and sensory integrative problems together often led to the very failure he so feared. Consequently, he gained neither skill nor a sense of capacity and efficacy. Moreover, the fear that something was very wrong with himself had increasingly taken on a life of its own and seemed to be growing as a dominant theme in Adam's emerging occupational identity.

Because Adam's volition was so dominated by his personal causation fears and anxieties, there was little opportunity for Adam to develop positive interests. Thus, he did not have strong attractions to occupations, nor did he experience much pleasure or satisfaction from performance. Adam desperately wanted to be like other children and to be a friend to his peers. He also wanted to be recognized as a good son to his parents. These values did not, however, serve as motives leading Adam toward positive activity and occupational choices. Rather, they served mainly as standards against which he judged himself a failure.

Adam's Therapy Goals

The therapist first shared with Adam and his mother her conceptualization of the situation, using terms that Adam could grasp and framing the situation as a problem they could readily address in therapy. She gave Adam a number of concrete examples of things he could learn how to do in therapy. By helping Adam envision therapy as an opportunity to learn things and feel better about himself, she pre-

pared him to engage in the next step of identifying some goals that could be used to show Adam, his mother, and the therapist that he was making progress. Collaborating together, the three of them arrived at the following goals:

- Each day, Adam will make positive activity choices related to situations and opportunities in school, home, and/or therapy
- Adam will develop more varied interests in play and social interaction within the school and home environments
- Adam will be able to successfully perform chores at home with the help of any adaptations he or his family need to make
- On a daily basis, Adam will be able to complete personal self-care routines successfully and without aversive responses
- Adam will demonstrate the ability to perform age-appropriate occupational forms in play.

Each week, short-term goals were identified in language Adam readily understood. These goals focused on what Adam would do outside therapy at home and school. The therapist provided consultation to the mother about ways to support Adam to achieve his weekly goals. This was particularly important to ensure that Adam could use skills learned in therapy at home and school.

Course of Therapy

The therapist focused on creating opportunities for Adam to be competent and independent within therapy and within his everyday environments. Early in the course of therapy, the therapist provided opportunities that were designed to encourage Adam's exploration and experimentation with different equipment and toys in the occupational therapy environment. Because beliefs about one's effectiveness in the environment are based on personal experience, the therapist wanted to focus first on providing for Adam a safe, playful environment, free from the pressure to perform or be good enough. She felt that, in this context, Adam needed special opportunities to take risks and experience success to develop his sense of capacity and efficacy. She wanted Adam to develop both the skills for and the belief that he was empowered to influence the physical and eventually the social environment.

Over the course of a few sessions, the therapist found Adam to become increasingly curious, articulate, and charming. Beneath his personal causation fears, it was important to Adam to do well. The therapist both validated how Adam felt about himself and his difficulties and constantly gave him feedback that reframed his interpretations of his performance by stressing his improvement and what he had learned. After 3 months, the therapist readministered the Pediatric Volitional Questionnaire by observing Adam in the same sensorimotor play context as she had done initially. As shown in *Figure 23-2*, Adam's volition had changed dramatically.

With Adam's volition so improved, the therapist sought to increasingly involve Adam in the decisions of what equipment to use, what games to play, and when to change to another activity as well as in the setting up and modifying of the equipment. With time, Adam and the therapist developed the ability to flow within and between different movement activities during the therapy sessions. As Adam was empowered to influence and control these therapeutic situations, he increased his readiness for coping with his sensory challenges in his other life environments.

On an ongoing basis, the therapist discussed with Adam's mother strategies for modifying the home and school environments to ensure Adam's success. For example, routines for completing self-care without undue emotion or stress were developed. As much as possible, Adam was encouraged to decide when he did certain self-care activities and the order in which he would do them. For example, he and his mother identified that taking a bath right before bedtime was too stressful and arousing for him. Adam decided that after dinner was a better time for his bath and washing his hair. He found that he was more relaxed and ready for sleep when bedtime rolled around. Although he was only 7 years old, the therapist carefully strove to facilitate in Adam an internalized sense of control over his own routine.

In working with Adam's mother, the therapist helped both her and Adam understand that Adam's performance difficulties were not the result of

FIGURE 23-2   Ratings and Comments on PVQ From the Second Observation of Adam.

Behavioral Indicators	Rating Scale				Comments
Explores novelty	P	H	I	**S**	Willingly tried a new motor task the therapist demonstrated
Initiates actions	P	H	I	**S**	When it was suggested what to do
Task-directed	P	H	I	**S**	Chose and stayed with motor tasks
Shows preferences	P	H	I	**S**	Still liked the suspended equipment best but enjoys other things
Tries new things	P	H	I	**S**	Invented new ways to use equipment
Stays engaged	P	H	**I**	S	Needed support to keep going
Expresses mastery pleasure	P	H	**I**	S	Shows pride when praised
Tries to solve problems	P	H	**I**	S	Able to problem-solve new movements with support
Tries to produce effects	P	H	I	**S**	Interested to see how high he could swing
Practices skills	P	H	**I**	S	Repeated new movements several times till he could do them effectively
Seeks challenges	P	H	**I**	S	With support
Organizes/modifies environment	P	H	I	**S**	Moved equipment around
Pursues activity to completion	P	H	I	**S**	Needed encouragement to keep going
Uses imagination/symbolism	P	H	I	S	Not observed
Key : **P** = Passive; **H** = Hesitant; **I** = Involved; **S** = Spontaneous					

Adam's not trying hard enough. Together, they examined the more stressful daily situations and identified the challenging sensory aspects of these situations to develop adaptations or modifications to ensure Adam's success.

The therapist coached Adam in how to attend to some of the details of the physical environment and how they differentially affected how he felt. Adam and his therapist explored various ways to modify the environment, such as optimal lighting and workspaces. Together, they identified calm, "get-organized" environments that Adam could use when he was feeling overwhelmed.

Throughout therapy, the therapist and Adam's mother worked together to give Adam the feedback that he was a good and valuable child. They were careful to offer Adam genuine praise for approximations of success and for his successful performance in daily tasks. Indeed, after several months in therapy, Adam spontaneously volunteered one day, "I knew I was really good inside after all! I am okay."

As Adam continued to improve, the therapist increased focus on his everyday role behaviors related to play, self-care, and peer interaction as well as on his routine organization of behavior. Although improvements in Adam's sensory integration and modulation were expected and observed over the course of therapy, the therapist also expected that Adam would not overcome all his sensory integrative difficulties. Most likely, he would always have some unique challenges related to sensory processing and motor performance in new, stressful situations.

The therapist strove to identify these likely challenges as part of how Adam, like everyone else, would have to adapt in life with his own unique strengths and weaknesses. This emphasized how Adam was like other children while highlighting his unique coping challenges. The therapist and Adam's mother discussed this together and determined on an ongoing basis what steps were important for enabling Adam to develop his own coping abilities.

Over time, Adam was offered even wider opportunities for developing new interests both in therapy and at home. Because the development of new and more varied interests was initially depen-

dent on Adam's experience during activities, he was provided as much variety within appropriate activities as possible. Natural extensions of the therapy experiences were built into his home and school environments. For example, as Adam became more organized and controlled in his gross motor play, Adam's parents took him regularly to a local park and playground where he could have appropriate experiences. When the weather became colder, Adam took advantage of the local children's indoor playground. Later, his father built a tree-house climbing structure in their backyard. This not only was a resource for playing with his newfound friends, but also an important symbol of Adam's accomplishments.

Adam's communication and interaction skills developed slowly within the home and school environments as his volition, sensory modulation, and physical capabilities improved. Through a combination of adaptation and successive interaction in progressively more complex social groups, Adam developed greater competence and belief in his own social skills and unique abilities.

One day while in therapy, Adam said, "You know I can do everything here. I think I don't need to see you so much anymore." After discussion and review of Adam's improvements, Adam, his parents, and the therapist agreed to cease direct treatment. The therapist continued to consult with the family and help them monitor Adam's ongoing development.

Adam in Perspective

This case underscores the value of paying particular attention to the negative synergy that can exist between performance difficulties and volition. As the case illustrated, Adam's volitional problems led him to make choices to do things that restricted his performance and led to further self-doubt and self-devaluation. To counter this process, the therapist created situations in which Adam's fears and anxieties could be minimized and in which he could be encouraged to make activity choices that would lead to positive sensory and motor experiences. The overall aim of therapy was to reverse the negative cycle of avoidance, performance during suboptimal emotional states, failure, and negative self-appraisal. Moreover, the therapist also followed the argument by Kielhofner and Fisher (1991) that change in sensory integration capacities requires the child to perform while in a positive volitional state.

Gaining Another Chance at Life

Employment Options[a] is a federally funded vocational rehabilitation program for persons living with AIDS and is operated by the Occupational Therapy Department at the University of Illinois at Chicago. In the program, initial evaluation is followed by a series of group sessions focused on return-to-work issues. During this first phase, clients also receive further evaluation and individualized therapy services. During a second phase, clients are placed in an internship or training program. Finally, clients are given support to find employment and offered follow-up support and services once employed. The case that follows tells the story of Dan, one of the clients in this program.

Dan

Dan heard about the Employment Options program from his case manager. He called the occupational therapist and was excited to learn he could join the program. On the appointed day of his intake evaluation, Dan showed up early and anxious to get started.

The therapist began by conducting an interview that combined the content of the Occupational Performance History Interview-II (OPHI-II) and the Worker Role Interview (WRI). These are routinely the first assessments given to clients in the program. Since the two are semi-structured interviews with overlapping content, it is possible to combine them into a single, longer interview after which the therapist completes the forms for both assessments. The following is the occupational narrative that Dan told during the interview.

[a]Employment Options is a Research and Demonstration grant funded by the U.S. Department of Education's Rehabilitation Services Administration (Grant #H235A980170).

Born in a small suburb south of Chicago, Dan was the youngest of five children. He had a strained relationship with his father, a strict disciplinarian, who spoke to him mainly when he wanted to point out that Dan had done something wrong. Pushed by conflict at home and worried over his family's acceptance of his homosexuality, Dan decided to start making his own life. When he was 13 years old, he lied about his age and began working as a busboy in a restaurant.

Three years later and still deeply frustrated with life at home, Dan moved to Colorado to live with his older sister. After what he described as a "wild and unsupervised time" finishing high school there, he moved back to Chicago and began working in a hotel restaurant. He routinely worked long hours at this and other part-time jobs.

Seeking to change his life, Dan moved to San Francisco where his older sister then lived. He worked in restaurants there, while attending technical school to learn video production. After the program, Dan completed a paid internship in a television studio. However, he became disillusioned with lack of job opportunities. He decided to return to Chicago and resume working in the food industry.

Dan worked mainly as a waiter, maintaining a reasonably satisfying lifestyle for the next few years. He generally found his work satisfying, although at times it was stressful due to the long hours and customer demands. His social life was limited because he mainly worked weekends and nights. On the other hand, he took advantage of having days off to stay in good shape by biking, jogging, and hiking. All in all, life was acceptable.

Three years before he came to the Employment Options program, Dan was employed as temporary help for a restaurant during the busy winter holidays. Working long hours almost daily, he started feeling ill. Soon, he was hospitalized with Pneumocystis pneumonia and was tested for HIV. The doctor came into his hospital room, announced that Dan had AIDS, and walked out of the room. Dan recalled, "I just wanted to turn over and die right then."

Dan admitted that he was only partly surprised. He explained, "Part of me always wondered anytime I got sick with anything because, being gay, that's just a part of life . . . When you see a lot of people around you die from AIDS and then you get the news, you feel like you're already gone." After recovering from pneumonia, Dan decided not to call his employer back because he expected that he would never be well enough to work again.

Dan decided to inform his widowed and aging mother that he had AIDS. She was shocked and troubled, but wanted to support Dan. When she invited him to live with her, Dan moved in. Dan's mother initially supported and helped him. As Dan's health improved, he increasingly became a caretaker for his mother.

On top of Dan's illness, he was plagued with economic and bureaucratic problems. Since he had neither health insurance nor income, he filled out the reams of paperwork necessary to receive public assistance and disability income. Dealing with the public aid system and his medical bills became a preoccupation and a major stress. For example, newly recovered from pneumonia, still feeling weak and reeling from news of his AIDS diagnosis, he received repeated calls from the hospital demanding payment. As Dan recalled, "I didn't even have a life anymore, and the person from the hospital wanted to know when I was going to pay twelve thousand dollars in hospital bills. I was beyond crying."

In the year that followed, Dan focused on stabilizing his health. He began a regimen of taking medications four times daily. He struggled with ongoing AIDS symptoms and medication side effects including drowsiness, diarrhea, fatigue, neuropathy, nausea, sleeplessness, and sweats. During this time, Dan also became quite depressed. He joined an AIDS support group. However, the members of the group were much more ill than Dan. Since it made him feel even worse, he quit.

With time, Dan began to slowly rebuild a routine to keep himself busy. Just before coming to the program, his routine included running errands, driving his mother places, and doing home management tasks. Feeling better, Dan had decided to explore the possibility of returning to work. As he put it, "I need a life again." Dan also was aware that he might lose his disability income since his health was improving. Mostly, however, Dan—who had been self-sufficient from such a young age—wanted to be productive.

At this juncture, Dan no longer wanted to work in the food industry because it was too physically demanding for him. Besides, he was hoping to find something new that he could enjoy, explaining, "When you've been on death's doorstep, you see things a lot differently." Dan's older sister worked in the computer industry and got Dan interested in learning computers. She bought him a computer that gave him e-mail and access to the Internet. Dan found that the computer opened up a whole new world for him. For example, through Internet chat rooms, he contacted others with HIV, creating a virtual support group for himself. Dan was unsure of what type of work he might do but he wanted it to involve computers.

As shown in *Figure 23-3*, Dan's occupational identity was largely intact, although his competence had been negatively affected by his illness, symptoms, and medication side effects. Similarly, his ratings on the Worker Role Interview (*Fig. 23-4*) indicated that Dan had many strengths for returning to work. These were highest in the areas of roles, values, and habits. Overall, the scores reflect Dan's strong work history and worker role identity. Finally, Dan's narrative slope (*Fig. 23-5*) illustrates his movement out of a difficult childhood and adolescence into adult employment, followed by his AIDS diagnosis and gradual recovery. He was beginning an upward slope that he hoped to continue by achieving employment.

When the therapist shared with Dan her understanding of his life from the interview, Dan agreed. They further discussed what might help or hinder his continuation on a positive trajectory. Dan saw the following barriers to getting back into work:

- Social prejudice and possible discrimination toward his HIV status
- Difficulties in maintaining insurance coverage
- His lack of specific job skills.

The major strength that he believed would get him back to employment was his sense of self-determination. Following his initial assessment, Dan sent his therapist an e-mail thanking her. This was the first of many examples of Dan's courteousness and concern for others.

FIGURE 23-3   Dan's Ratings on the OPHI-II.

Occupational Identity Scale	1	2	3	4
Has personal goals and projects			▨	
Identifies a desired occupational lifestyle			▨	
Expects success			▨	
Accepts responsibility			▨	
Appraises abilities and limitations			▨	
Has commitments and values			▨	
Recognizes identity and obligations			▨	
Has interests			▨	
Felt effective (past)			▨	
Found meaning and satisfaction in lifestyle (past)		▨		
Made occupational choices (past)		▨		

Occupational Competence Scale	1	2	3	4
Maintains satisfying lifestyle		▨		
Fulfills role expectations		▨		
Works toward goals		▨		
Meets personal performance standards		▨		
Organizes time for responsibilities			▨	
Participates in interests		▨		
Fulfilled roles (past)			▨	
Maintained habits (past)			▨	
Achieved satisfaction (past)		▨		

Occupational Behavior Settings Scale	1	2	3	4
Home-life occupational forms			▨	
Major productive role occupational forms		Not Applicable		
Leisure occupational forms			▨	
Home-life social group		▨		
Major productive social group		Not Applicable		
Leisure social group		▨		
Home-life physical spaces, objects, and resources			▨	
Major productive role physical spaces, objects, and resources		Not Applicable		
Leisure physical spaces, objects, and resources			▨	

Key : **4** = Exceptionally competent occupational functioning; **3** = Appropriate satisfactory occupational functioning; **2** = Some occupational dysfunction; **1** = Extremely occupationally dysfunctional

In a subsequent session, Dan completed the Role Checklist and the Occupational Self Assessment (OSA) as a prelude to setting long- and short-term goals. On the Role Checklist (*Fig. 23-6*), Dan indicated that most of his roles were interrupted. The roles he had kept all revolved around living with his mother, being a caretaker for her, and maintaining the home. His plans for the future included the possibility of returning to school, volunteering, and returning to work. He also identified that he very much wanted involvement in support groups, as he felt he needed more contact with others, and that

FIGURE 23-4 Dan's Ratings on the WRI.

Worker Role Interview Summary Scoring Sheet					
	4	3	2	1	N/A
Personal Causation					
Assesses abilities and limitations		▓			
Expectations of job success			▓		
Takes responsibility		▓			
Values					
Commitment to work		▓			
Work-related goals		▓			
Interests					
Enjoys work			▓		
Pursues interests					
Roles					
Identifies with being a worker		▓			
Appraises work expectations		▓			
Influence of other roles		▓			
Habits					
Work habits	▓				
Daily routines		▓			
Adapts routine to minimize difficulties		▓			
Environment					
Perception of work setting					▓
Perception of family and peers					▓
Perception of boss					▓
Perception of coworkers					▓

Key: **4** = Strongly support; **3** = Support; **2** = Interferes; **1** = Strongly interferes; **N/A** = Not applicable

he hoped to re-establish some of his old role as an outdoor exerciser. As discussed below, some of the same issues were identified in the OSA.

On the first part of the OSA (*Fig. 23-7*), Dan identified four problem areas:

- Physically doing what I need to do
- Having a satisfying routine
- Doing activities I like
- Effectively using my abilities.

In discussing his responses, Dan reported that he needed to get in better physical shape and become more involved in doing things he liked and valued. As he put it, "I need to sharpen my mind and body."

Regarding the environment section, Dan identified four problem areas:

- People who support and encourage me
- People who do things with me
- Opportunities to do things I value and like
- Places where I can go and enjoy myself.

In discussing this section, Dan noted that he felt isolated where he lived with his mother. His main concern was to find new friends.

Using the results of the OSA and the Role Checklist, Dan and his therapist identified the following long-term goals:

- Dan will improve his health by participating in a consistent exercise program for at least 2 months

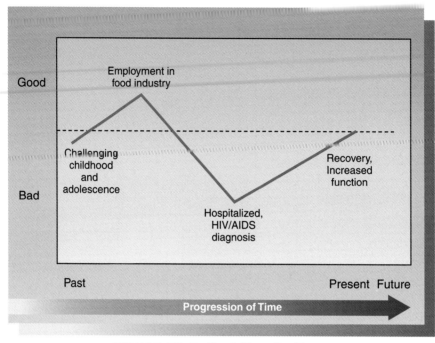

FIGURE 23-5   Dan's Narrative Slope.

FIGURE 23-6   Dan's Responses on the Role Checklist.

Role	Role Identity			Value Designation		
	Past	Present	Future	Not at all	Somewhat	Very
Student						
Worker						
Volunteer						
Caregiver						
Home Maintainer						
Friend						
Family Member						
Religious Participant						
Hobbyist/Amateur						
Participant in Organizations						
Other: Volunteer/Support Groups						

FIGURE 23-7 Dan's Responses on the OSA.

Myself	Competence				Values			
	Lots of problems	Some difficulty	Well	Extremely well	Not so Important	Important	More Important	Most Important
Concentrating on my tasks		▓			▓			
Physically doing what I set out to do	▓				▓			
Taking care of the place where I live			▓		▓			
Taking care of myself			▓		▓			
Taking care of others for whom I am responsible			▓		▓			
Getting where I need to go			▓		▓			
Managing my finances		▓						▓
Managing my basic needs (food, medicine)				▓				▓
Expressing myself to others			▓			▓		
Getting along with others				▓				▓
Identifying and solving problems			▓				▓	
Relaxing and enjoying myself		▓						
Getting done what I need to do								
Having a satisfying routine	▓					▓		
Handling my responsibilities			▓			▓		
Being involved as a student, worker, volunteer, and/or family member		▓			▓			
Doing activities I like	▓				▓			
Working towards my goals				▓				▓
Making important decisions based on what I think is important			▓				▓	
Accomplishing what I set out to do			▓					▓
Effectively using my abilities	▓				▓			
My Environment	**Environmental Impact**				**Value of Environment**			
	Lots of problems	Some problems	Good	Extremely good	Not so Important	Important	More Important	Most Important
A place to live and take care of myself		▓						▓
A place where I can be productive (work, study, volunteer)		▓			▓			
The basic things I need to live and take care of myself			▓					▓
The things I need to be productive		▓			▓			
People who support me and encourage me								▓
People who do things with me								▓
Opportunities to do things I value and like	▓							▓
Places where I can go and enjoy myself	▓						▓	

- Dan will learn Microsoft Word and Excel within 4 months
- Dan will work in an internship to gain computer skills within 3 months
- Dan will learn about (1) how employment would affect his health benefits and (2) his rights under the Americans with Disabilities Act (ADA)
- Dan will learn how to search for a job involving computers and to explain the hiatus in his employment to prospective employers.

Phase 1 of Dan's Therapy

Dan was early to the first group session and brought in magazines geared toward HIV education for other clients to read. He never missed a group session and actively participated and shared information with other members. During the sessions, Dan learned about health insurance benefits, legal issues concerning employment, and job search strategies.

Dan came to the program several hours each week to practice on the computer. He also participated in an Internet Workshop at the university library and made follow-up appointments with the instructor to further his education. He learned word processing and spreadsheet programs using an Internet tutorial and several books that he purchased.

Dan's physical status improved as he became more active. He attributed his increased level of activity to the structure of the program, noting, "Employment Options makes me get out . . . It's sort of like a job." Dan also reported that the program helped him manage his time more efficiently and feel more in control of his life.

Phase 2 of the Program

When Dan began the program, he considered attending school to further his computer skills. However, given his progress learning these skills on his own, he decided to do an internship instead of going back to school. Although ready to move into this next phase, Dan had a number of concerns that he shared with his therapist. He was afraid that he would not be able to physically tolerate the work and become ill as a result. He feared that his health care benefits would get "screwed up" if he went back to work in a job without a good health plan, while losing his public health benefits due to having

an income. The therapist validated Dan's concern and assured him that she would advise and coach him throughout the process to assure that he did not physically overtax himself or jeopardize funding for his health care.

Just as Dan was about to begin interviewing for an internship, he developed shingles. Determined not to let his condition deter him, Dan did his first interview even before he was completely recovered. This interview at an insurance broker's office turned out to be successful and Dan started interning for the broker the next week. He worked half days, three times a week.

The therapist provided job coaching to Dan. Mostly, he was anxious about whether he could manage it and needed encouragement. He was well organized and took notes on the therapist's suggestions concerning how to ask his supervisor for help and how to do his work in a more energy-efficient way. The internship went well, and Dan's supervisor gave him additional responsibility that boosted his sense of efficacy. After 2 months of the internship, Dan's boss offered him a full-time paid position.

Dan came to his therapist for advice. He generally liked the job, but was unsure if he should take it. The therapist suggested they do the Work Environment Impact Scale (WEIS) to assess how this work context was impacting Dan. The scores (shown in *Figure 23-8*) indicated that the work environment was generally supportive. As Dan reviewed the strengths of the work environment, he noted the following important features. The schedule was very flexible. He was comfortable working at a place where his supervisor knew he was HIV-positive. Finally, he felt that he had a good relationship with his supervisor.

The WEIS also helped identify four areas of concern. The first was the appeal of work tasks. Dan reported that some of the things that he had to do were tedious and boring. Dan said he was not sure if the type of work he was doing would be challenging enough for him in the long term. He also noted that his supervisor sometimes handled the more challenging occupational forms rather than taking the time to train Dan. The second problem area was the properties of objects. Dan identified that the computer at his desk was very outdated,

FIGURE 23-8 Dan's Response on the WEIS.

	1	2	3	4	N/A
Time Demands			■		
Task Demands			■		
Appeal of Work Tasks		■			
Work Schedule		■			
Coworker Interaction					■
Work Group Membership					■
Supervisor Interaction			■		
Work Role Standards			■		
Work Role Style			■		
Interaction with Others			■		
Rewards		■			
Sensory Qualities			■		
Architecture/Arrangement			■		
Ambience/Mood			■		
Properties of Objects		■			
Physical Amenities			■		
Meaning of Objects			■		

Key: **4** = Strongly Supports; **3** = Supports; **2** = Interferes;
1 = Strongly interferes; **N/A** = Not applicable

limiting what he could do. The third area was the job rewards. Dan was concerned that the job would not offer health benefits and his pay would not be very high. Dan's final concern was the demands of the full-time work schedule, given his continued fatigue. Although it had improved significantly since he began the program, he felt that he still could not handle a full-time job. He anticipated that he could increase beyond the hours that he worked as an intern, but not to 40 hours a week.

The therapist first identified that Dan could work for a period without jeopardizing his insurance and disability income. This would give him an opportunity to decide if he could handle the challenge of working. The therapist then coached Dan on how he could approach the boss about the other factors identified in the WEIS to ask him to consider making some adjustments. They decided together that the highest priority was to ask for fewer hours so that he could tolerate the job.

Dan successfully negotiated altered hours and opportunity to take on more challenges. He also suggested to his supervisor that he do some things at home so he could work at his computer, which had more capability than the one he used in the office. His supervisor approved the idea. Dan decided to take the job. He worked successfully at the insurance brokerage for 5 months. Unfortunately, he had to stop working because of severe neuropathy in his hands and feet.

Two months after leaving his position, Dan was feeling a little better and came to see his therapist for advice. They decided together that it might be best for Dan to do volunteer work, at least for a while. Together, they identified that Dan's first choice was volunteer work at a local AIDS organization. Eventually, he took on volunteer roles in two such agencies. Dan became very involved in support groups and other activities. Over time, he also made numerous friends with the staff and clients. Importantly for Dan, he no longer felt isolated. He also felt happy doing something that he enjoyed and found meaningful.

As time went on, Dan became more and more active as a volunteer. Eventually, he took on a leadership role in one organization. Using what he learned in the Employment Options program, Dan ran an educational group in which he shared information about disability benefits, rights under the ADA, and the intricacies of health insurance. Later, he initiated and helped organize a presentation to recruit clients for the Employment Options program for both of the organizations with which he was involved.

After a year of volunteering, Dan told the therapist that he was thinking about looking again for a part-time job. Before they could meet to discuss this plan, Dan called to say he was sick. Two months later, Dan died suddenly of congestive heart failure.

Dan in Perspective

Success in occupational therapy is often measured only in long-term positive outcomes. However, sometimes therapy accomplishes other things that are equally important. In this case, therapy enabled Dan to improve the quality of his last 2 years of life. Dan was able to gain new skills, work, volunteer, and become less isolated. In an article he wrote for the Employment Options client newsletter some months before he died, Dan said:

> I am seeing life as more of a positive challenge lately. Instead of just surviving, I am reaching for more, a little at a time, and am enjoying the people and friends along the way. Sure I am having rough times, but I am getting better and handling them and they make the good times seem a bit sweeter.

In that same article, he thanked the staff of the Employment Options program, noting that it was giving him "another chance at life."

Getting Control of Life

Paula was a 45-year-old woman who lived with her mother in the Cotswolds area of England. She had a mild learning disability, epilepsy, and a right-sided hemiparesis. Paula was referred to the occupational therapist because her mother was aging and Paula's sisters wanted her to become more independent in homemaking.

Paula

The therapist first made an informal home visit to discuss the referral with Paula and her mother. She also planned to begin collecting information informally and to identify the most appropriate formal assessment tools. It quickly became clear that her family determined Paula's routines. Her two sisters who lived nearby had set days for shopping, gardening, and visiting Paula and her mother. Paula had organized her schedule to fit in with the family's routines. She volunteered 2 days a week, but otherwise spent many hours alone in her room listening to music or watching videos.

Paula reported that she had mild right-sided weakness and had minor problems handling and gripping things with her dominant right hand. Her speech was unclear at times, especially when she was anxious. Paula reported that her difficulty pro-

nouncing words sometimes prevented her from communicating as freely as she would have liked. During this visit, the therapist asked Paula if she could observe her doing some household tasks, and Paula agreed. From the observation, Paula's process skills appeared adequate, although she complained that the medication (anticonvulsants) she took made her feel groggy and confused sometimes.

Although Paula showed no significant problems in performing, her mother intruded regularly, directing and correcting Paula throughout the task. The therapist could see that this was very frustrating for Paula. Moreover, it increased her anxiety, which made it harder for her to focus on her performance. Later, Paula complained, "This always happens." Despite her clear annoyance at her mother's intervention, Paula did not express to her mother her wish to continue alone in the task.

As a result of this visit, the therapist determined that Paula had the ability to self-report accurately and effectively and needed an opportunity to express her own views of her life. Consequently, the therapist decided to administer three assessments:

- The Occupational Self Assessment (OSA)
- The Occupational Performance History Interview–Second Version (OPHI-II)
- The Role Checklist.

The therapist explained to Paula that she wanted to meet with her alone the next time to ask her some questions and give her an opportunity to tell about her life. Paula liked this idea and agreed to an appointment time.

Occupational History

Paula responded to the OPHI-II interview with short but passionate responses. The life story she reported was as follows. Paula reported having motor and learning problems from an early age. Her first seizure occurred when she was 6 years old. She painfully recalled how, at school, her classmates ridiculed her because of her seizures and speech impediment. Things got somewhat better when she went to the senior school, because she found and confided in a supportive school counselor. This person helped Paula develop coping strategies and bolstered her self-confidence.

Paula left school at the age of 16. Some years later, she found a job in a warehouse. More than anything, working improved her life. She earned an income and felt capable and useful. Paula also made a number of friends at work with whom she shared hobbies and spent time.

Paula had always lived with her mother. Although Paula and her mother enjoyed a generally positive relationship, Paula felt that her mother dominated her decision-making. Moreover, her mother did most household tasks since she lacked confidence in Paula's abilities and worried about her having a seizure while doing something. Of late, Paula's seizures had become more frequent. Consequently, her mother pressured Paula to further diminish engagement in any household and leisure activities. For example, Paula had always used a bicycle as her major form of transportation, but she had also given it up at her mother's urging to avoid the possibility of having a seizure while riding.

The most critical event in Paula's life was the loss of her job a few months before. Paula had worked for 22 years in a warehouse where she operated light machinery. She had performed well at work. Despite occasional seizures, she had never had any injuries or problems. Paula's supervisors had been very supportive. Unfortunately, two events converged that led to her job loss. The first was a change in management structure that occurred when a larger corporation bought the company. The second was that Paula had a number of severe seizures at work. The new manager directed Paula's immediate supervisors to dismiss her on the grounds that her seizures made her an injury risk.

Paula was devastated by the loss of her job. She had begun to do volunteer work 2 days a week but deeply wanted to return to employment. Paula felt that she had lost the main area of her life in which she felt valued and effective. Moreover, her other occupational roles had been affected by her job loss. She lost friendships and leisure opportunities since most of her friendships and leisure pursuits had been shared with work colleagues. Her role within the family had reverted to being the disabled member, rather than a financial contributor. Her only interests at this point included listening to music and watching television. She spent long periods alone in her room, which contributed to her feeling increasingly isolated.

Paula's entire sense of efficacy was organized around her work in the past. Confined mostly at home where she had little access to the persons and things she had liked to do, Paula's life had taken a dramatic downward plunge as illustrated in her narrative slope (*Fig. 23-9*). She also had internalized

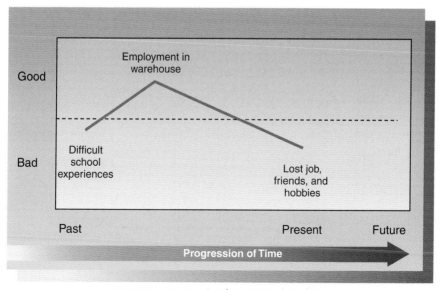

FIGURE 23-9 Paula's Narrative Slope.

many of the fears that her mother expressed about her becoming injured if she had a seizure. Although Paula had always managed life with some seizures, the consequences of her job loss, the increased frequency of seizures, and the growing concern expressed by her family led Paula herself to feel that everything was threatened by her seizures.

Paula had little control over her home environment. She felt hemmed in by expectations of her family members. For example, although Paula absolutely hated gardening, she was expected by her mother and sisters to maintain a large garden. Rather than create conflict or disappoint her family, Paula did the work without complaining.

FIGURE 23-10   Paula's Ratings on the OPHI-II.

Occupational Identity Scale	1	2	3	4
Has personal goals and projects			▓	
Identifies a desired occupational lifestyle				▓
Expects success		▓		
Accepts responsibility			▓	
Appraises abilities and limitations				▓
Has commitments and values				▓
Recognizes identity and obligations		▓		
Has interests				▓
Felt effective (past)				▓
Found meaning and satisfaction in lifestyle (past)				▓
Made occupational choices (past)				▓
Occupational Competence Scale	**1**	**2**	**3**	**4**
Maintains satisfying lifestyle	▓			
Fulfills role expectations	▓			
Works toward goals	▓			
Meets personal performance standards	▓			
Organizes time for responsibilities	▓			
Participates in interests	▓			
Fulfilled roles (past)				▓
Maintained habits (past)				▓
Achieved satisfaction (past)				▓
Occupational Behavior Settings Scale	**1**	**2**	**3**	**4**
Home-life occupational forms	▓			
Major productive role occupational forms	Not Applicable			
Leisure occupational forms	▓			
Home-life social group		▓		
Major productive social group	Not Applicable			
Leisure social group	▓			
Home-life physical spaces, objects, and resources		▓		
Major productive role physical spaces, objects, and resources	Not Applicable			
Leisure physical spaces, objects, and resources		▓		

Key : **4** = Exceptionally competent occupational functioning; **3** = Appropriate satisfactory occupational functioning; **2** = Some occupational dysfunction; **1** = Extremely occupationally dysfunctional

Paula acknowledged that her mother and sisters were the most significant people in her life. However, she felt very ambivalent her relationship with them. On one hand, she valued being part of the family group, but she also resented the restrictions and obligations put on her by her mother and sisters. She was also disturbed that her mother and sisters did not seem to recognize her abilities or place any value on her role within the family.

Paula's ratings on the OPHI-II are shown in *Figure 23-10*. Her occupational identity had been negatively affected by her loss of work and her competence was dramatically impacted as shown in the difference between the items reflecting the past and those reflecting the present. Finally, the negative impact of her environment is apparent in the ratings. She no longer had her work environment, and the opportunities for her occupational participation were quite constrained at home.

Paula filled out the Role Checklist and discussed it with the therapist. As shown in *Figure 23-11*, Paula's past roles were student, worker, friend, and hobbyist, to which she gave a value rating of very important. Her present roles were volunteer, home maintainer, and family member. Notably, she rated the volunteer role and family member role as only somewhat important. She explained that since the

work she did was unpaid, she was not contributing to the family budget as she always had.

In further discussing her responses, Paula noted that she desperately wanted to return to paid work. She also indicated somewhat guiltily that she wanted to move out of her mother's home and become a home maintainer in her own right. Paula also indicated that she wanted to get back to being involved in her roles as a friend and hobbyist. It was notable that she did not foresee a very significant involvement in the family member role. Paula explained that her mother was elderly and ill. Paula did not think she would have an ongoing close relationship with her sisters following her mother's death.

Occupational Self Assessment (OSA)

From the OPHI-II, it was clear that Paula felt she had lost control over her life. The therapist felt that it was important to begin giving control back to Paula. Therefore, when she presented the OSA to Paula, the therapist advised Paula that the OSA was her own assessment, since only Paula knew all the answers to the questions. The therapist also explained that in doing this assessment, Paula would be able to have a say in what she wanted her life to be and in the kind of services she received from the occupational therapist.

FIGURE 23-11 Paula's Responses on the Role Checklist.

Role	Role Identity			Value Designation		
	Past	Present	Future	Not at all	Somewhat	Very
Student	■					■
Worker	■					■
Volunteer		■			■	
Caregiver						
Home Maintainer		■				■
Friend	■					■
Family Member		■			■	
Religious Participant						
Hobbyist/Amateur	■					■
Participant in Organizations						

This was very empowering to Paula as she realized that she could influence the outcome of the assessment and the focus of her therapy. She worked through the forms eagerly with coaching from the therapist on how to complete them (see *Fig. 23-12* for her responses). In the discussion that followed, Paula wanted to talk about her total health needs and services. She was very concerned that her seizures were getting out of control. She felt isolated and increasingly self-conscious about her speech problems since he no longer had access to the coworkers who were accustomed and comfortable with her speech. She felt bored and useless. Finally, she felt very lonely, as she did not really see her mother and sisters as friends or companions with whom she could do leisure things. Together, the therapist and Paula set the following immediate goals:

- Get Paula's seizures better under control
- Get help to reduce her speech difficulties
- Increase her leisure activities, especially outside the home
- Identify companions with whom to spend time and make more friends.

The process of completing the OSA and setting goals empowered Paula to take more control over her health services. She attended a meeting of the interdisciplinary community team during which she asserted herself, expressing her own preferences and values.

The Therapist's Conceptualization of Paula's Situation

From the information gathered, the therapist constructed the following conceptualization of Paula's situation. Despite a previous pattern of positive occupational participation, Paula had recently experienced a contraction in all areas of participation. Paula had entered a negative spiral that began with the loss of her job and finding herself isolated back home where she had little control over her life.

Paula clearly knew what she valued, but because of her family's dominance of her decision-making and her own fears of being hurt during a seizure, she had increasingly restricted her participation in the things she most enjoyed and valued. The most significant limiting factor in her performance was her fear of doing things. Her family reinforced and maintained her anxiety and sense of inefficacy.

As Paula herself had identified on the OSA, her main priority was to undertake things that would increase her feeling of being capable of managing her life once again. When the therapist shared her conceptualization with Paula, she agreed and noted that she needed to "strengthen herself as a person" by undertaking things that she valued.

Intervention

Following the plan they had outlined when completing the OSA, the therapist and Paula began by addressing the medication issue. The therapist, working in conjunction with the community nurse, supported Paula in getting her medication adjusted. It was known from her previous medical history that Paula became stressed when a change in her drug therapy regimen was indicated. The therapist sought to put Paula in control as much as possible. The community nurse had advised Paula on how to chart her seizure activity. This identified that there was a definite pattern of seizure frequency during the month. Consequently, Paula and her therapist developed a schedule so that doing things that were new or potentially stressful was kept to the times of the month that were most likely to be seizure free.

Paula had told the therapist that her primary concern was that she might become injured from a seizure when using electrical equipment. Consequently, she had quit doing most household tasks that required use of such equipment. The therapist advised Paula that they would be able to find special appliances that would reduce this risk. However, as they explored purchasing such equipment, Paula decided that she wanted to use ordinary appliances, focusing instead on precautions that enhanced her safety. With support of the therapist, Paula planned a visit to a business that sold equipment with automatic electricity cut off.

The therapist next helped Paula refer herself to speech therapy. Since Paula had identified this as a problem she wanted to address, the therapist felt she would have a greater sense of control if she did a self-referral rather than simply finding a therapist for her. Paula found a therapist and began speech therapy. The speech therapist identified that Paula showed dysarthric and dyspraxic features in her speech. She developed a set of recommendations to help Paula

FIGURE 23-12 Paula's Responses on the OSA.

Myself	Competence				Values			
	Lots of problems	Some difficulty	Well	Extremely well	Not so Important	Important	More Important	Most Important
Concentrating on my tasks			■		■			
Physically doing what I set out to do		■			■			
Taking care of the place where I live		■					■	
Taking care of myself								■
Taking care of others for whom I am responsible			■					
Getting where I need to go						■		
Managing my finances			■			■		
Managing my basic needs (food, medicine)	■							■
Expressing myself to others	■							■
Getting along with others		■						
Identifying and solving problems		■			■			
Relaxing and enjoying myself			■					
Getting done what I need to do			■				■	
Having a satisfying routine		■						
Handling my responsibilities		■						
Being involved as a student, worker, volunteer, and/or family member								■
Doing activities I like			■				■	
Working towards my goals		■			■			
Making important decisions based on what I think is important			■					
Accomplishing what I set out to do			■				■	
Effectively using my abilities	■				■			

My Environment	Environmental Impact				Value of Environment			
	Lots of problems	Some problems	Good	Extremely good	Not so Important	Important	More Important	Most Important
A place to live and take care of myself	■							
A place where I can be productive (work, study, volunteer)			■			■		
The basic things I need to live and take care of myself				■				■
The things I need to be productive		■				■		
People who support me and encourage me			■					
People who do things with me							■	
Opportunities to do things I value and like							■	
Places where I can go and enjoy myself		■					■	

with her speech problems. She also gave Paula a set of exercises to improve her speech control.

Next, the therapist addressed Paula's last two goals of finding friends and increasing her leisure participation. The therapist accompanied Paula to a Disability Resource Center where they accessed a database. Paula had never used a computer before and was very proud of this achievement. In the database, they found information about local social clubs. Paula chose one to attend but expressed anxiety about going alone. The therapist accompanied her for the first three visits. Paula enjoyed this club and subsequently made arrangements to be picked up at her home by special transportation. In the next few months, she began to attend the group regularly and went on several trips with the group.

Coping With Life Changes

Paula's mother's health deteriorated to the point that she had to go into a nursing home. With the help of the therapist, Paula found a situation where she could live with a family as a paying guest. Paula hoped this would be temporary and that she could someday manage a household herself. Because she had not been given opportunities when living with her mother, Paula had not learned many of the necessary skills to live alone. Consequently, at the advice of the therapist, Paula began to attend a day center once a week where she had the opportunity to shop with others, plan, and cook lunch. The therapist also began working with Paula on other aspects of the homemaker role. Paula had identified ironing, sewing, and budgeting as areas she wanted to develop.

As her personal causation improved, Paula also identified that she would like to explore the possibility of working again. She expressed a desire to work in a library. The therapist helped Paula refer herself to an employment service for persons with learning disabilities. Paula soon began working two part-time jobs at a local university library and at the city library.

Shortly after she began working, the family with whom Paula was living moved to a nearby town and Paula moved with them. The distance required Paula to travel by bus to work and day care, which she found stressful. Also, another paying guest joined the family, and Paula felt this person intruded on her privacy. Finally, the teenage son in the household began to make fun of Paula, bringing back angry memories of her earlier victimization at school.

Paula's seizures began to increase as they did whenever she experienced stress. Paula was determined to find herself other accommodations and enlisted the help of the therapist. However, even before the therapist could assist her, Paula found a flat to rent. Although apprehensive about living alone, she decided that with some continued assistance from her therapist, she could manage.

Paula in Perspective

Paula's therapy exemplifies client-centered practice in which a therapist can empower a client to take control of life. It also illustrates how important it is for therapists to serve as advocates for clients when they are faced with social barriers. However well intentioned others' concerns about Paula were, she needed to be able to decide what reasonable risks she would take in her life. The therapist's most important role was to support Paula in making the decisions that put her in control of her life.

Conclusion

This chapter presented four cases that represented applications of MOHO in a community-based context. In presenting the cases, we sought to emphasize how therapists achieved client-centered practice that respected the client's views and desires. We also tried to point out how community-based practice inevitably draws therapists into dealing with the contexts in which clients work, play, and do their activities of daily living: home, school, neighborhood, community, and workplace.

Reference

Kielhofner, G., & Fisher, A. (1991). Mind-brain-body relationships. In A. Fisher, E. Murray, & A. Bundy (Eds.), *Sensory integration: Theory and practice* (pp. 27–45). Philadelphia: FA Davis.

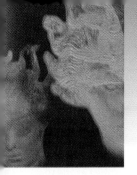

24

Enabling Clients to Reconstruct Their Occupational Lives in Long-Term Rehabilitation

- ● Gary Kielhofner
- ● Kathi Brenneman Baron
- ● Christiane Mentrup
- ● Daniela Schulte
- ● Jayne Shepherd

This chapter presents four cases from inpatient physical and psychiatric rehabilitation. A common theme throughout the cases is how therapy enabled these persons to envision and live their lives differently. While the nature of the clients' impairments varied, they shared a common challenge. Each had to reorganize volition, reconstruct habit patterns, revise or re-engage in life roles, and find new ways to effectively perform and participate in occupational life.

The therapists often had to gently nudge clients toward new ways of experiencing and seeing things, toward recognition of painful realities, and toward making hard decisions and compromises. They were able to help their clients to change through careful understanding of their situation made possible through the concepts and tools provided by MOHO.

Finding A Way To Trust Therapy

Clients do not always see the value of therapy. For a variety of reasons, they may feel that therapy is unnecessary or unhelpful. Fredrick, who is discussed below, came to therapy with serious doubts. Consequently, his therapist had to take special care to build a sense of trust and motivate him to collaborate in therapy. The case illus-

trates how MOHO provides a useful set of concepts and tools for understanding and building trust with a client who is not positively motivated toward therapy.

Fredrick

At age 23, Fredrick was admitted to a psychiatric ward of a general hospital in a small, northern German city. He was diagnosed with depression, which he had experienced since his childhood. Before this admission he had spent 3 weeks in a psychiatric ward of another local hospital, but left against medical advice. The next day he attempted suicide.

Fredrick had an understandably negative attitude toward psychiatric institutions. When Fredrick was 9 years old, his mother committed suicide while hospitalized in a psychiatric ward. The tragedy of his mother's death and doubts about the meaning of his own life dominated Fredrick's thoughts and feelings as a young man. Because he had little faith in the worth of psychiatric care, Fredrick had always been ambivalent at best about receiving psychiatric services. He regularly dismissed the advice of those attempting to provide him psychiatric services. He rarely followed through on their recommendations.

Guiding Questions and Initial Assessment

Fredrick's history suggested that he had long-standing problems of occupational adaptation. Therefore the therapist's main questions focused on understanding Fredrick's occupational identity and competence. Furthermore, she realized that his cooperation with therapy would depend on her understanding of his volition and being able to engage him in terms of his own view of himself and his world.

Because of Fredrick's history and perspective on psychiatric care, the occupational therapist was particularly concerned with beginning the process of assessment in a way that might build some trust and give him confidence in the therapist's genuine desire and ability to offer help to him. One advantage of MOHO-based assessments is that they focus on everyday occupational life rather than on illness or disability. Thus, they are aimed at revealing the client's unique perceptions, desires, and experiences. Using these assessments can often help to build trust and confidence.

The occupational therapist decided to begin assessment with the Occupational Performance History Interview-Second Version (OPHI-II). She reasoned that the interview would give Fredrick a chance to tell his own story and enable her to begin to build rapport with him. Also, it provides a level of detailed information that is often important to thoroughly understanding the perspective of a client.

At the beginning of the interview, Fredrick was aloof and skeptical. As he began to tell his occupational narrative and saw the interest of the therapist in his viewpoint, he became more open.

The OPHI-II pointed toward difficulties Fredrick had in enjoying life and feeling connected to roles. Therefore, the therapist decided to ask Fredrick to complete the Interest Checklist and the Role Checklist next. She chose these assessments because they allowed Fredrick to actively report about himself. To underscore this point, the therapist gave these assessments to Fredrick to fill out on his own. She explained them as opportunities for him to reflect on and record how he viewed these two important aspects of his life. The therapist also informally observed and had conversations with Fredrick on the ward and in occupational therapy. The sections that follow describe the assessment process and the understanding of Fredrick's occupational circumstances that the therapist was able to construct along with him.

Fredrick's Occupational Identity and Competence

Fredrick began his occupational narrative at the time he dropped out of high school. He saw no purpose and had no interest in school. For a while after leaving school he did nothing. Then he was accepted as a carpentry apprentice. A 3-year apprenticeship with a master carpenter is the traditional way to learn this trade in Germany. However, after only 4 weeks, Fredrick quit because he had second thoughts about whether he really wanted to learn carpentry.

Following this, Fredrick was unemployed. After almost a year, he decided to undertake training as a car mechanic. After successfully completing general mechanics training, he went on to take specialized courses in truck mechanics. Not long after he began employment as a mechanic, he quit the job. He was experiencing chronic back pain that he attributed to spending much of the day bent over his work. He was also disillusioned with his lack of satisfaction on this job.

Fredrick was unemployed for the next 6 months. During this time he sought treatment for his back pain at a German spa. Fredrick's physician also advised that he not return to mechanics because of his back problem. Thus, Fredrick began working as a janitor's assistant in an administration building complex. The pay was good, but he soon found himself once again disillusioned with his work. He quit the janitorial job, which was his last form of employment.

Fredrick related his occupational narrative as a series of failed attempts to find meaningful work. He complained of being unable to find enjoyment and satisfaction in what he did, even when he tried hard. He had not developed a clear sense of what he might find satisfying and had no clear identification with a work role or career. He lacked confidence in his ability to find something meaningful and stick with it. Along with the pattern of repeated unsuccessful attempts at work, Fredrick saw the future as gloomy. He expected more of the same and, accordingly, did not see a reason for trying.

Fredrick was convinced that any effort he made would ultimately result in the same disappointment and disillusionment as before. He could not recall a time in his life when things were really good. Most of his everyday life patterns had been bland and un-fulfilling to him. He could not imagine a life that he would find satisfying.

Along with his extreme difficulty in constructing an occupational identity, Fredrick had ongoing diffi-culty sustaining occupational competence (i.e., a pat-tern of everyday action that supported being pro-ductive and satisfied). His problems in occupational identity and competence are reflected in the first two scales of the OPHI-II as shown in *Figure 24-1*.

FIGURE 24-1 Fredrick's Ratings on the OPHI-II Scales.

Occupational Identity Scale	1	2	3	4
Has personal goals and projects	▓			
Identifies a desired occupational lifestyle		▓		
Expects success	▓			
Accepts responsibility		▓		
Appraises abilities and limitations			▓	
Has commitments and values			▓	
Recognizes identity and obligations				
Has interests				
Felt effective (past)	▓			
Found meaning and satisfaction in lifestyle (past)	▓			
Made occupational choices (past)	▓			
Occupational Competence Scale	**1**	**2**	**3**	**4**
Maintains satisfying lifestyle		▓		
Fulfills role expectations	▓			
Works toward goals	▓			
Meets personal performance standards		▓		
Organizes time for responsibilities	▓			
Participates in interests		▓		
Fulfilled roles (past)	▓			
Maintained habits (past)	▓			
Achieved satisfaction (past)	▓			
Occupational Behavior Settings Scale	**1**	**2**	**3**	**4**
Home-life occupational forms		▓		
Major productive role occupational forms	▓			
Leisure occupational forms			▓	
Home-life social group				▓
Major productive social group		▓		
Leisure social group				
Home-life physical spaces, objects, and resources				▓
Major productive role physical spaces, objects, and resources		▓		
Leisure physical spaces, objects, and resources				▓

Key : **4** = Exceptionally competent occupational functioning; **3** = Appropriate satisfactory occupational functioning; **2** = Some occupational dysfunction; **1** = Extremely occupationally dysfunctional

FIGURE 24-2   Fredrick's Responses on the Interest Checklist.

Activity	What has been your level of interest						Do you currently participate in this activity?		Would you like to pursue this in the future?	
	In the past ten years			In the past year						
	Strong	Some	No	Strong	Some	No	Yes	No	Yes	No
Gardening/yardwork			X			X		X		X
Sewing/needlework		X				X		X		X
Playing cards			X					X	X	
Foreign languages	X					X		X		X
Church activities			X			X		X	X	
Radio					X		X			X
Walking					X		X		X	
Car repair			X			X		X		X
Writing			X	X				X		X
Dancing			X	X				X	X	
Golf			X			X		X		X
Football						X		X		X
Listening to popular music		X				X		X		X
Puzzles			X			X		X		X
Holiday activities	X			X				X	X	
Pets/livestock			X			X		X		X
Movies		X				X		X	X	
Listening to classical music			X			X		X		X
Speeches/lectures			X			X		X		X
Swimming			X			X		X	X	
Bowling			X			X		X		X
Visiting		X				X		X	X	
Mending			X			X		X		X
Checkers/chess			X			X		X		X
Barbecues			X			X		X	X	
Reading			X			X		X		X
Traveling			X			X		X	X	
Parties		X				X		X		X

(continued)

FIGURE 24-2 (Continued)

Activity	What has been your level of interest						Do you currently participate in this activity?		Would you like to pursue this in the future?	
	In the past ten years			In the past year						
	Strong	Some	No	Strong	Some	No	Yes	No	Yes	No
Wrestling										
House cleaning										
Model building										
Television										
Concerts										
Pottery										
Camping										
Laundry/ironing										
Politics										
Table games										
Home decorating										
Clubs/lodge										
Singing										
Scouting										
Clothes										
Handicrafts										
Hairstyling										
Cycling										
Attending plays										
Bird watching										
Dating										
Auto racing										
Home repairs										
Exercise										
Hunting										
Woodworking										
Pool										
Driving										

(continued)

FIGURE 24-2 (Continued)

Activity	What has been your level of interest						Do you currently participate in this activity?		Would you like to pursue this in the future?	
	In the past ten years			In the past year						
	Strong	Some	No	Strong	Some	No	Yes	No	Yes	No
Child care										
Tennis										
Cooking/baking										
Basketball										
History										
Collecting										
Fishing										
Science										
Leatherwork										
Shopping										
Photography										
Painting/drawing										

Fredrick's Volition

During the OPHI-II interview, Fredrick initially expressed skepticism about the merits of occupational therapy. The therapist offered to show him the areas where therapy took place and the things that were available there for him to do. He agreed to take a look. When he saw the therapy crafts room, he indicated that he had always had an interest in arts and crafts, but never an opportunity to follow up on this interest. With encouragement from the therapist, he decided to work on some clay projects during an open activity group.

His attraction to doing creative activities was also reflected in his responses to the Interest Checklist (*Fig. 24-2*). Similarly, during the OPHI-II interview he had mentioned creative interests, but again noted that he had never followed up on them. The Interest Checklist also indicated that Fredrick was inclined toward sports, arts, and culture.

During the OPHI-II interview, Fredrick indicated that his personal values included having freedom to make his own choices and making good use of his leisure time. Nevertheless, he noted that he lacked confidence in his own decision-making ability and had not used his leisure time well for a long time. It was also clear that he wanted to have a work career but felt very defeated in reaching this goal after all his failures.

Fredrick showed very poor personal causation. He doubted his capacity and felt he had been very ineffective in the past. Fredrick felt no control over the events in his life. He was quite hopeless about the possibility of success in the future. His long history of difficulties and failures left him with little motivational energy to try anything new or to work toward goals.

Fredrick's Habituation

Fredrick indicated on the Role Checklist (*Fig. 24-3*) that he moderately to strongly valued the roles he had occupied recently and that he planned to fulfill them in the future. These included his roles as a friend, as a sportsman in an athletic club, and occasionally as a caretaker (baby-sitter) for his sister's children. For many years, Fredrick had been living with a group of four friends in a rented house. He was very satisfied with this living arrangement and was accepted by the friends. This positive environmental impact is noted in his OPHI-II ratings shown in Figure 24-1. Fredrick's family member role involved some contact with his sister, who lived 20 km away. He saw his father infrequently. Otherwise, he reported no other friends or social contacts. He felt his friend role was limited and expressed a longing to be able to have more intense human contact and to build up an extended circle of friends. Fredrick wanted to re-enter the worker role in the future,

FIGURE 24-3 Fredrick's Responses to the Role Checklist.

Role	Role Identity			Value Designation		
	Past	Present	Future	Not at all Valuable	Somewhat Valuable	Very Valuable
Student						
Worker						
Volunteer						
Caregiver						
Home Maintainer						
Friend						
Family Member						
Religious Participant						
Hobbyist/Amateur						
Participant in Organizations						
Other						

and hoped to find a job that would fulfill him more than the others had.

Fredrick was dissatisfied with his former habits, which he described as lacking structure. The only scheduled activities he indicated were attending karate class 3 times a week and meeting friends once a week. However, for some time before his admission, he was not doing either of these things.

Fredrick's Performance Capacity, Performance, and Skill

Fredrick did not report any major limitations of capacity. He complained about mild back pain, but it did not interfere with his performance. He also noted that attending the karate class had had a relaxing and pain relieving effect on it. He wanted to reinitiate his involvement in karate.

Fredrick chose to begin doing ceramics in occupational therapy. His therapist observed his performance informally to note whether he had any identifiable performance problems. Initially, Fredrick worked slowly, but this appeared related mainly to his continued depression. Nonetheless, he worked on his clay projects independently. Despite his stated desire to be involved in creative activities, Fredrick approached the tasks rather mechanically and without any obvious creative expression. Moreover, when he encountered problems with a new activity, he was reluctant to ask for help or information from the therapist or others.

Goal Setting

The occupational therapist shared her understanding of Fredrick's situation with him and to a large extent he agreed. Fredrick clearly recognized that the therapist had made an earnest and successful effort to understand his perspective and to make sense of his circumstances. Consequently, he agreed that he would be willing to work with the therapist to accomplish some goals. The following long-term goals were identified by Fredrick and the therapist together and shared with the multidisciplinary team:

- Fredrick will develop new perspectives for restructuring his occupational identity
- Fredrick will undertake vocational retraining in a more creative and less physically demanding area

- Fredrick will experience a greater degree of satisfaction in everyday life
- Fredrick will increase the number of his friends and increase his involvement with others.

To work toward these long-term goals, the therapist and Frederick developed short-term goals and a plan of therapy. These were refined as the course of therapy unfolded.

Course of Treatment and Outcome

Fredrick remained in psychiatric rehabilitation for 10 weeks. Consistent with his history, he periodically expressed his ambivalence about psychiatric care through sarcastic remarks and through challenging hospital staff. Fredrick did participate in occupational therapy throughout this period. Initially, however, he was wary and his attitude toward therapy was inconsistent.

Four weeks after admission he attempted suicide again, by cutting a gash in his neck. Immediately after harming himself, he panicked and sought nursing assistance. Following this incident, Fredrick was transferred to a more structured rehabilitation unit. This event proved to be a turning point for Fredrick. He began to recognize that he needed to do something to change his life. With encouragement, he slowly began to open up to the possibility that with help he might be able to improve his life. Since the occupational therapy department provided services to clients in several units, Fredrick was able to continue with the same therapist and the same therapy plan. Over the next 6 weeks, Fredrick became increasingly invested in occupational therapy.

Fredrick attended craft groups regularly, working with clay. He became more able to accept coaching and feedback from the therapist to improve his performance. On his own, he chose to start reading books about working with clay. With time, his technique improved and he became more relaxed and creative when he worked with the clay. He also learned to seek advice and suggestions and to ask for help when he encountered a new problem. As a result, he was able to produce pottery objects that he found pleasing. His sense of efficacy in doing something of value increased over time. He began to feel a sense of pleasure and satisfaction in doing something that he had experienced before.

During this time, Fredrick expressed concern to the therapist about his difficulties interacting with others. Based on his concerns and her own observation of his tendency to isolate himself, the therapist informally interviewed him about this aspect of his performance. Fredrick admitted that he was greatly distressed and felt very uncomfortable around people, with the exception of the long-term friends with whom he lived. He was also able to recognize that this discomfort was an obstacle to his goal of establishing new friends and intensifying his social contacts.

Fredrick identified that he felt very insecure about his skills for interacting with others. At this point, the therapist advised Fredrick that the Assessment of Communication and Interaction Skills (ACIS) could help identify his social strengths and weaknesses. Fredrick acknowledged that while he lacked confidence in his social skills, he had no idea what his strengths and weaknesses were. He agreed that such information would be useful.

They decided on the following approach. As noted above, Fredrick had developed some good skills for working with clay. The therapist suggested that it would be a good learning experience for him to lead a small ceramics group. Fredrick was reluctant at first but then agreed to do it. The therapist and Fredrick decided to videotape the group so that they could review his performance afterward. Fredrick was able to lead the group, giving initial instructions and supporting the other clients when they needed it.

Afterward, Fredrick and the therapist together used the ACIS to rate his communication/interaction skills while watching the videotape. Because of Fredrick's history of distrust of therapy, the therapist administered the ACIS in this way to give Fredrick a greater sense of control and responsibility for recognizing his own strengths and weaknesses. She invited Fredrick to rate himself and then offered to compare his views with hers. To allow Fredrick to do the rating, the therapist explained the meaning of each item.

Figure 24-4 shows both the therapist's and Fredrick's ratings, illustrating that they were in close agreement. Using the ACIS in this way allowed Fredrick to concretely see his own limits in sustaining communication and in providing verbal support and information to others. He recognized some of his challenges to being able to engage and respond to other persons' needs. On the other hand, the occupational therapist gave him feedback concerning strengths that he showed in this situation. Fredrick considered this exercise a success since it reassured him of social abilities he did possess and gave him some concrete feedback on areas to improve. He was proud to have done it despite his initial reservations. Moreover, he found it a very positive experience to see himself on videotape successfully leading the group.

The assessment exercise increased his confidence in his social skills. He came to recognize that even with some weaknesses, he could get along with people. At the same time, he became aware of the fact that he needed some time to retreat and that, when he allowed this for himself, he was more motivated and able to interact with others. He identified a necessary rhythm between doing solitary things and being socially involved.

Fredrick collaborated with the occupational therapist to examine his habit patterns and to plan for a more productive and satisfying use of his time. At first, Fredrick was unable to plan for himself, so he agreed to allow the occupational therapist to structure a weekly plan with him that reflected things that had been positive for him in the past. Then, they worked together to see how this schedule could be modified to reflect his growing interests, role involvement, and occasional need for some private space. By the time the team was planning discharge with Fredrick, he had completely taken over responsibility for sustaining his daily structure. He was highly motivated to keep planning and sustaining his daily routine.

Over the course of therapy, Fredrick showed increased efficacy, enjoyment, and satisfaction with his performance. He was able to plan and expect success in projects. As he became more regularly involved in performance and experienced success, he

FIGURE 24-4 Therapist Ratings and Fredrick's Self-Ratings on the Assessment of Communication/Interaction Skills.

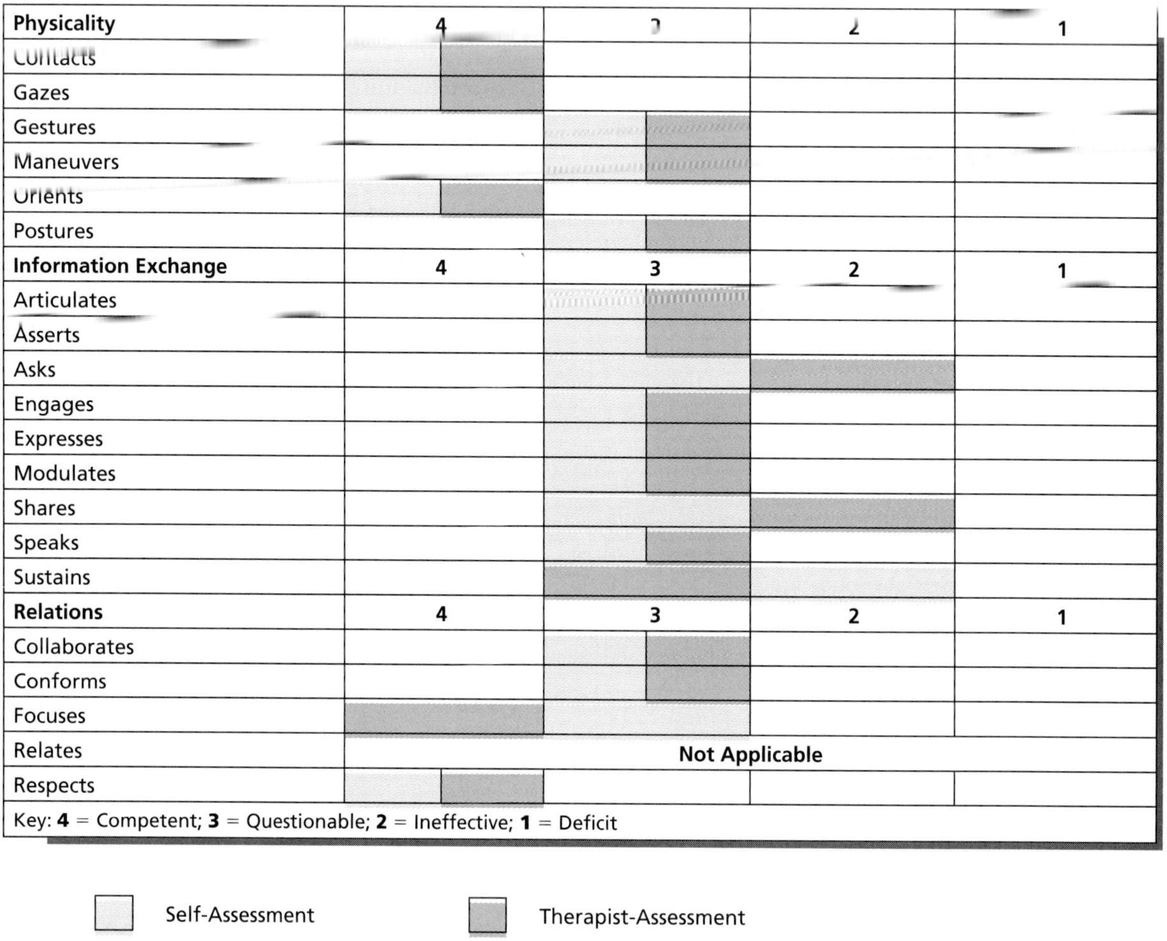

Physicality	4	3	2	1
Contacts	▇			
Gazes	▇			
Gestures		▇		
Maneuvers		▇		
Orients	▇			
Postures		▇		
Information Exchange	**4**	**3**	**2**	**1**
Articulates		▇		
Asserts			▇	
Asks			▇	
Engages			▇	
Expresses			▇	
Modulates			▇	
Shares			▇	
Speaks			▇	
Sustains		▇		
Relations	**4**	**3**	**2**	**1**
Collaborates		▇		
Conforms		▇		
Focuses	▇			
Relates	Not Applicable			
Respects	▇			

Key: **4** = Competent; **3** = Questionable; **2** = Ineffective; **1** = Deficit

☐ Self-Assessment   ▣ Therapist-Assessment

was able to identify an increasing range of interests and to explore new things. By the time of his discharge, he showed markedly improved personal causation. As Fredrick put it, he realized that he "had adequate skills, but just didn't use them."

Fredrick also came to realize how much his preoccupation with anxiety about performance and his conviction that life had no meaning had interfered both with his performance and enjoyment of the things he did. He focused on approaching performance with a positive attitude and on relaxing and enjoying what he did. In collaboration with Fredrick, the therapist used his responses on the Interest Checklist as a guide for him to try out new things. Fredrick realized that many of the things that he thought he might like to do he had never or only partly experienced. Consequently, he explored a variety of interests during his hospitalization and was able to identify the things that were most enjoyable to him.

As his confidence increased and as he identified things that he enjoyed, he was able to identify three major goals for himself to pursue after discharge. These were to improve his karate skills, to learn to play a musical instrument, and to learn a second language. Before discharge, Fredrick, in collaboration with the social worker and the occupational therapist, took the initiative to contact the local labor department for an appointment. There, he began to plan for future vocational training in an area that would allow him more creativity. He identified getting this training as another major goal to pursue after discharge.

Fredrick in Perspective

Fredrick began therapy with a very poor occupational identity. It included feelings of inability, lack of interest and enjoyment in life, difficulty identifying goals combined with limited role involvement, negative experiences in the worker role, and an unsatisfying daily routine. All these elements of occupational identity were woven into a narrative in which the dominant theme was a series of failed attempts with no prospect for a positive future. This narrative also included a viewpoint that therapy would not help him.

The therapist was able to successfully earn Fredrick's trust and engage him by giving him a voice and a degree of control. She initially did this by engaging him in assessments that allowed him to tell his story and write down his own view of things. Moreover, her interest in learning how he saw things and her efforts to understand his situation helped to win Fredrick's trust.

One notable strategy was the therapist's use of the ACIS. Engaging the client in completing the ratings with her was not only a good way to enable him to have a voice, but also an effective means to involve him in developing a more realistic understanding of his strengths and weaknesses. In fact, it was not his lack of skills that primarily isolated him, but rather his sense of incapacity and inefficacy in interacting with others. Once he was able to change his thoughts and feelings about his social effectiveness, the problem of social isolation was largely ameliorated. In addition, he had an awareness of areas of weakness that he would attempt to improve.

Clients should never be written off as uncooperative and noncompliant. They are always acting from their own narratives and with the rationale those narratives provide. Successful therapy means giving those narratives voice and working within them. This, of course, is almost always a difficult task that requires tact and patience on the part of the therapist. The potential payoff of such efforts is made apparent by this case. Once the therapist earned Fredrick's trust and respect, he was able to begin to recognize and to address each of his problems and challenges. He was able to begin to develop a positive occupational narrative for himself in which there was hope for the future. That is, he came to envision himself as enjoying life, finding satisfying work, and developing more friendships and social involvement. Finally he identified personal projects for himself (learning a language, being involved in karate, and learning to play a musical instrument). Constructing an occupational identity that envisioned a positive future was a major accomplishment for Fredrick. Although much of the challenge of enacting this identity (i.e., occupational competence) remained to be realized after discharge, he had a story to realize—something that was formerly absent.

Rebuilding Life Following Spinal Cord Injury

Persons with spinal cord injury face sudden and life-shattering changes in their performance capacity. The biomechanical model (Kielhofner, 1997; Trombly, 1995) provides concepts for understanding and addressing the movement problems due to spinal cord injury. A number of physiologic challenges, such as losing bowel and bladder control and being prone to infection and pressure sores, require special dietary and hygienic practices. These and other changes require the person with spinal cord injury to alter most aspects of everyday performance.

Persons with spinal cord injury also face major challenges in continuing their occupational identity and competence. To achieve a satisfying pattern of occupational participation, persons with traumatic spinal cord injury will often need to completely reorganize volition, habituation, and performance capacity. For example, they have to develop a new sense of capacity and efficacy. They may need to alter values and interests. They may lose or have dramatically altered a number of life roles. They must completely reorganize their habit patterns. They must relearn motor skills and learn to substitute process, communication, and interaction skills for lost motor skills. Moreover, their social and physical environments often must undergo tremendous changes. MOHO can be helpful in addressing these and other related aspects of the necessary adjustment to spinal cord injury. The following case illustrates how MOHO can be used to guide this aspect of therapy.

Alex

Alex was 30 years old when he sustained a complete C7 spinal cord lesion as a result of diving into an unexpectedly shallow creek near his home in rural Missouri. After 4 weeks of acute care, he was transferred to a rehabilitation unit in a halo vest. At the time, his condition was complicated by sacral pressure sores, a urinary tract infection, and orthostatic hypotension. This discussion of his occupational therapy begins in the rehabilitation unit.

Initial Information Gathering and Therapeutic Reasoning

Alex was still experiencing high fevers and unstable blood pressure, so the occupational therapist began the process of gathering information at bedside. Since Alex identified his major life role as a worker supporting a family, the therapist chose to conduct the Worker Role Interview (WRI) to assess Alex's work history. The interview was administered very informally over two sessions since Alex's endurance and attention were limited due to continuing medical problems. Alex tended to give brief, unelaborated responses. Nonetheless, the therapist was able to put together a reasonable picture of his unfolding history as a worker and complete the WRI ratings as illustrated in *Figure 24-5*.

The therapist next asked Alex to complete the Role Checklist (*Fig. 24-6*). Since Alex lacked the motor skills to complete the form and since the therapist wanted to use it as a basis from which to learn more about Alex, she administered it as a semi-structured interview. Since Alex was not very verbal, the detailed structure and partial redundancy of the WRI and the Role Checklist helped elicit a more comprehensive understanding of Alex. What the therapist learned is summarized below.

Alex's Work History and Plans

Alex dropped out of school after 10th grade to start earning money. He first went to work on a maintenance crew for the county and later was hired by a road construction firm. During this time, Alex became heavily involved in using drugs. The problem grew until he was unable to work and realized he needed help. He accepted hospitalization and was treated in an inpatient substance abuse unit. Alex's experience in drug rehabilitation introduced him to a new way of thinking about himself and relating to others. He began to identify with others' struggles to overcome substance abuse problems. Following his rehabilitation for substance abuse, he entered a federally funded, on-the-job training program, wherein he worked as a counselor. Alex tremendously enjoyed this kind of work.

Unfortunately, due to a cut in federal funding for the program, Alex's training was terminated. Realizing that his status as a high school dropout disadvantaged him and discouraged by the loss of opportunity for training, he reluctantly returned to a physical labor job. Alex worked as a plumber's apprentice for 6 months. However, disinterested in this line of work, he quickly became disillusioned with his coworkers and with the tediousness of the job, so he quit. Left with narrowing options, he next found employment as a stock clerk for a large supermarket. He was working at this job at the time of his injury.

Alex still had a very strong desire to pursue a counseling career, but he was uncertain of what would be possible for him. Although still denying the permanency of his paralysis, he realized that he faced some sort of impairment that might limit his work possibilities. He realized that his work history was sporadic and that he had had difficulty keeping a job. He also recognized that his limited education was a deterrent to a career. However, he was still able to envision some possibilities and was willing to investigate and pursue training options.

Alex's Other Occupational Roles

Alex's other major life commitments related to family and friends. Before his accident, Alex lived with his wife, their 3-year-old son, and two children from her previous marriage. At the time of the accident, they were expecting another child. Alex identified

FIGURE 24-5 Alex's Ratings on the Worker Role Interview (WRI).

Variable Definitions	Ratings				
	4	3	2	1	NA
Personal Causation					
Assesses abilities and limitations		▓			
Expectation of job success			▓		
Takes responsibility		▓			
Values					
Commitment to work	▓				
Work-related goals		▓			
Interests					
Enjoys work			▓		
Pursues interests	▓				
Roles					
Identifies with being a worker	▓				
Appraises work expectations		▓			
Influence of other roles		▓			
Habits					
Work habits			▓		
Daily routines			▓		
Adapts routine to minimize difficulties			▓		
Environment					
Perception of work setting					▓
Family and peers			▓		
Perception of boss					▓
Perception of coworkers					▓

Key: **4** = Strongly supports; **3** = Supports; **2** = Interferes; **1** = Strongly Interferes; **NA** = Not applicable

FIGURE 24-6 Alex's Responses on the Role Checklist.

Role	Role Identity			Value Designation		
	Past	Present	Future	Not at all Valuable	Somewhat Valuable	Very Valuable
Student						
Worker						
Volunteer						
Caregiver						
Home Maintainer						
Friend						
Family Member						
Religious Participant						
Hobbyist/Amateur						
Participant in Organizations						
Other						

being a family member and a friend as his only surviving roles. Moreover, these roles had been altered radically. He was very concerned that his family role had changed from being a provider and caregiver to his child and wife to being cared for and dependent on others.

Being a caregiver and being a family member were very valuable roles to Alex and were closely related to his working role. In Alex's Midwestern, working class view of the world, he should work hard and support his family. His perspective on life also stressed physical strength and prowess. His strong leisure interests had been in sports and other physically demanding occupations. Being paralyzed was not something he could fully comprehend or imagine as part of his life. Indeed, Alex persisted in announcing that he would walk out of the hospital. Alex had only just begun to realize what it meant to be in his vastly altered body and had yet to find out what gains in capacity would result from therapy.

One of Alex's immediate concerns was how his son would react to him in a wheelchair. He was very attached to his son, and feared he would be frightened or reject him. Moreover, he was also worried about his own ability to care for both his son and the new baby. In many ways, the future of his being a father was very vague and uncertain for Alex.

Alex's Motor Skills

Alex's motor skills were extremely limited. He did not have a measurable grip in either hand and he had difficulty doing fine motor tasks (e.g., he could not dial a phone or manipulate money). His endurance for activity was low; he could only do an upper extremity activity for 5 minutes before needing a rest or experiencing dizziness. With built-up handles and someone's assistance in setting up necessary objects, Alex could wash his face and arms, brush his teeth, and feed himself (although he did not have the endurance for an entire meal). He could not dress himself or bathe his lower body. He had no bowel and bladder control. He needed assistance to transfer with a sliding board and to roll from side-to-side. Alex's sitting balance in his wheelchair was precarious, and with great effort, he could slowly propel his wheelchair about 150 feet on a flat surface before becoming fatigued.

Alex's Overall Occupational Situation

The therapist formulated the following understanding of Alex's situation. Alex's spinal cord injury occurred on the heels of a sporadic work history complicated by previous substance abuse problems. Despite this, Alex had begun to develop a positive occupational identity and make efforts toward achieving competence by fulfilling his work and family roles. The injury and radical loss of capacity that followed it had impacted Alex's competence and threatened his occupational identity. He was not yet fully aware of the extent or permanency of his motor skill limitations. As these became more apparent, his feelings of inefficacy could be exacerbated.

Intervention

Given her understanding of Alex, the therapist reasoned that engaging Alex in occupational forms that gave him some control and that allowed him to recapture aspects of his previous occupational participation was a necessary first step. Also, the therapist expected that such engagement would give Alex experiences that would help him develop a realistic awareness of his capacities.

The therapist began by advising Alex about his medical status and necessary self-care. She coached him on how to direct others to undertake his care (since he was still in a halo vest, he needed complete assistance for most self-care). By receiving this information and being given the responsibility to direct others in his care, Alex began to experience a limited feeling of efficacy.

Nonetheless, Alex complained that he felt that his whole day was controlled by others or by his medical conditions (e.g., if his skin was too red, if his blood pressure dropped, if he spiked a fever, or if he had a bowel accident, the whole routine changed). He depended on others for his self-care, transfers, and being wheeled to therapies. Therefore, what he did and when he did it depended on them. Even his visitors came when they wished. Consequently, the therapist validated Alex's feelings and coached him in planning a schedule for daily routine care and leisure time. Alex was put in charge of his schedule and given responsibility for adhering to it.

Later, Alex shifted from directing others to care for him to performing his own care as he acquired the necessary skills. These steps put Alex back in control of parts of his life. Additionally, it provided Alex with a new routine for which he was responsible. The latter assisted him in developing the habits to accommodate his changed capacities.

Since Alex had a number of concerns about his role as a parent, and had lost the capacity to pursue most of his previous interests, his occupational therapist carefully selected occupational forms which appealed both to his role as a father and to his male-oriented interests. For example, with therapist guidance, Alex chose to make a wooden toy truck for his new son. This occupation also provided him opportunity to address biomechanical goals of increasing upper extremity strength and endurance. He used the bilateral sander with weights, a paintbrush, hammer and nails, glue, and a wax dabber while constructing this truck.

He planned and practiced how to stabilize and position himself and the wood, how to use the tools, how to sequence the construction steps, and how to maneuver his wheelchair to gather needed items. Consequently, the occupational form of woodworking gave him opportunities to redevelop some motor skills and substitute process skills for motor skills when necessary.

In other occupational therapy sessions, Alex learned how to use such adapted equipment as a reacher, a long-handled sponge, a long and short transfer board, a button hook, a zipper pull, an adaptive can holder/dispenser, and wheelchair gloves to perform necessary mobility and self-care. By learning how to incorporate these new objects into old and new occupational forms, he became more skillful in his performance.

The therapist also continued to discuss with Alex where he saw his life headed and what was important to him. Together they translated Alex's ideas into long-term goals, which were reviewed periodically. They also worked together to develop short-term goals for each week.

Ongoing Information Gathering

Observation of and discussion with Alex about his progress in occupational therapy were constant sources of information for his therapist. As he could feel more control over his life situation, Alex worked hard in therapy and made good progress in his self-care, transfers, mobility, and fine motor manipulation. He was gaining a sense of efficacy in his ability to manage his routine and perform self-care tasks. His interest in these and leisure activities showed a generally optimistic view toward his future.

The therapist did a home visit with Alex in anticipation of his discharge. The therapist observed that Alex and his wife had difficulty controlling their son when he misbehaved. Their frustration level was clearly high. It was also apparent that Alex and his wife had difficulty working together. On the other hand, Alex's son interacted with him quite naturally. He talked with Alex while sitting on his lap. He got items that Alex requested, and he kissed his father affectionately. Alex also held his second son (who was born during Alex's rehabilitation) and spontaneously played peek-a-boo with him. Alex's warm and spontaneous connection with his children contrasted with the strained interaction with his wife.

After discharge, Alex planned to share his two-bedroom apartment with his wife, her brother, her two children from a previous relationship, their 3-year-old son, and their 2-month-old second child. The entrance to the apartment was wheelchair accessible, but the bedrooms and bath were up 14 steps. Consequently, Alex planned to live in the living room, sleep on the couch, have a bedside commode, and wash in the kitchen sink. Unfortunately, there was no way to divide the small crowded living room to give Alex some privacy. Alex did not have the financial resources for a better arrangement.

Preparation for the Return Home

The occupational therapist discussed information from the home evaluation with Alex. Together, they decided to focus during the remainder of therapy on Alex's re-entering his roles as a father and homemaker. The following are examples of the kinds of sessions that occurred in therapy. Alex first practiced how to diaper a baby, how to discipline a child, and how to react to emergency situations. Alex's two children were then brought into therapy where he was responsible for their care. These sessions occurred in a private environment and began with Alex using a doll for diapering and dressing.

During the first three sessions with his own children, the therapist stayed with Alex, made suggestions, modeled appropriate disciplinary action, and provided immediate feedback to Alex. Later, Alex cared for the children himself, first in the hospital setting and then when he went home for the weekend. Alex also practiced homemaking tasks such as cooking, cleaning, and laundry. He went out in the community for grocery shopping, went to the store, and used a local public transportation system for disabled persons.

Alex's functional abilities for being able to return home were progressing well. However, Alex's relationship with his wife was deteriorating. He confided that before his injury, they had had difficulty getting along and, in particular, coping with their extremely active 3-year-old son. Through the course of his hospitalization, their relationship had grown increasingly stormy, with frequent disagreements and periods of not talking to each other. As Alex's discharge date came closer, they appeared to move increasingly apart, and began to speak of the other as a former or lost spouse. Both were beginning to express a sense of defeat about being able to preserve their relationship.

As Alex's return to his wife and children began to look less promising, it became necessary to explore alternatives. Finding an alternative scenario for Alex's discharge was helped by the fact that Alex's family was very supportive. His parents, younger brother, and a married sister participated in occupational therapy to be trained in Alex's care. His parents offered their house as an alternative living situation for Alex in the event that things did not work out with his wife. As it turned out, Alex did move to his parents' home.

At the time of his discharge, Alex's performance in such areas as wheelchair mobility, transfers, handwriting, and manipulating money and letters improved to the point that he had reached the maximal independence expected for a person with his level of spinal lesion. Alex lived in the hospital apartment for 1 week before discharge home. This environment more nearly simulated his expected conditions after discharge and allowed Alex to gain a more realistic picture of his capacities and needs. He was able to do almost all self-care independently. He dressed, cooked, cleaned, made his bed, did laundry, took his medicines, and kept his own schedule independently.

The occupational therapist observed as the week went on that Alex increasingly resorted to talking others into assisting him in these activities. When the therapist gave this feedback to Alex he expressed concern over whether his energy level was sufficient to be independent in all activities and he noted that he found it comforting to get some assistance. Consequently, the therapist and Alex agreed that some reliance on others was ideal for him. Alex and his parents and siblings came to therapy together in a subsequent session, and they identified activities in which assistance could be given if both parties were agreeable at the time.

Throughout therapy, Alex grew firmer in his desire to enter the counseling field. As it became clear that Alex did not see himself returning for a lengthy education, alternatives were explored. Alex agreed that some form of shorter-term vocational training to prepare him for work with disabled persons would be acceptable, so this option was pursued. Following discharge, Alex went to another facility for vocational training. Three months later, he began work for Goodwill Industries as a cashier and assisting in the supervision of workers.

A few months after discharge, he was happily working at Goodwill Industries. He pursued interests as a sports spectator, did some woodworking, and swam regularly at a local YMCA. He was on the waiting list for an apartment designed for disabled persons and hoped to move to these more accessible quarters within a few months. Alex studied for and successfully passed the test for a learner's permit for driving. He completed his behind-the-wheel training at the vocational center and was successful in learning to drive with hand controls. This represented one more step in Alex's plan to eventually live on his own.

Although his marriage ended in divorce, he received joint custody of his children. He both visited his children at his ex-wife's apartment and had them over to his parents' home where he baby-sat them regularly. He looked forward to a time when he could have them to his apartment for more extended visits. He met new friends and renewed friendships, which was extremely important to him.

Although Alex continued to maintain hope for more improvement and occasionally spoke of being able to walk again, he began to develop and pursue a realistic occupational narrative for himself. Overall, Alex felt confident in his capabilities and saw himself as pursuing the life he desired.

Alex in Perspective

Alex exemplifies two important issues in physical rehabilitation. First, while the onset of a physical disability requires and draws attention to the plethora of challenges and necessary changes in physical capacity and motor aspects of performance, these must be situated in the client's larger occupational life. Success in learning and carrying on new areas of occupational performance depends on their integration into an occupational narrative that the client must construct. Recrafting this occupational narrative is ordinarily more complex and challenging than the reorganization of everyday performance.

Second, the challenges that people face are frequently complicated by factors that proceed and follow the acquisition of the disability. Alex's history of substance abuse and his divorce are not factors separate from his rehabilitation needs. Rather, they are part of a total package of life events to which he had to adjust. His therapy was successful because it took into consideration the full range of human events and struggles that made up his life.

Re-entering Life Following Brain Injury

Jessy was 22 years old when she sustained a closed head injury in an automobile accident. She was initially referred to occupational therapy 7 days after the accident while still in the intensive care unit (ICU). As sequelae to left intracerebral hemorrhage, Jessy experienced right hemiparalysis, aphasia, and multiple contractures. She remained comatose for 4 weeks and

semicomatose and confused for 7 weeks while in acute care. Because of the nature of problems Jessy experienced from the head injury, the therapist used the biomechanical, motor control, and cognitive-perceptual models (Katz, 1992; Kielhofner, 1997; Mathiowetz & Haugen, 1994; Trombly, 1995) to guide much of therapy as it pertained to Jessy's performance capacity throughout her rehabilitation. The therapist used MOHO as an overall framework to guide efforts to help Jessy reclaim elements of her former occupational life and to fashion a new occupational identity and competence. The discussion below illustrates how her therapist incorporated MOHO concepts and tools throughout Jessy's therapy.

Jessy

Initial Information Gathering and Intervention During Acute Care

The therapist began by interviewing Jessy's family members and some visiting friends to get information on Jessy's interests and valued activities, roles, and routines. They described Jessy as an attractive, intelligent, and active young woman who enjoyed rock music and cared about animals and nature.

Since Jessy was still minimally responsive, her therapist's first goal for her volition and habituation was to provide an enriched environment that would begin to orient her to the external rhythm and structure of everyday life. Her therapist developed a program of environmental stimulation using rock music as well as objects and pictures of animals and nature. The therapist taught the nursing staff and family members how to most effectively position Jessy and how to provide her this environmental stimulation.

Initially, Jessy was dependent on others for all aspects of her care including feeding, bathing, toileting, dressing, bed mobility, and transfers. She made no attempt to speak; her only expression was that she often cried. She was unable to sit up for more than 5 minutes without going into a pattern of total extension and sliding out of the chair. Jessy had to be restrained as she often thrashed her body around and would fall out of bed. Initially, Jessy did not respond to any sensory stimuli except pain.

As she became semicomatose, Jesse remained in decorticate posturing with marked spasticity and contractures of all extremities. Hence, she was still severely limited in performing any voluntary, controlled movement. However, she did begin to show favorable responses to visual, auditory, and tactile stimulation. She was still very confused and could not follow one-step instructions. When possible during therapy, her restraints were removed or she was seated in a chair.

The therapist initiated a swallowing and feeding program, coaching Jessy on how to eat with adaptive equipment. The therapist also began to engage Jessy in completing simple self-care, which was soothing to her since it evoked familiar habits. As she progressed, Jessy was able to express herself with the aid of a picture communication chart. Toward the end of her stay in acute care, Jessy could attend to a task for 2 to 3 minutes, following one-step verbal directions approximately 50% of the time. She also began to use facial expressions and other physical gestures to communicate. Finally, Jessy could perform some basic self-care with assistance and supervision.

Information Gathering and Intervention During Rehabilitation

When Jessy was medically stable she was transferred to a rehabilitation center in the same facility. In the rehabilitation phase, Jessy's therapist first gathered data through informal observations that revealed the following. Jessy often dropped items, was unable to write with her left hand, and could not button even large buttons. Her dominant right hand was severely limited by a frozen shoulder that hurt with any movement. She could roll side-to-side in bed using the bed rails but could not sit up on her own. She required assistance to transfer. The left side of Jessy's face was paralyzed and she drooled constantly.

Because her skills were initially so limited, Jessy's therapist informally observed her motor, process, and communication/interaction skills as she worked with her each day. Her reacquisition of skills was uneven, and her performance thus required constant surveillance, structuring, and coaching. For example, as she was relearning to eat, her therapist observed that with a scoop dish and a built-up spoon, Jessy was able to feed herself, but she needed coaching and encouragement to stay focused on the task and to properly grip the spoon and her cup. Otherwise, Jessy would be easily distracted or might drop the spoon or cup. Jessy was still experiencing flexion contractures, spasticity, incoordination, and poor balance which severely constrained her motor skills in other self-care activities such as bathing and dressing. Her occupational therapist first focused on having Jessy cooperate with these occupational forms. As she observed any progress, she encouraged Jessy to begin doing small steps.

Jessy initially communicated by gesturing, shaking, or nodding her head or by pointing to objects, letters, words, or pictures. Her awareness of the environment increased daily. With time, Jessy could attend to simple activities for about 10 minutes. Beyond this, she easily became agitated and frustrated. Because of her limited tolerance for performance, the therapist saw Jessy for 10 to 15 minutes, 2 to 4 times a day. Jessy still sometimes became confused and had difficulty heeding the goal of even simple two-step tasks. Approximately half the time she did not get to the second step. An illustration of her process skill difficulties at the time is that Jessy could gather the items needed to brush her teeth but could not sequence the steps of this occupational form correctly.

At this point, Jessy's performance was also impaired because she was so often emotionally agitated. For example, she was constantly moving around and would often be crying with her hand on her forehead. Clearly, her sense of capacity and efficacy was severely shaken. Consequently, she had a low frustration tolerance and would give up on tasks that were difficult for her. Furthermore, she seldom initiated anything because of her feelings of limited capacity. For example, because communication posed such a challenge for her, she would not initiate interaction with others.

Even as Jessy progressed, the effects of her altered sense of personal causation were apparent. For example, although Jessy's communication skills improved and she was able to speak, her interactions with others were very helpless and child-like. She became embarrassed easily and often giggled nervously. When she had difficulty expressing her feelings, she resorted to crying, pouting, or yelling. It was clear that these behaviors were not consistent with what she deeply desired. For example, despite often acting helpless, it was clear she resented being "bossed around" (as she called it) when others sought to assist or direct her. This was a tumultuous time marked by irregular progress. For example, when she became very distressed, Jessy developed migraine headaches that kept her in bed for up to 2 days at a time.

Discovering the Original Jessy

Once Jessy had sufficient communication skills to tell her therapist about her life before the accident and could tolerate it emotionally and cognitively, the therapist interviewed her using the Occupational Performance History Interview-Second version (OPHI-II). This assessment helped identify both Jessy's previous occupational life and how her life had been altered since her injury. The therapist also asked Jessy to fill out the Role Checklist and they later discussed it. Together, these assessments provided the following picture of Jessy before her accident.

Jessy was a bright and high-achieving student who completed high school with honors. She was a senior at a prestigious New England university, majoring in chemistry at the time of her accident. During college, she had worked part-time for 3 years as a waitress in a restaurant. Jessy had previously worked as a baby-sitter, a sales clerk, and a housekeeper to earn money. She had enjoyed all of the above jobs, as she liked working with people. Jessy had planned to be a chemist, working in a university laboratory doing research. She saw her accident as delaying this goal but not obliterating it. Jessy's strong interests included crafts, nature, animals, cooking, and socializing.

Jessy was the oldest of three children. Before entering college, she often spent time baby-sitting her 9-year-old brother. She had lived with her brothers, mother, and stepfather until 2 years ago when she moved out of the house. Before her acci-

dent, she lived on campus in an apartment with her boyfriend, and they shared financial costs and household chores. Her choice to live with her boyfriend in defiance of her parents' desires evidenced Jessy's strong-willed nature. In addition to working in a fast-food restaurant, Jessy volunteered at the local humane society, worked on the school newspaper, and maintained a high grade point average. All in all, her occupational history revealed a talented, willful, and energetic young woman with a strong past occupational identity.

As shown in *Figure 24-7* Jessy still retained many elements of her past occupational identity, but it had been dramatically impacted by her trauma and its sequelae. She had all but lost her sense of efficacy, feeling very out of control. While hoping to reconstitute the life she previously lived, her ability to envision how realistic it was or how she would go about reestablishing her life was extremely limited. Her personal causation was particularly affected as she had no clear idea of what her future capacities would be and was very unsure of what success she would have in the future. Jessy's occupational competence, which had been strong, was severely compromised.

Figure 24-8 summarizes Jessy's responses on the Role Checklist. While the pattern of role change tells a story of its own, discussion of Jessy's responses gave her therapist useful insights into the transformation that had taken place following the accident. What follows is a summary of their discussion.

Whereas Jessy had previously been actively involved in a number of roles, the accident had removed her from all those roles and placed her in a dependent patient role. Moreover, Jessy felt that she no longer had control over any of her previous role responsibilities. For example, her parents had been appointed by the court as her legal guardians during her comatose and semicomatose periods, and consequently, they controlled her finances. They also controlled other details of her life such as who her visitors were and when they came, as well as what mail and phone calls she received.

Before the accident, Jessy was extremely active. Her typical day included getting up at 6:00 a.m., studying, going to classes or work, volunteering, or

FIGURE 24-7   Jessy's Ratings on the OPHI-II Scales.

Occupational Identity Scale	1	2	3	4
Has personal goals and projects			▓	
Identifies a desired occupational lifestyle			▓	
Expects success		▓		
Accepts responsibility		▓		
Appraises abilities and limitations	▓			
Has commitments and values				▓
Recognizes identity and obligations			▓	
Has interests			▓	
Felt effective (past)				▓
Found meaning and satisfaction in lifestyle (past)				▓
Made occupational choices (past)				▓
Occupational Competence Scale	1	2	3	4
Maintains satisfying lifestyle	▓			
Fulfills role expectations	▓			
Works toward goals	▓			
Meets personal performance standards	▓			
Organizes time for responsibilities	▓			
Participates in interests	▓			
Fulfilled roles (past)				▓
Maintained habits (past)				▓
Achieved satisfaction (past)				▓

Key : **4** = Exceptionally competent occupational functioning; **3** = Appropriate satisfactory occupational functioning; **2** = Some occupational dysfunction; **1** = Extremely occupationally dysfunctional

working on the school paper. She had no set times for meals or household chores, and she saw her boyfriend erratically as he also had a part-time job. Jessy's day was now dictated by the hospital routine. She was awakened at 6:00 a.m. She was then bathed, dressed, and given breakfast. For 8 hours, she attended therapies. She had only 30 minutes of free time during the day, but evenings were generally free except for 45 minutes of self-care activities before bedtime.

Jessy's view of her previous life is highlighted by the four things she valued most in the following order of importance: independence, being with her boyfriend, having pets, and living away from home. In many ways she was a typical young adult involved in the transition toward constructing her own inde-

pendent life and moving toward family roles of her own. In addition, her priorities also showed what a high premium she placed on her independence and self-reliance. In this context, the impact of her current situation became more apparent. Jessy had been robbed of what she most valued. The life of independence and self-reliance she had been living had come to a halt. She was forced to depend on others for almost all aspects of her life. Overall, she felt severely constrained and confined. Most of all she felt, as she put it, "like a prisoner" in her own body. Her occupational narrative was clearly one of entrapment.

Jessy fiercely wanted to be released from her confinement. With coaching and encouragement from her therapist, Jessy was able to translate this

FIGURE 24-8 Jessy's Responses on the Role Checklist.

Role	Role Identity			Value Designation		
	Past	Present	Future	Not at all Valuable	Somewhat Valuable	Very Valuable
Student						
Worker						
Volunteer						
Caregiver						
Home Maintainer						
Friend						
Family Member						
Religious Participant						
Hobbyist/Amateur						
Participant in Organizations						
Other						

desire into concrete goals. Jessy's long-term goal was to walk on her own in 6 months. Her immediate goals were to be able to wash and dress herself and to have a weekend pass to her apartment. Jessy recognized that her valued life of independence and self-reliance could only be reestablished after she could care for herself and walk on her own.

While Jessy recognized the importance of these goals, her immediate sense of efficacy was, nevertheless, still a problem for her. Jessy repeatedly complained of her lack of control over her life. She felt as if she had lost her past 2 years of independence from her family and had been returned to the situation of child-like dependence. She was plagued with anxieties that she would be permanently limited, dependent on others, and incapable of taking control of the direction of her life.

Regaining Control

As her attention span and concentration level increased, Jessy came to occupational therapy twice a day for 90-minute sessions. Therapy initially took place in a room where distractions were eliminated as much as possible to enhance Jessy's ability to attend. Also, because of her limited ability to heed the purpose of a task, brief activities were used and a

new task was introduced about every 20 minutes. This structuring of the environment also gave Jessy a greater feeling of control. Being able to successfully complete a task helped eliminate her frustration and agitation.

The occupational forms used to help Jessy increase her range of motion, coordination, and strength were based on Jessy's previous interests and her personal concerns. For example, early on Jessy engaged in rolling cookie dough and sanding a project to increase voluntary control, strength, and range of motion. These activities reflected her interest in crafts and cooking and therefore also had the effect of enhancing her enjoyment in therapy and giving her experiences which helped reinforce the idea that she was, by degrees, beginning to re-enter the kind of life she previously had. Later, as more voluntary movement returned, new activities that still reflected her interests but provided more appropriate motor challenges were used. For example, Jessy practiced motor and process skills in occupational forms such as cross-stitching, preparing meals, and doing leatherwork. Slowly, Jessy could manage a wider range of occupational forms including such things as cooking. She practiced tuning out distractions and attending to performance for longer periods.

The therapist and Jessy set and reviewed goals weekly according to Jessy's improvements and her personal desires. Throughout this process the therapist was careful to give Jessy opportunities to be in control and to have her desires validated. The following illustrates this. One day, 1 month into rehabilitation, the therapist asked Jessy what she wanted to cook. She indicated sugar cookies. When the therapist offered her a sugar cookie mix, Jessy became horrified. She had been a gourmet cook and would not think of using a mix! The therapist validated her desire to bake cookies from scratch. Although she struggled with process skills limitations that made following the recipe difficult, her volition counterbalanced these difficulties. When the cookies were finished Jessy was clearly bolstered by the fact she was able perform according to her own standards.

Jessy continued to become upset at times when she encountered her limitations and what felt to her like painfully slow progress. Her therapist worked to encourage her, to give feedback on her progress, to underscore the times that were enjoyable, and to celebrate the small triumphs that came when she mastered something that she could not previously do. These efforts helped to locate Jessy in a narrative in which she could see herself progressing toward a life she wanted. They also helped reduce her frustration about the distance she still needed to go. For example, when Jessy's ataxia decreased, she was once again able to write; however, it was initially inaccurate. To reduce her frustration over the discovery that her writing was impaired, it was important to give her feedback that reframed it as sign of progress, since she could not write at all previously. The therapist also helped her to envision her impaired writing as a phase on the way to being able to write competently. By helping Jessy interpret her experience this way, her therapist enabled Jessy to feel a greater sense of efficacy even while her capacities were still limited. Eventually, Jessy's right arm became sufficiently coordinated so she could write effectively.

Throughout this phase of therapy Jessy experienced simultaneous, although uneven, gains in a number of areas. Each week brought new surprises and new frustrations. With her therapist's assistance, she was able to place all these experiences in a larger story in which she was making her way back toward a way of life she enjoyed and valued.

As Jessy's process skills improved, her therapist modified occupational forms and environmental support to give her more challenge. Her therapist also provided necessary memory aids. As Jessy's motor skills increased, she was able to do such things as dress, bathe, style her hair, brush her teeth, and shave her legs. However, for quite some time she required stand-by assistance for all transfers as she often lost her balance when standing.

Jessy progressed from living with a roommate to modified independent living and finally to staying in the hospital's apartment before discharge. Jessy was given increasing responsibility for more of her own care and worked with her therapist to develop and follow a routine that allowed her to establish new workable habits. This routine included making her bed, doing her laundry, keeping her room organized and clean, making and keeping her own appointments, taking her own medicine on schedule, and cooking one meal a day. Mnemonic aids were still necessary to assist Jessy in carrying out this routine. In the last 3 weeks of her hospitalization, Jessy planned her own schedule, setting up her own therapies, bedtime, self-care, and leisure time.

Jessy persisted in wanting to return to her previous lifestyle. In particular, it was important to her to be in control and self-sufficient. Therefore, the occupational therapist collaborated with Jessy to develop an inventory of all her previous responsibilities. Together Jessy and her therapist put them in order of priority, considering both the importance and the feasibility of each. Following the creation of this priority list, Jessy began to work toward recapturing her previous responsibilities.

For example, Jessy had lost control of her own finances when her parents took over that responsibility. Consequently, regaining financial responsibility became a goal. Jessy and her therapist agreed to tackle this initially through simulating the kind of financial responsibilities she had when living on her own. To this end, her therapist and Jessy worked out a hypothetical budget and Jessy had to "pay weekly bills" to different people for the following things: rent, food, electricity, water and sewage, phone, therapies, entertainment, clothes, toiletries, transportation, and savings. Her therapist monitored and gave Jessy feedback on her ability to follow through on these financial management activities. At the time of discharge, Jessy was writing checks correctly and balancing her checkbook, although she continued to forget payments unless reminded or sent an overdue bill.

In similar fashion, Jessy and her therapist identified a host of objects and occupational forms, large and small, that she sought to master once again. For example, she practiced the use of such objects as a phone book, newspaper, a dictionary, an encyclopedia, and a vending machine. She engaged in occupational forms such as filling out a job application, doing functional mathematics, filing paperwork, reading maps, giving directions, writing letters, and reading bus schedules. She also practiced performing in occupational settings such as the library and supermarket.

By the time she was discharged, Jessy's performance in a range of occupations was greatly improved. However, Jessy still had difficulty attending and noticing. Moreover, she sometimes became flustered, which further impaired her performance. While Jessy desperately wanted total control of her life, she had to accept that her memory loss and process skill deficits meant that she needed some supervision. Moreover, she also required stand-by assistance when she walked because she was still unsteady and at risk to fall.

Jessy was still having difficulty communicating and interacting with others. Sometimes she was too passive to get her needs met or to receive necessary assistance. Other times she lost control and had outbursts with those around her. Jessy's therapist worked with her to identify and practice appropriate assertiveness and socially appropriate behavior. This was done in a variety of settings with Jessy's therapist giving her instruction and feedback. Jessy relearned how to initiate conversations in different situations and how to effectively participate in community outings to a variety of occupational behavior settings. Jessy was a naturally engaging person. Consequently, as she relearned expected behavior, she readily became friends with numerous patients and staff members. She often advocated for and encouraged other patients.

One of the biggest challenges for Jessy was to come to grips with what her discharge status would likely be. Her ongoing impairments limited how much independence and self-reliance was safe for her. To ease Jessy toward acknowledging and accepting this reality, she went on numerous weekend trips home before discharge. Jessy's therapist gave her family a list of things Jessy could do independently so they would both allow and expect her to do them. This helped ensure that Jessy's most important social group at the time, her family, would support and expect the level and kind of occupational performance of which Jessy was capable. Additionally, the therapist worked with Jessy and her family to develop a schedule for her at home. This schedule allowed Jessy to do what was most important to her and provided structure for both Jessy and her family so that she could be supervised without too much interference.

Re-entering Occupational Life

Jessy returned to live at home with her parents and brothers. She was followed up as an outpatient in occupational therapy. As part of that follow-up, the therapist decided to readminister the Role Checklist to see whether Jessy was re-entering roles as she had intended. The checklist and subsequent discussion indicated that Jessy had not followed through on her plans to re-enter the student and volunteer roles (i.e., she had planned to enroll in a community college class and volunteer at the local humane society). Her therapist learned that Jessy was also having difficulty structuring her day.

On the positive side, Jessy had become reacquainted with some old friends and had gone to the movies and out to eat with them. She had pursued her leisure interest of cross-stitching and frequently played games with her younger brothers. Nonetheless, Jessy felt she could do more than her parents were allowing her to do. She felt that her occupational competence was being limited by her parents.

While Jessy clearly knew how she wanted her life to turn out, she was quite unsure of the immediate future. Therefore, therapy focused on helping Jessy develop a clearer idea of what she wanted her life at the time to be and on prioritizing short-term goals. Jessy would make a list of what she wanted to achieve by her next scheduled therapy, when she would report her accomplishments or problems to the therapist. She developed lists incorporating her values and interests and became increasingly realistic about her capabilities.

As time went on, Jessy decided she wanted some kind of vocational training that would allow her to obtain a job. She also wanted to pursue opportunities to live somewhere other than at home. With help from her therapist she found and began attending a vocational training center, where she could live in a dormitory. During this time, she continued to return for periodic follow-up in occupational therapy. At the vocational training center, she received 6 months of training in computer skills. She continued to practice her habits and skills and worked toward her goal of personal independence. She was able to take over her personal finances at this point, including managing the investment of funds she had received from an insurance settlement related to her accident. During this time, in occupational therapy, she learned to drive again.

Reinventing Her Occupational Narrative

A year and a half after her head injury, Jessy had partially reclaimed her previous life. Importantly, she was also able to recraft her occupational narrative in necessary ways. Jessy had largely come to grips with much of the reality of her continuing limitations. Considering these, she felt she had rebuilt some significant portions of her previous life. Still, there were losses. Her old boyfriend was unable to handle all the changes in Jessy, and their relationship had ended. Jessy realized that she would never become the chemist she had aspired to be before the accident.

Jessy became increasingly reconciled to the fact that she was not exactly the same person she had been. Her right hand was still impaired. She could walk on her own but needed a cane. She was able to do all her self-care and basic homemaking and had developed new habits that supported her daily living tasks and work. However, she continued to have some trouble with process skills. This required her to accept minimal supervision for daily tasks.

Jessy moved to a group of supervised living apartments where she had her own room and shared household chores with other residents. She took the bus to her part-time job as a computer operator. She continued to make friends easily and had a new boyfriend. She lobbied those in charge of the supervised living apartments to secure permission for residents to have pets; this was a big accomplishment for her.

Jessy felt that her schedule allowed a level of activity that she could handle and that she had a good mix of work and leisure time. She talked with her family on a bimonthly basis and had demonstrated to their satisfaction that she could be semi-independent. Although Jessy had to relinquish the image of herself as a chemist–researcher, she was inventive in sustaining involvement in chemistry as part of her life story. She volunteered as a technical aide in a junior high school chemistry club.

Jessy was content with the life she had managed to compose for the time being. Nonetheless, in her future story she would be living on her own. In that story she would get around in her own car with her cocker spaniel in the back seat!

Jessy in Perspective

Jessy's course of therapy involved a long and complex process of change. While much of the therapy involved restoration of her motor, process, and communication/interaction skills, it was equally important that her volition be supported throughout and that necessary changes in personal causation and values were also attended to in therapy. Finally, the redevelopment of her habits and roles was essential.

Like many persons who incur permanent and significant impairments, Jessy was not able to return to the life she had previously lived and desired. Therefore, successful therapy had to enable her to reconstruct her occupational identity and build a new occupational competence that was possible given her remaining abilities and lingering limitations. By doing this, therapy enabled Jessy to be living an occupational narrative that she could accept and find satisfying. Happily, several years later, Jessy was working 30 hours per week as a computer operator doing data entry and basic analysis for a researcher at a research center. She had held the job for 5 years, needed only minimal job coaching, and was considered an extremely reliable worker. She was trying to piece together her experience of trauma and recovery and planned to write about it for others so they would know what the experience is like. She had four pets!

From Running Away to Joining Life

Kim was 16 years old when she was referred for an inpatient psychiatric admission by her social worker because she was threatening suicide. Just before admission, Kim and some friends with whom she was living were picked up by the police in a stolen car. Kim was placed on 1 year's probation and ordered to live at home. Kim's admission came within a few days of being at home with her mother. She was diagnosed with major depression. Because Kim had a history of heavy drinking, she was given detoxification status.

Kim was admitted to a small diagnostic unit in a large New England hospital for adolescents and children. The basic philosophy of this unit is that each patient should receive a thorough workup by each team member.

Kim

A Brief Life History

The admitting psychiatrist and social worker interviewed Kim and shared the following history with the team. Until age 7, Kim grew up in an intact family consisting of her father, mother, and two older brothers. Her father was a severe alcoholic, and Kim witnessed several episodes of his constant physical abuse of her mother. When Kim was 7, her father was found in the street in the early morning hours with a severe head injury. Since then, he has been confined to a nursing home, partially paralyzed and cognitively impaired. Kim's only memories of her father were as a heavy-drinking and abusive man. At the time her father was injured, police investigated Kim's mother as a suspect. While no formal charges were brought and her mother had made no public

admission, Kim and her brothers speculate that their mother was somehow involved in their father's fate.

In the years that followed her father's abrupt departure from the household, Kim's two brothers moved out of the home. One brother moved to Chicago. The other left to live with his paternal grandmother.

During this time, Kim was showing all the outward signs of being deeply disturbed. Previously a competent student, Kim barely managed to complete the 9th grade and was truant for most of 10th grade. Kim also began to openly discuss with her mother and her friends the possibility of overdosing on aspirin. Kim's mother, who by this time was very depressed herself, was unable to deal with Kim's behavior in any way. The school counselor and a social worker became involved. Legal steps were taken to transfer guardianship to her aunt; however, this never occurred because Kim's condition deteriorated rapidly, and she was placed in a foster home. At the same time, Kim reported hearing voices and was seen at a community mental health center by a psychiatrist who prescribed medication for her. Shortly thereafter, when she no longer heard the voices, she discontinued the medication and stopped seeing the psychiatrist.

A few months later, after a breakup with her boyfriend, she overdosed on the medication she still had. At that time, she was admitted to an intensive care unit at a large public hospital in New York. Thereafter, she bounced from home to home of different relatives and friends. While living with her grandmother, Kim took a bottle of her grandmother's penicillin tablets in an apparent suicidal gesture. She was admitted to a psychiatric hospital then and subsequently was referred to a mental health center. There, she was scheduled to be seen as an outpatient. Before outpatient therapy could get underway, Kim was arrested for being in a stolen car, leading to her return home and subsequent hospitalization.

Initial Information Gathering

After hearing Kim's history in the team meeting, Kim's occupational therapist was concerned about the disruptiveness and chaos of Kim's life. It was clear that she faced a major challenge in restoring any order to it. The therapist's impression was that Kim's occupational narrative had taken on the theme of a frantic flight or escape, which is not unusual for someone growing up in an abusive environment. Finding a new occupational narrative would require identification of a new theme.

In deciding how to gather information from Kim, the therapist chose to give the occupational therapy information gathering and intervention a strong focus on doing to balance the strong verbal orientation of the unit. Therefore, the therapist chose a number of data gathering instruments that Kim could complete on her own and that could serve as the basis for collaboration to achieve an understanding of her situation. The therapist decided to ask Kim to complete the Role Checklist and the Interest Checklist to gather data on her roles, values, and interests along with an activity configuration (i.e., an informal report of how she typically spent her time during the day) to give information about Kim's habits. The therapist observed Kim doing things to informally screen her for problems in motor, process, and communication/interaction skills. Finally, Kim completed the Occupational Self Assessment (OSA), which provided information about how Kim saw herself and served as a basis for negotiating goals for therapy.

Kim appeared both frightened and distrustful. Consequently, the occupational therapist approached the information gathering process with the intention to set up a collaborative atmosphere that would provide Kim with a sense of control. The therapist informed Kim that she wanted to get to know her and that she would need Kim's help to gather some information. She then gave Kim the choice to start out by either filling out forms or undertaking a craft project (the latter being the basis for observing Kim's skills).

When she showed Kim the occupational therapy workshop, Kim saw other adolescent patients active, comfortable, and successful in the workshop and this relaxed her. When other patients informed Kim that if she got the forms finished she could go on to do fun things, she chose to complete the assessments first. When she had completed the assessments, the therapist met with Kim to review the data from each tool and to give her feedback. This process also gave the therapist an opportunity to cross-check and add necessary data.

On the Interest Checklist (*Fig. 24-9*) Kim was able to clearly indicate her preferences. Overall, her pattern of interests did not provide opportunities for skill development or a sense of competence. When discussing her responses, it also became clear that Kim did not follow through on all her interests, particularly interests such as needlework, cooking, and photography, which could provide opportunity for her to develop skills. It also became evident that Kim's interest involvement tended to center on drinking-related leisure pursuits such as music, dancing, singing, and drinking games (e.g., quarters).

Kim's responses on the Role Checklist (*Fig. 24-10*) show her alienation from ordinary adolescent roles. She had quit school, never wanted to be a caregiver, and did not see herself in or value the family member, religious participant, or hobbyist/amateur roles. When her occupational therapist discussed her responses on the Role Checklist and their apparent meaning, Kim acknowledged that she had a sense of failure about the student role and that she was aware of having withdrawn from other roles as well. Moreover, she related that she did not have much expectation for the future and, therefore, did not imagine herself in many roles. The data from this instrument reinforced that Kim's occupational narrative did not place her in an ordinary continuum of role development. For adolescents, in particular, the ordinary succession of roles provide benchmarks of one's progress and an image of an unfolding future.

Kim's reports of a typical weekday and weekend day (*Fig. 24-11*) indicated that she lacked a satisfying routine and instead organized her leisure time around the habit of drinking. Moreover, it confirmed that she was not pursuing any of her skill-based interests nor did it involve any personal responsibility. By her own admission, her schedule was that of a person "headed nowhere." None of her activities had a future orientation, instead reflecting her theme of flight and escape.

A screening observation of Kim's performance doing crafts revealed no problems with motor or process skills. In the area of communication and interaction skills, she had difficulty with the skills of

FIGURE 24-9 Kim's Responses on the Interest Checklist.

	Strong Interest	Casual Interest	No Interest		Strong Interest	Casual Interest	No Interest
Camping	■			Laundry			■
Television	■			Yoga			■
Writing		■		Antiques			■
Travelling	■			Academics	■		
Pets	■			Personal appearance	■		
Team sports			■	Roller skating			■
Clerical	■			Cycling		■	
Conversations	■			Boating	■		
Clothes	■			Backgammon			■
Movies	■			Politics			■
Shopping	■			Winter sports			■
Walking			■	Car repair			■
Organization	■			Swimming	■		
Languages	■			Jogging		■	
Dating	■			Ping-Pong			■
Business			■	Bridge			■
Religion			■	Painting	■		
Dining		■		Woodworking			■
Crafts			■	Tennis			■
Art	■			Cooking	■		
Solitaire			■	Bowling			■
Chess			■	Dancing	■		
Picnic		■		Ceramics			■
Golf			■	Reading		■	
Checkers			■	Singing	■		
Home repairs			■	Photography			■
Skiing		■		Fishing			■
Music listening	■			Sewing			■
Puzzles			■	Sculpting			■
Needlework		■		Gardening		■	
Acting			■	Model building			■
Collecting			■	Weight lifting			■
Cleaning			■	Playing instruments			■

respecting others and asserting herself. For example, she was sometimes abusive and aggressive toward her peers. She also had difficulty sharing her thoughts and expressing feelings.

As the therapist shared the information that came from Kim's self-reports and the therapist's ob-

servations and discussed it with her, Kim volunteered that self-control was hard for her. Kim was very troubled and ambivalent about the issue of personal control. She lacked a sense of power to act on those things within her control, such as pursuing her education and leisure interests. When her ther-

FIGURE 24-10   Kim's Responses on the Role Checklist.

Role	Role Identity			Value Designation		
	Past	**Present**	**Future**	**Not at all Valuable**	**Somewhat Valuable**	**Very Valuable**
Student		Quit	Not going back			
Worker	Quit	Looking	Full time			
Volunteer	Never done it	Never done it	Never done it			
Caregiver	Babysat	No	No			
Home Maintainer	Clean house	No	Yes			
Friend	Go out drinking *	Go out drinking *				
Family Member						
Religious Participant						
Hobbyist/Amateur						
Participant in Organizations						
Other						

* Kim originally wrote "go out drinking" and then crossed this out.

apist gave her feedback that she also repeatedly lost control through alcohol and substance abuse, Kim was reluctant to see it as losing control. Kim also had difficulty accepting those things that were not in her control such as her court placement with her mother.

Therapist's Conceptualization of Kim's Occupational Circumstances

The therapist put together the following conceptualization of Kim's occupational circumstances. Kim came from an obviously turbulent and abusive family context, leaving her distrustful of others and alienated from mainstream social values and roles. Kim also came from a family in which members were unable to control themselves. Her father could not control his drinking or his temper, and her mother could not exercise her parental responsibilities. Not surprisingly, Kim's personal causation was dominated by her belief that she could not control herself. Together Kim's values and personal causation suggested that she had no vision of where she should take her life and no real hope that she could effectively steer her life in a direction if she chose one.

FIGURE 24-11   Kim's Report of a Typical Weekday and Weekend Day.

Time period	Weekday	Weekend
8:00am–10:00am	Sleep	Sleep
10:00am–12:00pm	Sleep	Go to the beach at 11:00
12:00pm–2:00pm	Get up at 1:00	Beach
2:00pm–4:00pm	Take a shower at 2:30	Come home at 3:30
4:00pm–6:00pm	Call my boyfriend 5:00	Take shower
6:00pm–8:00pm	Play quarters* w/friends	Play quarters
8:00pm–10:00pm	Still playing quarters	Play quarters
10:00pm–12:00pm	11:00 go out to meet boyfriend	Play quarters 12:00 go out to meet boyfriend

* A drinking game in which an individual bounces a quarter off the table attempting to make it into a glass. When the individual does make it, he/she chooses someone to drink. If the individual does not make it, he/she must drink.

Kim's interests did not reflect opportunities for developing capacity and efficacy and, instead, were related to drugs and alcohol. This interest pattern (and even more so, her interest involvement) was consistent with a life in which capacity did not matter and in which escape and immediate gratification were guiding principles.

Overall, Kim's occupational narrative appeared dominated by a theme that life was out of control, that she was alienated from the values of her environment, and that she did not belong to the ordinary stream of life as represented in a sequence of roles. Instead, Kim was in a state of flight, trying to escape potentially harmful others and painful feelings. Her desperation to escape was reflected in floating from home to home, fleeing into substance abuse, and flirting with suicide. Kim had been making activity and occupational choices that had taken her away from ordinary roles and activities and toward increasingly self-destructive and socially problematic behaviors. She had substituted chemical dependency for life satisfaction. Her life had become a downward tumble that culminated in her involvement in an auto theft. As a consequence of her choices, Kim's habituation was marked by an interruption of adolescent life roles and a problematic use of time, centered on drug and alcohol use.

Despite these serious problems, Kim's skill level was generally good. One area of concern was that her communication and interaction skills were limited by her abrasive street behavior and by her difficulty in expressing emotion and thought. However, these problems appeared more related to Kim's exposure to street life than to an innate problem of communication and interaction. Finally, because of her poor choices, she had not had the opportunity to develop her ability to perform in leisure or academic contexts, which would be a basis for success in characteristic adolescent roles. The most important conclusion to be drawn from available data was that Kim was clearly the product of disorganized environments.

Negotiating for Therapy to Enter Kim's Life

The therapist and Kim together examined the OSA that Kim had completed (*Fig. 24-12*). Since the OSA required Kim to reflect on the same issues that her occupational therapist was considering, it enabled them to compare their respective views of her

strengths and weaknesses and to negotiate treatment priorities. They both agreed to focus on the following three goals that were derived from the OSA:

- Doing activities I like
- Effectively using my abilities (to feel more personal control)
- Making decisions based on what I think is important (before acting impulsively).

Based on this agreement and her conceptualization of Kim, the occupational therapist planned the following approach to intervention. First, she would try to enhance Kim's knowledge of capacity and sense of efficacy by giving her opportunities to try out various occupational forms in the occupational therapy workshop.

The therapist anticipated that Kim would need substantial feedback to guide how she interpreted her performance, since Kim's tendency was not to expect or recognize her own competence. The occupational therapist also planned to support Kim in being in control of herself and in achieving good outcomes. This would require that she help Kim to plan before she acted and to pause to consider what would be the consequences of her actions.

Finally, the therapist wanted to offer Kim opportunities to increase her role functioning as a student, hobbyist, and family member. Overall, she envisioned occupational therapy as helping Kim decide how to join rather than run away from life. Joining life would also require that Kim learn a new habit pattern that would reflect reinvolvement in her interests.

Realizing the impact of dysfunctional social environments on Kim, her occupational therapist planned for therapy to provide a different kind of environmental context to help shape the organization of her behavior in new directions. Caught up in the cascade of her flight, living for the moment, and heading nowhere in the future, Kim had found no real satisfaction or control in her life. The challenge to therapy was to find a way back into a life that could offer Kim some control, some value, and some enjoyment.

Kim's therapist wanted to structure an environment that would give opportunities and resources as well as expect behavior quite different from that to which Kim had become accustomed. Such an en-

FIGURE 24-12 Kim's Responses on the Occupational Self Assessment.

Myself	Competence: Lots of problems	Competence: Some difficulty	Competence: Well	Competence: Extremely well	Values: Not so Important	Values: Important	Values: More Important	Values: Most Important
Concentrating on my tasks	■					■		
Physically doing what I set out to do		■			■			
Taking care of the place where I live		■				■		
Taking care of myself	■						■	
Taking care of others for whom I am responsible	Not Applicable							
Getting where I need to go	■						■	
Managing my finances	■				■			
Managing my basic needs (food, medicine)	■					■		
Expressing myself to others			■		■			
Getting along with others		■			■			
Identifying and solving problems	■				■			
Relaxing and enjoying myself	■						■	
Getting done what I need to do	■					■		
Having a satisfying routine	■						■	
Handling my responsibilities	■					■		
Being involved as a student, worker, volunteer, and/or family member	■				■			
Doing activities I like	■							■
Working towards my goals	■						■	
Making important decisions based on what I think is important	■							■
Accomplishing what I set out to do	■							■
Effectively using my abilities	■							■

My Environment	Environmental Impact: Lots of problems	Environmental Impact: Some problems	Environmental Impact: Good	Environmental Impact: Extremely good	Value of Environment: Not so Important	Value of Environment: Important	Value of Environment: More Important	Value of Environment: Most Important
A place to live and take care of myself	■							■
A place where I can be productive (work, study, volunteer)	■							■
The basic things I need to live and take care of myself		■						■
The things I need to be productive	■							■
People who support me and encourage me	■					■		
People who do things with me		■						■
Opportunities to do things I value and like	■							■
Places where I can go and enjoy myself		■						■

vironment would be supportive yet expect appropriate behavior. It would also demand competent performance while giving Kim the opportunity to experience self-control. Additionally, the environment would have to provide models and experiences of a kind of life that could be in control, valuable, and enjoyable. Unless Kim could begin to experience an alternative way of participating in life and receive support and rewards for doing so, she could never successfully put forth all the necessary efforts that change would require.

Recognizing that detoxification from alcohol is a painful process, Kim's therapist also resolved to validate her struggle. Kim could be nasty, abusive, and street-wise. As she detoxified from alcohol, she became increasingly irritable. The occupational therapist was understanding, provided Kim choices and options, and sought to stay out of control struggles. Since Kim had been chronically robbed of control by her environments and since she was very unsure of her ability to have control, this was an especially sensitive area for her. Moreover, Kim needed to begin to feel that she could be in control. At the same time, the environment needed to convey messages about what was proper behavior, that is, what was valued. Thus, Kim's therapist set firm limits when appropriate (e.g., when Kim was abusive to her peers).

Using Social Groups and Occupational Forms in Kim's Therapy

The occupational therapist used groups as the primary method of Kim's therapy. Her introduction of appropriate occupational forms into the group was important. Since occupational forms carry cultural meanings and evoke personal reactions based on each individual's narrative (Helfrich & Kielhofner, 1994; Nelson, 1988), the kinds of occupational forms introduced were very consequential. For Kim, whose occupational forms (e.g., playing quarters) had come to represent escaping and being outside of the mainstream life, it was important to select forms that would draw her in, challenge her to become involved, and provide new pleasures to replace old habits of substance abuse. Knowledge of Kim's volition provided important clues as to how she might react to various occupational forms.

Since the peer group is the most important socializing influence on adolescents, it was natural and

most effective to use the group to engage adolescents together in various occupational forms and for a context of productivity, pleasure, and competence. Since most adolescents in the group struggled with their sense of control, satisfaction, and value in productive action, it was important to process feedback about what went on in the group. The therapist used a variety of means (as we will see) to encourage and coach adolescents to talk about their experiences, share feelings, support each other, and problem solve together. The therapist also used discussions at times when it seemed necessary to tie together doing, thinking, and feeling or to relate experiences in therapy to daily function outside.

Course of Kim's Therapy

The following are some highlights of Kim's experiences in occupational therapy. Kim's therapist introduced crafts to Kim since they are occupational forms that provide opportunities for skill building and success. Kim initially stated that she did not find crafts interesting. However, she quickly came to like their nonthreatening quality. She particularly liked being able to learn without getting graded. Kim also benefited from doing crafts in a small group with her peers. The activities evoked a sense of calm and togetherness. The group members often discussed difficult things while working on their projects. Initially, Kim could not share her feelings but could respond to her peers' feelings.

As Kim became reinvolved in activities and developed new interests that could contribute to a more adaptive habit structure, her occupational therapist decided to move Kim toward more effective management of her time in everyday life. She reviewed with Kim the importance of having a balance between time spent in school, leisure, self-care, and rest. The occupational therapist coached Kim to visually portray how she would like to spend her time by constructing a pie chart that represented the 24 hours of the day. This helped her better grasp the idea of time management and lifestyle balance. While Kim was able to plan for a more adaptive use of time, it was clear that she had no idea about how to actually go about implementing such a schedule.

Her therapist anticipated that it would be very difficult for Kim to change her lifestyle so radically and to not spend her time drinking. Consequently, she felt it would be important for Kim to begin to regularly practice this new schedule and take responsibility for how she used her time. To this end, the occupational therapist shared Kim's Interest Checklist with her nurse, who then supported Kim to make activity choices for what to do in her free time in the evenings and on weekends. Soon, Kim began to use her occupational therapy sessions to choose activities and to prepare supplies that she would utilize in her free time. She was eventually more comfortable being responsible for and involved in her own interests. New habits were becoming more natural and familiar to her.

In the craft group, the therapist noticed that Kim was consistently seeking out projects far below her own skill level. When the occupational therapist gave Kim this feedback, she protested that she did not perceive herself as being able to do more difficult projects. The therapist began to give Kim consistent feedback about her skill level and to negotiate with her to choose tasks slightly more difficult than the ones she ordinarily selected. At first Kim refused, so the therapist decided to focus on the process of having fun by trying something new. The occupational therapist reasoned that if Kim could be persuaded to try something new for the fun of it, she might discover that she could do and, in fact, enjoy tasks more closely related to her skill level.

The therapist utilized a group session to engage participants to do a craft that none of the group members had tried. Throughout the activity participants were asked to write down how they felt about doing something new, and then group members discussed what they wrote. Before starting the task, Kim wrote "this is dumb and it's too hard for me." Her peers gave her feedback that she would probably do well, based on what they had seen her do in the past. Halfway through the activity, Kim wrote "fun." Upon completion of the craft, Kim was feeling more comfortable and wrote down "fine." Over time, new activities became easier for her and Kim gradually progressed to higher-level projects that challenged her and gave her a greater sense of efficacy.

At this point, the occupational therapist felt that she had a good rapport with Kim. This was necessary to begin tackling the alienation reflected in Kim's values and roles. Since this would be a sensitive issue, the therapist felt that it would be best for Kim to have some privacy. Consequently, a one-to-one session was arranged with Kim. With some support, Kim admitted that she did see some value and importance to school. However, she reported feeling very insecure about being able to return successfully to it. It became clear that rejection of the student role allowed Kim to protect herself from the fear of failing in that role. Kim's therapist gave her feedback about her high level of skills and assured her that these would support her success in school. Kim then shared that her home life interfered with her ability to go to school.

At this point, Kim blurted out that she drank because she felt depressed and she did not have support at home to overcome the depression. It became apparent to both Kim and the occupational therapist that to stop drinking and go to school, she would need a lot of support, which she was not getting at home. After more discussion, Kim was able to say that she would like to be able to go to school if she felt she had some way to succeed. The therapist told Kim that she would like to share their talk with the team, so they could discuss how best to help her. Kim agreed.

The next day at morning rounds, the occupational therapist reported on her meeting with Kim. The therapist strongly recommended that Kim be referred to a residential alcohol treatment program for adolescents that could provide both support for her drinking problem and help her to be able to succeed at school. The treatment team decided to find this type of program to which she could be discharged.

As Kim continued to attend craft workshop sessions in occupational therapy, the group members, including Kim, were becoming increasingly supportive of and open with each other. The therapist decided to foster and capitalize on their cohesiveness by facilitating a discussion on each person's goals. The group members were each given their OSA forms and asked to choose two goals that they were working on and that they felt comfortable sharing with the group. Group members, after hearing each other's goals, identified how they could support each other in reaching them.

Kim was very disruptive throughout this session and in the week to follow. Her behavior suggested that it was still very hard for her to choose a direction for herself and feel hope that things would turn out as she wanted. She seemed to be struggling with imagining a positive identity and choosing goals for herself. These feelings were intensified by her knowledge that she was being referred to an adolescent alcohol treatment center.

Around the same time, many members of the unit were being discharged. Kim was having such difficulty separating from them that the occupational therapist planned a "goodbye book" activity in which each member was to write a page to each of the others, wishing them well and telling them something inspirational or something they wanted them to remember. Each member collected the pages they received into a book. After this activity, Kim was much calmer and seemed to adjust to the discharge of several peers.

A few days before Kim's discharge, the occupational therapist met with Kim to review her progress. Both agreed that Kim had experienced an improved sense of her ability to control herself, which enhanced her confidence that she could be effective. Kim had also increased her involvement and enjoyment in interests. She had become aware of how her new habits were affecting the quality of her life. Kim acknowledged that she had a new appreciation for the importance of the student role in her life.

Before Kim's discharge, the therapist made a number of recommendations to Kim. First, she suggested Kim continue to practice lifestyle balance and monitor her own routine using methods she learned in therapy. Second, she advised Kim to become involved in interests as a source of gratification and to refer to the Interest Checklist she completed for ideas. Third, she recommended that Kim seek out the support of the teacher in the alcohol treatment center to begin to successfully function in the student role.

Kim seemed proud of her achievements and thanked the occupational therapist. She expressed feeling scared to go, but ready. Kim was discharged to an alcohol treatment center for adolescents. She continued to call the hospital occasionally to report on her good grades and sobriety.

Kim in Perspective

Kim represents a challenging type of client who can readily fail to benefit from therapy because her own occupational narrative is so at variance with the ordinary vision of therapy. Kim's understandable distrust of adults, her theme of escape, and her alienation from mainstream values are all barriers to actively engaging in the therapy process. The occupational therapist had to first understand how Kim made sense of her life in order to allow therapy to enter into Kim's life and have an impact. In this regard, the case exemplifies one of the most important values of MOHO. It provides a way to comprehend a client's experiences and to think about how to work within those experiences to achieve change.

Conclusion

As noted at the outset of this chapter, the cases described herein represent complex challenges. Because of the difficulty and painful issues faced by each client, success in therapy was far from guaranteed. The successes that occurred in each case reflect the fact that the therapist took the time and used the necessary tools to fully understand clients and how best to approach them. Thus, the cases represent good examples of how to actively use MOHO to make sense of clients' circumstances and to devise a thoughtful approach to the therapy process.

References

Helfrich, C., & Kielhofner, G. (1994). Volitional narratives and the meaning of therapy. *American Journal of Occupational Therapy, 48,* 319–326.

Katz, N. (1992). *Cognitive rehabilitation: Models for intervention in occupational therapy.* Boston: Andover Medical Publishers.

Kielhofner, G. (1997). *Conceptual foundations of occupational therapy* (2nd ed.). Philadelphia: FA Davis.

Mathiowetz, V., & Haugen, J. B. (1994) Motor behavior research: Implications for therapeutic approaches to central nervous system dysfunction. *American Journal of Occupational Therapy, 48,* 733–745.

Nelson, D. (1988). Occupation: Form and performance. *American Journal of Occupational Therapy, 42,* 633–641.

Trombly, C. (1995). *Occupational therapy for physical dysfunction* (4th ed.). Philadelphia: FA Davis.

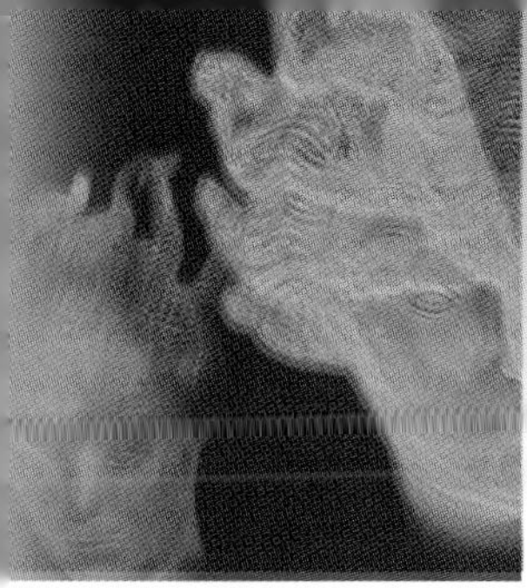

25 Use of MOHO to Complement Other Models of Practice

- Gary Kielhofner
- Gloria Furst
- Victoria Goldhammer
- Deborah K. Roitman
- Camille Skubik-Peplaski
- Cynthia Stabenow
- Noga Ziv

This chapter contains four cases that illustrate the use of MOHO to complement other practice models. In each case, the client's impairment indicated the need to employ the biomechanical, cognitive-perceptual, motor control, and/or sensory integration models (Abreu & Toglia, 1987; Ayres, 1979; Fisher, Murray, & Bundy, 1991; Katz, 1992; Mathiowetz & Haugen, 1994; Trombly, 1995). In discussing each case, it is only briefly indicated which of these other models was used to address the client's problems of performance capacity. The focus is on how MOHO complemented these models to achieve a more comprehensive and effective approach to addressing the clients' occupational needs and problems.

Volition and Habituation Considerations For a Person With an Upper Extremity Injury

Sometimes upper extremity impairments that are temporary can be effectively addressed with the biomechanical model (Kielhofner 1997; Trombly, 1995). However, when such impairments seriously affect the client's occupational life and/or when motivational problems affect client progress, therapists may need to complement the biomechanical model with MOHO concepts. The case that follows illustrates such a circumstance.

Fabrecio

Fabrecio was a 40-year-old, Hispanic man attending outpatient occupational therapy 3 days per week. While working as a cable TV installer in Chicago, he fell from a ladder and broke his left wrist. Following surgery, Fabrecio developed a severe case of complex regional pain syndrome. After his cast was removed, his biomechanical-based therapy consisted of fluidotherapy that alleviated some of his pain, followed by very light stretching and doing fine motor movements. While motivated to regain use of his hand, Fabrecio was preoccupied with fear of reinjury and of exacerbating his pain. As a result, he was extremely guarded when asked to begin using his hand to do things in therapy. He reported avoiding its use at home. Despite encouragement to use his injured hand in therapy and advice to do so at home, Fabrecio made no progress. Instead, he became increasingly distressed. The discussion below indicates how the therapist used assessments and approaches based on MOHO to address Fabrecio's situation.

The therapist concluded that Fabrecio's lack of progress in regaining use of his hand was clearly being impacted by his personal causation (i.e., his fear of stimulating pain and worsening his condition by using the hand). Therefore, she decided to gather information on other aspects of his volition that might be used as resources in therapy. She began by asking Fabrecio to complete the Interest Checklist. The therapist administered the assessment orally while Fabrecio was in the fluidotherapy machine, which gave them ample opportunity to talk about his interests. The Interest Checklist indicated that Fabrecio had given up almost all of his interests (*Fig. 25-1*). For example, playing pool was one of the past activities he regretted having to give up. He indicated that he could play pool one-handed. However, he avoided the pool hall because he was afraid someone might hurt his arm.

The Interest Checklist also identified Fabrecio's strong interest in cooking. He explained that he had worked as an assistant chef for approximately 12 years, but had taken a job as a cable installer to earn more money. However, he still loved to cook. Before the injury he often prepared meals at home.

When the therapist attempted to further examine Fabrecio's past occupational participation, he indicated that he did not want discuss any "psychological stuff." Given his response, the therapist decided that the Occupational Self Assessment (OSA) would be a good assessment to use next because the items are concrete and easy to understand and, therefore, would not be threatening to Fabrecio.

At the next therapy session, the therapist and Fabrecio completed the assessment together while he was using the fluidotherapy machine. When they discussed his responses on the OSA (*Fig. 25-2*), Fabrecio acknowledged that he had many areas that were both problematic and of importance to him. He indicated that he was managing to do what he had to do because he had learned to compensate by using his right hand for most tasks. However, he became very frustrated when he was unable to do things the way he used to do them. Moreover, although he could compensate, it took him much longer to do things. Every aspect of everyday life

had been affected in some way. For example, he was only able to wear certain types of clothes that were easier to put on using one hand. This had been disturbing because personal appearance was very important to him.

Fabrecio explained his difficulties concentrating, noting that the pain "dominates me mentally." He acknowledged that he had become very forgetful. As a way of maintaining control, he tried to "keep the pain in my head" and, consequently, did not attempt to participate in many activities at home. He admitted that he did not try activities with his left hand because he was very afraid of reinjury and potentially "losing my arm." Due to his need to maintain control over the pain and his fear of reinjury, he had given up all his prior activities and interests and stayed home watching TV. He wanted to be able to relax, but could not as he was always focusing on maintaining control over the pain.

As a result of the stress and frustration, Fabrecio had developed a very short temper and tended to yell at his family. He lived with his siblings in a house and they, along with his girlfriend, took care of many things for him. He appreciated this support but was anxious to be able to do things for himself again.

The two assessments confirmed that Fabrecio's condition was affecting much of his life and, in particular, eroding his sense of capacity and feelings of efficacy, his enjoyment, and his ability to do what was important to him. Clearly, the functional status of his arm was creating major stressors not only because of pain, but also because of its effect on his whole occupational life. His participation in work, leisure, and self-care were all extremely disrupted.

Taking advantage of the forum the OSA presented for a practical discussion of what he faced in his life, the therapist was able to persuade Fabrecio to collaborate with her to identify priorities for change. With her encouragement, Fabrecio chose, in order of priority, the following areas to change:

- Physically doing what I need to do
- Relaxing and enjoying myself
- Taking care of myself.

FIGURE 25-1 Fabrecio's Responses on the Interest Checklist.

Activity	What has been your level of interest						Do you currently participate in this activity?		Would you like to pursue this in the future?	
	In the past ten years			In the past year						
	Strong	Some	No	Strong	Some	No	Yes	No	Yes	No
Gardening/yardwork			X			X		X		
Sewing/needlework						X		X		
Playing cards		X					X		X	
Foreign languages		X				X	X		X	
Church activities			X			X		X		
Radio								X	X	
Walking		X					X			
Car repair		X				X		X		
Writing			X			X		X		
Dancing						X		X	X	
Golf			X			X		X		
Football								X		
Listening to popular music			X				X			
Puzzles			X			X		X		
Holiday activities	X			X			X			
Pets/livestock	X					X		X		
Movies	X						X		X	
Listening to classical music			X			X		X		
Speeches/lectures			X			X		X		X
Swimming			X			X		X		X
Bowling						X		X		X
Visiting		X					X			X
Mending			X			X		X		X
Checkers/chess			X			X		X		X
Barbecues			X				X		X	
Reading						X		X		X
Traveling		X				X		X		X
Parties	X				X			X		X

(continued)

FIGURE 25-1 (Continued)

Activity	What has been your level of interest						Do you currently participate in this activity?		Would you like to pursue this in the future?	
	In the past ten years			In the past year						
	Strong	Some	No	Strong	Some	No	Yes	No	Yes	No
Wrestling			■			■				■
House cleaning			■			■		■		■
Model building		■				■		■		■
Television			■		■		■			■
Concerts			■			■		■		■
Pottery			■			■		■		■
Camping			■			■		■		■
Laundry/ironing			■			■		■		■
Politics			■			■		■		■
Table games			■			■		■		■
Home decorating			■			■		■		■
Clubs/lodge			■			■		■		■
Singing			■			■		■		■
Scouting			■			■		■		■
Clothes	■			■					■	
Handicrafts			■			■		■		■
Hairstyling			■			■		■		■
Cycling	■				■			■		■
Attending plays			■			■		■		■
Bird watching			■			■		■		■
Dating			■			■		NA		■
Auto racing			■			■				■
Home repairs			■		■			■	■	
Exercise			■			■		■	■	
Hunting			■			■		■		■
Woodworking			■			■		■		
Pool	■				■		■			
Driving		■			■		■			

(continued)

FIGURE 25-1 (Continued)

Activity	What has been your level of interest						Do you currently participate in this activity?		Would you like to pursue this in the future?	
	In the past ten years			In the past year						
	Strong	Some	No	Strong	Some	No	Yes	No	Yes	No
Child care	■		■			■		■		■
Tennis			■			■		■		■
Cooking/baking				■			■		■	
Basketball		■			■			■		■
History			■			■		■		■
Collecting			■			■		■		■
Fishing			■			■		■		■
Science			■			■		■		■
Leatherwork			■			■		■		■
Shopping		■			■			■	■	
Photography			■			■		■		■
Painting/drawing			■			■		■		■

FIGURE 25-2 Fabrecio's Responses on the OSA–Myself Section.

Myself	Competence				Values			
	Lots of problems	Some difficulty	Well	Extremely well	Not so Important	Important	More Important	Most Important
Concentrating on my tasks	X							X
Physically doing what I set out to do	X							X
Taking care of the place where I live		X				X		
Taking care of myself	X							X
Taking care of others for whom I am responsible	Not Applicable							
Getting where I need to go		X						X
Managing my finances		X				X		
Managing my basic needs (food, medicine)		X						
Expressing myself to others	X						X	
Getting along with others		X						
Identifying and solving problems		X						
Relaxing and enjoying myself		X						
Getting done what I need to do		X						
Having a satisfying routine							X	
Handling my responsibilities		X						
Being involved as a student, worker, volunteer, and/or family member	X							
Doing activities I like		X						X
Working towards my goals			X			X		
Making important decisions based on what I think is important		X						
Accomplishing what I set out to do	X							X
Effectively using my abilities	X							

Therapeutic Reasoning and Intervention

The therapist decided it was important to reinvolve Fabrecio in an occupation that he found important and interesting. However, she was concerned about him getting frustrated at not being able to perform an activity, resulting in an even lower sense of self-efficacy. Therefore, the therapist validated his concerns and frustrations, suggesting that they together explore doing things of his choice to "see how it goes." This approach conveyed to him that the therapist was going to give him control over what he chose to do and at the same time would support him.

Fabrecio was initially hesitant. The therapist gently suggested that they consider cooking together. At first reluctant, Fabrecio became involved and relaxed as they talked about a potential menu, should he decide to cook. In their conversation the therapist mentioned that she ate lots of rice and beans because she was vegetarian. At that, Fabrecio offered to teach her how to make Puerto Rican rice and beans. As they made the list of necessary ingredients, Fabrecio decided that rice and beans alone would not be a complete meal, concluding that they needed to have fish as well. By the time they finished planning the meal and making the shopping list, Fabrecio was palpably excited. They agreed to cook the meal the following week. Fabrecio was to bring the ethnic spices and the therapist would provide the rest of the ingredients.

Fabrecio arrived early for the cooking session. While he was preparing the meal, the therapist encouraged him to try to use his left hand as an assist whenever possible. After approximately 15 minutes she no longer needed to remind him. Fabrecio sustained the effort to use his hand. As he cooked, Fabrecio took pride in teaching the therapist how to prepare the food. The therapist took on the student role, helping Fabrecio only when he requested it. Two hours later, they had a delicious meal. The other therapists in the clinic sampled it as well, and everyone enjoyed the food. Fabrecio was especially happy to have impressed all the therapists with his cooking prowess. While they were eating, the therapist and Fabrecio discussed how the cooking went. At first, Fabrecio indicated that he felt disappointed, because he needed the therapist's help. She gave him feedback, reminding him of how little she did. At this point, he reframed the situation, recognizing that he had done most of it himself. As he discussed and thought about it more, he recognized that even if he could not do things exactly as before, he could still enjoy doing things. Fabrecio was very appreciative of the experience and the therapist's encouragement. He noted that it "felt good" to cook again after 6 months.

The cooking session was a pivotal event for Fabrecio. Not only had he begun to use his left hand, but he was able to reframe his situation. His volition had been dominated by fears of pain and reinjury and by the feeling of loss of enjoyment and value. Through the cooking experience, he became aware that he could resume participation in past occupations. He left the session motivated to try cooking at home. He continued to have significant pain and some fear of reinjury. Consequently, he used the structure of the therapy context to explore new occupational forms before doing them at home. Although he continued to have pain in his hand and wrist, Fabrecio continued to progress, participating in an increasingly wider range of occupations.

Fabrecio in Perspective

This case illustrates how MOHO and related assessments can be useful for clients who require a biomechanical approach. In this case, it was important to address the fact that the biomechanical problem greatly impacted on Fabrecio's occupational life. Also, MOHO pointed out that his personal causation interfered with Fabrecio's progress in therapy. The Interest Checklist revealed another element of volition (the value and interest he attached to cooking) that could counterbalance the personal causation problems in therapy. By thus understanding his volition, the therapist was able to address Fabrecio's problem, engaging Fabrecio in a meaningful occupational form that became a turning point for him. Additionally, the OSA helped the therapist to engage Fabrecio as a collaborator in addressing his problem in a practical way without raising his concerns about therapy getting too psychological. This approach enabled him to achieve greater occupational participation despite ongoing pain.

Overcoming Entrapment

When Esther was 79 years old, she had a cerebrovascular accident (CVA) that resulted in spastic hemiplegia of her left side and severe sensory impairment. She also had very obvious perceptual deficits, especially in the areas of spatial perception and body scheme. She was dependent in almost all areas of basic self-care.

Esther had undergone initial, short-term rehabilitation before returning home for a brief period with her husband. She was then placed in a skilled nursing facility (SNF) in Ramat Gan, Israel. She had been placed in the facility at the request of her husband, who was unable to care for her in their apartment. In addition to her functional limitations, one of the key considerations was that Esther was incontinent. In the SNF, Esther began receiving individual occupational therapy services at bedside. The therapist addressed Esther's motor control and perceptual problems using the cognitive-perceptual and motor control models (Abreu & Toglia, 1987; Trombly, 1995). The discussion below illustrates how the therapist also used MOHO to address the psychosocial challenges that Esther faced.

Esther

Esther seemed extremely unhappy and distressed regarding her current situation, although highly motivated to participate in therapy. The occupational therapist decided to evaluate Esther using the Occupational Performance History Interview-Second Version (OPHI-II). She anticipated that the OPHI-II would help make sense of the apparent discrepancy between Esther's high level of motivation for therapy and her depressed mood. She also chose this assessment as a means of learning about Esther's occupational history and her views of her current situation. The therapist expected that the OPHI-II would address concerns she had about Esther's adjustment to being placed in the facility.

Esther's ratings on the three OPHI-II scales are shown in *Figure 25-3*. They indicated that the stroke and placement in the SNF had some impact on Esther's occupational identity, although important elements such as what she desired in life were still intact. Esther's occupational competence was severely restricted, and she perceived the SNF as having a very negative effect on her occupational life.

Esther's Occupational Narrative

The occupational narrative Esther told was organized around the metaphor of entrapment. She found herself constrained by her physical condition and placement in an environment in which she was extremely unhappy. *Figure 25-4* shows her narrative slope. It illustrates her feeling of having fallen into an extremely bad time, characterized by being "trapped" in the SNF.

Esther had a successful career as an office clerk, having been promoted a number of times because of her excellent performance. Her work career had been fulfilling to her and she was very proud of it. After retirement, Esther also had an equally fulfilling routine that included traveling, attending the theater and concerts, and visiting museums. She described this period of her life as "very busy." She and her husband did most everything together. They lived a full life, according to Esther.

Before her stroke, Esther lived with her husband in the adjacent assisted living section of the nursing home complex. Their apartment was small but comfortable. Esther described her retirement years with her husband before her stroke as the most positive period of her life. The brief period after the stroke, when she still lived in the apartment, was difficult but still satisfactory to her. She saw her current situation as intolerable.

Esther felt that she was being held against her will in the nursing home. At the time of the transfer she believed that being in the SNF was only temporary. She wanted to be in the apartment where her husband still resided. The negative feelings she expressed were so strong that she even admitted considering suicide, saying, "Maybe I should stop taking my medications, so that everyone would be relieved of me."

Esther emphasized how much she missed being able to manage her daily routines as she did when she lived in the apartment. She longed to do even the simple things like heating up the meals on wheels and washing the dishes. Instead, she described her routine as follows:

> I wake up in the morning. I get dressed with the help of the staff. I try hard to minimize the amount of help that I need. I ask for help to get dressed. I shower, I go outside, I eat breakfast, do exercise in a group, or hear a lecture . . . .go to the crafts room and do needlepoint. My personal caregiver comes. We go for a walk, sometimes we go as far as my apartment, but my husband isn't always there. I read. Eat lunch. Rest. My husband comes and we have tea . . . Sometimes I have therapy. Sometimes, I go out to walk again. Sometimes I sit in the lobby and talk to someone. I have supper early, read, and go to sleep.

In telling about her routine, Esther stressed the extent to which she was dependent on others and desired to be more independent. Esther's most important value was to receive as little assistance as possible and to do as much as she could. Especially evident throughout the interview was that Esther was highly motivated to minimize the effort for the staff that cared for her. As she saw it, she had to work hard to overcome her limitations in order "not to be humiliated."

Intervention

Based on the insight that the OPHII interview gave to Esther's occupational identity and competence

FIGURE 25-3 Therapist's Ratings and Comments Concerning Esther on the OPHI-II.

Occupational Identity Scale	1	2	3	4	Comments
Has personal goals and projects			▓		Wants to be as independent as possible
Identifies a desired occupational lifestyle		▓			Dislikes nursing facility; wants to live with husband
Expects success			▓		Willing to work hard to make gains
Accepts responsibility			▓		Willing to work hard as a patient
Appraises abilities and limitations	▓				Unrealistic expectations
Has commitments and values					
Recognizes identity and obligations			▓		Main role now is patient role and she works hard to be a good patient
Has interests				▓	
Felt effective (past)				▓	
Found meaning and satisfaction in lifestyle (past)				▓	
Made occupational choices (past)				▓	
Occupational Competence Scale	**1**	**2**	**3**	**4**	
Maintains satisfying lifestyle	▓				
Fulfills role expectations		▓			Patient role yes, but has not occupational role
Works toward goals			▓		Works hard to her goal to recover function
Meets personal performance standards	▓				Unable to perform independently as she wishes
Organizes time for responsibilities					Not Applicable
Participates in interests	▓				Extremely limited
Fulfilled roles (past)				▓	
Maintained habits (past)				▓	
Achieved satisfaction (past)				▓	
Occupational Behavior Setting Scale	**1**	**2**	**3**	**4**	
Home-life occupational forms		▓			Very little for her to do in SNF
Major productive role occupational forms					Not Applicable
Leisure occupational forms		▓			Very little for her to do in SNF
Home-life social group		▓			Husband and staff her only social contact
Major productive social group					Not Applicable
Leisure social group		▓			Husband and staff her social contact
Home-life physical spaces, objects, and resources			▓		
Major productive role physical spaces, objects, and resources					Not Applicable
Leisure physical spaces, objects, and resources		▓			

Key : **4** = Exceptionally competent occupational functioning; **3** = Appropriate satisfactory occupational functioning; **2** = Some occupational dysfunction; **1** = Extremely occupationally dysfunctional

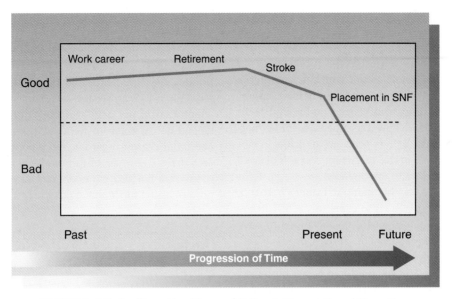

FIGURE 25-4 Narrative Slope of Esther's Occupational Narrative.

and her view of the nursing home environment, the therapist felt it was critical to address the most realistic of Esther's desires. The therapist reasoned that if Esther could make some gains in an area important to her, she might accept and adjust to the remaining limitations and to her SNF placement. The nature of her need for support and her husband's own limitations made it impossible to consider her return to live in the apartment.

The therapist began by concentrating on the area of bed mobility. The goal, with which Esther agreed, was to reach maximum independence and minimal need for assistance. This was an area of performance that would give Esther the most immediate sense of freedom and independence. The ability to transfer from supine to sitting at the edge of the bed was within her capacity, especially if she could learn to compensate for her perceptual difficulties. Thus, although the goal for Esther was simply stated as "sitting up in bed," her therapist realized that this goal was attached to Esther's need to be as independent as possible and to maintain personal dignity.

Because of Esther's motor and perceptual difficulties, progress toward this goal was slow and required Esther to practice repeatedly with coaching

and support from the therapist. Eventually, the goal was achieved, and Esther was pleased with her new ability to sit at the edge of the bed whenever she wished. She described with a sense of satisfaction that she could greet her caretakers in a sitting position, making their work even easier.

Intervention continued in this vein and emphasized goals that increased Esther's performance in her daily routines and that enriched her environment. The therapist reasoned that meeting realistic goals in these two areas would have a positive effect on Esther's well-being and would provide opportunities for Esther to feel effective and to find meaning in her present life situation.

With that reasoning in mind, the therapist targeted three areas:

- The time Esther spent with her personal caregiver
- Esther's daily routines that involved her husband and their apartment
- The meaning and significance of the occupational forms in which Esther was engaged in the crafts room.

With her consent, the therapist advised Esther's personal caregiver on how to better spend their time together. The following are some examples of the changes that the therapist recommended and the caretaker implemented. When they took a walk as far as the apartment, Esther took a rest in her bed at the apartment, prepared light food items to share with her husband, or dusted the furniture or did other light household chores with the care-giver's help. These activities also provided needed opportunities for Esther to practice one-handed techniques and to learn how to compensate for her perceptual deficits. Esther took great pride in her accomplishments in the apartment and was pleased to report successes to the therapist.

Encouraged by the therapist, Esther's husband, whose daily routine was to come to the SNF in the afternoon to join Esther for tea, arranged to have tea in their own apartment, at least once a week. This weekly afternoon tea became a very special time for Esther. She was bolstered by her husband's attention and looked forward to having tea at home.

Finally, the therapist evaluated Esther's involvement in the crafts room. Esther had been doing simple weaving on a frame loom. The weavings she produced were collected by the crafts teacher and then sold. The therapist asked the crafts teacher to have Esther create samples of her weaving that she could distribute to interested residents in the SNF. This change allowed Ether to gain a greater sense of productivity since she could show others the kinds of weavings she was creating. This was very important to Esther since being productive and not being a burden was such a strong value. Finally, showing her weaving to others allowed her to get to know more residents, something she was willing to do in a context in which she could display her competence.

Esther in Perspective

The therapist's primary focus in direct intervention was focused on remediating and minimizing the impact of Esther's motor, cognitive, and perceptual impairments. However, the therapist's use of MOHO:

- Allowed her to gather critical information and undertake indirect interventions (e.g., consulting with Esther's caregiver and the craft teacher) that ad-

dressed factors impacting on Esther's occupational adaptation
- Helped her decide functional priorities in direct interventions.

Notably, the OPHI-II provided insights that informed interventions to improve Esther's quality of life and her adaptation to her new living setting. These changes helped her to come to terms with her new environment. Her distress regarding her placement decreased, as did her sense of entrapment in the SNF. These changes in her occupational identity were just as important as the functional gains she made.

Increasing Volition During Sensory Integration Intervention

David was a 9-year-old boy with a diagnosis of developmental delay. Whereas David achieved early developmental milestones on schedule, he had always tired easily, talked constantly, and was impulsive. His parents noted that David still was very clumsy and had a poor attention span. He was very uncomfortable with any changes in his routines and had difficulty learning new tasks. Finally, David's parents described him as fearful of being hurt in everyday situations that were not actually physically threatening. David attended a regular third grade class and received speech therapy services in school. There had been discussion of holding him back in school due to his fine motor deficits.

David was seen privately by his occupational therapist. His parents had sought out occupational therapy services to address problems stemming from David's sensory integration difficulties. The therapist initially assessed David with a battery of motor and perceptual assessments and an observational guide generated for use with the sensory integration model. When evaluated from the perspective of sensory integration (Ayres, 1979; Fisher, Murray, & Bundy, 1991), David displayed auditory, gustatory, and tactile defensiveness. This meant he had difficulty integrating sound, taste, and touch senses and perceived these sensory stimuli as uncomfortable and threatening. He was hypersensitive to many forms of sensory stimulation such as loud noises. His diet was limited to a small range of foods he could tolerate (i.e., pasta, hamburgers, creamy peanut butter, white bread, and ketchup). He was unable to eat most anything that was firm or crunchy.

David also displayed gravitational insecurity and vestibular deficits. For example, he was very uncomfortable doing anything that involved moving away from the ground such as climbing or swinging. Merely watching a merry-go-round would make him dizzy. He avoided most playground equipment. As a consequence of these limitations of performance capacity, David's performance was quite restricted. For example, he could not manipulate buttons or tie his shoes. Moreover, David's handwriting was very poor.

The following discussion illustrates how the occupational therapist also employed MOHO concepts as a component of her therapy. Sensory integrative difficulties are typically interwoven with volitional problems (Kielhofner & Fisher, 1991). Moreover, as discussed in Chapter 6, there is also a lived body experience of having these difficulties. Finally, the long-term impact of therapy on a child like David must involve enabling him to make choices to do things that facilitate sensory processing and to learn habits and bodily strategies for minimizing the interference of sensory challenges with performance.

Therefore, while his therapist used sensory integrative principles and strategies as the major focus of David's therapy, MOHO concepts were also used. Because our aim is to show how MOHO supported and complemented the sensory integrative approach, we will only discuss those details of the sensory integrative approach that were most intertwined with the therapist's use of MOHO.

David

The therapist began to evaluate David's volition through informal observation. Since therapy involved engaging David in various sensorimotor activities, the therapist had constant opportunity to observe David's volition in action. Additionally, discussions with David's parents provided information about David's volition, especially his sensorimotor likes and dislikes.

In the area of personal causation, David was keenly aware that he lacked skills that other children possessed. He had an especially difficult time in

gym class, where his poor coordination made him stand out. David had little that was positive to say about his capacities. As his parents had indicated, David was extremely fearful of occupational forms that required him to do motor actions.

David had few interests. His main pastimes were playing Nintendo and watching TV. Because David had difficulty performing in a wide range of contexts, he attempted to dismiss as unimportant many of the things that other children his age found meaningful and valuable. For example, he disavowed any interest in going to the playground in the local park. However, he was also very aware of being "different" from other children in other ways. For example, he was unable to tolerate or manipulate ordinary clothes, so he wore sweat clothes and sneakers with Velcro closures. David was clearly disturbed by these differences as he very much valued being like other children.

David made very restricted decisions for engaging in ordinarily childhood occupations. In particular, he avoided participating in games with other children that involved gross movement. He did not participate in any of the childhood sports that his peers enjoyed. Clearly, David's volitional problems included:

- Feelings of lack of control, especially in motor performance
- Lack of a feeling of enjoyment in performance and failure to develop a range of age-appropriate interests
- Attempts to avoid the pain of not being able to do things valued by others by disavowing their importance
- Feeling threatened by sensory stimulation from his environment.

These problems were critical to address because they affected David's quality of life.

Any changes he might achieve in his performance capacity would depend on David choosing to perform in ways that would enable him to develop his capacity and skills.

Intervention

David attended occupational therapy once a week. His therapist engaged him in doing things that were indicated from a sensory integrative perspective. At the same time, the therapist also focused on the goals that David would:

- Demonstrate that he felt in control and expected to succeed while engaging in ordinary childhood occupations that involved motor challenges
- Show greater enjoyment and a greater desire to do things involving motor challenges
- Be able to do more things that he valued and found meaningful.

Because David's volition was so limited, the therapist began all intervention at the exploration level and progressed toward competence and achievement—the continuum of change discussed in Chapters 10 and 18.

David's therapy began with simple movement patterns on objects that were close to the ground and had small radiuses of movement (i.e., therapy ball, platform swing, scooter boards). To address David's volition, these movement activities were integrated into games that the therapist created and played with him. These games were designed to allow David to physically explore the environment in a safe context with minimal performance demands. To maximize his feeling of control, David was allowed to make up the "rules" of the games. Over time, David showed increasing enjoyment in his therapy sessions and was able to make up new games.

After a period of therapy, David cautiously expressed an interest in sports. In response the therapist began to incorporate basketball and baseball themes into the same kind of safe therapy games. As he became more comfortable with gross motor games, David played with increasing ease and intensity, willingly choosing to do such things as swinging, rolling in barrels, and jumping off a loft into foam pillows. During this phase, the therapist coached David's parents to replicate some of the same safe opportunities for exploration at home and the local playground. She also began to explore new foods with him and helped David's mother figure out ways to allow him to explore different foods at home. His diet became more diverse and he was increasingly willing to try new foods.

Given David's progress in the gross motor area coupled with his increased sense of efficacy, the therapist decided to address some of the fine motor

challenges that he faced. Concurrent with this change, the therapist recognized that David's performance capacity and volition had improved to the point that he could handle competency level demands. During the competency stage of change, she expected David to begin to handle greater performance demands by improving his performance. As noted in Chapter 10, striving for competence leads to skill development and the organization of these skills into habits. Competency affords an individual a growing sense of personal control. As persons strive to organize their performances into routines of competent behavior that are relevant to their environment, they immerse themselves in a process of becoming, growing, and arriving at a greater sense of personal mastery.

David's therapist began by adding performance demands requiring fine motor capacity. For example, she suggested that they play Star Wars and "dress up" using costumes. This allowed her to introduce the manipulation of buttons to David. David started with oversize buttons and then progressed to being able to handle more typical buttons. During this phase, she also negotiated with David's parents to work with David to practice things he was learning in therapy.

The therapist initiated a program aimed at enhancing David's handwriting performance. This program used principles consistent with the lived body concept discussed in Chapter 6. In the program (Benbow, 1990), the therapist gave David visual and verbal feedback so that he could feel each letter as he wrote it. The therapist developed and taught David to do a warm up exercise program before writing in school that prepared his hands for handwriting. Over time, he was able to copy sentences from a paper and then from the chalkboard, with improving accuracy. Eventually, David's handwriting improved significantly and he found that it took much less effort to write. David was especially excited when he realized that the improvement in his handwriting had contributed to the decision not to hold him back in school.

The therapist also initiated a program to help David learn to monitor, maintain, and change his level of alertness in different situations. The program helped David become more aware of his inner experiences and to control them. This allowed him to better attend and learn in the classroom and to interact more effectively with other children. David actively worked to learn to do this as it gave him a greater sense of control. With time and practice, the handwriting warm up exercise and the self-monitoring of his alertness became habits.

Next, David began to show signs of moving to the achievement level (i.e., being able to face greater challenges and risks). For example, David found ways to vary his performance and challenge himself to do more than what he was already able to do. He increasingly attempted new things he had never done before. As he saw peers in therapy do something he had not yet done, he would want to do it.

Achievement also means having greater control and integrating new skills and habits for managing everyday life. David was showing signs of this as well. For example, he increasingly sought out his therapist's advice and coaching to help him improve his performance in areas of daily life.

Recognizing David's readiness for the achievement level, the therapist decided to offer David even more control over the aims of therapy. She invited David to complete the Child Occupational Self Assessment (COSA). In addition to giving him a voice in stating how he saw himself and what he most wanted to address in therapy, the COSA would also allow David to see the progress he had made in therapy.

The therapist administered the COSA verbally to David. He was initially shy when asked the COSA questions, but as the assessment progressed, he was able to identify how he felt about his performance and what was important to him. His responses are shown on *Figure 25-5*. The assessment provided an important opening to set goals that David found important. On the COSA David identified many areas wherein he had some problems. However, the COSA did provide him an opportunity to note some areas that were okay and others in which he had strengths.

Together the therapist and David discussed his responses on the COSA. In this discussion David identified that he felt his relationships with his peers would be improved if he could do more of the things they did and was able to dress like them. As a result they developed three new goals for therapy:

- To manage a button and zipper independently so he could wear jeans like his peers
- To tie his shoes independently so he could have the special kind of sneakers that many of his peers wore
- To learn and use strategies that would help him calm down to learn at school.

The therapist's acknowledgment of these goals as being important to David, and her assurance that they would work toward them in therapy, was highly motivating for David.

The therapist worked out a plan with David's parents in which they progressively bought him new clothes. David brought the clothes into therapy to work on necessary skills for getting them on. David learned to mange his button and zipper and to tie his shoes over the next 2 months. In another month he learned to tie double knots. His mother then purchased him a pair of the fancy sneakers his peers were wearing. Throughout this stage of therapy, David increasingly felt effective in accomplishing goals.

As his personal causation was enhanced, David continued to identify new occupational forms that he wanted to learn in therapy. When he did so, the therapist allowed him to work on these self-initiated goals. In this way, David began to direct his own therapy. For example, he identified that he wanted to be able to make his own snack. Thus, in therapy he practiced making a peanut butter sandwich until he mastered it.

Near the end of therapy, David told the therapist he wanted to have his birthday party at a local indoor play area since his peers were having their parties there also. He shared his concern over whether he would be able to handle himself okay on the playground. In response, the therapist secured approval from the insurance company to do a therapy session at this play area. With his therapist's encouragement and coaching, David tried each play apparatus (e.g., climbing tube, rope ladders, ball pits, drawbridge, and swings). With practice David managed to master each piece of equipment during the session. Importantly, this gave him confidence

FIGURE 25-5 David's Initial Responses on the COSA.

Myself	I HAVE A BIG PROBLEM DOING THIS	I HAVE A LITTLE PROBLEM DOING THIS	I DO THIS	NOT SO IMPORTANT	IMPORTANT	REALLY IMPORTANT
Keep my mind on what I am doing	☹					★★
Make my body do what I want it to do		☹				★★
Dress myself	☹					★★
Brush my teeth	☹			★		
Bathe myself	☹			★★		
Get my homework done	☹				★★	
Get myself a snack	☹			★		
Keep my room clean	☹				★★	
Keep my desk neat	☹			★★		
Get my chores done	☹			★★		
Get around in my neighborhood	☹			★★		
Buy things by myself	☹			★★		
Answer questions in school	☹					★★
Tell others my ideas and they understand	☹				★★	
Get along with my classmates		☹				★★
Ask the teacher questions when I do not understand something	☹					
Think of other ways to do things when I have a problem	☹			★		
Calm down when I am having a problem	☹					★★
Do things that make me happy	☹				★★	
Do things I am good at	☹			★		
Finish my work in school on time	☹				★★	
Have enough time to do things I like	☹				★★★	
Follow classroom rules		☹			★★	
Be a good friend		☹			★★	
Do what my parents ask	☹					★★
Do activities in school	☹					★★
Do activities in my neighborhood	☹				★★★	
Do things with friends		☹			★★	
Keep working on something even when it gets hard		☹			★★	
Make my mind on important things		☹			★★	
Try my best		☹			★★	

FIGURE 25-6 David's Final Responses on the COSA.

Myself	I HAVE A BIG PROBLEM DOING THIS	I HAVE A LITTLE PROBLEM DOING THIS	I DO THIS	NOT SO IMPORTANT	IMPORTANT	REALLY IMPORTANT
Keep my mind on what I am doing			☺	★★★		
Make my body do what I want it to do		☺		★★★		
Dress myself			☺	★★★		
Brush my teeth		☺		★		
Bathe myself			☺	★		
Get my homework done			☺		★★	
Get myself a snack			☺		★★	
Keep my room clean		☺			★★	
Keep my desk neat		☺		★		
Get my chores done			☺			
Get around in my neighborhood		☺		★	★★	
Buy things by myself			☺	★★★		
Answer questions in school		☺		★★★		
Tell others my ideas and they understand		☺			★★	
Get along with my classmates				★★★		
Ask the teacher questions when I do not understand something			☺		★★	
Think of other ways to do things when I have a problem		☺		★★★		
Calm down when I am having a problem			☺	★★★		
Do things that make me happy			☺		★★	
Do things I am good at			☺	★		
Finish my work in school on time		☺		★★★		
Have enough time to do things I like		☺		★★★	★★	
Follow classroom rules		☺		★★★		
Be a good friend		☺			★★	
Do what my parents ask	☺			★★★	★★	
Do activities in school		☺		★★★		
Do activities in my neighborhood				★★★	★★	
Do things with friends	☺			★★★		
Keep working on something even when it gets hard			☺		★★	
Make up my mind on important things			☺		★★	
Try my best			☺	★★★		

to go ahead with the birthday party. During his birthday party, he was able to enjoy himself and use all the equipment along with the other children.

Also near the end of therapy, the therapist readministered the COSA to review progress with David and to identify goals David would continue to work on himself. As shown in *Figure 25-6,* most areas were now adequate and he was able to identify a number of strengths. He noted only two areas in which he still had some problem: doing what his parents told him and playing with friends.

In the follow-up discussion with the therapist, he identified two goals for his future. He noted that he wanted to improve his ability to "shift his engine to just right" to better:

- Finish school work in allotted time
- Adjust his behavior to play with other kids.

David was able to plan how to address both of these goals. This included, for instance, using sour candy to "shift his engine."

By the time therapy came to an end, David had successfully played baseball on a school team. He preferred basketball because he was the best player on the court for his age. When terminating therapy, David's final comment on how things had gone in therapy was he could "do lots of stuff." David also announced that he had decided to become an artist when he grew up. As noted in Chapter 10, one of the important developmental steps for latency age children is occupational choice. It requires that the child have both interests and some sense of efficacy. Before he began therapy David rarely picked up a pencil or crayon.

David in Perspective

David's therapy illustrates how MOHO can be readily integrated within therapy designed around a sensory integration perspective. This case emphasized the concept of volition, since for David it was so critical. However, habituation, lived body, and environmental concepts were also used to guide the therapy process. The concept of volition was critical because it illuminated an area in which David needed to achieve changes and because the volitional process was important for the

success of the sensory integrative aspects of the therapy. A child can only benefit from sensory integrative strategies when the child is volitionally engaged (Kielhofner & Fisher, 1991).

David's therapy also illustrates how client-centered therapy takes on different forms over time. In the early stage of his therapy, David was unable to choose goals for therapy because he did not believe in his ability to achieve goals. Consequently, the therapist needed to understand David's volition and his limitations of performance capacity to set goals on his behalf. Only later, when David's volition had improved, was he able to actively participate in deciding what the goals would be in therapy.

Choosing and Organizing Life Occupations

Sally was a 37-year-old, college-educated homemaker who formerly taught in elementary school. She had been diagnosed with rheumatoid arthritis 5 years earlier. Sally's impairments had progressed to the point at which she became an outpatient at a rehabilitation facility. At the time, Sally had pain and swelling in her wrists, fingers, knees, ankles, and feet. The progressive nature of her arthritis and the failure of medication to place the disease in remission meant that Sally would have to find a lifestyle in which she could successfully cope with her limitations. The first hint that Sally was having difficulty coping came from her social worker, who expressed concern that Sally was depressed.

Because Sally's disease attacks the musculoskeletal system, Sally's occupational therapist used the biomechanical model (Kielhofner, 1997; Trombly, 1995) complemented by the MOHO to guide the data gathering process and the planning and implementation of therapy. The discussion below details the MOHO-related aspects of her therapy.

Sally

Sally's therapist was concerned about the impact of the disease on her interests, values, and feelings of personal causation. He wanted to know what changes had taken place in Sally's volition and to understand how these may have influenced her activity and occupational choices. Moreover, the occupational therapist wanted to know how Sally's roles and habit patterns had changed and what the consequences were for Sally's lifestyle.

Since Sally was a bright and articulate woman, information gathering was done so as to maximize her role in shaping an understanding of her situation. Sally's therapist interviewed her using the OPHI-II. In addition, Sally was given the Modified Interest Checklist and the National Institutes of Health Activity Record (NIH-ACTRE) to take home and complete.

"Making Do"

In the OPHI-II interview, Sally remarked about having to "make do" when her arthritis prevented her from performing an activity as it "should have been done." In many ways, this comment summarized what Sally's occupational narrative had become. She had routinely found herself unable to carry out the occupational forms she valued and enjoyed. Being a practical person who readily acquiesced to such problems, she routinely compromised and found a way to get by. In this way, she had changed much of her life to accommodate her pain and limitations. However, her life had also lost much of its spontaneity and joy and was instead characterized by a series of losses and compromises. Formerly a sports enthusiast, she talked about the bowling ball and tennis racket hidden away in the attic and a bicycle reluctantly retired since she could no longer safely operate the hand brakes.

Sally was a trained and credentialed primary and secondary educator who interrupted her career to become a full-time homemaker, rearing her two children. She had planned to return to teaching after her teenage children were grown. Sally had taken on the homemaker role full-time because of strong family and religious values. She had a sense of obligation to devote most of her attention to raising her children. While Sally valued her caretaking role, the occupational forms that the role required were not those most satisfying for her. Sally's voluntary exit from work, along with her forced discontinuation of sports, had created a major loss of identity and satisfaction.

Sally had been an active volunteer in her church, running an education program for senior citizens. Volunteering was quite satisfying and important to her. However, as the arthritis progressed, she had also been forced to relinquish the volunteer role (another major loss) and to concentrate her efforts on the homemaker and patient roles.

Sally acknowledged that her teenaged children would soon be gone from home and that she would then be without any major occupational role. She had some vague ideas about returning to teaching as a substitute since her arthritis made full-time teaching impossible. However, the future mainly seemed very uncertain and gloomy to her.

Sally also indicated in the OPHI-II that the arthritis interfered with many of her routines and posed constant problems for undertaking ordinary activities. She described a series of small incidents in which she performed an ordinary task, like making breakfast, where some simple action like stirring eggs suddenly brought on severe pain. She also related incidents in which her pain or motor limitations meant she could not finish an activity. While Sally was resourceful in making the best of her limitations and finding a way to get through most activities, her sense of efficacy had been eroded by the barrage of small things that gotten the best of her. She always performed under the threat of not being able to manage things. She repeatedly needed to stop or change course when confronted with her pain, weakness, or fatigue.

Overall, Sally told and lived an occupational narrative in which she had many losses, managed to barely hold on and make do, and lived under the constant threat of being unable to manage. Finally, her narrative did not include a clear or hopeful future. Rather, if the future promised anything it was more losses.

As *Figure 25-7* illustrates, both Sally's occupational identity and competence had been affected by her arthritic condition. In contrast to her past, Sally's identity was now marked by uncertainty of what she could accomplish and what she wanted in life. Her competence was affected, especially in her ability to meet her own performance standards and participate in interests. Sally's environmental impact was marked by the loss of involvement in a major productive role and the lack of available objects and occupational forms that would support her

FIGURE 25-7   Sally's Responses on the OPHI-II.

Occupational Identity Scale	1	2	3	4
Has personal goals and projects		▨		
Identifies a desired occupational lifestyle			▨	
Expects success		▨		
Accepts responsibility			▨	
Appraises abilities and limitations				
Has commitments and values				▨
Recognizes identity and obligations			▨	
Has interests			▨	
Felt effective (past)				▨
Found meaning and satisfaction in lifestyle (past)				▨
Made occupational choices (past)			▨	
Occupational Competence Scale	**1**	**2**	**3**	**4**
Maintains satisfying lifestyle		▨		
Fulfills role expectations			▨	
Works toward goals		▨		
Meets personal performance standards	▨			
Organizes time for responsibilities			▨	
Participates in interests	▨			
Fulfilled roles (past)				▨
Maintained habits (past)				▨
Achieved satisfaction (past)				▨
Occupational Behavior Settings Scale	**1**	**2**	**3**	**4**
Home-life occupational forms		▨		
Major productive role occupational forms	Not Applicable			
Leisure occupational forms	▨			
Home-life social group			▨	
Major productive social group	Not Applicable			
Leisure social group		▨		
Home-life physical spaces, objects, and resources		▨		
Major productive role physical spaces, objects, and resources	Not Applicable			
Leisure physical spaces, objects, and resources			▨	

Key : **4** = Exceptionally competent occupational functioning; **3** = Appropriate satisfactory occupational functioning; **2** = Some occupational dysfunction; **1** = Extremely occupationally dysfunctional

functioning. Sally's family was generally supportive but unaware of ways in which they might best help her. Sally had lost contact with friends for leisure as she could no longer do the things they had done before.

Loss of Satisfaction and Self

On the Modified Interest Checklist (*Fig. 25-8*), Sally indicated that she had 11 strong interests in the past 10 years. In the year previous to the evaluation, Sally had maintained a strong interest in only two of

FIGURE 25-8 Sally's Responses on the Modified Interest Checklist.

| Activity | What has been your level of interest | | | | | | Do you currently participate in this activity? | | Would you like to pursue this in the future? | |
| | In the past ten years | | | In the past year | | | | | | |
	Strong	Some	No	Strong	Some	No	Yes	No	Yes	No
Gardening/yardwork										
Sewing/needlework										
Playing cards										
Foreign languages										
Church activities										
Radio										
Walking										
Car repair										
Writing										
Dancing										
Golf										
Football										
Listening to popular music										
Puzzles										
Holiday activities										
Pets/livestock										
Movies										
Listening to classical music										
Speeches/lectures										
Swimming										
Bowling										
Visiting										
Mending										
Checkers/chess										
Barbecues										
Reading										
Traveling										
Parties										

(continued)

FIGURE 25-8 (Continued)

Activity	What has been your level of interest						Do you currently participate in this activity?		Would you like to pursue this in the future?	
	In the past ten years			In the past year						
	Strong	Some	No	Strong	Some	No	Yes	No	Yes	No
Wrestling			X			X		X		X
House cleaning	X				X		X		X	
Model building			X			X		X		X
Television		X			X		X		X	
Concerts			X			X		X		X
Pottery			X			X		X		X
Camping			X			X		X		X
Laundry/ironing	X				X		X		X	
Politics			X			X		X		X
Table games		X			X		X		X	
Home decorating			X			X		X		X
Clubs/lodge			X			X		X		X
Singing			X	X			X		X	
Scouting			X			X		X		X
Clothes		X			X		X		X	
Handicrafts			X			X		X		X
Hairstyling			X			X		X		X
Cycling			X			X		X		X
Attending plays			X			X		X		X
Bird watching			X			X		X		X
Dating			X			X		X		X
Auto racing			X			X		X		X
Home repairs		X			X		X		X	
Exercise		X			X		X		X	
Hunting			X			X		X		X
Woodworking		X			X		X		X	
Pool			X		X		X		X	
Driving			X			X	X		X	

(continued)

FIGURE 25-8 (Continued)

Activity	What has been your level of interest						Do you currently participate in this activity?		Would you like to pursue this in the future?	
	In the past ten years			In the past year						
	Strong	Some	No	Strong	Some	No	Yes	No	Yes	No
Child care		■				■		■		■
Tennis		■				■		■		■
Cooking/baking		■			■		■		■	
Basketball			■			■		■		■
History			■			■		■		■
Collecting								■		■
Fishing								■		■
Science			■		■			■		■
Leatherwork					■	■		■		■
Shopping					■	■				
Photography			■			■		■		■
Painting/drawing			■							■

those areas, singing and mending. The Checklist confirmed Sally's interview report that many of her strong interests involved physical activity and, consequently, had been dropped. Sally also confirmed that many of the interests she had been forced to relinquish had previously provided her with social contact she enjoyed. She had lost not only those activities but also the connection with others.

According to Sally she had only acquired one new interest, swimming. She was quick to point out that swimming was "therapy" for her arthritis. When Sally discussed swimming, it was clear she felt unworthy to pursue her own interests, since she was barely able to discharge her homemaker role. According to Sally's world view (i.e., her religious views and her image of what it means to be a good mother) it was important to meet the needs and demands of her children, church, and community and to give priority to these needs over her own. This view of life had previously worked fine for Sally, but now it seemed to contribute to her story of loss. She seemed sadly resigned to the idea that she should just bear the losses herself and devote her remaining resources to her obligations.

Sally reported her roles on the Role Checklist (*Fig. 25-9*). She had been able to maintain continuous friend, family, home maintainer, and religious participant roles. Both the student and worker roles were not part of her current life and she did not in-

dicate them for the future. The volunteer role that was very important to Sally was interrupted, but she planned to return to this role. Sally found completing the checklist and the information it automatically provided to be helpful. It confirmed for her what she had managed to hold on to and what she wanted for the future.

Reports on the NIH-ACTRE can be summarized as shown on *Figure 25-10*. This summary shows Sally's time use in terms of the percentage of waking hours she spent doing things she enjoyed, valued, and felt competent to do. Overall, Sally's days appeared deficient in activities that provided a feeling of value, personal causation, and interest. She rated only about one-third of the activities in her day as related to major life roles. She had several long periods of rest, but did not routinely rest during activities. Finally, she experienced a moderate amount of pain and difficulty in her daily activities.

The NIH-ACTRE provided a wealth of detail about Sally's routines. For example, it allowed her occupational therapist to identify particular activities that were not valuable or interesting to Sally. Such information was very useful when Sally and her therapist worked to plan and implement a more adaptive daily routine.

The therapist and Sally together reflected on her performance in a range of daily living tasks to identify the motor skills with which she had the

FIGURE 25-9   Sally's Responses on the Role Checklist.

Role	Past	Present	Future	Not at all Valuable	Somewhat Valuable	Very Valuable
Student						
Worker						
Volunteer						
Caregiver						
Home Maintainer						
Friend						
Family Member						
Religious Participant						
Hobbyist/Amateur						
Participant in Organizations						
Other						

FIGURE 25-10 Sally's NIH Activity Record Results.

System Components	Percent Waking Hours	
	Initial	Discharge
VOLITION		
Personal Causation		
How well done		
Very poorly	0	0
Poorly	19	0
Average	79	83
Well	1	16
Interests		
Time in recreation and leisure	22	32
Enjoyment of activities		
Not at all	3	0
Very little	21	0
Some	51	61
A lot	24	39
Values		
Meaningfulness of activities		
Not meaningful	8	0
Slightly meaningful	6	0
Meaningful	69	76
Very meaningful	16	23
Value of activities to others		
Not at all	5	0
Very little	3	0
Some	35	95
A lot	56	5
HABITUATION		
Roles		
Role-related activities	30	44
Habits		
Rest during activities	1	22
PERFORMANCE		
Level of difficulty		
Very difficult	5	0
Difficult	6	0
Slightly difficult	41	40
Not difficult	46	59

most difficulty. These observations revealed that Sally consistently had the most problems with reaching, transporting, lifting, and gripping. She also had difficulty manipulating because of pain and limited range in her hands. Finally, Sally's endurance was sometimes limited by pain. The consequence of

Sally's impaired motor skills was that she had difficulty with a range of self-care tasks such as buttoning her clothes, using zippers, brushing her teeth, and caring for her hair. Household activities, especially cooking, were also difficult for Sally.

Collaborating with Sally to Create an Understanding of Her Situation

After all the information was collected, Sally's therapist shared his understanding of her situation. As part of this discussion, he introduced Sally to MOHO so that she could appreciate better how the therapist was making sense of her situation. Sally then responded to his evaluation from her own perspective. Together, Sally and the therapist arrived at the following, final conceptualization of her situation.

Pain and other symptoms often determined Sally's activity choices and forced her to alter her routine. Sally had been resourceful in figuring out ways to deal with her limits, but her knowledge of the disease process and ways to manage its symptoms had come from trial and error. Consequently, her strategies were not always optimal. In addition, her progressive symptoms meant that she had given up a former lifestyle of sports involvement and volunteerism to focus on being a homemaker. This transformation in Sally's daily routine and lifestyle had resulted in important decrements in her life satisfaction. Her daily routine reflected a lack of opportunities for exercising feelings of competence and enjoyment. She had also lost roles that gave her a sense of identity and worth.

Sally's view of her life situation had been that she should simply accept all her losses and focus on doing her best in her role as a homemaker. Yet, she often did not feel competent or in control of these responsibilities. Together, the sense of loss, the feeling of being out of control, the pain, and the erosion of her quality of life contributed to her feeling depressed. As Sally became more and more depressed, her energy level was lower. This exacerbated her functional problems and made it even more difficult for her to carry on with daily life. Sally had recognized her life was getting steadily worse, but the process had been gradual and seemed inevitable. Therefore, she had very little sense that she could do anything with it except endure it and "make do" with what she had remaining. More-over, because things were gradually getting worse for Sally, she only imagined that they would continue to do so.

Together Sally and the therapist agreed that her occupational narrative had contributed to the downward slide in her life. She needed to reframe and re-think her life—to retell her occupational narrative. The story she and the therapist headed toward was one in which Sally would have more control, find a way toward a more satisfying daily life, and be able to imagine and work toward a positive future.

Therapeutic Goals and Strategies

Sally and her therapist identified the following goals for her therapy. First, Sally needed to gain more information and to learn ways to be more in control of the symptoms and compensate for the limits imposed by her arthritis. This would potentially help her to function better and enhance her sense of efficacy. Second, Sally wanted to improve the quality of her everyday life. Completing the NIH-ACTRE had been an eye-opening experience for Sally, and she was able to see both how her overall pattern of activity was less than optimal and how some of her activities offered her no satisfaction or meaning. Third, Sally agreed that she needed to look at her choices in life. She recognized that al-though she believed it was important to devote most of her energies to her family, it was also im-portant to consider how her activity choices af-fected her mood. Sally also recognized that she needed to prepare to make an occupational choice for the future. This was important in a practical way, since her children would soon leave home and her homemaking would both diminish and take on less importance for her. It was also symbolically impor-tant that she begin to imagine a future for herself that was not dominated by the unknown progress of her arthritis.

The first emphasis in therapy was to diminish the influence of Sally's impairments through adapted equipment as well as strategies of energy conservation and joint protection. The therapist an-ticipated that reducing constraints imposed by im-pairments would be a first step for Sally to experi-ence a greater sense of efficacy.

Since the arthritis had been and would likely continue to be progressive, the therapist recognized that Sally would need to learn how to compensate for her impairments. Additionally, it was important that Sally learn to have some control over symptoms and over how they influenced her everyday func-tion. Achieving this would enhance Sally's sense of personal causation.

Sally's biomechanical interventions included such things as instruction in an active range of mo-tion program for both upper extremities. Sally was also provided splints to decrease the pain and in-crease the stability of her wrists during performance and resting hand splints for nighttime or rest peri-ods to maintain hand and wrist alignment. Sally was given the opportunity to explore various adaptive devices that would allow her to perform maximally even with her limited strength and range of motion.

While these biomechanical-guided interven-tions provided a measure of control over symptoms and compensation for limitations, Sally's therapist also recognized that Sally would need to use both process skills and communication and interaction skills (e.g., asserting her needs for rest and asking for help) to compensate for motor skill decrements. Consequently, Sally and her therapist collaborated together to identify which of her daily routines needed rethinking. The NIH-ACTRE, in which she recorded her level of pain in each activity, was very helpful for this purpose. They singled out a number of troublesome spots in Sally's routine and together explored how the occupational forms she was hav-ing trouble with could be reorganized to be more manageable. Once the appropriate mix of skills for successful completion of an occupational form was identified, Sally practiced to establish new habits.

Sally enrolled in a joint protection and energy conservation program. This program provided infor-mation on the disease process and offered Sally op-portunities to learn how to do an activity analysis to plan how to perform and how to stop and reflect on alternatives when she found herself in trouble. In this way she could adjust her performance when she had more pain or other limitations. Moreover, by being in a group with others who were coping with similar problems, she received both encouragement and helpful suggestions.

The next step was to look at her routine. Having been taught MOHO in a very basic way, Sally could see the interrelationship of her performance, habits, roles, values, interests, and personal causation. She recognized that she had already developed an increased sense of efficacy and that her awareness of her limitations was not so overwhelming if she felt she could compensate for them. She came to see how exercising more control over symptoms and maximizing her function would give her more discretionary time. She also saw how her occupational and activity choices, while they were affected by her strong values, were leading her into a lifestyle with little for herself (i.e., little enjoyment or satisfaction and little sense of efficacy). She recognized that if she was more satisfied and optimistic, she would have more to offer her family. She also allowed herself to recognize that with all her losses, she needed to devote the same attention to figuring out how she could recapture some interest in her life. As Sally engaged in this volitional process, she was increasingly able to make activity and occupational choices that enhanced the quality of her everyday routines.

Sally began to explore some old interests in therapy to see if she could adapt them and still enjoy them. She also began to try new things. Eventually, using the NIH-ACTRE as a guide, she was able to restructure her routine to incorporate some interests and to give herself more sense of efficacy while still undertaking the things that were most important for her family.

When Sally terminated outpatient therapy she had accomplished a number of notable changes. She was able to identify that she was quite competent in managing her arthritic condition while still maintaining major life roles. Sally recognized that her true interests were in the areas of science and health care and had begun exploring opportunities for education and volunteer work related to these interests. Sally improved her ability to analyze and plan her

daily activities and to carry them out so as to minimize her pain and maximize her functional ability.

Some of the changes in Sally's life were reflected when she completed the Activity Record for a second time at discharge. As Figure 25-10 shows, Sally increased interests, values, and feelings of competence in her routine. She also increased the amount of time she spent in leisure and in role-related activities.

Sally in Perspective

When Sally was preparing for discharge from the program and discussing her progress with her therapist, she identified the following as important to her. First, Sally felt that she had learned in therapy how to give herself permission to enjoy life. Previously, she had been so dominated by feelings that she could not adequately respond to others' needs (especially her family) that she could not allow herself opportunity to seek enjoyment. This added to her sense that her life was out of her control. By reclaiming her right to find satisfaction in her occupational participation, she not only increased enjoyment in her life, but also took control of it again. A second major area of concern for Sally had been her general anxiety over being out of control that was reflected in her everyday routines. By reorganizing her habits, Sally was much more able to fulfill roles by still controlling her pain and fatigue. According to Sally, her life felt like it was back in control and had a degree of order, which she needed. Finally, Sally had begun to see the future with a sense of hope. At the time of discharge, she had not made final plans but was actively exploring alternative scenarios for her future occupational narrative.

Conclusion

This chapter presented four cases in which MOHO was used as a complement to other models of practice. As noted throughout this text, MOHO will often be used in combination with other models. MOHO readily complements models that focus on the motor, sensory, perceptual, and cognitive aspects of performance capacity. These cases illustrate that MOHO can be particularly useful in:

- Identifying when progress in change in performance capacity is being affected by factors such as volition and the environment
- Suggesting alterative ways of thinking about what to do with a client when there are limits to improvements that can be achieved in performance capacity

- Offering enriched perspectives for how to go about achieving change in performance capacity.

The cases in this chapter illustrate that models of practice are not simply used side by side with one model illuminating one set of problems and an another model illuminating other problems. Rather, the concepts from the models work in synergy to provide a deepened appreciation of key problems and challenges for a client.

References

Abreu, B. C., & Toglia, J. P. (1987). Cognitive rehabilitation: A model for occupational therapy. *American Journal of Occupational Therapy 41,* 439.

Ayres, A. J. (1979). *Sensory integration and the child.* Los Angeles: Western Psychological Services.

Benbow, M. (1990). *Loops and other groups.* Tucson, AZ: Therapy Skill Builders.

Fisher, A., Murray, E., & Bundy, A. (Eds.). (1991). *Sensory integration: Theory and practice.* Philadelphia: FA Davis.

Helfrich, C., & Kielhofner, G. (1994). Volitional narratives and the meaning of therapy. *American Journal of Occupational Therapy, 48,* 319–326.

Katz, N. (1992). *Cognitive rehabilitation: Models for inter-vention in occupational therapy.* Boston: Andover Medical Publishers.

Kielhofner, G. (1997). *Conceptual foundations of occupational therapy.* Philadelphia: FA Davis.

Kielhofner, G., & Fisher, A..G. (1991). Mind-brain-body relationships. In A. G. Fisher, E. A. Murray, & A. C. Bundy (Eds.), *Sensory integration: Theory and practice.* Philadelphia: FA Davis.

Mathiowetz, V., & Haugen, J. B. (1994). Motor behavior research: Implications for therapeutic approaches to central nervous system dysfunction. *American Journal of Occupational Therapy, 48,* 733–745.

Trombly, C. (1995). *Occupational therapy for physical dysfunction* (4th ed.). Philadelphia: FA Davis.

IV

Program Development, Research, and Further Resources

Introduction to Section IV

This final section of the book includes two chapters. It also provides information about additional resources that can be accessed by persons interested in learning more or finding out the latest about MOHO theory, research, and application.

Chapter 26 discusses how MOHO can guide the program development process. Three examples of programs developed in the United States, Canada, and Chile are provided. The chapter is also a resource for understanding how a conceptual practice model is used in program development. The examples illustrate different ways that MOHO can be used to create programs in both institutional and community-based settings.

Chapter 27 discusses MOHO-based research. This chapter begins by providing an overview about why research is important to a conceptual practice model and what types of research are typically undertaken to examine and develop a model. Then, the types of research that have been completed on MOHO are discussed and exemplified through brief presentations of studies. A comprehensive bibliography of published research with brief study abstracts is contained at the end of the chapter. This chapter is a detailed resource for anyone who wishes to understand the research base of MOHO and anyone who is considering undertaking research related to MOHO.

The next part of this section is a guide to the Model of Human Occupation Clearinghouse Web site. The clearinghouse was established a number of years ago to serve as a repository of information on MOHO and to distribute information related to the model. The web site is one of the key elements of the clearinghouse. It provides a range of up-to-date information and resources. As noted in this guide, there is also a MOHO listserv that can be an excellent vehicle for discussion of MOHO. Educators, researchers, and practitioners from throughout the world belong to the listserv and regularly contribute to discussing issues and questions raised by members. A final resource is a comprehensive MOHO bibliography. The bibliography contains English language articles, books, and chapters that discuss MOHO. The body of more than 220 citations is constantly growing. This bibliography is updated monthly, and a current bibliography can be found on the web site.

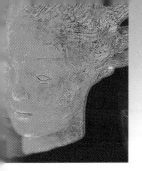

26

Program Development

- **Brent Braveman**
- **Gary Kielhofner**
- **René Bélanger**
- **Carmen Gloria de las Heras**
- **Veronica Llerena**

The contexts in which occupational therapists work have become progressively complex and demanding. There is increased pressure and scrutiny by consumers, employers, third-party payers, and accrediting bodies to provide high-quality services that are effective and provided at the lowest possible cost. As a result, therapists must be able to propose, create, implement, and evaluate service programs that are efficient and effective.

Program development refers to creating and evaluating an approach to service delivery for a defined client group. Developing a program involves such things as:

- Specifying clients' needs for occupational therapy
- Indicating the aims or intended outcomes of the program
- Providing a rationale for and detailing the kinds of services that will be included
- Establishing the steps, stages, or processes involved in clients' progression through the program
- Determining how the program will be evaluated.

Completing these and other aspects of developing a program of services can be greatly enhanced when one makes explicit use of a conceptual practice model. A model can enable the program development process by providing:

- A theoretical context for framing client problems and for conceptualizing the services and their intended impact

- Empirical evidence to back claims about the relevance and likely impact of services
- Assessments for use in client evaluation and in determining the outcomes of the program
- Protocols of service that can be emulated or adapted in the proposed program.

This chapter focuses on how therapists can use MOHO to develop occupational therapy programs. It briefly overviews the steps of program development to provide a context for discussion. Readers looking for in-depth guidance about the steps involved in developing a program are encouraged to use existing resources with that focus (Braveman, 2001; Braveman, Sen, & Kielhofner, 2001; Brownson, 2001; Youngstrom, 1999).

Program Development Process

Discussions of program development in the occupational therapy literature (Brownson 2001; Grossman & Bortone, 1986; Youngstrom, 1999) propose similar steps and associated tasks. Building on these works and, for the purposes of discussion here, the basic steps of program development include:

- Needs assessment
- Program planning
- Program implementation
- Program evaluation.

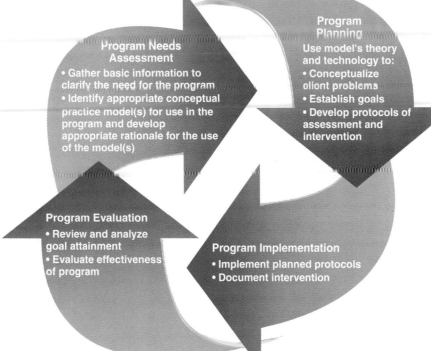

FIGURE 26-1   The Process of Program Development.

As shown in *Figure 26-1*, these steps are part of an ongoing process that involves constantly evaluating and improving how the program meets client's needs by offering the most relevant and effective services. The components of each step identified in Figure 26-1 are those that most pertain to selecting, creating a rationale for, and implementing a conceptual practice model. This chapter does not focus on financial, logistical, or organizational aspects of program development, which are also essential to a successful program.

As Figure 26-1 shows, the first step of program development includes selecting and creating the rationale for the model(s) that will inform and shape each subsequent step. Therefore, it is important to determine that one has selected the appropriate model(s) to address clients' needs. Selecting and justifying the conceptual practice model(s) can be facilitated when one reflectively addresses key questions along the way.

Questions to Guide Selecting and Justifying a Conceptual Practice Model

Program development requires active reasoning. In fact, there are parallels between the therapeutic reasoning process discussed in Chapter 11 and program development. The main difference is that the former is concerned with a single client, whereas the latter addresses an entire client group.

This section poses and discusses a series of questions to guide thinking about the model(s) one selects and uses in program development. Answering these questions can:

- Shape the initial choice of the appropriate conceptual practice model(s) for a program
- Validate the choice as the program development process unfolds
- Generate a thorough rationale for the model(s) selected.

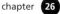

> - *Does the model specify the underlying mechanisms of action necessary to deal with the occupational problems and challenges faced by the client group?*
> - *Is there sufficient evidence to support application of the model to the client group and the occupational problems that they experience?*
> - *Does the model fit with the social, cultural, political, professional, or financial contexts in which the program must be implemented?*
> - *Does implementation of programming based on the model have any special requirements for space, equipment, or personnel?*

Question 1: Does the Model Specify the Underlying Mechanisms of Action Necessary to Deal with the Occupational Problems and Challenges Faced by the Client Group?

When developing a program, it is important to specify how the services included will achieve changes to address the client's problem and challenges. Therefore, one must consider the underlying mechanism(s) of action of an intervention (Gitlin et al., 2000). The **mechanism of action** refers to the theoretical and empirical account of how a particular change occurs as a consequence of participating in an intervention. The mechanism of action should delineate:

- How change proceeds
- Conditions under which an intervention achieves beneficial results
- Why a change may occur for certain groups of participants and not others.

A conceptual practice model provides the structure for identifying specific pathways by which interventions may function.

Sometimes more than one model may be chosen because a single model does not adequately address all the necessary mechanisms of action. Consider, for example, a program for persons with head injury that is designed to address problems of motivation, occupational lifestyle, and impairments of performance capacity due to neurologic impairments. MOHO would provide accounts for how motivation and lifestyle change through the concepts and propositions associated with volition and habituation. However, it would not provide sufficient guidance for structuring aspects of intervention meant to remediate neurologic impairments of performance capacity. In such an instance, MOHO must be used in conjunction with another conceptual practice model that more specifically addresses the mechanisms of action related to facilitate change in nervous system functioning.

Question 2: Is There Sufficient Evidence to Support Application of the Model to the Client Group and the Occupational Problems that They Experience?

Those who receive and pay for occupational therapy services increasingly expect that occupational therapy practice will be evidence-based. **Evidence-based practice** refers to conscientiously, explicitly, and systematically using available evidence in deciding the kinds of services that will be provided to individuals (Sackett, Rosenberg, Gray, Haynes, & Richardson, 1996). Before basing programming on a conceptual practice model, one must be sure that there is evidence to support its use with the target client group. Such evidence may exist in the literature. It may reflect others' experience in using the model with a similar client group. Sometimes it is generated through pilot work that precedes developing the program.

Excellent resources to guide practitioners in finding and evaluating published evidence are now available (Holm, 2000; Taylor, 2000). Basically, evidence-based practice involves considering whether:

- Others have successfully used the model with the target client group
- Others have successfully used the model to address the same kinds of problems faced by the target client group
- There is evidence that the model is effective with the target client group or with the kinds of problems faced by the target group.

Whereas not all these criteria may be met, there should be some form of evidence that the model will be relevant to and potentially effective for the target client group.

A variety of resources exist for therapists who are considering the use of MOHO for program development. As will be discussed in Chapter 27, there is a substantial research base. Moreover, a wide range of programs using MOHO has been described in the literature. These include, for example, programs for such diverse clients groups as those with chronic pain (Gusich, 1984; Padilla & Bianchi, 1990), traumatic brain injury (DePoy, 1990), Alzheimer's dementia (Oakley, 1987; Olin, 1985), acquired immune deficiency syndrome (AIDS) (Pizzi, 1984, 1989, 1990a, 1990b; Schindler, 1988), and borderline personality disorder (Salz, 1983). MOHO has guided programs for persons who are homeless and mentally ill (Kavanaugh & Fares, 1995), for battle-fatigued soldiers (Gerardi, 1996), for emotionally disturbed children and adolescents (Reekmans & Kielhofner, 1998; Sholle-Martin, 1987; Weissenberg & Giladi, 1989), and for children with attention deficit hyperactivity disorder (Woodrum, 1993). Moreover, there have been MOHO-based programs described for a range of specific contexts, such as a day hospital (Gusich & Silverman, 1991), a work rehabilitation program (Mentrup, Niehaus, & Kielhofner, 1999), prison and correctional settings (Michael, 1991; Schindler, 1990), and early intervention contexts (Schaaf & Mulrooney, 1989).

The MOHO bibliography presented at the end of Section IV is a useful resource for identifying publications relevant to a specific target group or context. These publications are often valuable not only because they provide some evidence about others' experiences in using MOHO, but they also provide a wealth of ideas and strategies for building a program for a given client group or context. Additionally, the MOHO Clearinghouse distributes manuals with detailed program protocols. Finally, the MOHO listserv is an excellent resource for communicating with others who have relevant program development experiences. The bibliography is maintained in updated form, and information about the manuals and listserv may be found on the MOHO Web site. Information on the Web site is provided at the end of Section IV on page 556.

Question 3: Does the Model Fit with the Social, Cultural, Political, Professional, or Financial Contexts in Which the Program Must Be Implemented?

In selecting a conceptual practice model, one must consider whether contextual factors will support or hinder developing the kind of programming necessary to implement the model. For example, reimbursement or funding for the program might limit the type, frequency, or intensity of intervention, influencing how a model can be implemented in a given context. Cultural groups with particular values or expectations may influence how the program can be delivered and whether the concepts of a model are relevant to their concerns. The theories and approaches used by other professionals in the program or in the larger context may or may not be compatible with a particular model. Consideration of such factors can both assure that one selects a model that fits with the context and takes necessary action to introduce the model appropriately to the context.

Question 4: Does Implementation of Programming Based on the Model Have any Special Requirements for Space, Equipment, or Personnel?

Before proceeding with program development, practitioners should be aware of the resources required to adequately implement an effective program based on the chosen model. A conceptual practice model may have implications for such things as space, equipment, personnel, or training. For example, MOHO stresses the importance of doing therapy using culturally relevant occupational forms and, when possible, natural contexts for intervention. This may mean creating the organizational structure and resources for making a range of meaningful occupational forms and social groups available.

Another consideration is whether therapists have adequate training and knowledge to implement a model. Moreover, one needs to ask whether assessments or necessary client written materials are available that fit the setting (e.g., will they need to be adapted or translated to suit the language/culture of the clients). Thinking about such issues helps to anticipate the necessary resources and activities for implementing a model successfully.

Three Examples of Program Development

The following sections provide three examples of the authors' experiences using MOHO to develop occupational therapy programming. The first example is Employment Options, a vocational rehabilitation program for clients living with AIDS. This program was developed with federal grant funding and its aim was to create, study, and disseminate a model service. The second example is Reencuentros, a community-based day program in Santiago, Chile. This private occupational therapy program serves clients with a range of diagnoses who have difficulties with occupational life. The third example is Programme Spécifique d'Intervention, Premier Épisode (PSI), (Specific Intervention Program, First Episode). PSI was developed at the Hôtel-Dieu de Lévis Hospital in Quebec City, Quebec, Canada. This program offers specialized and integrated services for young clients with schizophrenia. Occupational therapy services are an essential component of this interdisciplinary program.

In each of these instances, using MOHO provided a systematic basis for such things as:

- Providing a rationale for why the program is needed or for why it should be organized in a particular way
- Informing constituencies about the components of a program and how they are intended to work
- Convincing others of the value of investing in the program or including one's concepts and approaches in the program.

Each of the three programs initially had to address lack of knowledge or skepticism about occupational therapy services. To develop these programs successfully, the trust and confidence of multiple constituencies had to be gained. Although MOHO was not a guarantee of success, it provided a variety of resources that ultimately helped to shape each program's success.

The following sections describe each program, following the four basic steps of program development shown in Figure 26-1. The discussion focuses on those aspects of each program that demonstrate how MOHO was used and what its contributions were to the nature and success of the program.

Example 1: Employment Options

In 1997, the Department of Occupational Therapy at University of Illinois at Chicago approached Howard Brown Health Center (HBHC), a community-based health center serving Chicago's gay and lesbian population, to explore whether occupational therapy services may benefit HBHC clients. There were no occupational therapy services and very little knowledge about occupational therapy at the center.

The staff at HBHC asked whether occupational therapy could provide services for an increasing number of their clients with AIDS who were expressing interest in returning to work. Some of these clients had previously developed serious symptoms and received the recommendation to leave their jobs and receive private or public disability to assure adequate medical coverage until their deaths. Other clients, who were unemployed when diagnosed with AIDS, were not encouraged to pursue employment, given their prognoses. However, new pharmacologic treatments had substantially decreased HIV-related mortality rates while improving health and function, making consideration of work possible for these clients (Feinberg, 1996; Hogg et al., 1997).

Program Needs Assessment

To gain a clearer understanding of their needs, a survey was conducted on 55 HBHC clients. The average respondent was 38 years old and last employed 3.5 years earlier. Eighty-two percent of respondents had already discussed returning to work with their case managers, although none had yet returned to any form of employment.

Respondents identified a number of important barriers to re-entering the workplace, including uncertainty over whether:

- Their functional capacity was adequate
- Working might negatively impact their health status
- They could maintain the routine of full-time employment

- Returning to work might negatively affect their health insurance benefits or future eligibility for disability income.

In addition, most respondents described experiencing significant inertia secondary to prolonged illness and interruption of work. They also voiced concerns about how to address the gap in their employment history, facing prejudice because of their AIDS diagnosis, and how workplaces would react to their need to manage ongoing symptoms and complex medication regimens.

Since the issues raised by these clients are addressed by MOHO concepts, a pilot program of vocational services based on MOHO was developed and implemented at HBHC with funding from the National Aids Fund. Twenty clients were enrolled in the pilot program that included group education sessions and individual occupational therapy. More than 40% of members of the pilot program returned to work within 5 months, and a waiting list soon developed for the program. It became clear that an ongoing service was needed for this client group. Moreover, the pilot program provided evidence that the kind of program envisioned had potential to meet the needs of the clients for vocational services. At the same time, it was clear from communication with other agencies throughout the country that the situation at HBHC reflected a national trend of persons with AIDS wanting services to assist them to return to work. The Department of Occupational Therapy at UIC and HBHC agreed to enter into a partnership to seek federal funding for a large demonstration program.

Rationale for Selecting MOHO

To obtain federal funding in a research and demonstration grant competition, it was necessary to articulate and justify to an interdisciplinary audience why and how MOHO was to be used as the conceptual practice model for the program. Because of previous applications of MOHO at UIC and elsewhere, it was possible to document that MOHO had been:

- Applied to the study of injured/disabled workers (Azhar, 1996; Corner, Kielhofner, & Lin, 1997; Corner, Kielhofner, & Olson, 1998; Kielhofner & Brinson, 1989; Mallinson, 1995; Munoz & Kielhofner, 1995; Olson, 1995; Salz, 1983; Velozo, Kielhofner, & Fisher, 1998)

- Used for more than a decade to design work-related rehabilitation programs (Mallinson, 1998; Olson, 1998)
- Used to incorporate variables that had been shown to predict success in return to work (Braveman, 1999)
- Applied to rehabilitation services for persons with HIV/AIDS (Pizzi, 1989, 1990a, 1990b; Schindler, 1988, 1990).

These previous applications of MOHO for clients with AIDS and for addressing return to work issues, together with data from the pilot study, were used to justify MOHO as the model for the proposed program. This argument was also complemented by a demonstration that MOHO could effectively be used to conceptualize the problems and needs of the clients and how they would be addressed in the program.

Conceptualizing the Client Group from a MOHO Perspective

The following is a brief overview of how MOHO was used to conceptualize the factors that would influence work success of persons with AIDS. Data from several sources—including the HBHC survey, the pilot study, literature review, and information from HBHC case managers—were used to inform this conceptualization. *Table 26-1* summarizes these factors and shows them in relationship to program goals that will be discussed later.

Volition

The target client group was extremely diverse in culture, socioeconomic status, educational background, and work history. Consequently, the role of work in these persons' lives and the identity that they had formed as workers were also extremely diverse. Many persons living with AIDS whose functional capacity had increased through new medications expressed a desire to return to being self-sufficient and productive. They missed the stimulation, challenges, and feelings of positive self-esteem they experienced at work. Despite their desires for work, most were unsure of their capacity for and had a limited sense of efficacy for returning to work. Many felt they could no longer handle the stress of their former jobs and wondered what new form of work might interest and be meaningful to

TABLE 26-1 MOHO-Based Conceptualization of Factors Influencing Vocational Success of Persons Living with AIDS and Corresponding Program Services

	Factors Influencing Vocational Success of Persons Living with AIDS	Employment Options Program Services
Personal Factors	**Volition** • Lack of or need to change work-related interests • Concerns about personal capacity for work and impact of work on health status • Concerns about coping with challenges (e.g., disclosure) • Concerns for optimizing values (i.e., being productive, economic sustenance, maintaining health)	• Self assessment of work interests • Assessment/review of functional capacity • Training and group sessions on coping in the workplace • Economic counseling, benefits management • Peer mentoring and support
	Habituation • Long-term work role disruption • Identification with work versus sick role • Challenges of role transitions • Absence of a functional routine • Routine requirements for managing illness	• Opportunity to reacquire a productive role though volunteer positions, internships, and temporary work experiences • Job coaching to facilitate adjustment to worker role • Structured program schedule to support development of a functional routine
	Performance Capacity • Impairments related to disease, symptoms, and drug side effects • Limited motor, process, and communication/interaction skills	• Support client in identification and request for reasonable accommodations • Skill-building group sessions, volunteer positions, internships and temporary work placement, job coaching, and referral for job training
Environmental Factors	**Workplace** • Negative attitudes/prejudice toward persons with AIDS • Reluctance to accommodate to the challenges of a worker with chronic disability	• Education/consultation for potential/actual employers of clients • Offering employers the National AIDS Fund's "A Positive Workplace" training program (Breuer, 1997)
	Community • Lack of peer network and social support for work • Negative influence of drugs, crime, and poverty • Complicated system of health and social policy	• On the Job Club (drop-in availability for clients to socialize with other clients and program staff) • Determination of economic benefit/impact of returning to work along with counseling and advocacy to ensure continuous medical benefits

them. Others, with sporadic work records and histories of relying on public assistance, had never developed strong vocational interests, succeeded in establishing a stable work career, or found meaning in work.

Regardless of background, most shared fears about whether working would negatively influence their health status. They worried about the impact that returning to work would have on their social and health benefits, especially given the costly nature of their life-sustaining medications. They were apprehensive about how peers or supervisors would relate to them and their illness. All these factors strongly influenced whether they would make the occupational choice to work.

HABITUATION

Clients' work histories varied tremendously, as did their development of worker roles. Many clients had limited experience and were in the second or third generation of their family who had relied on public assistance. Even clients who had successful work histories had spent significant time in the sick role, which made return to work a difficult role transition. All clients had to face and overcome the barrier of inconsistent work histories or gaps in employment that affected their public identities as workers. Clients in established relationships with partners or families had to renegotiate roles with significant others who had already made substantial sacrifices to accommodate their illnesses.

Clients faced the challenge of overcoming the inertia of habitual inactivity and reinstituting a routine to support working. Clients who had been habituated to nonproductive lifestyles complicated by drug habits faced achieving a productive routine for the first time. The challenge of instituting productive habits was complicated by ongoing symptoms, drug side effects, impairments, and needs to maintain a medication routine.

PERFORMANCE CAPACITY

As noted previously, it was the resurgence of capacity for many persons with AIDS that opened the possibility for returning to work. Nonetheless, many persons had some ongoing impairments. Many experienced periodic illness and medication side effects such as nausea and diarrhea. A common problem, fatigue, was complicated by deconditioning due to prolonged illness and inactivity. Some had neuropathies and mild cognitive impairments.

Together, these underlying impairments and symptoms adversely affected clients' motor and process skills. Many clients lacked the communication/interaction skills required in nearly any form of employment. These limitations were complicated by the fact that entering the workplace as a person with AIDS posed its own special interpersonal challenges. Persons faced the issues of disclosure, dealing with stigma and prejudice, and the need to negotiate accommodations. Those with poor work histories lacked knowledge and abilities for any specific type of work.

ENVIRONMENT

The context of the workplace could present attitudinal and other barriers to return to work (Weitz, 1990). Although many of the clients were not visibly disabled, they had to disclose their HIV status to request the reasonable accommodations they required to successfully maintain a worker role. By disclosing their HIV status, they increased the visibility of their disease and hence risked the discrimination associated with the stigma of AIDS.

Other contextual factors were community and organizational challenges. Many persons had lost touch with working peers and lacked support networks for work. For many persons, the neighborhood presence of drugs, crime, and poverty were potential barriers to achieving self-sufficient lifestyles (Billingsley, 1988; Stack, 1974). While facing these hurdles, persons with AIDS had to navigate a jungle of poorly coordinated systems and service agencies that sometimes functioned at cross-purposes, creating disincentives to self-sufficiency and work.

Program Planning

Once MOHO was used to conceptualize the occupational problems faced by the target client group, it was possible to specify mechanisms of action, that is, to spell out how services would address client problems and how they would contribute to clients' successful return to work. Table 26-1 shows the factors just discussed that influence vocational success and the corresponding program services designed to address each factor. After identifying these program services, it was necessary to consider how they would be organized and sequenced in the program.

The program was organized in four phases to support clients moving through a continuum of development of volition, habituation, and performance capacity. Each of these stages also had different implications for the kind of environments in which service would take place and the kinds of supports clients needed. *Figure 26-2* shows the four phases of the program that are briefly described in the following sections.

PHASE 1

Clients were initially screened to establish appropriateness of the program for them and to determine neces-

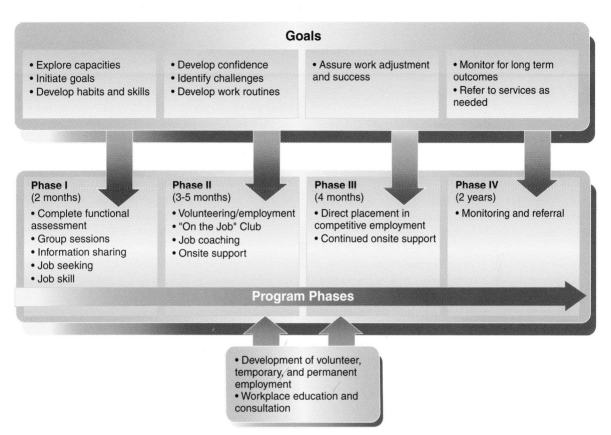

FIGURE 26-2 Continuum of Employment Options Services.

sary problem solving and resources to support program attendance (e.g., child care, transportation). On entry into the program, the client participated in a comprehensive assessment process including:

- The Occupational Performance History Interview-Version 2.0 (OPHI-II)
- The Worker Role Interview (WRI)
- The Occupational Self Assessment (OSA)
- The Assessment of Communication and Interaction Skills (ACIS)
- A fatigue scale.

These evaluations were used in such a way that the therapist and client together formed an appreciation of the client's potential for work and individual needs for services to support return to work.

During this phase, clients also attended individual and group sessions designed to help them explore and develop both work skills and the daily habits needed to support a vocational role. Group sessions included:

- Self-assessment exercises
- Vocational planning exercises
- Information sharing related to economics, benefits, the Americans with Disabilities Act (ADA), and other logistics of return to work
- Job search and job skill development exercises
- Peer support groups
- Work task experiences.

Individual therapy sessions addressed each client's unique needs.

The aim of phase 1, which lasted 8 weeks, was to provide:

- An opportunity for self-assessment and strengthening and refinement of vocational choice

- A structured routine to develop habits of promptness, consistency, and a commitment to the program
- A forum for sharing critical information about returning to work
- A community of emotional support for return to work
- A context wherein factors that impact on work readiness were identified and addressed
- Opportunities to develop job-relevant skills.

PHASE 2

During this phase, the client began participation in volunteer work, an internship, or placement in temporary employment. These opportunities were developed by partnering with businesses in Chicago and were planned to be part-time and combined with continued participation in some components of the group program outlined in phase 1. The duration and intensity of this phase were variable and adjusted to the clients' needs, but typically ranged from 1 to 3 months.

This phase of the program was designed to assist clients to develop confidence in their ability to manage the routine of working. During this phase, the OSA was repeated with clients to allow for self-assessment in this new phase of change and to identify further individualized goals.

This phase was also designed to allow clients to face and cope with the challenges associated with working with a chronic disability. Each work, training, or volunteer placement was designed so that clients received assessment and feedback concerning job performance. Project staff worked closely with the volunteer or work supervisor in these placements to assure that the client was receiving appropriate supervision and to support the supervisor in responding to any challenges.

PHASE 3

In this phase, clients were placed in paid jobs developed by the project or were assisted by project staff to apply for and secure employment. Job analysis and adaptation, as well as on-site job coaching of the client, were provided as needed. Each client participated in the Work Environment Impact Scale at this stage to assess how the work context was influencing the client's performance and well-being. Information gained from this interview was used to assist the client in making personal adjustments to the workplace and in requesting reasonable accommodations.

In addition, employer education, consultation, and trouble-shooting support for the supervisor and coworkers of the client were provided. Clients in this phase could still take advantage of individual meetings with project staff for ongoing support and training. The intensity and duration of this phase varied, but was planned to average 4 months.

PHASE 4

This phase consisted of long-term follow-up and support. Because AIDS is a chronic condition and periods of illness or functional limitation may occur, it was considered important that project staff be able to intervene and provide support as needed. Consequently, ongoing contact and periodic support through group meetings with others and/or with staff was to be maintained.

Program Implementation

The plan of the program as discussed above was developed as part of the proposal that was funded as a national research and demonstration project for 3 years by the U.S. Department of Education's Rehabilitation Services Administration.[a] Following funding, implementation of Employment Options required developing the specifics of the program, identifying and training appropriate staff, and coordinating and documenting activities to facilitate program evaluation.

As the program was implemented, two occupational therapists already familiar with MOHO were hired. They were provided with training and education to assure their competence in using MOHO concepts and assessments. For example, one staff member was already certified in the Assessment of Motor and Process Skills, but the second one had to receive training and certification. Early in the project the therapists presented cases and received supervision from the first two authors of this chapter. A third key member, the vocational placement specialist, was not an occupational therapist. Therefore, specific efforts were made throughout the program planning and implementation to orient her to MOHO and its constructs. As she

---

[a]Employment Options: Grant #H235A980170, Rehabilitation Services Administration, U.S. Department of Education.

became more familiar with how clients were conceptualized from the perspective of MOHO and occupational therapy, she was able to provide helpful observations about the clients that related to key concepts of MOHO. For example, she was able to postulate how a particular client's inaccurate knowledge of capacity, poor sense of self-efficacy, and lack of structured habits and routines acted in combination to prevent the client from following through on recommendations she made. With time, the entire team functioned as a whole to assure optimal implementation of MOHO-based strategies.

Program Evaluation

Since this program was funded specifically to investigate its process and outcomes, an extensive program evaluation was designed. It included both a qualitative study of the program implementation and a quantitative study of outcomes. The qualitative component took place within the framework of participatory action research (PAR), a strategy for conducting research that involves persons being studied to be involved in all phases of research that affects them (NIDRR, 1995). Data collection for this evaluation ranged from simple strategies, such as conducting client evaluations after every group session to obtain client feedback, to more complicated strategies, such as conducting periodic interviews with clients and their case managers. This component of the program evaluation allowed staff to constantly improve services to better meet the clients' needs. At this point, near the end of the 3 years, the program has been refined and is being prepared as a manual for dissemination to those who wish to replicate the program.

The second element of the program evaluation was to determine the impact of the program on clients. To this end, data were collected throughout the project on the following outcome indicators:
- Percentage of program clients who returned to volunteer work or internships
- Percentage of clients who entered formal education or vocational training programs
- Percentage of clients who returned to part-time or full-time paid employment
- Percentage of clients who chose not to return to work but reported increased satisfaction with their life routines and occupational performance.

At the time of this writing, the Employment Options program is in the final stage of implementation. Based on evolving results, it appears that approximately 80% of clients who completed the program will achieve employment. A local agency serving people living with AIDS was so impressed with the program that it has hired its first full-time occupational therapist, who is implementing programming that includes all the components of the Employment Options Program.

While there were very positive outcomes from clients who completed the program, approximately 28% of initially enrolled clients dropped out of the program within the first 8 weeks because they lacked the prerequisite volitional and habituation strengths to consistently attend the program. Therefore, program evaluation also focused on examining this client group in detail to see why the program was not meeting their needs. This subgroup tended to be persons whose life situations were even further complicated by cumulative effects of poverty, homelessness, mental illness, and histories of substance abuse.

This information led to beginning the cycle of program development again, this time leading to a proposal for a program based in residential, supportive living settings where many of these types of clients reside. Once again MOHO was used to conceptualize the needs and the kinds of services that might effectively address them. In the proposed program, components of Employment Options were combined with additional services and resources that would be needed to allow these more severely disabled clients to participate and benefit.

Example 2: Reencuentros

Seven years ago, in Santiago, Chile, at the end of a presentation for persons with schizophrenia, several attendees asked the speaker, an occupational therapist, if she would help them develop a self-help group. Over time, the therapist worked with these and other clients to plan, organize, and obtain a government-funded community center. Pressure from family members who were uncomfortable with their relatives with severe mental illness being in a program aimed at community integration resulted in the program being redirected to become a sheltered workshop. Disappointed with the program change, the majority of clients approached the occupational therapist, with the request that she help develop a new, independent center. Without funds or any other resources, the therapist and clients began to work together to develop what would become a private, community-based day program, Reencuentros (Reencounters).

Needs Assessment

Because a private program had to rely on self-pay and insurance for income, Reencuentros was designed for adolescents, adults, and elders primarily from the middle and upper class in Santiago. The program's clients were still predominantly persons with mental illness. However, the program broadened its intake to include clients who were facing occupational challenges or problems for any reason. For example, the program has served clients with impairments that range from visual impairments, neurologic and other physical disabilities, as well as vocational and familial crises precipitated by environmental conditions.

A common denominator of all the clients was that they needed:

- A sense of social belonging
- Support for being self-directed
- Opportunities to participate in meaningful occupation.

The founding occupational therapist chose to base Reencuentros on a combination of the Clubhouse Model (Flannery, Glickman, Fuller, & Torrey, 1996) and MOHO.

The Clubhouse Model includes the following tenets:

- The Clubhouse belongs to clients who take on active roles in shaping what it is
- All clients are made to feel that their presence is expected daily and is important
- Clients participate together with staff in a cooperative effort to design all program components
- The Clubhouse satisfies the basic human need to be needed and to be an important part of a group.

While the Clubhouse Model provided organizational framework for the program, MOHO provided the concepts, tools, and strategies for designing the content of the program's services, including the:

- Types of assessments used
- Opportunities for client occupational engagement that would be provided
- Strategies to be used by therapists
- Overall process by which clients achieved the change necessary to reach individual goals.

The Clubhouse Model and MOHO complemented each other, resulting in a comprehensive and client-centered program for community integration.

Conceptualizing the Client Group from a MOHO Perspective

All clients at Reencuentros share a common occupational problem: a lack of occupational adaptation following disruption of participation in occupational roles such as worker, family member, self-maintainer, and friend. MOHO enabled a conceptualization of the factors contributing to the breakdown of occupational adaptation that guides the program at Reencuentros. This conceptualization is briefly discussed in the following sections.

VOLITION

Clients' volitional problems stemmed from debilitating symptoms of mental illness and other impairments and from experiences of failure in significant life roles. Many adolescents, for example, had faced ridicule or rejection by peers in classroom settings or had been so sheltered by parents that they lacked a realistic sense of their capabilities. Although they longed to have satisfying peer interaction and to test their independence, they were often hindered by fear of failure or rejection. Some adults had been successful workers before their illness and wished to return to more productive lives. Still others, who were most severely affected by illness, struggled to cope with lost roles and the need to identify new interests and alternatives for participation. For all, uncertainty about personal capacity and the need to discover or rediscover strengths and limitations in various environmental contexts was central.

HABITUATION

Most clients had experienced a severe loss of roles or had never developed meaningful role patterns in their lives. Many were struggling to maintain a basic family member role, having lost roles in the larger community context such as worker or student. They also struggled with the need to identify social groups and to build friendships in the community. Many adults who previously had a worker role faced the challenge of adjusting to changes in performance capacity. Often, they needed training in a different, less demanding job. Adolescents needed to explore the options of returning to a student role or pursuing skill development toward a worker role.

All clients had problems with habits. Most faced the need to create new daily routines. For some people this meant finding a better balance of occupational participation. For others it meant overcoming years of unstructured, passive daily living.

PERFORMANCE CAPACITY AND SKILL

The range of capacities among clients was wide. Although most had sufficient motor skills to perform their daily routines, many had severely limited process and communication/interaction skills. Some individuals were incapable of verbal communication beyond the most basic monosyllabic answers to questions. Others were extremely articulate verbally, but lacked other skills which often hindered their social acceptance. Process skill limitations, for some, meant they could only perform tasks with a maximum of three steps.

ENVIRONMENTAL CONTEXTS

Clients varied in their exposure to environmental contexts. Some had a wide variety of past experience in community roles, while others had never spent time away from their homes and families. Some struggled to simply find a place for themselves in their homes. This was often complicated by the family's misconception that the client was incapable of contributing to the family. In some circumstances, families struggled to understand and accept the new limitations the client now faced. In both circumstances, family expectations were unmatched with the client's actual potential to play a role in this social sphere.

Most clients had at least some difficulty functioning outside the home. Consequently, they needed supports within each new environment where they hoped to participate. Due to the level of impairment for many individuals, they were often poorly understood and stigmatized in the community.

Program Planning

Reencuentros' professional staff consisted of five full-time occupational therapists. A bookkeeper and an artist were also contracted part-time. In keeping with the Clubhouse philosophy, the professional staff together with clients shared responsibility for initially planning the program. As Reencuentros continues to evolve, staff and clients work together to plan how the program can be improved.

In keeping with MOHO, Reencuentros was designed to address the challenges faced by its clients by creating a dynamic context that allowed individuals to develop interests, values, a sense of capacity and efficacy, roles, habits, and skills. It was envisioned that clients would come to Reencuentros during the day, dividing their time among the center's components. The components, which are discussed later, evolved to constitute a dynamic and integrated group milieu within which each client's unique needs are met. While clients would begin their occupational engagement within Reencuentros, they would gradually extend it to other contexts with support of the program. Consequently, Reencuentros was designed as a transitional facility, acting as a stepping-stone for individuals to reintegrate into their homes and community in ways suited to their capacities and personal desires.

An important part of the planning was to select a site for the program. Reencuentros is located in a large rented house in a pleasant Santiago neighborhood within walking distance of many businesses and shops. The location was chosen because it created a context in which clients could begin to interact with the community in natural ways (e.g., purchasing needed supplies). Clients and staff worked together to organize, decorate, and fix up the house to their liking. This house provides the physical space for the majority of the Reencuentros programs.

Program Implementation

The occupational therapists at Reencuentros were initially trained by its founder in both MOHO and the Clubhouse Model. Overall program goals were established, and MOHO assessments to be used were translated into Spanish. Forms were created for documenting client participation and progress. Since Reencuentros is a comprehensive day program, a wide range of resources had to be created for ongoing operations.

As already noted, clients and staff worked together to design and implement the actual components of the program. These components evolved over time. Reencuentros currently consists of six interactive components that are discussed below. Together, these components create a dynamic environment of naturally occurring occupational forms and groups in which clients participate. Each component is discussed below.

PRACTICAL OCCUPATIONS

Practical occupations make up the largest program. They include tasks necessary to keep the center in working order, such as the administrative work in the office, cleaning and maintenance tasks, preparing lunch and snacks in the kitchen, and gardening. They also include creative projects such as painting, music, and creative writing. A carpentry shop, art room, computer lab, and library were created to support them. Many of the practical occupations are also designed to serve public relations and education purposes. For example, artistic exhibitions and presentations, educational workshops, and the two literary magazines produced at the center serve to provide information to the community at large about disability to reduce misconceptions and stigma about Reencuentros and its mission. Such efforts serve to better integrate Reencuentros and its members into the larger community.

Practical occupations occur simultaneously and allow individuals opportunities for choosing how to structure their daily routine according to their own needs and interests. For example, many of the administrative tasks, like banking errands, are done in the morning at the same time that lunch preparation takes place. Members chose which team, office or kitchen, they would participate in, and on what days. Similarly, theatre projects, art, and music are generally scheduled to overlap.

Clients are expected and supported to contribute to a group project to the extent they are able. For example, some members who come to the office are able to perform a variety of functions such as answering phones and running errands. Others with limited tolerance for social contact might work individually preparing pamphlets for an event. Regardless of what clients do, they are all regarded as valuable contributors.

Practical occupations also provide opportunities for all clients to:

- Develop commitment and responsibility
- Practice making decisions and solving problems
- Participate in diverse roles
- Develop new skills.

Moreover, each participant works on individual goals within practical occupations. For example, working in the kitchen might be a step toward reassuming the role of mother, learning an occupational form necessary to live independently, developing a new leisure interest, or preparing for a job in a restaurant.

One of the most important characteristics of the practical occupations at Reencuentros is that they present opportunities to genuinely contribute to the Reencuentros community. For example, the occupational forms performed in the office are necessary to assure that finances are in order, supplies are available, and organized records are kept. Filing, taking inventory, organizing cabinets, creating computer documents, and writing checks are examples of occupational forms necessary to maintain office functions. Moreover, roles are naturally created around office operations. For example, members take turns serving as receptionists.

In the same way, the kitchen involves occupational forms to assure that clients could eat lunch at the center every day. A team working in the kitchen has to plan a menu every Friday for the upcoming week. A daily trip to the grocery store is made to obtain needed ingredients. Along with preparing the food, the team also sets tables, serves food, and collects lunch money from clients. Roles around the necessary kitchen tasks include shoppers, cooks, waiters, and cashiers.

Other groups, like the musical group, are shaped by clients' interests and talents. The broad goal of this group is to communicate with the larger community by performing at children's homes, hospitals, and other locations. The group chooses which songs to practice, where they wish to perform, and other details. Within the group different roles are also assumed as members plan and carry out performances.

In sum, practical occupations are founded on real interests and needs of the center. They require collaboration of Reencuentros' clients while allowing flexibility in member participation through diverse roles. They allow creativity while still demanding that deadlines be met and necessary tasks performed. They require that members cooperate with one another. Finally, they produce tangible or visible results by which clients can judge their own individual and collective accomplishments.

INDIVIDUAL COUNSELING SESSIONS

The second component of the Reencuentros program is individual counseling provided by an occupational therapist. Counseling sessions allow the individual member and therapist to collaboratively examine the client's needs and progress. Clients are supported to reflect on their experiences and to identify strengths, weaknesses, and critical areas for development.

EDUCATIONAL AND VOCATIONAL PROGRAMS

This component supports members to assume satisfying roles in the larger community. Two separate group modules, one educational and one vocational, take place regularly and serve to facilitate clients' planning and problem-solving for pursuing educational or vocational goals. In the group modules, clients examine their own expectations, interests, and goals. They consider what demands they would face in work or school environments and how adequate their own habits and skills are for meeting those demands. In this way, they can set more realistic goals and/or plan to develop necessary skills and habits and take steps for achieving their educational and vocational goals.

Therapists facilitate these groups, and members serve as sources of information, ideas, and support for one another in the group. Each group has some standard components that are offered, such as sessions on study habits and note taking for school and sessions on interviewing and preparing resumes for work.

Along with the group modules, therapists meet with clients on an individual basis to evaluate, discuss, and plan how to accomplish each client's educational and/or vocational goals. Members ordinarily begin to address their goals through structured participation in practical occupations within Reencuentros. Later, they transition to participating in community businesses and agencies outside of Reencuentros.

EDUCATIONAL SELF-HELP AND PEER SUPPORT GROUPS

Self-help and peer support groups met every weekday at Reencuentros. These groups encourage peer contributions and are facilitated by staff members. Clients attend those groups that best met their needs. The groups deal with five general themes:

- Achieving personal goals
- Solving problems and making decisions
- Managing free time
- Improving social skills
- Maintaining healthy lifestyles.

FAMILY EDUCATION AND COUNSELING

Families of each client are offered individual family education to help support the client's progress. Families were oriented and educated in:

- Managing their family member's illness
- Developing realistic expectations about their family member's performance and participation
- Stress management
- Strategies for facilitating their family member's progress.

Sessions with each family take place according to family needs. Additionally, educational lectures and support groups are held for families once a month.

YOUNG PEOPLE'S CLUB

Adolescents and young adults in the program need to have a space where they can share ideas and support one another in keeping with cultural norms of youth. They created a special space in the garage where they met to plan projects, produce their literary magazine, and generate ideas.

Individualization of Client Services

MOHO stresses that each client's unique characteristics must be considered when deciding appropriate services. In keeping with this view, each new client initially works with a therapist to outline a plan to meet personal goals. This process begins with assessment. A wide range of MOHO assessments are used in Reencuentros. *Table 26-2* lists the assessments most frequently used and notes how they are ordinarily employed in the program. In addition to the formal assessments, a range of informal observation and interviewing are also used to continuously collect information on clients. Since therapists are in constant contact with clients individually or in groups during the day, they gain a wealth of information on clients.

TABLE 26-2 Formal Assessments Most Frequently Used at Reencuentros

Assessment	Use/Focus
Occupational Performance History Interview-Version 2.0 (OPHI-II)	Used as an initial assessment If a member is unable to self-report, interviews with family members are conducted
Occupational Self Assessment (OSA)	Used as part of an initial assessment battery and to guide the goal setting process Repeated throughout intervention
The Volitional Questionnaire (VQ)	Ordinarily used as an initial assessment Tool may also be taught to members who reach a level where they can self-monitor their own progress
Role Checklist	Often used in initial assessment
Assessment of Communication and Interaction Skills (ACIS)	Administered through observation of a social interaction mutually agreed on by the client and therapist Completed in a variety of contexts for each member as needed to indicate the client's skill in that context
Worker Role Interview (WRI)	Used as needed with members who wish to be employed in community settings
Work Environment Impact Scale (WEIS)	Used when members are working in the community

Which assessments are used and when they are used depends on each client's needs. Completing assessments, considering what they reveal about the client, and translating the findings into client goals are done collaboratively by the client and the occupational therapist. Moreover, clients are invited to be active participants in the process of assessment, including interpretation of findings from assessments. Clients are taught MOHO concepts at a basic level that they can understand, and many clients learn to apply assessments or informal data gathering to monitor themselves.

Once the therapist and client use the assessment information to establish goals together, the therapist assists the client in deciding what components of Reencuentros best facilitate meeting those goals. For example, a client may decide to divide her time in the practical occupations of working in the office, art, a note-taking class (which is offered as part of the educational program), and gardening. Individual goals for this client may be to show an increase in volition by spontaneously choosing occupations of interest and developing productive habits, such as timeliness and following through on commitments. These goals may be realized through practical occupations by choosing an office project, by completing a work of art, by com-

pleting homework in class, and by showing up on time.

Another client may have simpler goals based on his level of functioning. He may not be able to communicate verbally with the occupational therapist, and an assessment of his interests and needs may be done based on observation. This client may be observed smiling as the musical group sings or spontaneously helping to wash vegetables with the kitchen team. This individual's goals would include participation in occupations that appear to give him pleasure and fulfillment to the greatest extent possible. As the examples illustrates, the therapist will set client goals when the client is not able to collaborate in doing so. However, as soon as the client is capable, the process becomes collaborative.

As clients progress through the program, they begin to participate more and more in the larger community outside of Reencuentros (e.g., working, going to school, volunteering). Consequently, they spend less time at the house. However, ongoing support is provided in the form of support groups and individual follow-up. *Figure 26-3* shows how each client progresses through the program at Reencuentros. The case of Claudio, presented in Chapter 21, is an example of a client at Reencuentros.

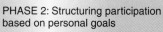

PHASE 1: Initial evaluation and introduction to the center

GOAL: Explore opportunities, develop interests with sense of security and acceptance.

1. **Formal Assessment**

2. **Informal Observation:** Members are invited to participate in practical occupations. Information is gathered based on member's performance.

3. **Exploration of Practical Activities:** Members participate in or observe practical activities at the center in an unstructured manner to facilitate choice.

PHASE 2: Structuring participation based on personal goals

GOAL: Identify strengths and weaknesses, increase confidence and skills, and develop necessary habits to obtain future goals.

1. **Individual Counseling:** Client and therapist identify interests and personal goals based on initial observations and assessments.

2. **Educational or Vocational Goal Setting:** Specific skills related to educational or vocational goals are identified and plans made to develop them.

3. **Structured Participation in Practical Occupations:** Client, with assistance of therapist, develops a daily and weekly schedule for participation.

4. **Participation in Educational Groups:** Members choose to participate in educational groups based on interest and goals.

5. **Reevaluation:** In individual counseling, client and therapist examine client's experiences, successes, challenges, strengths, and weaknesses, determining any need to readjust goals.

6. **Assuming Increased Responsibility as Goals Are Met:** Clients assume increased responsibility in accordance to their level of functioning.

7. **Ongoing Family Education and Counseling:** Occurs throughout Phase 2 as needed.

PHASE 3: Exploring alternatives for participation in other contexts

GOAL: Participate in a satisfying routine using skills and abilities in a meaningful context.

1. Test skills and abilities in different contexts in the community through employment, internship, volunteering, or student roles. Members still receive support from Reencuentros as needed.

2. Participate in self-help groups run by peers monthly.

3. Ongoing self-evaluation using VQ, OSA, and other tools.

4. Seeking additional assistance as needed.

5. Ongoing family education and counseling occurs throughout Phase 3 as needed.

FIGURE 26-3   Typical Client Progression Though Reencuentros.

Program Evaluation

Because of the client-centered nature of Reencuentros, a critical dimension of program evaluation is client progress and satisfaction. Assessments that are used for initial client evaluation are routinely repeated to monitor individual client progress. These include the Volitional Questionnaire (VQ) and the OSA. To the extent possible, clients are educated about the meaning of assessment tools and are encouraged to engage in a process of self-evaluation. Client satisfaction with their own progress is an important measure of impact of services.

In keeping with Reencuentros' mission to facilitate community reintegration, the following outcomes are considered indices of program success:

• Being involved in work, school, and leisure in the community outside of Reencuentros
• Meeting individual goals to increase participation in areas of interest or meaningful roles
• Achieving a satisfying daily routine

- Increasing family satisfaction with the client's performance and participation at home.

Data on these outcomes are routinely kept, and percentages calculated to monitor the extent to which the program is meeting its goals. These data are also useful to document the value of the program to professionals and families who refer clients to the program.

Reencuentros is a thriving private program whose success is recognized by many professionals throughout metropolitan Santiago. Moreover, it has gained a strong reputation among many family groups. As a result, there are always ample referrals for new clients. The program has also captured the attention of a number of corporations that provide scholarships for clients to attend Reencuentros. In sum, the program offers a unique service meeting the needs of a client group that otherwise would have difficulty integrating into community life.

Example 3: PSI

The Programme Spécifique d'Intervention, Premier Episode (PSI) was initiated in 1997 in Quebec City in the Province of Quebec, Canada. It is an interdisciplinary program for young clients experiencing their first psychotic episode. This example illustrates how MOHO was used to develop the occupational therapy component of this program.

Program Needs Assessment

The program was developed at Hôtel-Dieu de Lévis Hospital, a general hospital with psychiatric units. Before the PSI program came into existence, there was not a well-coordinated structure between the different multidisciplinary interventions at the hospital. There was also difficulty coordinating the various services offered for schizophrenic clients by other institutions in the region. Some received very specific attention with long-term rehabilitation, whereas others received only little help or no services at all. Moreover there were no valid, quantitative, and objective data to measure the effects of interventions. The hospital has a mandate for research and teaching and therefore supported the psychiatric department in the idea of developing a program that would represent best practice and assess its own outcomes.

Several other factors also influenced the development of the PSI program. In the development of specialized services for clients with psychosis, analytical approaches have given way to the development of cognitive therapy approaches and brief intervention therapies. Moreover, a new generation of anti-psychotic medications enables better control of the disabling symptoms of schizophrenia, allowing greater expectations for client functioning. Since family members of schizophrenic clients often want to play a more active role in the recovery process, education and support groups have had to be developed. Finally, various community groups supporting the rights for persons with mental illness were lobbying for services to allow the clients to be better informed about their diseases and to actively participate in the intervention process.

As a consequence of these factors, a decision was made to create a specialized program. Three interdisciplinary teams refer clients to the PSI program. Each of these teams works with clients who have a variety of psychiatric problems. When a client meets PSI criteria (first psychotic episode), he or she is referred to the PSI program at discharge. Each of the referring teams continues to work with clients after discharge. There is careful coordination between PSI program services and other services given by the referring team.

Assessing the Needs of the Client Group

Although the program officially began in 1997, the groundwork was laid as early as 1995. A literature search was conducted on early intervention for young psychotic and schizophrenic clients, and a study on client demographics in the area covered by the hospital was undertaken. The literature clearly indicated that schizophrenia is a disease of the brain, genetically influenced and characterized by cognitive deficits, low self-esteem, difficulties in daily functioning, and poor social integration (Brenner et al., 1994; Green, 1996; Harding, 1988; Kaplan, 1994; Mawrer & Häfner, 1995; Nicole et al., 1999). The social, economic, and human costs of schizophrenia are high, and it is an extremely difficult illness to treat.

The literature review also identified several important points that had to be addressed to make the program efficient and effective:

- Early intervention helps to limit or avoid neurologic deficits, social repercussions, and the progressive de-

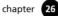

generation associated with the disease (Harding, 1988; Mawrer & Häfner, 1995; Wyatt, 1991)

- It is important to reduce the period between the appearance of the symptoms of disease and effective therapy (Beiser, Erickson, Fleming & Iacono, 1993; Falloon, 1992; Johnstone, Crow, & Johnson, 1986)
- The complexity of the disease and its multiple facets require an interdisciplinary structure of intervention and specialized care (Nicole et al., 1999).

The PSI program was developed according to guidelines suggested by evidence found in the literature. The goal of the PSI program was to develop a state-of-the-art, specialized, and integrated approach for schizophrenic clients to benefit them during the initial phase of the disease and subsequent recovery. To accomplish this, it was decided the program should include an optimal combination of interdisciplinary treatment interventions that would:

- Intervene early after the first psychotic episode
- Maintain continuity of care
- Provide innovative and relevant services
- Integrate elements from traditional approaches with newer treatments
- Promote new kinds of therapies as much as possible
- Use standard clinical tools
- Make optimal use of resources.

Every member of the multidisciplinary team was asked to propose standardized evaluations that would objectify and contribute to understanding the biological, psychological, and social components of each client's condition and to propose corresponding interventions to address identified problems. Within the interdisciplinary team, psychiatrists and nurses covered the biological areas, psychologists covered the neurocognitive and personality areas, social workers covered family history, and occupational therapists covered occupational problems. It was within this general context of program development that the occupational therapy approach, based on MOHO, was developed. Importantly, the incorporation of MOHO into the overall program meant that other members of the team had to understand and accept MOHO concepts and that MOHO contributions to the overall program had to be integrated with other theories and approaches used in the interdisciplinary program. This meant that the occupational therapists had to provide an overview of

MOHO and its potential contributions to the program for the interdisciplinary team. This served to initially introduce the team to the ideas and to secure their support for including MOHO as an essential component of this interdisciplinary program.

RATIONALE FOR SELECTION OF MOHO

MOHO was chosen as the framework for the occupational therapy component of the PSI program because it:

- Furnishes a detailed framework of the occupational functioning of the individual (Hagerdon, 1992)
- Enables precise measurement and useful description of the client's occupational characteristics
- Provides clear links between the occupational problems it helps identify and the intervention strategies to address them (Bonder, 1991)
- Gives specific and detailed guidelines and tools for evaluating a client, a specific language for describing the difficulties/challenges encountered, and a framework for setting treatment goals and selecting the most appropriate strategy to achieve the desired level of change
- Allows for a flexible approach to individualize therapy for a client and provides a comprehensive picture of the occupational functioning of the person
- Provides a conceptualization of the process and stages of change that was useful for guiding the sequence of therapy (including deciding when a client is ready to move from one level of change to another)
- Offers a solid theoretical view of occupation that clearly helps to explain the occupational functioning of a client faced with his or her first psychotic episode through clearly identified concepts that have been shown to predict later functioning (Henry, 1994; Henry & Coster, 1996).

MOHO is also compatible with cognitive-behavioral and psychoeducational approaches used by other disciplines in the program. Further, MOHO allows the occupational therapist to make valuable, distinct, and specific contributions to the team. For example, MOHO allowed the team to distinguish between the disappearance of the disease's psychotic symptoms and the return to a functional level of occupation. MOHO-based research indicates that remittance of psychotic symptoms does not ensure a return to premorbid levels of functioning (Henry, 1994).

Program Planning

The interdisciplinary team decided to develop the PSI program to include two sequential modules. The first module includes evaluating and developing a specific intervention plan. The second module includes intervention. The first step in developing the occupational therapy component of both modules was to use MOHO to conceptualize a client's occupational situation and to develop related goals.

Conceptualizing the Client Group from a MOHO Perspective

MOHO provided a framework for structuring the information gathered from the interdisciplinary team's literature review and survey, as well as practice experiences with this client group, to create a conceptualization of the occupational problems, challenges, and needs of this population. The following is a brief discussion of how MOHO was used to conceptualize the occupational situation of clients following a first psychotic episode. *Table 26-3* summarizes this information and also shows the major goals of the occupational therapy component of the program.

Volition

Problems with motivation are extensively documented in the description of symptoms of schizophrenia (Kaplan, 1995; Lalonde & Greenberg, 1988; Nicholi, 1999). There is a decline in motivation, difficulty in self-determination, loss of interest, and feelings of inadequacy stemming principally from past negative occupational experiences. All these come to influence volition.

As a result of the disease, clients often have difficulty in evaluating their actual capacity. Clients may be vaguely conscious of their problems, especially those related to communication and social interaction. Clients tend to feel very ill at ease managing everyday social interaction that involves emotional content. As a consequence, they often make choices to avoid interaction and isolate themselves from others. Many have difficulties initiating action. They typically shun everyday responsibilities and cannot set life goals for themselves. They often have extreme difficulty achieving a sense of meaning and purpose in their occupational lives.

Habituation

Roles and habits are ordinarily very disturbed in these clients, although the extent will vary from one client to another. Clients often feel a painful sense of loss and emptiness when they have relinquished roles and been deprived of the many elements of their daily routine. Productive work is almost always absent from their lives. Their participation in occupations in the home is often minimal. Their leisure tends to be solitary, passive, and requiring minimal organization and planning. Performance of activities of daily living can also degenerate in these clients, although it is variable. Finally, the general routine of these clients tends to be bland and discouraging. Many of these clients have reversed day/night cycles that serve to further isolate them from others. Finally, they have difficulty imagining themselves in a variety of roles and do not have an image of the kind of life they would like to lead.

Performance Capacity and Skills

Clients experience a range of impairments, especially in the area of cognitive processing including difficulties with attention, memory, concentration, and problem solving (George & Neufeld, 1985). In more than three quarters of clients, basic communication and social skills are severely affected (Brenner et al., 1994). They particularly have difficulty in exchanging information and adjusting their behavior to others. However, clients' communication/interaction skills vary widely, which makes it critical to do a precise evaluation of these skills with each client.

In many young psychotic clients, process skills are severely constrained within daily tasks. The skills most affected are related to adaptation, temporal organization, spatial organization, and energy level maintenance. All these skill problems can make daily activities laborious and difficult.

Environmental Contexts

These clients are often faced with incomprehension on the part of their families and loved ones. Since the disease may not be physically visible, people with schizophrenia are often misunderstood and accused of being unmotivated or uncooperative. The family is often rendered impotent to deal with the disorganized behaviors and often does not know how to respond to these situations in a helpful way. The family's expectations of the client are not always appropriate given the nature of the disease. Sometimes the family is overstimulating, whereas in other families clients are more or less abandoned. The emotional intensity of some families can also adversely affect clients.

T A B L E 26-3 Conceptualization of Client Problems and Related Strategies to Address Them Within the PSI Program

MOHO Component	Problems and Challenges of Clients	Occupational Therapy Goals
Volition • Personal causation • Values • Interests	• General decline in motivation and loss of interest • Feelings of inadequacy stemming from failures • Difficulty evaluating actual capacity (abilities and limitations), underconfident or overconfident • Vague awareness of problems may lead to choices that isolate self • Difficulty achieving a sense of meaning and purpose in their occupational lives • Difficulty in initiating action and self-determination • Avoidance of responsibilities • Difficulty setting and prioritizing goals • Inability to prioritize among what is important • Avoid decisions to engage in occupations • Difficulty seeking assistance appropriately • Poor concentration leading to difficulty in occupational forms	• Greater expectation of success for engagement in occupational forms • Increase confidence to approach tasks within one's capacity • Develop realistic understanding of abilities and limitations along with acceptance of them • Identify areas in which person can feel sense of accomplishment and meaning • Support choices to engage in occupations with meaning, interest, and social involvement • Develop sense of basic responsibility for self and for productivity according to capacity • Set and pursue realistic life goals • Stimulate interest and desire to do things • More willingness to ask for help when needed • Increase tendency to sustain efforts to realize goals • Increase the ability to identify what is important in a situation • Increase satisfaction and self-esteem from realizing goals • Increase participation in things of interest
Habituation • Roles • Habits	• Roles and habits disturbed • Poor role script • Difficulty meeting role expectations • Sense of loss and emptiness due to lost/absent roles and limited routine • Absence of productive occupation • Minimal participation in home occupational forms • Leisure activities solitary, passive, and simple • Activities of daily living degenerate • Routine bland and discouraging • Difficulty structuring the day due to lack of roles • Reversed day/night cycle isolates self from others • Difficulty imagining self in a variety of roles and kind of life desired • Structured program schedule to support development of a functional routine	• Increase perception of self as involved with roles that are necessary and desirable • Improve organization of daily routine • Improve awareness of responsibilities associated with success in various roles • Increase effectiveness in meeting multiple role expectations of realistic role responsibilities • Increase effectiveness in completing a specific occupation due to acquisition/change in habitual way of doing it

continued

TABLE 26-3 (Continued)

MOHO Component	Problems and Challenges of Clients	Occupational Therapy Goals
Performance Capacity and Skills	• Range of impairments, especially in the area of cognitive processing, attention, memory, concentration, logic inference, and anticipation • Communication/interaction skills affected • Process skills constrained within daily tasks • Performing daily activities is laborious and difficult	• Improve visual perception in social conditions • Develop social adaptive mechanisms to make up for cognitive deficits • Improve skills of the physical domain • Improve capacity to receive, give, and exchange daily information • Improve skills of the relational domain • Improve repertoire of social competence skills • Develop preventive strategies of management of emotions during more intense daily situations • Develop alternative solutions for daily problems encountered
Environment	• Incomprehension, misunderstanding, and impotence to deal with disorganized behaviors on the part of their families and loved ones • Inappropriate family expectations of the client • Overstimulating or abandoning home environment • Negative influences of drugs, alcohol, and physical and psychological abuse • Stigma and prejudice associated with mental illness	• Improve the capacity of the client to express his or her need for assistance and to locate daily difficulties • Improve client's knowledge about the negative effects of drugs and alcohol on psychosis • Improve competence of the client to set limits and to say no • Teach the client how to distinguish and explain to his or her entourage the difference between psychosis and madness

The clients are often affected by negative influences in their environment such as drugs, alcohol, or physical and psychological abuse (Bennet, Bellack, & Gearon, 2001). Consumption of drugs and alcohol has an adverse affect on psychotic processes. The stigma and prejudice associated with mental illness in all sectors of society also presents barriers for these clients.

Translating the MOHO Conceptualization into Contributions to Program

Since the program was interdisciplinary, the conceptualization of client problems from a MOHO perspective served to identify problems that occupational therapists could address in the program. Corresponding intervention strategies to be used by therapists to address these problems were also identified. They are shown in Table 26-3. With this information, the therapists were able to

negotiate their contributions to the assessment and intervention modules of the PSI program.

MODULE 1: ASSESSMENT

As noted above, occupational therapy assessment was designed to be part of the first module of the PSI program, as shown in *Figure 26-4*. It is a collaborative, interdisciplinary assessment process. In the first module of the program, a comprehensive assessment of the client includes a measure of premorbid adaptation:

• A systematic family interview
• A longitudinal clinical history
• A psychiatric state examination and a standardized psychiatric interview of all the symptomatology of the disease
• Biological testing, including such laboratory tests as an electroencephalogram

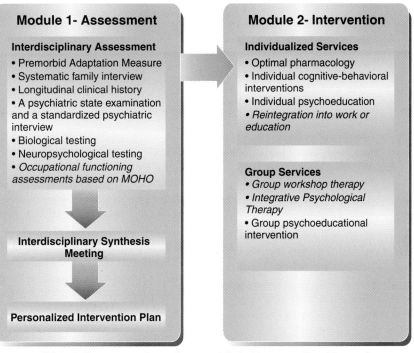

Module 1- Assessment

Interdisciplinary Assessment
• Premorbid Adaptation Measure
• Systematic family interview
• Longitudinal clinical history
• A psychiatric state examination and a standardized psychiatric interview
• Biological testing
• Neuropsychological testing
• *Occupational functioning assessments based on MOHO*

Interdisciplinary Synthesis Meeting

Personalized Intervention Plan

Module 2- Intervention

Individualized Services
• Optimal pharmacology
• Individual cognitive-behavioral interventions
• Individual psychoeducation
• *Reintegration into work or education*

Group Services
• *Group workshop therapy*
• *Integrative Psychological Therapy*
• Group psychoeducational intervention

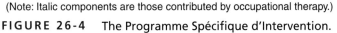

(Note: Italic components are those contributed by occupational therapy.)

FIGURE 26-4 The Programme Spécifique d'Intervention.

• Neuropsychological testing including cognitive tests, personality tests, diagnostic classification, and intelligence quotient
• Occupational functioning assessments based on MOHO.

The assessments that make up the final component during the assessment module are:

• Occupational Performance History Interview-Version 2.0 (OPHI-II)
• Assessment of Motor and Process Skills (AMPS)
• Activity Configuration (Mosey, 1986).

The activity configuration was chosen for getting a picture of the client's daily life pattern, after initially piloting the Occupational Questionnaire and finding that it was too complex for the clients to complete at this early stage following the first psychotic episode.

Once the assessment process is complete, members of the interdisciplinary team gather for a synthesis meeting that includes the referring psychiatrist and other professionals working with the client. During this meeting, each professional summarizes the assessment results, and the team together develops a specific interdisciplinary intervention plan to decide the combination of treatment interventions that will be most beneficial to the client.

Module 2: Intervention

As with assessment, the occupational therapy component of the intervention is fully integrated with the entire interdisciplinary PSI program. Therefore, the entire structure of the PSI intervention module is presented below and shown in Figure 26-4. While the components of the program are standard, they are tailored to each client as a result of the personalized plan of intervention developed during the synthesis meeting.

MOHO is an important component of the intervention module of the PSI program. MOHO provides specific guidelines for goals of treatment and helps identify the strategies to be undertaken to achieve client change. Additionally, MOHO integrated well with the other theories and approaches that are used in the program such as Integrated Psychological Therapy, a cognitive approach developed by Brenner et al. (1994), and individual cognitive-behavioral intervention developed by Kingdon and Turkington (1994), Jackson et al. (1998), Haddock, Morrisson, Hopkins, Lewis, and Tarrier (1998), and Kuipers et al. (1998).

The treatment module includes individual interventions and group interventions. Individual interventions include:

- Optimal pharmacology directed by the psychiatrist and designed to assure the best medication approach is used with the client
- Individual cognitive-behavioral interventions given by psychiatrists and psychiatric nurses. This intervention is aimed at reducing the impact of positive symptoms of schizophrenia (e.g., delusions or hallucinations) by giving clients cognitive strategies for managing them. Occupational therapy assessment is often used to inform the psychiatrists and nurses of how any symptoms are interfering with performance
- Individual psychoeducation (Liberman et al., 1993) that covers the disease (psychosis) and pharmacology is provided on an individual basis by nurses to clients and their families
- Reintegration into work or education is an individualized component of the program offered by social workers. This component is usually a follow-up service for clients who have progressed through the group components of the program and are ready to cope with productive objectives.

In addition to these individualized services, clients can participate in the following group services.

Group Workshop Therapy

Occupational therapy operates group workshop therapy for two to eight people at a time. This group meets for 90 minutes. Clients engage in occupational forms that are personally meaningful to them. The aims of this group are to:

- Mobilize the client in a significant activity related to his or her current life and stimulate volitional thoughts and feelings
- Identify basic challenges he or she may wish to undertake

- Activate motor, process, and communication/interaction skills.

During this workshop, clients are invited to stop and reflect on the effects of what they do to identify the most appropriate actions that will give satisfactory results. Clients often begin in this group when they are too unstable to handle the demands of the next group, integrative psychological therapy.

Integrative Psychological Therapy

Integrative psychological therapy (IPT) is a group intervention based on the combined principles of the cognitive-behavioral work of Pomini, Neis, Brenner, Hodel, and Roder (1995) and on MOHO. The group focuses simultaneously on difficulties in cognitive functioning, social skills, and emotion management. This group consists of 7 to 10 clients. The program comprises six different modules of exercises, organized hierarchically into increasing levels of complexity. In this manner, the amount of social interaction and emotional content is gradually increased. This program addresses and is designed to enable the clients to improve skills in the following areas:

- Social perception
- Verbal communication
- Social skills
- Emotional management
- Problem solving.

The program begins with the first two areas in which the client aims to improve the quality of data processing and perception. The training then proceeds to more complex verbal competency, social skills, and finally to problem solving. This group is directed by two occupational therapists over 8 months. It meets twice a week for 1.5-hour therapy sessions.

MOHO was especially helpful for the design of this group because it integrated well with the IPT principles and gave specific assessments and strategies that were not adequately specified in this model. For this group, the ACIS and the VQ are used to identify specific client motivation and communication/interaction skill problems from which treatment objectives are developed for each client. These assessments also provide a means of measuring client change.

Group Psychoeducational Intervention

This is a group for families of young psychotic clients, (Anderson, Hogarty, & Reiss, 1980). Four 2-hour sessions are held by two social workers. Goals of the group are to decrease family isolation and help them to have a positive and active role during treatment and disease evolution.

Program Implementation

All key decision-makers in the hospital and in the Provincial Ministry of Health strongly supported the PSI program. A detailed plan was needed to lay the groundwork for the program, which required personnel training and new equipment and space. The team was designed to be composed of two psychiatrists, two psychiatric nurses, two neuropsychologists, one social worker, and three occupational therapists, each of whom devotes about half-time effort to the program. Not all members of the team work exclusively in this program.

Various members of the team received additional training and certifications to assure that they had the most appropriate competencies for the program. For the occupational therapists involved, the planning and preparation focused on training in MOHO and the cognitive-behavioral approaches that were to be integrated with it.

MOHO experts provided guidance and consultation to the Quebec team on use of the model and its tools. Two training sessions were implemented in Quebec (a total of 4 days) on MOHO. In addition to receiving training in the use of MOHO and relevant assessments, the team received guidance in making translations of the assessments for use in French-speaking Quebec. At the time of this writing, future plans are to evaluate the psychometrics of the translations. Practical experience with them suggests the translated assessments are very effective. The occupational therapists in the PSI program were already certified in AMPS training, so additional training in this area was not necessary. The occupational therapists, along with most other interdisciplinary staff, received training from a team of experts in implementing the cognitive-behavioral approach.

For each of the individual and group interventions, protocols were developed to assure the quality of the sessions. At this stage, the incorporation of MOHO into the overall program structure called attention to the importance of volition and of the client's interests, values, and personal causation being considered thoroughly in intervention planning. This element served to enhance clients' feelings that they were truly involved in the treatment. Another important element of MOHO, recognized by the interdisciplinary team, was the extent to which assessments like the VQ, AMPS, and ACIS provided very precise descriptions of volition and skill that could be used to establish specific objectives for the clients in therapy.

Another important step in implementation was to integrate the therapists' use of MOHO with the total team. As noted earlier, the occupational therapists initially presented MOHO concepts to the team during the program planning phase. This served to garner initial support, but as some team members remained skeptical and others had very little appreciation of MOHO, it was the therapist's contributions to the team in actual implementation (i.e., demonstration of what information the assessments yielded and demonstration of how MOHO was used in intervention) that served to inform the team more fully about MOHO, to make them comfortable with its terminology and concepts, and to eventually secure strong support for it as an integral part of this interdisciplinary program.

Program Evaluation

One component of the evaluation of the PSI program involves taking clinical measurements at the beginning and end of the intervention to evaluate the therapeutic effects of the components of the programs, such as the IPT. MOHO assessments are used principally for the measurement of the effects of the IPT. The ACIS and VQ are used to measure the effects of the Brenner IPT group therapy. Measurements are taken at the beginning and at the end of the group.

In 1998, research and measurement components were added to begin to evaluate the PSI program. This involved establishing a longitudinal database that describes in detail the clients who enter the program and that tracks them at 18 and 36 months following entry into the program (Nicole et al., 2000). The data are collected by the psychiatrists, neuropsychologists, and occupational therapists involved in the program. The fact that occupational therapists are involved in data collection for the longitudinal database reflects the respect that MOHO assessments are accorded by the interdisciplinary team.

Part of the goal of the database is to identify initial characteristics of the clients that predict how clients will fare over time. The descriptive evaluation includes data on sociodemographic information, history of the client, symptomatology, neuropsychological functioning, job adaptation and housing, occupational functioning, quality of the client's life and that of his or her family, and the amount and type of services offered to the client.

The research questions that the team aims to answer in the next few years are:

- What are the sociological, neuropsychological, and functional characteristics of the clients when they are first referred to the PSI program?
- How do these characteristics evolve over the course of 18 months and 36 months in clients referred to the PSI program?
- What factors (including interventions) predict future outcomes for clients?

As answers to these questions are found, the PSI program will further evolve to better meet the needs of its clients.

Conclusion

This chapter outlined a process of program development that emphasized the importance of using a conceptual practice model. It offered a set of questions to guide the selection and justification of the model(s) to be used in a program. It also indicated four major steps that are ordinarily undertaken in program development. Finally, the authors illustrated how MOHO can be used to guide programs through three detailed examples. These examples illustrated different situations in which MOHO was used to systematically plan, implement, and evaluate occupational therapy services.

Key Terms

Evidence-based practice: Conscientiously, explicitly, and systematically using available evidence in deciding the kinds of services that will be provided to individuals.

Mechanism of action: Theoretically and empirically

accounting for how a particular change occurs as a consequence of participating in an intervention.

Program development: Creating and evaluating an approach to service delivery for a defined client group.

References

Anderson, C. M., Hogarty, G. E., & Reiss, D. J. (1980). Family treatment of adult schizophrenic patients: A psychoeducational approach. *Schizophrenia Bulletin, 6* (3), 490–505.

Azhar, F. T. (1996). *The relevance of worker identity to return to work in clients treated for work related injuries.* Unpublished master's thesis, Department of Occupational Therapy, University of Illinois at Chicago.

Beiser, M., Erickson, D., Fleming, J. A. E., & Iacono, W. G. (1993). Establishing the onset of psychotic illness, *American Journal of Psychiatry, 150,* 1349–1354.

Bennet, M. E., Bellack, A. S., & Gearon, J. S. (2001). Treating substance abuse in schizophrenia. An initial report. *Journal of Substance Abuse & Treatment, 20* (2), 163–175.

Billingsley, A. (1988). *Black families-white America.* New York: Simon & Schuster.

Bonder, B. R. (1991). *Psychopathology and function.* Thorofare, NJ: Slack.

Braveman, B. (1999). The model of human occupation and prediction of return to work: A review of related empirical research. *Work: A Journal of Prevention, Assessment & Rehabilitation, 12* (1), 13–23.

Braveman, B. H. (2001). Development of a community-based return to work program for people living with AIDS. *Occupational Therapy in Health Care. 13* (3–4), 113–131.

Braveman, B. H., Sen, S., & Kielhofner, G. (2001). Community-based vocational rehabilitation programs. In M. Scaffa (Ed.), *Occupational therapy in community-based practice settings* (pp.139–162). Philadelphia: FA Davis.

Brenner, H. D., Roder, V., Hodel, B., Kienze, N., Reed, D., & Liberman, R. P. M. (1994). *Integrated psychological therapy for schizophrenic patients (IPT).* Toronto, Canada: Hogrefe.

Breuer, N. (1997). *The positive workplace: Managing HIV at work.* Washington, DC: National AIDS Fund.

Brownson, C. (2001). Program development for community health: Planning, implementation, and evaluation strategies. In M. Scaffa (Ed.), *Occupational therapy in community-based practice settings* (pp. 95–116). Philadelphia: FA Davis.

Corner, R., Kielhofner, G., & Lin, F. L. (1997). Construct validity of a work environment impact scale. *Work, 9,* 21–34.

Corner, R., Kielhofner, G., & Olson, L. (1998). *Work Environment Impact Scale (WEIS). (Version 2.0).* Chicago: Model of Human Occupation Clearinghouse, Department of Occupational Therapy, College of Applied Health Sciences, University of Illinois at Chicago. (Translated and published in Finnish, German, and Swedish).

DePoy, E. (1990). The TBIIM: An intervention for the treatment of individuals with traumatic brain injury. *Occupational Therapy in Health Care, 7* (1), 55–67.

Falloon, I. R. H. (1992). Early intervention for first episodes of schizophrenia: A preliminary exploration. *Psychiatry, 55,* 4–15.

Feinberg, M. B. (1996). Changing the natural history of HIV disease. *Lancet, 348,* 239–246.

Flannery, M., Glickman, M., Fuller, E., & Torrey, M. D. (1996). Fountain House: Portraits of lives reclaimed from mental illness. Center City, MN: Hazelden.

George, L., & Neufeld, R. W. (1985). Cognition and symptomatology in schizophrenia. *Schizophrenia Bulletin, 11* (2), 264–285.

Gerardi, S. M. (1996). The management of battle-fatigued soldiers: An occupational therapy model. *Military Medicine, 161* (8), 483–488.

Gitlin, L. N., Corcoran, M., Martindale-Adams, J., Malone, M. A., Stevens, A., & Winter, L. (2000). Identifying mechanisms of action: Why and how does intervention work? In R. Schulz (Ed.), *Handbook of dementia caregiving: Evidence-based interventions for family caregivers* (pp. 225–248). New York: Springer Publishing.

Green, M. F. (1996). What are the functional consequences of neurocognitive deficits in schizophrenia? *American Journal of Psychiatry, 153,* 321–330.

Grossman, J., & Bortone, J. (1986). Program development. In S. C. Robertson (Ed.), *SCOPE: Strategies, concepts and opportunities for program development and evaluation* (pp. 91–99). Bethesda, MD: American Occupational Therapy Association.

Gusich, R. (1984). Occupational therapy for chronic pain: A clinical application of the model of human occupation. *Occupational Therapy in Mental Health, 4* (3), 59–73.

Gusich, R. L., & Silverman, A. (1991). Basava day clinic: The model of human occupation as applied to psychiatric day hospitalization. *Occupational Therapy in Mental Health, 11* (2/3), 113–134.

Haddock, G., Morrisson, A. P., Hopkins, R., Lewis, S., & Tarrier, N. (1998). Individual cognitive-behavioural interventions in early psychosis. *British Journal of Psychiatry Supplement, 172* (33), 101–106.

Hagerdon, R. (1992). *Occupational therapy: Foundation for practice, models, frame of reference and care skills.* New York: Churchill.

Harding, C. (1988). Course types in schizophrenia: An analysis of European and American Studies. *Schizophrenia Bulletin, 14* (4), 633–643.

Henry, A. D. (1994). *Predicting psychosocial functioning and symptomatic recovery of adolescents and young adults with a first psychotic episode: A six-month follow-up study.* Unpublished doctoral dissertation, Boston University.

Henry, A., & Coster, J. (1996). Predictors of functional outcome among adolescents and young adults with psychotic disorders. *American Journal of Occupational Therapy, 50* (3), 171–181.

Hogg, R. S., O'Shaugnessy, M. V., Gatarac, N., Yip, B., Craib, K., Schecter, M. T., & Mantaner, J. S. (1997). Decline in deaths from new antiretrovirals [letter]. *Lancet, 349,* 1294.

Holm, M. (2000). Our mandate for the new millennium: Evidence-based practice. *American Journal of Occupational Therapy, 54* (6), 575–585.

Jackson, H., McGorry, P., Edwards, J., Hulbert, C., Francey, S., Maude, D., Cocks, J., Power, P., Harrigan, S., & Dudgeon, P. (1998). Cognitively-oriented psychotherapy for early psychosis (COPE): Preliminary result. *British Journal of Psychiatry Supplement, 172* (23), 93–100.

Johnstone, E. C., Crow, T. J., & Johnson, A. L. (1986). The Northwick Park study of first episode schizophrenia: Presentation of the illness and problems relating to admission. *British Journal of Psychiatry, 148,* 115–120.

Kaplan, H. I., Sadock, B. J., Grebb, J. A., (1994). *Synopsis of Psychiatry; Behavioral Sciences Clinical Psychiary,* 7th ed. Baltimore MD: Williams & Wilkins.

Kavanaugh, J., & Fares, J. (1995). Using the model of human occupation with homeless mentally ill patients. *British Journal of Occupational Therapy, 58* (10), 419–422.

Kielhofner, G., & Brinson, M. (1989). Development & evaluation of an aftercare program for young chronic psychiatrically disabled adults. *Occupational Therapy in Mental Health, 9,* 1–25.

Kingdon, D., Turkington, D., & John, C. (1994). Cognitive-behavioral therapy of schizophrenia. *British Journal of Psychiatry, 165* (5), 695.

Kuipers, E., Fowler, D., Garety, P., Chisholm, D., Freeman, D., Dunn, G., Bebbinton, P., & Hadley, C. (1998). London-East Anglia randomised controlled trial of cognitive-behavioural therapy for psychosis: Follow-up and economic evaluation at 18 months. *British Journal of Psychiatry, 173,* 61–68.

Lalonde, P., & Grunberg, F. (1988). *Psychiatry clinique approche bio-psycho-sociale*, Québec, Canada: Gaëtan Morin Éditeur.

Liberman, R. P., Wallace, C. J., Blackwell, G., Eckman, T. A., Vaccaro, J. V., & Kuehmel, T. G. (1993). Innovations in skills training for the seriously mentally ill: The UCLA social and independent living skills module. *Innovations and Research, 2* (2), 43–59.

Mallinson, T. (1998). *Work rehabilitation in mental health programs:* A companion manual to the videotapes "Working it out" and "The write stuff". Chicago: Model of Human Occupation Clearinghouse, Department of Occupational Therapy, College of Applied Health Sciences, University of Illinois at Chicago.

Mawrer, K., & Häfner, H. (1995). Methodological aspect of onset assessment in schizophrenia. *Schizophrenia Research, 15,* 265–267.

Mentrup, C., Niehaus, A., & Kielhofner, G. (1999). Applying the model of human occupation in work-focused rehabilitation: A case illustration. *Work: A Journal of Prevention, Assessment & Rehabilitation, 12* (1), 61–70.

Michael, P. S. (1991). Occupational therapy in a prison? You must be kidding! *Mental Health Special Interest Section Newsletter, 14,* 3–4.

Mosey, A. C. (1986). *Psychosocial components of occupational therapy*. New York: Raven Press.

Munoz, J., & Kielhofner, G. (1995). Program development. In G. Kielhofner (Ed.), *A model of human occupation: Theory and application* (2nd ed.). Baltimore: Williams & Wilkins.

National Institute on Disability and Rehabilitation Research (NIDRR). (1995, April). *Forging collaborative partnerships in the study of disability: A NIDRR conference on participatory action research*. Washington, DC.

Nicholi, A. M. (1999). *The Harvard guide to psychiatry* (3rd ed.). Cambridge, MA: The Belknap Press of Harvard University Press.

Nicole, L., Pires, A., Routhier, G., Bélanger, R., Bussière, G., L'Heureux, S., Gingras, N., Rivard, P., Chabot, P., Descombes, J., Sylvain, C., Abdal-Baki, A., Duval, N., Vignola, A., & Rhéaume, J. (1999). Schizophrénie, approche spécialisée et continuité de soins: Le programme spécifique d'intervention premier épisode de l'Hôtel-Dieu de Lévis. *Santé Mentale au Québec, XXIV* (1), 121–135.

Nicole, L., Routhier, G., L'Heureux, S., Duval, N., Vignola, A., Rivard, P., Abdal-Baki, A., & Bélanger, R. (2000). *Clinical characteristics of a group of patients with a first psychotic episode*. Acta Psychiatrica Scandinavia (suppl.), Abstract book from the 13th International Symposium for the Psychological Treatments of Schizophrenia and Other Psychoses, *102,* 67–68.

Oakley, F. (1987). Clinical application of the model of human occupation in dementia of the Alzheimer's type. *Occupational Therapy in Mental Health, 7* (4), 37–50.

Olin, D. (1985). Assessing and assisting the person with dementia: An occupational behavior perspective. *Physical & Occupational Therapy in Geriatrics, 3* (4), 25–32.

Olson, L. (1998). *Work readiness: Day treatment for the chronically disabled*. Chicago: Model of Human Occupation Clearinghouse, Department of Occupational Therapy, College of Applied Health Sciences, University of Illinois at Chicago.

Padilla, R., & Bianchi, E. M. (1990). Occupational therapy for chronic pain: Applying the model of human occupation to clinical practice. *Occupational Therapy Practice, 1* (3), 47–52.

Pizzi, M. A. (1984). Occupational therapy in hospice care. *American Journal of Occupational Therapy, 38,* 252–257.

Pizzi, M. A. (1989). Occupational therapy: Creating possibilities for adults with HIV infection, ARC and AIDS. *AIDS Patient Care, 3,* 18–23.

Pizzi, M.A. (1990a). The model of human occupation and adults with HIV infection and AIDS. *American Journal of Occupational Therapy, 44,* 257–264.

Pizzi, M. A. (1990b). Occupational therapy: Creating possibilities for adults with human immunodeficiency virus infection, AIDS related complex, and acquired immunodeficiency syndrome. *Occupational Therapy in Health Care, 7* (2/3/4), 125–137.

Pomini, V., Neis, L., Brenner, H. D., Hodel, B., & Roder, V. (1995). Thérapie psychologique des schizophrénies, Version francaise révisée. Liège, Belgique: Mardaga Presses.

Reekmans, M., & Kielhofner, G. (1998). Defining occupational therapy services in child psychiatry: An application of the model of human occupation. *Ergotherapie, 5,* 6–13.

Sackett, D. L., Rosenberg, W. M. C., Gray, J. A. M., Haynes, R. B., & Richardson, W. S. (1996). Evidence-based medicine: What it is and what it isn't. *British Medical Journal, 312,* 71–72.

Salz, C. (1983). A theoretical approach to the treatment of work difficulties in borderline personalities. *Occupational Therapy in Mental Health, 3* (3), 33–46.

Schaaf, R. C., & Mulrooney, L. L. (1989). Occupational therapy in early intervention: A family centered approach. *American Journal of Occupational Therapy, 43,* 745–754.

Schindler, V. J. (1988). Psychosocial occupational therapy intervention with AIDS patients. *American Journal of Occupational Therapy, 42,* 507–512.

Schindler, V. P. (1990). AIDS in a correctional setting. *Occupational Therapy in Health Care, 7 (2/3/4),* 171–183.

Sholle-Martin, S. (1987). Application of the model of human occupation: Assessment in child and adolescent psychiatry. *Occupational Therapy in Mental Health, 7* (2), 3–22.

Stack, C. B. (1974). *All our kin.* New York: Harper and Row.

Taylor, M. C. (2000). *Evidence-based practice for occupational therapists.* London: Blackwell Science.

Velozo, C., Kielhofner, G., & Fisher, G. (1998). *A user's guide to the Worker Role Interview (WRI). (Version 9.0).* Chicago: Model of Human Occupation Clearinghouse, Department of Occupational Therapy, College of Applied Health Sciences, University of Illinois at Chicago.

Weissenberg, R., & Giladi, W. (1989). Home economics day: A program for disturbed adolescents to promote acquisition of habits and skills. *Occupational Therapy in Mental Health, 9* (2), 89–103.

Weitz, R. (1990). Living with the stigma of AIDS. *Qualitative Sociology, 13* (1), 23–28.

Woodrum, S. C. (1993). A treatment approach for attention deficit hyperactivity disorder using the model of human occupation. *Developmental Disabilities Special Interest Section Newsletter, 16* (1), 1–2.

Wyatt, R. J. (1991). Neuroleptics and the natural course of schizophrenia. *Schizophrenia Bulletin, 17,* 325–351.

Youngstrom, M. J. (1999). Developing a new occupational therapy program. In Jacobs, K., & Logigian, M. K.(Eds.), *Function of a manager* (3rd ed.). Thorofare, NJ: Slack.

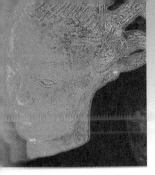

27

Research: Investigating MOHO

● Gary Kielhofner

● Anita Iyenger

Since MOHO was first published more than 20 years ago, over 80 studies based on the model have been published. The majority of these studies were completed in the past decade (*Fig. 27-1*), indicating an accelerating growth in research on MOHO. It is not possible to synthesize this diverse body of research in a single discussion. Therefore, this chapter aims to characterize the kinds of research that has investigated MOHO and place it in a framework for thinking about what research is needed to examine any conceptual practice model. This chapter addresses the following questions:

● Why is research important to a conceptual practice model like MOHO?

● What kinds of research had been undertaken to study MOHO?

● What kinds of evidence have MOHO-based studies provided about the model and its application in practice?

● What kind of research is needed in the future?

In answering these questions, the authors refer to many published studies. To aid the reader in identifying the full range of research related to MOHO, an appendix is included at the end of this chapter which contains brief abstracts of all published MOHO-based studies.

Drawing Conclusions From Research: Rigor and Cumlative Evidence

In the current brief presentation of studies to characterize types of MOHO-based research, we will focus on what the findings have revealed and how they have been used to further develop theory and practice. We will not discuss the details of research designs, statistics, or other methodological issues that bear on the rigor of

the studies. Nonetheless, methodological rigor is critical to consider in deciding how much credibility to give any study. The findings from any investigation must always be looked at in light of its methodology. There are excellent resources for critiquing studies and their relevance to occupational therapy practice (see, for example, Crombie, 1996; Helewa & Walker, 2000; Holm, 2000; Taylor, 2000). An evaluation of evidence from studies of MOHO should always consider the strengths and limitations of each investigation.

It is also important to keep in mind that no single study provides definitive evidence. Rather, conclusions can only be drawn from cumulative findings across many studies with different research designs, methods, and samples. With the growing research base of MOHO, it is increasingly possible to consider the results from several studies that have addressed a given issue in different ways.

Thus, it is both the rigor of individual studies and the consistency of cumulative evidence across studies that ultimately determines what research has to say about MOHO. Whenever evidence has been used to alter some aspect of MOHO, it has been based on whether the evidence is both sound and consistent across studies. In fact, as we will demonstrate, a model represents a dynamic and evolving body of theory and practice that constantly changes in response to what research reveals.

Integration of Applied and Basic Research Within Conceptual Practice Models

As discussed in Chapter 1, conceptual practice models like MOHO offer theory to explain certain phenomena. Additionally, each model generates a technology for

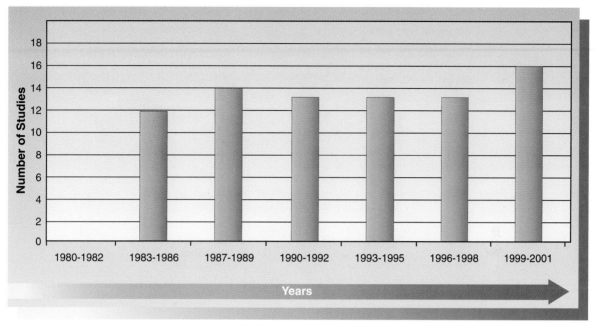

FIGURE 27-1 Published Research Studies Based on MOHO.

application (e.g., assessments and intervention strategies) for use in practice. As shown in *Figure 27-2*, research within a model includes both the testing of a model's theoretical accuracy and the examination of its practical utility. Consequently, the research can be referred to as encompassing both basic and applied aims. Basic research aims to test the explanations offered by a theory, whereas applied research examines the practical results of using theory to solve problems (Mosey, 1992a, 1992b).

As illustrated in Figure 27-2, a model naturally integrates basic and applied research concerns. We will use the term **basic research** to refer to investigations or aspects of investigations that aim to test the theoretical arguments proposed in MOHO. Such research examines whether the concepts and propositions of the theory are supported by evidence. This kind of research yields findings that may lead one to have confidence in the theory and/or to eliminate, change, or expand a concept and/or proposition. Thus, basic research is ordinarily guided by the following broad questions:

- Is there evidence for the model's concepts?
- Is there evidence for the model's propositions?

- What does new evidence say about the theory and does it point to the need to change concepts and propositions?

These types of questions are concerned with testing and improving the accuracy and adequacy of the explanations offered in the model's theory.

We will refer to investigations or aspects of investigations that aim to test the practical utility of the theory and related technology for application as **applied research**. Such studies ordinarily address the following types of broad questions, as shown in Figure 27-2:

- Do assessments based on a model provide dependable and useful information when applied in practice?
- How do a model's concepts influence therapeutic reasoning?
- When the model's concepts are operationalized in practice, how do they shape what occurs in therapy?
- What outcomes are achieved from therapy based on the model?

As can be seen from these questions, applied studies are primarily concerned with how well a model works in practice.

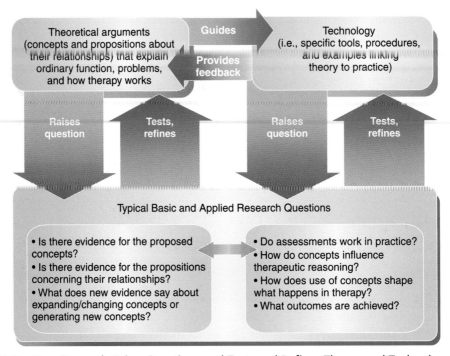

FIGURE 27-2 How Research Raises Questions and Tests and Refines Theory and Technology in a Conceptual Practice Model.

Although we can distinguish basic from applied research purposes in studies that have examined MOHO, it is important to recognize that:

- Many MOHO-based studies incorporate both basic and applied research aims
- When studies are undertaken within the framework of a conceptual practice model, they tend to have both applied and basic relevance, no matter what their primary aim.

For example, some studies that primarily sought to examine the dependability of an assessment tool have identified new concepts that were later incorporated into the theory. One instance is a study by Mallinson, Mahaffey, and Kielhofner (1998) that sought to understand how the Occupational Performance History Interview rating scales worked. This study provided the first evidence for the concept of occupational identity that was subsequently added to MOHO theory. Thus, while the original purpose of the study was applied, it yielded findings relevant to basic research concerns.

In similar fashion, studies that have had as their primary or sole purpose the testing or development of theory have contributed to applied concerns. For example, some MOHO-based research has concerned itself with the nature of occupational narratives and how they are shaped over time. These studies, which will be discussed in more detail later, were primarily concerned with examining occupational identity and its development. However, the findings of these studies about how occupational narratives are shaped and change have implications for how therapists might best support clients to change and develop their narratives in therapy. Thus, whereas the main aim of the research was basic, the findings have immediate applied relevance.

Therefore, as shown in Figure 27-2, basic and applied research overlap and interact within a model. Many studies will explicitly incorporate both basic and applied purposes. Moreover, when studies are undertaken with primarily applied or basic aims, their findings will tend to be relevant for both applied and basic purposes. Thus, the studies we later discuss as examples of either basic or applied research often have broader aims and relevance.

Types of Basic Research on MOHO

As noted above, the purpose of basic research on a model is to test and develop theory. Within a theory, the web of concepts and propositions create a logically interconnected explanation of the phenomena addressed by the theory. Since no study can ever test all the concepts or propositions of MOHO theory at once, studies necessarily partition chunks of the theory and derive research questions from it. Translating theory into testable research questions can be done by asking whether evidence exists for the concepts included in the theory and for the postulated relationships between the concepts. It also involves asking whether the theory can account for and predict the kinds of phenomena it seeks to explain. Therefore, basic research on MOHO includes the following kinds of studies:

- Construct validity studies that seek to verify MOHO concepts
- Correlative studies that examine the accuracy of relationships between constructs proposed in MOHO theory
- Studies comparing groups on concepts from MOHO theory to test whether they explain group differences
- Prospective studies that examine the potential of MOHO concepts and propositions to predict future behavior or states
- Qualitative studies that explore MOHO concepts and propositions in depth.

Over time as the evidence accumulates across such studies, informed judgments can be made about the theory and its accuracy. Moreover, findings from such research lead to alterations in the theory to create a more accurate explanation. In the following sections, each of the above types of studies are discussed and illustrated.

Construct Validity Studies

One of most fundamental tasks of any theory is to clearly identify the concepts that make up the theory. In early stages of theory development, concepts may be in-

completely defined, too narrow, or too broad. Additionally, theories may include unnecessary concepts or fail to include concepts that capture critical phenomena.

In any theoretical tradition, empirical study of the concepts requires that methods to gather information on the construct be developed. Such studies usually have an applied purpose since they examine tools that are designed to capture information on the intended construct. Nonetheless, these studies are equally important for validating the underlying concept (Benson & Schell, 1997). Consequently, they address the basic scientific purpose of gathering evidence about how well a concept corresponds to the phenomenon it references.

Studies that were part of developing measures of MOHO concepts have been critical to generating evidence about the concepts. In many instances, these studies have led to refinement in the definitions of the concepts. Occasionally, such studies have even pointed toward new concepts. We already noted one example of how the concept of occupational identity emerged from research that was also designed to examine the Occupational Performance History Interview (Mallinson, Mahaffey, & Kielhofner, 1996). In that case, the research pointed out that the concept of occupational adaptation actually encompassed two discrete phenomena that were later represented in the concepts of occupational identity and competence.

Some further examples are as follows. Early research on the AMPS (Doble, 1991; Pan & Fisher, 1994) resulted in a critical change in the concept of skill. Originally, skill was equated with underlying capacity, but the research efforts in developing measures of skill resulted in a redefinition of skill as a quality of the performance itself. The research that was part of developing the Role Checklist (Oakley, Kielhofner, Barris, & Reichler, 1986) helped refine the definition of role and the range of roles identified in the theory.

Many of the studies listed in the appendix of this chapter are primarily characterized as psychometric or instrument development studies. Most of these studies have also substantially contributed to testing and clarifying concepts. Moreover, in the earlier stages of developing a conceptual model of practice, it is important to do such research since it not only refines concepts, but also creates operational measures of concepts that can be used in other types of basic studies.

Correlational Studies

MOHO theory specifies relationships between variables that can be tested in research. The following is an example. Volition includes the concepts of personal causation, values, and interests. A proposition of MOHO theory is that a person's values, interests, and personal causation lead to activity and occupational choices. The theory also proposes that, over time, these choices result in a pattern of occupational participation. As shown in *Figure 27-3,* one can logically derive from these two propositions that one's personal causation, values, and interests should bear a relationship to one's pattern of occupational participation.

An example of a study that tested this relationship is Neville-Jan's (1994) examination of the correlation between volition and patterns of occupation among 100 individuals with varying degrees of depression. This study found, as expected, a relationship between the adaptiveness of the subjects' routines and measures of their personal causation and interests. Another example is a study by Peterson et al. (1999) that examined the relationship between personal causation (feelings of efficacy related to falling) and pattern of occupational engagement in 270 older adults. They found, as expected, that lowered falls self-efficacy was related to reduced leisure and social occupations, mediated by the elders' choices to restrict what they did.

These two studies thus provided evidence in support of the propositions noted above.

Correlational studies are also helpful in identifying concepts that do not hold up under scrutiny. For example, the concept of values previously included a subconcept, temporal orientation (Kielhofner, 1985). The study by Neville-Jan (1994) failed to find an expected relationship between extent of future orientation and adaptiveness in the subjects' occupational participation. Kavanaugh (1982) also failed to find a relationship between future orientation and interaction with the environment among adults with mental retardation. The findings of these two studies, combined with those of other basic and applied studies (Duellman., Barris, & Kielhofner, 1986; Muñoz, Lawlor, & Kielhofner, 1993), led to the elimination of temporal orientation from the concept of values.

Correlational research also has important implications for intervention. When the concepts in a theory have been shown to be important in explaining actions that may be targets of intervention, therapists can have greater confidence that it is worth their efforts to evaluate and address them in therapy. For example, evidence that falls self-efficacy leads to decisions to unnecessarily curtail doing things suggests that assessing and addressing the fear of falling could have a positive impact on persons' occupational participation.

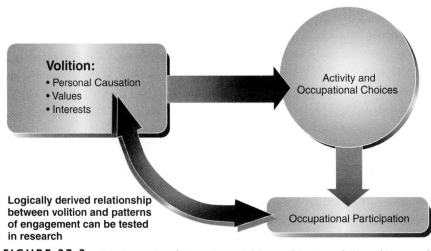

FIGURE 27-3   An Example of Questions Addressed in Correlational Research.

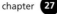

Comparative Studies

Comparative studies test the explanatory value of MOHO concepts by asking whether distinctly different groups differ on variables derived from these concepts. The logic of such studies derives from the fact that MOHO concepts are aimed at explaining occupational adaptation. For example, MOHO argues that environmental impact, volition, habituation, and performance capacity (and their subconcepts) contribute to occupational adaptation. Therefore, groups whose occupational adaptation is clearly different should demonstrate some differences on environmental impact, values, personal causation, interests, roles, habits, and performance capacity.

When such hypothesized differences are found, they lend support to the explanatory value of the concepts. When differences are not found, the evidence can suggest that the theory is not useful for explaining why the individuals belonging to the two or more groups differ in their occupational adaptation. Also, when groups are compared on several variables derived from MOHO, the fact that some concepts distinguish the groups while others do not can be helpful in refining how the theory is used to explain the occupational adaptation of particular groups.

The following are some examples of comparative studies. Dickerson and Oakley (1995) compared 1020 community-living adults with 292 adults who had physical or psychological impairments. They found that persons with disabilities had fewer roles and fewer anticipated future roles. Ebb, Coster, and Duncombe (1989) compared 18 nondisabled male adolescents with 15 who had psychosocial impairments. They also found differences between the groups in the number of current and anticipated future roles. Lederer, Kielhofner, and Watts (1985) compared 15 delinquent and 15 nondelinquent adolescents and found that fewer delinquent adolescents valued student and worker roles highly and that more delinquents assigned no value to the volunteer and home maintainer role. These studies support the MOHO assertion that problems of occupational adaptation involve a disruption or failure of roles.

Barris, Dickie, and Baron (1988) compared 66 adolescents and young adults who had chronic physical impairments, psychiatric impairments, or eating disorders with 86 adolescents and adults who did not have impairments. They found differences in personal causation, values, roles, and family environment impact across these groups. Barris, Kielhofner, Burch, Gelinas, Klement, and Schultz (1986) studied 30 adolescents. Two groups had either psychophysiologic illness or psychiatric diagnoses. A third group included subjects not being treated currently for any medical or emotional problems. Personal causation, values, roles, and habit patterns were shown to be factors that effectively discriminated between the three groups. These two studies provided evidence for expected differences in volition and habituation and indicated that MOHO concepts can effectively explain differences in the occupational adaptation of groups.

In addition to studies that examine different groups of persons, some studies examine the same group across time to compare when they did and did not have disabilities. For example, Davies Hallet, Zasler, Maurer, and Cash, (1994) examined 28 adolescents and adults following traumatic brain injury, comparing their roles before and after the onset of disability. They found that subjects tended to lose the worker, hobbyist, and friend roles, although some subjects also gained the roles of home maintainer, family member, and religious participant. Studies such as this one are useful for revealing information about the kinds of disability-related changes that occur over time.

Although aimed at testing and refining theory, these types of studies have important implications for practice. They constitute a form of needs assessment. That is, they identify areas of likely problems in certain client groups. This information is helpful for knowing what needs to be addressed in therapy. For example, the study of adolescents indicates that adolescents who are identified as being delinquent tend to experience alienation from roles valued by most members of society. This information suggests that a program for such adolescents should consider addressing the development of role identification.

Predictive Studies

Predictive studies ask whether MOHO concepts can explain and anticipate future behavior or states in subjects. The logic of these studies is similar to that of correlational studies. Predictive studies are generally more rigorous tests of theory than correlational studies, since they add the element of temporal directionality to the questions. Such studies test whether the current status of a variable derived from MOHO concepts can accurately predict what a client will do or what kind of status a subject will have at a later time.

For example, Rust, Barris, and Hooper (1987) found that roles and leisure values, along with an exercise-specific variable derived from the concept of personal causation, were predictors of women's exercise behavior. A further example of this type of research is Henry's (1994) follow-up study of adolescents and young adults following a first psychotic episode. She found that occupational adaptation (OPHI) and a self report checklist predicted psychosocial functioning and symptomatic recovery of subjects 6 months later. In another predictive study, Chen, Neufeld, Feely, and Skinner (1999) asked whether volition, habituation, and performance capacity variables would predict compliance in 62 outpatient clients at an orthopedic upper extremity rehabilitation facility. They found that while roles and physical capacity were not related, personal causation-related variables (perceived self efficiency and health locus of control) were predictors of compliance.

Studies such as the last two, which examine the ability of MOHO concepts and explain and predict health-related or intervention-related outcomes, are also important to inform intervention. For example, if personal causation is consistently shown in ongoing research to predict compliance, then it would follow that outpatient services that rely heavily on client compliance might improve their impact by addressing personal causation in intervention. Similarly, if occupational adaptation, as captured by the OPHI-II and client self-report, predicts psychosocial functioning and symptomatic recovery, practitioners might be encouraged to administer the OPHI-II and self reports such as the OSA in practice to identify and focus on remediating specific problems of occupational adaptation that might otherwise compromise a client's later functioning.

Qualitative Research That Examines and Explicates Theory

Whereas most quantitative studies are designed to test whether concepts hold up under empirical scrutiny, qualitative studies often seek to go beyond this aim.

That is, they also examine phenomena in depth to see how adequately a theory explains it. Such research then often tends to further explicate theory. That is, it reveals a richer, deeper dimension to the phenomena addressed by the theory, thereby allowing the theory to be altered to better fit the phenomena. Such research leads to expanding or refining concepts and postulates. It can also result in new concepts and postulates.

The following three investigations that are part of a longitudinal, qualitative study exemplify this approach. As shown in *Figure 27-4*, the studies were concerned with the role of narrative in occupational adaptation. The central postulate that the studies examined was that persons understand their occupational lives in terms of narrative and seek to influence how their occupational narrative unfolds.

In this longitudinal, multiple-year study, Jonsson, Kielhofner, and Borell (1997) first examined a group of 32 older persons just before retirement. The study underscored two things. First, the way that elders anticipated retirement could be seen as progressive (things will get better after retirement), regressive (things will get worse), or stability (things will be the same) narratives. Second, the kind of narrative with which each person anticipated retirement was closely tied to work experience. For example, someone who did not like work was likely to tell a progressive narrative in which retirement would be a release from a negative experience. This study lent support to the hypothesis that persons made sense of their occupational lives in terms of narratives and provided some insight into how persons formed their occupational narratives.

In the next investigation, Jonsson, Josephsson, and Kielhofner (2000) examined how these narratives shaped and were, in turn, influenced by what happened as these persons retired. They found that the direction that retirees' lives took reflected an interaction between their original narrative and unfolding events and circumstances. Subjects' narratives readied them to respond in particular ways to what happened. At the same time, what happened could also nudge the narrative in one direction or another. Although occupational narratives tended to be resilient—that is, to maintain their own plot—they could also change in response to changed circumstances. The study also identified that some persons were much more active in at-

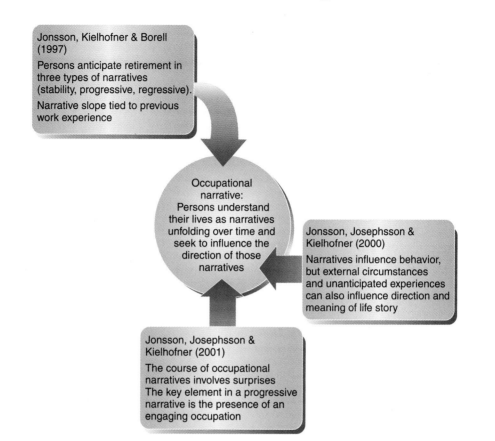

FIGURE 27-4 An Example of Theory Explicating Research: Three Sequential Studies of Occupational Narratives.

tempting to change the shape of their narrative (e.g., avoid an undesired outcome or affect a desired one) than others. Thus, the original postulate that persons seek to continue their narratives was somewhat attenuated by this finding. In fact, the extent to which persons are motivated by their narratives appeared to vary depending on whether their tendency was to actively shape versus respond to the events of their lives.

The third study (Jonsson, Josephsson, & Kielhofner, 2001) that followed the subjects further into retirement yielded two findings. First, elders' narratives often had to deal with surprising turns of events. Things happened that were quite unanticipated by each person's narrative. This included not only events but also how some persons felt about their situations. Interestingly, elders were often surprised at their own reactions and experiences. One example is that elders

had anticipated being highly motivated to do things once they could do only what they wanted. Paradoxically, they found it more difficult to find the energy to get things done.

The second major finding of this study was that constructing a positive life story required these elders to find and participate in an engaging occupation. Engaging occupations evoked a passion or strong feeling and were a central feature in occupational narratives. They were infused with positive meaning connected to interest (i.e., pleasure, challenge, enjoyment), personal causation (i.e., challenge, indication of one's competence), and value (i.e., something worth doing, something important, a contribution to family or society). This study thus provided more information about how narratives unfold and about what is critical to the construction of a positive narrative.

Taken together these three studies validated the postulate that persons made sense of their lives and anticipated their futures through narrative. Even more importantly, the studies offered additional insights into how occupational narratives figure in persons' lives and into how they are constructed. In this way, the studies provided information that enriched and allowed the theory to be extended further. Finally, the studies' findings provided information useful to therapists who were attempting to help their clients construct positive occupational narratives.

Types of Studies Characterizing MOHO-Based Applied Research

Studies with applied research purposes address questions on a continuum of events that occur in providing individual services or in a program, as shown in *Figure 27-5*. This means that the types of applied research fall in the following categories:

- Psychometric studies leading to development of structured assessments
- Studies of how concepts influence therapeutic reasoning and practice
- Studies that examine what happens in therapy
- Outcomes studies.

Each of these types of applied research are examined below.

Psychometric Studies Leading to Development of Structured Assessments

As discussed in Chapter 12, research that supports development of structured assessments seeks to assure the dependability of those methods (Benson & Schell, 1997). A dependable information-gathering method is reliable and yields consistent information in different circumstances, at different times, with different clients, and when different therapists administer it. For example, Biernacki (1993) examined the inter-rater reliability of the WRI by comparing the ratings of three different therapists who interviewed 30 adults receiving rehabilitation. She also interviewed 20 of the subjects a second time to test retest reliability. The study found the assessment to have good inter-rater and test-retest reliability.

A dependable information-gathering method must also be valid, that is, provide the information it is intended to provide. MOHO concepts point toward certain phenomena. To be valid, assessments must capture information on these specific phenomena.

Validity studies often begin by examining whether the content of an assessment is coherent and representative of what is intended to be gathered (i.e., content validity). Thus, items on an assessment may be examined for the extent to which they cohere to reflect the underlying concept. Sometimes this is done by gathering the opinions of experts. For example, Brollier, Watts, Bauer, and Schmidt (1989) examined content va-

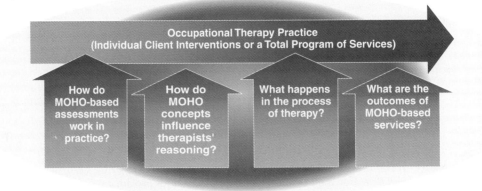

FIGURE 27-5   Applied Research Questions.

lidity of the AOF by asking 15 occupational therapists to match the 25 items in the assessment to MOHO concepts of volition, personal causation, interests, roles, habits, and skills. Based on the responses of these therapists, they concluded that the AOF adequately covered the domain of content of the six concepts.

Another approach to examining the content validity is statistical analysis of the items to determine whether the items coalesce to identify an underlying trait. Forsyth, Lai, and Kielhofner (1999) examined 52 therapists' ratings of 117 subjects and found evidence that the items on the ACIS coalesced well to capture this area of skill. As noted earlier in the discussion of basic research, studies such as these also serve to provide evidence about the underlying concept the assessment is designed to capture. Thus, they have both the applied purpose of developing an assessment for use in therapy and the basic purpose of providing evidence about the concept on which the assessment gathers information.

Other research that examines validity asks whether the assessments correlate with measures of concepts which are expected to concur and whether it diverges from those with which no relationship is expected. Brollier, Watts, Bauer, and Schmidt (1989) demonstrated that the AOF was correlated, as expected, with a well-known measure of adaptation, the Global Assessment Scale (GAS), when both were administered to 41 persons with a primary diagnosis of schizophrenia.

Another way of examining the validity of assessments is to determine whether they can differentiate between different groups of people. An example of this type of study is an investigation by Viik, Watts, Madigan, and Bauer (1990) in which the AOF was administered to 24 adults undergoing inpatient treatment for alcoholism and 24 adults with at least 1 year of alcohol abstinence and attendance at Alcoholics Anonymous meetings. The rater who scored the AOF was unaware of the subjects' group membership. AOF scores correctly discriminated all but 3 of 48 subjects into the correct group.

In addition to studies that examine reliability and validity, some studies examine the clinical utility of assessments. For example, Fossey (1996) examined the use of the Occupational Performance History Interview by British therapists who were assessing persons who

had psychiatric disabilities. She concluded that the therapists found the interview useful for planning intervention, but also made recommendations for improving the utility of the assessment.

The development of any MOHO assessment ordinarily involves a series of studies. These studies not only provide evidence about the reliability, validity, and utility of each assessment, but also contribute to the ongoing improvement of the assessment. Some of the assessments are quite extensively studied, whereas others are still in the process of development, as was noted in Chapters 13 through 16.

Studies of How MOHO Theory Influences Therapeutic Reasoning

Chapter 11 emphasized that therapists should actively use MOHO theory and technology in their therapeutic reasoning. An important area of research is to examine how therapists use the theory and related tools in practice. One example of such an investigation is a survey by Muñoz, Lawlor, and Kielhofner (1993). The study examined the use of MOHO among 50 skilled occupational therapists and identified which concepts therapists most actively used in their practices.

A study by Oakley, Kielhofner, and Barris (1985) examined how information from MOHO-based assessments influenced therapists' ability to make judgments about clients. In this study, the results of a battery of MOHO-based assessments on 30 persons hospitalized due to psychiatric illness were given to a therapist, who was blind to the identities of the clients.

The therapist reviewed the assessment results and rated each subject on a scale of adaptiveness. The therapist's judgment was found to be an excellent predictor of the patients' adaptive behaviors as rated by nursing staff. This study provides evidence that therapists who use MOHO concepts and assessments can effectively discriminate between levels of adaptive potential in clients.

Studies that scrutinize the use of theory by therapists examine how the theory impacts practice. These studies also highlight which concepts in the theory are most helpful to therapists. Thus, such studies provide critical information about how the theory can be altered to be more relevant to practitioners.

Studies That Examine What Happens in Therapy

It is important not only to understand whether interventions based on a model of practice work, but also to know why they do or do not work. Studies that examine the impact of interventions increasingly focus on identifying the underlying mechanism of change (Gitlin et al., 2000). Examining what goes in therapy to improve services before they are more formally tested is often an important prelude to designing intervention outcome studies.

The following are two examples of studies that examined what happened in the process of therapy. Helfrich and Kielhofner (1994) examined how client occupational narratives influenced the meaning they assigned to occupational therapy. This study showed how the meanings of therapy intended by therapists were often not received by or in concert with clients' meaning. The study findings underscored the importance of therapists having knowledge of the client's narrative and organizing therapy as a series of events that enter into that narrative.

Kielhofner and Barrett (1997) examined occupational therapists' use of goal setting in therapy. Their findings illustrate that therapists actively worked both to give substance to the occupational form of goal setting and to surround it with an implied progressive narrative in which the client makes short-term efforts to impact the long-term outcomes of the narrative. At the same time, clients' assigned meaning to the therapy process is based on their own narratives. When the two narratives did not coincide, therapists ended up encouraging clients toward attitudes and performances that did not resonate with their experience of reality.

Studies such as those just presented illuminate, from the perspective of MOHO concepts, aspects of the dynamics of therapy. They provide specific information about how therapy can be improved to better meet client needs and support clients to achieve desired change. More studies that carefully examine what goes on in therapy are needed to better illuminate the dynamics of therapy and more clearly illuminate the nature of client change.

Outcomes Studies

Outcomes research is concerned with the results of applying MOHO in practice. Such studies examine whether therapy based on the model's theory and technology for application produces desirable outcomes. A limited number of such studies have been reported in the literature. The following are examples.

Josephsson, Backman, Borell, Nygård and Bernspång (1995) examined the effectiveness of a MOHO-based intervention to improve occupational performance among four clients with dementia. They found that three of four clients showed gains in performance. The study underscored the importance of attending to volition and habituation to achieve increases in observed skill in performance.

Kielhofner and Brinson (1989) developed and studied an aftercare program for young adults with psychiatric disabilities. Twenty randomly assigned subjects received a 12-week aftercare program based on MOHO, and 14 randomly assigned subjects served as controls. Although the study found lower rates of recidivism and higher functioning among those who received the MOHO-based services, these differences were not statistically significant. The lack of significance was likely due to the small sample size.

These studies underscore an important issue about outcomes research. The design, funding, and conduct of rigorous outcomes research with adequate sample sizes present a substantial challenge (Bland & Schmitz, 1987, Holcomb & Roush, 1988; Watson, 1990).

The development of outcomes studies follows a process (Case-Smith, 1999) in which a variety of the research strategies are integrated over time into an ongoing program of research, culminating in large-scale studies. The following is an example of this process.

At the University of Illinois at Chicago, investigators began several years ago developing measures of psychosocial and environmental factors relevant to work success (Haglund, Karlsson, Kielhofner, & Lai, 1997; Kielhofner, Lai, et al., 1999; Velozo et al., 1999). They developed, implemented, and documented work programs based on MOHO (Kielhofner, Braveman, et al., 1999; Mallinson, LaPlante, & Hollman-Smith, 1998; Mentrup, Neihaus & Kielhofner, 1999; Olson & Kielhofner, 1998). With funding from the American Occupational Therapy Foundation, a preliminary outcomes study of one of these work programs was conducted (Barrett, Beer, & Kielhofner, 1999; Kielhofner & Barrett, 1997). Subsequently, another foundation grant supported a pilot project that applied and investigated the approach with persons living with AIDS. Building on the experience and expertise developed over several years, investigators undertook a federally funded, multi-year research and demonstration project to investigate the process and efficacy of a MOHO-based work program, Employment Options.[a] In this program, 110 clients use a multi-method action research design that uses ongoing findings to inform program development and that involves clients as active participants in generating and analyzing the data as well as considering its practical implications (Heron, 1988; Jensen, 1989; Reason 1988; Sanford, 1981; Torbert, l981). This study is currently being completed (see Chapter 26 for a discussion of this program).

Another example of large-scale studies that examine the impact of services based on aspects of MOHO are two multi-year investigations being undertaken by Laura Gitlin[b,c] at Thomas Jefferson University, Philadelphia, Pennsylvania, each funded by the National Institute on Aging. One study examines the effectiveness of an occupational therapy home-based intervention for family caregivers of individuals with dementia. The other study tests a similar intervention for physically frail elders. Both studies use many of the environmental concepts from MOHO.

Discussion

This chapter sought to identify why research on a conceptual practice model is important and to characterize the kinds of studies that have examined and contributed to the development of MOHO. In the course of the discussion, types of both basic and applied research that examine MOHO were identified. Only some of the published studies were used as examples.

Anyone who wishes to have a fuller appreciation of the research that has been completed in a particular area should review the relevant studies directly. At the end of this chapter is an appendix that lists all the published MOHO-based studies. A brief summary of each

[a]Employment Options: A Program Leading to Employment of Persons Living with AIDS (Rehabilitation Services Administration, U.S. Department of Education, Grant no. DED H235A980170-00).
[b]Project ABLE: Advancing Better Living among Elders (National Institutes of Aging, Grant no. RO1 AG13687).
[c]Environmental Skill-building Program for Families of Persons with Dementia (National Institutes of Aging, Grant no. U01-AG13265).

study is provided. Finally, the studies are coded to indicate what type of research the study represents.

One of the most important things about MOHO research, as with research undertaken within any model, has been the establishment of a tradition of research. Within a research tradition, two important things occur:

- Findings are cumulative
- The approach to conducting research on the model is refined and becomes more sophisticated.

Cumulative Findings

As repeatedly noted, no single study can ever provide the definitive evidence to answer a research question. Therefore, it is important to generate cumulative findings (Christiansen, 1981, 1990). Over time, a growing body of evidence can be used to scrutinize and refine the theoretical arguments and the various technologies for application. This results in:

- More and more accurate explanations of the phenomena the model addresses
- Greater effectiveness in the model's application.

In the end, this is the fundamental purpose of research on a model. It improves the ability of the model to explain some phenomena and to generate practical actions to address those phenomena.

Refinement of Research Methodologies

More than 20 years ago when MOHO was first introduced, it was not clear how it would be studied. The kinds of research that have been generated by a wide range of investigators have demonstrated a variety of ways in which the model can be studied. For example, the previous discussions illustrate that MOHO is being studied with a range of quantitative and qualitative research methods and that the body of research includes a number of different kinds of studies that address both basic and applied questions. The fact that many different research strategies are being used to investigate this model is a definite strength. Different research approaches provide different kinds of evidence that, when taken together, provide greater scrutiny of and insight into MOHO.

Over time, MOHO-based research has grown more sophisticated and rigorous. As one develops a tradition of research within a model, studies are able to build on the findings of previous studies, refine their approaches and methods, and provide more precise results. For example, early studies often used instruments to gather data that were relevant to but not specifically developed to capture MOHO concepts. Now that many tools have been developed for gathering data on MOHO concepts, more precise studies are possible.

Another example of the growing sophistication of the research tradition is that more and more MOHO research is taking place across national and cultural boundaries. This has allowed the examination of the relevance of MOHO across differences in culture. A number of the studies have, for example, specifically examined how assessments work in different languages and cultural contexts. Some cross-cultural research has begun to examine whether MOHO concepts have equal relevance across cultures.

Need for Further Research

We have repeatedly noted that any single study cannot stand alone as a test of theory or utility of a model. Rather, the strength of the research on any model is found in the accumulation of evidence across studies and in the quality and rigor of the studies. MOHO-based research represents an ongoing and maturing process of refining methods and accumulating findings.

Many of the earlier and continuing studies have focused on validation of MOHO concepts and assessments. Studies that examine the therapy process and the outcomes of therapy are less well represented in the body of research. Of course, this represents a natural sequence as shown in *Figure 27-6*. When a conceptual practice model is being developed, early efforts ordinarily focus on refining concepts and developing technology of practice (including assessments and intervention strategies). Later studies examine and refine the use of the theory and technology in practice. Studies of therapeutic effectiveness tend to come last.

It is difficult to identify a single priority for future research. All the kinds of research discussed in this chapter are important to making MOHO a more effective model, that is, they enhance the ability of the model to guide the provision of services that achieve good outcomes. However, at this stage in the development of the model, some important directions for future research can be identified. For example, it would be particularly useful to have further examination of the process of therapy to:

- Determine more accurately the mechanisms of change that underlie MOHO-based therapy
- Determine therapist and client actions involved in the change process as well as process variables such as the structure, timing, and mode of intervention that contribute to change.

This book represents the first attempt to describe in detail the factors that influence change in therapy. For example, Chapter 18 discussed the change process and pro-

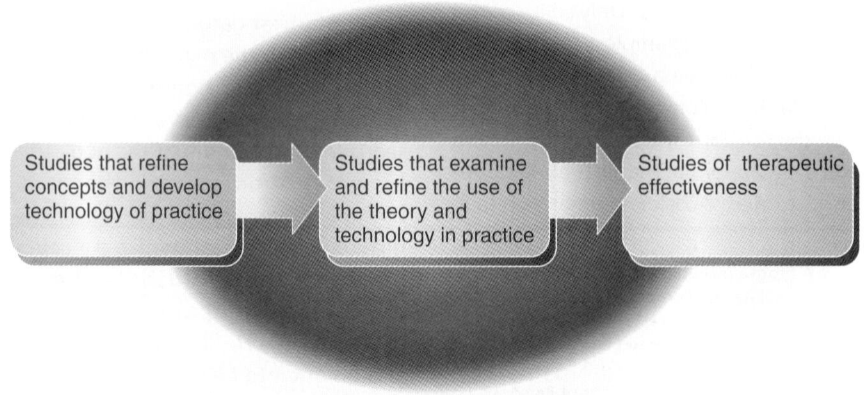

FIGURE 27-6   A Typical Sequence of Research for Studying a Conceptual Practice Model.

posed a taxonomy of client occupational engagement that drives change. Chapter 19 proposed a taxonomy of therapist strategies that support client occupational engagement and change. An important future research topic will be to examine and expand these taxonomies and to study the relationship of specific forms of client occupational engagement and therapist strategies to outcomes.

A final important direction for future research is outcomes studies. The ultimate value of MOHO depends on whether services based on its concepts and technology produce results. Although much anecdotal data, including cases and programs of intervention presented in this book and elsewhere, suggest that the model guides effective therapy, additional evidence is needed. Particularly important will be the funding and implementation of multi-year studies that combine large sample sizes with methodological rigor. Once again, no single study will answer the question of what outcomes emanate from MOHO-based services. The answer to that question will require the cumulative evidence from many studies.

Conclusion

The MOHO-based research that has been reported in the literature constitutes a useful body of evidence concerning the model. It also provides important resources for guiding future research. Moreover, new studies are always expanding the ways that MOHO is investigated. For example, Christine Helfrich at the University of Illinois at Chicago is conducting a longitudinal study (funded by the U.S. Department of Education, National Institute on Disability and Rehabilitation Research) of women who have experienced domestic violence. In this study, women initially participate in the OPHI-II and several other MOHO-based assessments that are being used to describe their occupational performance and participation. The study then follows these subjects for 2 years to understand their service utilization and how well their occupational needs are met. This study will contribute in new ways to illustrating how MOHO can be used to frame the occupational adaptation of a new target group.

If the growing base of MOHO research over the past decade is any indication of the future, we can look forward to an increasing number of studies that will shed light on and further refine and improve MOHO. The quality of studies underway at the time of this writing also indicates that increasingly complex and rigorous research will be reported in the future. As these studies are reported in the literature, they will contribute to the further refinement of MOHO theory and to the improvement of its utility in practice.

Key Terms

Applied research: Investigations or aspects of investigations that aim to test the practical utility of the theory and related technology for application.

Basic research: Investigations or aspects of investigations that aim to test the theoretical arguments proposed in the model.

References

Barrett, L., Beer, D., & Kielhofner, G. (1999). The importance of volitional narrative in treatment: An ethnographic case study in a work program. *Work: A Journal of Prevention, Assessment & Rehabilitation, 12* (1), 79–92.

Barris, R., Dickie, V., & Baron, K. (1988). A comparison of psychiatric patients and normal subjects based on the model of human occupation. *Occupational Therapy Journal of Research, 8*, 3–37.

Barris, R., Kielhofner, G., Burch, R. M., Gelinas, I., Klement, M., & Schultz, B. (1986). Occupational function and dysfunction in three groups of adolescents. *Occupational Therapy Journal of Research, 6*, 301–317.

Benson, J., & Schell, B. A. (1997). Measurement theory: Application to occupational and physical therapy. In Van Deusen J., & Brunt D. (Eds.), *Assessment in occupational therapy and physical therapy*. Philadelphia: WB Saunders.

Biernacki, S. D. (1993). Reliability of the Worker Role Interview. *American Journal of Occupational Therapy, 47*, 797–803.

Bland, C. J., & Schmitz, C. C. (1987). Characteristics of the successful researcher and implications for faculty development. *Journal of Medical Education, 61*, 22–31.

Brollier, C., Watts, J. H., Bauer, D., & Schmidt, W. (1989). A content validity study of the Assessment of Occupational Functioning. *Occupational Therapy in Mental Health, 8* (4), 29–47.

Case-Smith, J. (1999). Developing a research career: Advice from occupational therapy researchers. *American Journal of Occupational Therapy, 53,* 44–50.

Chen, C., Neufeld, P. S., Feely, C. A., & Skinner, C. S. (1999). Factors influencing compliance with home exercise programs among patients with upper-extremity impairment. *American Journal of Occupational Therapy, 53,* 171–180.

Christiansen, C. (1981). Toward resolution of crisis: Research requisites in occupational therapy. *Occupational Therapy Journal of Research, 1,* 115–124.

Christiansen, C. (1990). The perils of plurality. *Occupational Therapy Journal of Research, 10,* 259–265.

Crombie, I. K. (1996). *The pocket guide to critical appraisal.* London, UK: BMJ Publishing Group.

Davies Hallet, J., Zasler, N., Maurer, P., & Cash, S. (1994). Role change after traumatic brain injury in adults. *American Journal of Occupational Therapy, 48,* 241–246.

Dickerson, A. E., & Oakely, F. (1995). Comparing the roles of community-living persons and patient populations. *American Journal of Occupational Therapy, 49,* 221–228.

Doble, S. E. (1991). Test-retest and inter-rater reliability of a process skills assessment. *Occupational Therapy Journal of Research, 11,* 8–23.

Duellman, M. K., Barris, R., & Kielhofner, G. (1986). Organized activity and the adaptive status of nursing home residents. *American Journal of Occupational Therapy, 40,* 618–622.

Ebb, E. W., Coster, W., & Duncombe, L. (1989). Comparison of normal and psychosocially dysfunctional male adolescents. *Occupational Therapy in Mental Health, 9,* 53–74.

Forsyth, K., Lai, J., & Kielhofner, G. (1999). The assessment of communication and interaction skills (ACIS): Measurement properties. *British Journal of Occupational Therapy, 62* (2), 69–74.

Fossey, E. (1996). Using the occupational performance history interview (OPHI): Therapists' reflections. *British Journal of Occupational Therapy, (5) 59,* 223–228.

Gitlin, L. N, Corcoran, M., Martindale-Adams, J., Malone, M. A., Stevens, A., & Winter, L. (2000). Identifying mechanisms of action: Why and how does intervention work? In R. Schulz (Ed.), *Handbook of dementia caregiving: Evidence-based interventions for family caregivers.* New York, Springer Publishing.

Haglund, L., Karlsson, G., Kielhofner, G., & Lai, J. S. (1997). Validity of the Swedish version of the Worker Role Interview. *Scandinavian Journal of Occupational Therapy, 4* (1–4), 23–29.

Helewa, A., & Walker, J. M. (2000). *Critical evaluation of research in physical rehabilitation: Towards evidence-based practice.* Philadelphia: WB Saunders.

Helfrich, C., & Kielhofner, G. (1994). Volitional narratives and the meaning of occupational therapy. *American Journal of Occupational Therapy, 48,* 319–326.

Henry, A. D. (1994). *Predicting psychosocial functioning and symptomatic recovery of adolescents and young adults with a first psychotic episode: A six-month follow-up study.* Unpublished doctoral dissertation, Boston University.

Heron, J. (1988). Validity in co-operative inquiry. In P. Reason (Ed.), *Human inquiry in action.* London: Sage Publications.

Holcomb, J. D., & Roush, R. E. (1988). A study of the scholarly activities of allied health faculty in southern academic health science centers. *Journal of Allied Health, 17,* 277–293.

Holm, M. (2000). The 2000 Eleanor Clarke Slagle Lecture. Our mandate for the new millennium: Evidence-based practice. *American Journal of Occupational Therapy, 54,* 575–585.

Jensen, U. J. (1989). From good medical practice to best medical practice. *International Journal of Health Planning and Management, 4,* 167–180.

Jonsson, H., Josephsson, S., & Kielhofner, G. (2000). Evolving narratives in the course of retirement: A longitudinal study. *American Journal of Occupational Therapy, 54,* 463–470.

Jonsson, H., Josephsson, S., & Kielhofner, G. (2001). Narratives and experience in an occupational transition: A longitudinal study of the retirement process. *American Journal of Occupational Therapy, 55,* 424–432.

Jonsson, H., Kielhofner, G., & Borell, L. (1997). Anticipating retirement: The formation of narratives concerning an occupational transition. *American Journal of Occupational Therapy, 51,* 49–56.

Josephsson, S., Backman, L., Borell, L., Nygård, L., & Bernspång, B. (1995). Effectiveness of an intervention to improve occupational performance among persons with dementia. *Occupational Therapy Journal of Research, 15,* 36–49.

Kavanaugh, M. (1982). *Person-environment interaction: the model of human occupation applied to mentally retarded adults.* Unpublished Masters Thesis, Virginia Commonwealth University.

Kielhofner, G. (1985). *A model of human occupation: Theory and application* (2nd ed.). Baltimore: Williams & Wilkins.

Kielhofner, G., & Barrett, L. (1997). Meaning and misunderstanding in occupational forms: A study of therapeutic goal-setting. *American Journal of Occupational Therapy, 52* (5), 345–353.

Kielhofner, G., Braveman, B., Baron, K., Fischer, G., Hammel, J., & Littleton, M. (1999). The model of human occupation: understanding the worker who is injured or disabled. *Work: A Journal of Prevention, Assessment & Rehabilitation, 12* (1), 3–11.

Kielhofner, G., & Brinson, M. (1989). Development and evaluation of an aftercare program for young and chronic psychiatrically disabled adults. *Occupational Therapy in Mental Health, 9* (2), 1–25.

Kielhofner, G., Lai, J. S., Olson, L., Haglund, L., Ekbadh, E., & Hedlund, M. (1999). Psychometric properties of the work environment impact scale: A cross-cultural study. *Work: A Journal of Prevention, Assessment & Rehabilitation, 12* (1), 71–77.

Lederer, J., Kielhofner, G., & Watts, J. (1985). Values, personal causation and skills of delinquents and non delinquents. *Occupational Therapy in Mental Health, 5,* 59–77.

Mallinson, T., Kielhofner, G., & Mattingly, C. (1996). Metaphor and meaning in a clinical interview. *American Journal of Occupational Therapy, 50,* 338–346.

Mallinson, T., LaPlante, D., & Hollman-Smith, J. (1998). *Work rehabilitation in mental health programs.* Chicago: Model of Human Occupation Clearinghouse, Department of Occupational Therapy, College of Applied Health Sciences, University of Illinois at Chicago.

Mallinson, T., Mahaffey, L., & Kielhofner, G. (1998). The occupational performance history interview: Evidence for three underlying constructs of occupational adaptation. *Canadian Journal of Occupational Therapy, 65,* 219–228.

Mentrup, C., Niehaus, A., & Kielhofner, G. (1999). Applying the model of human occupation in work-focused rehabilitation: A case illustration. *Work: A Journal of Prevention, Assessment & Rehabilitation, 12* (1), 61–70.

Mosey, A. C. (1992a). *Applied scientific inquiry in the health professions: An epistemological orientation.* Rockville, MD: American Occupational Therapy Association.

Mosey, A. C. (1992b). Partition of occupational science and occupational therapy. *American Journal of Occupational Therapy, 4,* 851.

Muñoz, J., Lawlor, M., & Kielhofner, G. (1993). Use of the model of human occupation in psychiatric practice: A survey of skilled therapists. *Occupational Therapy Journal of Research, 13,* 117–139.

Neville-Jan, A. (1994). The relationship of volition to adaptive occupational behavior among individuals with varying degrees of depression. *Occupational Therapy in Mental Health, 12,* 1–18.

Oakley, F., Kielhofner, G., & Barris, R. (1985). An occupational therapy approach to assessing psychiatric patients' adaptive functioning. *American Journal of Occupational Therapy, 39,* 147–154.

Oakley, F., Kielhofner, G., Barris, R., & Reichler, R. K. (1986). The Role Checklist: Development and empirical assessment of reliability. *Occupational Therapy Journal of Research, 6,* 157–170.

Olson, L. M., & Kielhofner, G. (1998). *Work readiness: Day treatment for persons with chronic disabilities.* Chicago: Model of Human Occupation Clearinghouse, Department of Occupational Therapy, College of Applied Health Sciences, University of Illinois at Chicago.

Pan, A. W., & Fisher, A. G. (1994). The assessment of motor and process skills of persons with psychiatric disorders. *American Journal of Occupational Therapy, 48,* 775–780.

Peterson, E., Howland, J., Kielhofner, G., Lachman, M. E., Assmann, S., Cote, J., & Jette, A. (1999). Falls self-efficacy and occupational adaptation among elders. *Physical & Occupational Therapy in Geriatrics, 16,* 1–16.

Reason, P. (1988). The co-operative inquiry group. In P. Reason (Ed.), *Human inquiry in action.* London: Sage Publications.

Rust, K., Barris, R., & Hooper, F. (1987). Use of the model of human occupation to predict women's exercise behavior. *Occupational Therapy Journal of Research, 7,* 23–35.

Sanford, N. (1981). A model for action research. In P. Reason & J. Rowan (Eds.), *Human inquiry. A source book of new paradigm research.* Chichester, England: Wiley.

Taylor, M. C. (2000). *Evidence-based practice for occupational therapists.* Osney Mead, Oxford: Blackwell Science.

Torbert, W. R. (1981). Why educational research has been so uneducational: The case for a new model of social science based on collaborative inquiry. In Reason, P., & Rowan, J. (Eds.). *Human inquiry: A sourcebook of new paradigm research.* Chichester, England: Wiley.

Velozo, C., Kielhofner, G., Gern, A., Lin, F-L., Azhar, F., Lai, J-S., & Fisher, G. (1999). Worker Role Interview: Validation of a psychosocial work-related measure. *Journal of Occupational Rehabilitation, 9,* 153–168.

Viik, M. K., Watts, J. H., Madigan, M. J., & Bauer, D. (1990). Preliminary validation of the Assessment of Occupational Functioning with an alcoholic population. *Occupational Therapy in Mental Health, 10* (2), 19–33.

Watson, P. G. (1990). Faculty research skills development. *Journal of Allied Health, 19,* 25–37.

Appendix: Research Abstract Abbreviations

COR = correlation
CV = concept validation
GC = group comparison
OR = outcomes research
POT = processes that occur in therapy

PD = predictive
PSU = psychometric and studies of the utility of assessments
QET = qualitative study explicating theory
TR = therapeutic reasoning

1. Aubin, G., Hachey, R., & Mercier, C. (1999). Meaning of daily activities and subjective quality of life in people with severe mental illness. *Scandinavian Journal of Occupational Therapy, 6* (2), 53–62. (COR)
This correlation study examined the relationship between the meaning of daily activities (i.e., perceived competence, value, and pleasure) and the subjective quality of life in 45 people with severe and persistent mental illness. The results suggest that perceived competence in daily tasks and rest as well as pleasure in work and rest activities are positively correlated with subjective quality of life.

2. Barrett, L., Beer, D., & Kielhofner, G. (1999). The importance of volitional narrative in treatment: An ethnographic case study in a work program. *Work: A Journal of Prevention, Assessment & Rehabilitation, 12* (1), 79–92. (POT)
This qualitative study intensively examined a single subject over a period of months before, during, and after her treatment in the work program. The study examined the process of therapy and illustrated how knowledge of a client's narrative and life world can shed light on difficulties that arise in the course of intervention.

3. Barris, R., Dickie, V., & Baron, K. (1988). A comparison of psychiatric patients and normal subjects based on the model of human occupation. *Occupational Therapy Journal of Research, 8* (1), 3–37. (GC)
In this study, data were collected from 152 subjects (young adults with chronic conditions, patients with eating disorders, adolescents hospitalized for psychiatric disorders, and graduate students) on values, personal causation, roles, skill, the environment, and role performance. The four groups differed on most measures of personal and environmental characteristics. Combinations of different variables explained variance in social role performance in each group.

4. Barris, R., Kielhofner, G., Burch, R. M., Gelinas, I., Klement, M., & Schultz, B. (1986). Occupational function and dysfunction in three groups of adolescents. *Occu-*

pational Therapy Journal of Research, 6 (5), 301–317. (GC)
This study compared characteristics of groups of adolescents with psychophysiologic illness (n = 10), with psychiatric diagnosis (n = 10), or without identified medical or emotional problems (n = 10). Data were collected on the volition and habituation variables. Taken together, locus of control, self ratings of competence and importance of activities in a typical day, number of not valued roles, time spent in work, play, and activities of daily living best discriminated the three groups.

5. Biernacki, S. D. (1993). Reliability of the Worker Role Interview. *American Journal of Occupational Therapy, 47* (9), 797–803. (PSU)
This psychometric study examined the inter-rater and test-retest reliability of the Worker Role Interview (WRI). Based on data from 30 adults who were receiving rehabilitation after an upper extremity injury and 3 therapist raters, the WRI showed good inter-rater and test-retest reliability.

6. Bränholm, I., & Fugl-Meyer, A. R. (1992). Occupational role preferences and life satisfaction. *Occupational Therapy Journal of Research, 12* (3), 159–171. (COR)
This correlation study examined the relationship between fulfillment of occupational roles and life satisfaction. The study included 214 men and women aged 25, 35, 45, and 55 years old. The subjects were asked to complete a version of the Role Checklist modified to be suitable for a Swedish population. The role profiles appeared similar for each gender at all ages. Factor analysis showed roles were clustered into the following areas: family, leisure, vocational, and organizational participant. Of the four, only vocation was age dependent. Fulfillment of different occupational roles was correlated with life satisfaction.

7. Bridle, M. J., Lynch, K. B., & Quesenberry, C. M. (1990). Long term function following the central cord syndrome. *Paraplegia, 28,* 178–185. (GC)
This study included 18 adults with spinal cord injury 2

to 9 years after injury. The Occupational Performance History Interview (OPHI) was used to capture an individual's process of adapting in everyday occupational performance. The results on the OPHI indicated that the central cord injury significantly and negatively affected occupational performance in the areas of organization of daily living routines, maintenance of life roles, identification and enactment of interests, and perception of ability and responsibility.

8. Brollier, C., Watts, J. H., Bauer, D., & Schmidt, W. (1988a). A concurrent validity study of two occupational therapy evaluation instruments: The AOF and OCAIRS. *Occupational Therapy in Mental Health*, *8* (4), 49–60. (PSU)

This psychometric study examined the concurrent validity of the Assessment of Occupational functioning (AOF) and Occupational Case Analysis Interview and Rating Scale (OCAIRS) using the Global Assessment Scale (GAS). Forty-one psychiatric patients (24 male, 17 female) with a primary diagnosis of schizophrenia were the subjects of the study. The OCAIRS and the AOF were correlated, as expected, to the GAS.

9. Brollier, C., Watts, J. H., Bauer, D., & Schmidt, W. (1988b). A content validity study of the Assessment of Occupational Functioning. *Occupational Therapy in Mental Health*, *8* (4), 29–47. (PSU)

This psychometric study examined the content validity of the Assessment of Occupational Functioning (AOF). A content validity questionnaire consisting of the AOF items in a scrambled order was administered to 15 occupational therapists who were asked to match model components—volition, personal causation, interests, roles, habits, and skills—to the 25 items on the questionnaire. The AOF was found to adequately cover the domain of content of the six model components.

10. Brown, T., & Carmichael, K. (1992). Assertiveness training for clients with psychiatric illness: A pilot study. *British Journal of Occupational Therapy*, *55* (4), 137–140. (OR)

This study examined the outcome of a 7-week assertiveness training program, based on MOHO and social learning theory, for clients with a psychiatric illness. The one group, pre-test/post-test design study indicated that the 33 participants exhibited a statistically significant increase in assertive behavior and self-esteem.

11. Chen, C., Neufeld, P. S., Feely, C. A., & Skinner, C. S. (1999). Factors influencing compliance with home exercise programs among patients with upper-extremity impairment. *American Journal of Occupational Therapy*, *53* (2), 171–180. (PR)

This study examined factors from three models (MOHO, Health Belief Model, and Health Locus of Control Model) to identify those that predicted increased compliance and satisfaction with home exercise programs in 62 outpatient clients at an orthopedic upper extremity rehabilitation facility. Results suggested that volition was a good predictor of increased compliance and satisfaction with home exercise programs.

12. Chern, J., Kielhofner, G., de las Heras, C., & Magalhaes, L. (1996). The volitional questionnaire: Psychometric development and practical use. *American Journal of Occupational Therapy*, *50* (7), 516–525. (CV, PSU)

Two psychometric studies of the Volitional Questionnaire (VQ) are reported. In the first study, data from 43 women and men in a long-term psychiatric facility indicated that the VQ items worked well together to define the construct of volition. Based on this study, the scoring criteria were modified. In the second study, observations of 18 persons with psychiatric illness and developmental disabilities indicated that the revised scoring system improved inter-rater reliability.

13. Corner, R., Kielhofner, G., & Lin, F. L. (1997). Construct validity of a work environment impact scale. *Work*, *9* (1), 21–34. (PSU)

This psychometric study examined the construct validity of the Work Environment Impact Scale (WEIS). Data from 20 individuals with psychiatric illness indicated that the items worked well together to define the construct of environmental impact. The WEIS also was shown to provide clinically relevant information for planning work-related interventions or reasonable accommodations.

14. Davies Hallet, J., Zasler, N., Maurer, P., & Cash, S. (1994). Role change after traumatic brain injury in adults. *American Journal of Occupational Therapy*, *48* (3), 241–246. (GC)

This group comparison study examined changes in adult life roles after a severe traumatic brain injury. The Role Checklist was given to 28 adults with traumatic brain injury who had been in the community for more than 8 months before the study. Their main role change was role loss. Role losses were mainly those of worker, hobbyist, and friend. Role gains were mainly those of home maintainer, family member, and religious participant.

15. DeForest, D., Watts, J. H., & Madigan, M. J. (1991). Resonation in the model of human occupation: A pilot study. *Occupational Therapy in Mental Health*, *11* (2/3), 57–71. (OR)

This outcomes study asked whether successful perfor-

mance of craft activities would positively influence sense of capacity. Six adolescents who were in a juvenile corrections facility participated in three craft activities: leather, wood, and clay. The results provided evidence that performance skill enhanced the person's sense of capacity.

16. Dickerson, A. E., & Oakely, F. (1995). Comparing the roles of community-living persons and patient populations. *American Journal of Occupational Therapy , 49* (3), 221–228. (GC)
This group comparison study contrasted the occupational role profile of 1020 community-living adults without disabilities to 393 adults with psychosocial or physical disabilities. Persons with disabilities identified fewer present roles and also anticipated participation in fewer future roles than community-living adults with no disabilities.

17. Doble, S. E. (1991). Test-retest and inter-rater reliability of a process skills assessment. *Occupational Therapy Journal of Research, 11* (1), 8–23. (PSU)
This psychometric study studied a process skills assessment by observing 93 subjects undergoing psychiatric treatment. The data indicated that the instrument had good test-retest reliability if the same task was given to clients during retest. Inter-rater reliability was moderate.

18. Duellman, M. K., Barris, R., & Kielhofner, G. (1986). Organized activity and the adaptive status of nursing home residents. *American Journal of Occupational Therapy, 40* (9), 618–622. (COR)
This correlation study examined whether the environment influences the adaptive status of elderly people. The amount of organized activities in 3 nursing homes was found to be related to 44 residents' perceptions of their roles in the present and the future.

19. Ebb, E. W., Coster, W., & Duncombe, L. (1989). Comparison of normal and psychosocially dysfunctional male adolescents. *Occupational Therapy in Mental Health, 9* (2), 53–74. (GC)
This group comparison study asked whether MOHO variables (personal causation, values, interests, roles, habits, communication/interaction skills, and process skills) would discriminate between 18 nondisabled and 15 psychiatrically disabled adolescents. The number of current and anticipated roles and the presence of strong interests discriminated between the groups.

20. Egan, M., Warren, S. A., Hessel, P. A., & Gilewich, G. (1992). Activities of daily living after hip fracture: Pre and post discharge. *Occupational Therapy Journal of Research, 12* (6), 342–356. (GC)
This study asked whether anticipated role loss would

be predictive of levels of activities of daily living function in 61 older adults. As expected, there was no relationship.

21. Elliott, M., & Barris, R. (1987). Occupational role performance and life satisfaction in elderly persons. *Occupational Therapy Journal of Research, 7* (4), 215–224. (COR)
This correlation study examined the relationship between occupational role performance (number and meaningfulness of roles performed) and life satisfaction in 185 noninstitutionalized older persons (older than 65 years of age). There was a positive relationship between life satisfaction and both the number of roles performed and involvement in meaningful roles.

22. Evans, J., & Salim, A. A. (1992). A cross-cultural test of the validity of occupational therapy assessments with patients with schizophrenia. *American Journal of Occupational Therapy, 46* (8), 685–695. (COR, GC)
In this correlation and group comparison study, a battery of assessments including MOHO-based interview designed for the study was administered to 50 African patients with schizophrenia and 10 nondisabled subjects. The MOHO-based interview discriminated between the two groups and was correlated with functional performance and with two of three history variables indicating the seriousness of the disability. The authors underscore the importance of cultural relevance in assessment.

23. Forsyth, K., Lai, J-S., & Kielhofner, G. (1999). The assessment of communication and interaction skills (ACIS): Measurement properties. *British Journal of Occupational Therapy, 62* (2), 69–74. (CV, PSU)
This study examined the psychometric properties of the ACIS. Ratings obtained from 52 occupational therapists and 117 clients were examined. Results supported construct and person response validity of the instrument as well as inter-rater and intra-rater reliability.

24. Fossey, E. (1996). Using the occupational performance history interview (OPHI): Therapists' reflections. *British Journal of Occupational Therapy, 59* (5), 223–228. (PSU, TR)
This qualitative study describes four therapists' experience using the Occupational Performance History Interview with clients referred to a psychiatric day hospital service. The study provides insight into the process of clinical interviews with a semi-structured tool and describes the clinical reasoning, interactive reasoning, and professional values that may guide the conduct and interpretation of such interviews.

25. Gerber, L., & Furst, G. (1992). Validation of the NIH Ac-

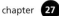

tivity Record: A quantitative measure of life activities. *Arthritis Care and Research, 5,* 81–86. (PSU)

This psychometric study examined the use of the NIH Activity Record (ACTRE) with 21 adults diagnosed with rheumatoid arthritis. The clients were also given the Activity Lifestyle Index from the Stanford Health Association Questionnaire (ALI), Pain Disability Index, Ritchie Articular Index (AI), and the Psychosocial Adjustment Illness Scale (PAIS). Pain scores on the ACTRE showed positive correlation with disability from pain on the PDI, measures of pain on the ALI, and tenderness on the AI. There was positive correlation between fatigue on the ACTRE and fatigue on the FTC. Difficulty with self-care positively correlated with difficulty and pain on the ALI.

26. Gregory, M. (1983). Occupational behavior and life satisfaction among retirees. *American Journal of Occupational Therapy, 37* (8), 548–553. (COR)

This correlation study examined the relationship between occupational participation (type, amount, and meaningfulness of activities) and life satisfaction among 79 retirees. Life satisfaction positively correlated with the index of occupational behavior. Occupational behavior was found to play an important role in affecting life satisfaction among retirees.

27. Hachey, R., Jumoorty, J., & Mercier, C. (1995). Methodology for validating the translation of test measurements applied to occupational therapy. *Occupational Therapy International, 2* (3), 190–203. (PSU, COR)

This psychometric study examined the test-retest reliability of the French translation of the Role Checklist. Fifty-one clients with schizophrenia completed the Role Checklist twice. Results indicated that the French version had good test-retest validity. A further correlation analysis indicated that there was good concordance among the English and French versions.

28. Haglund, L. (1996). Occupational therapists' agreement in screening patients in general psychiatric care for occupational therapy. *Scandinavian Journal of Occupational Therapy, 3* (2), 62–68. (PSU, TR)

This study examined therapists' reasoning process about whether to include clients in therapy. Two methods of interviewing (a traditional interview and the Occupational Case Analysis Interview and Rating Scale [OCAIRS]) were used. No difference in therapist decisions about whether to include the client in therapy was found between the two methods.

29. Haglund, L., & Henriksson, C. (1994). Testing a Swedish version of OCAIRS on two different patient Groups. *Scandinavian Journal of Caring Sciences, 8* (4), 223–230. (PSU, TR)

This study examined psychometric properties of the Swedish version of the OCAIRS. Six occupational therapists rated videotaped interviews of 12 clients (6 patients with psychiatric illness and 6 patients with chronic muscular pain). The OCAIRS had reasonable inter-rater reliability. The content validity study indicated the need for further research.

30. Haglund, L., Karlsson, G., Kielhofner, G., & Lai, J. S. (1997). Validity of the Swedish version of the Worker Role Interview. *Scandinavian Journal of Occupational Therapy, 4* (1–4), 23–29. (PSU)

This study examined the psychometric properties of the Swedish Worker Role Interview (SWRI) with persons with psychiatric disabilities. Results indicated that the Swedish instrument is a valid measure of psychosocial capacity for work.

31. Haglund, L., Thorell, L., & Wälinder, J. (1998a). Assessment of occupational functioning for screening of patients to occupational therapy in general psychiatric care. *Occupational Therapy Journal of Research, 18* (4), 193–206. (PSU)

This psychometric study studied the inter-rater reliability of the Swedish version of the Occupational Case Analysis Interview and Rating Scale (OCAIRS) with 145 patients. Therapists using the OCAIRS showed good agreement in determining whether clients should be included or excluded from occupational therapy services or should be monitored further.

32. Haglund, L., Thorell, L., & Wälinder, J. (1998b). Occupational functioning in relation to psychiatric diagnoses: Schizophrenia and mood disorders. *Nordic Journal of Psychiatry, 52* (3), 223–229. (GC)

This group comparison study examined 18 persons with schizophrenia, 20 persons with major depression, and 22 persons with bipolar disorder using the Occupational Case Analysis Interview and Rating Scale (OCAIRS). Persons with schizophrenia and bipolar disorder tended to get similar scores on the OCAIRS. However, these two groups differed with the group with major depression on most variables tapped by the OCAIRS.

33. Hammel, J. (1999). The Life Rope: A transactional approach to exploring worker and life role development. *Work: A Journal of Prevention, Assessment & Rehabilitation, 12* (1), 47–60. (QET)

This qualitative study described the role changes of 16 persons with spinal cord injury (SCI). Multiple data were gathered over 4 years. Findings showed that individuals formed multiple strands within their role repertoires at any point of time. After a SCI, the worker role becomes an elective role strand that often unravels first with breakdowns in more basic survival roles.

34. Helfrich, C., & Kielhofner, G. (1994). Volitional narratives and the meaning of occupational therapy. *American Journal of Occupational Therapy, 48* (4), 319–326. (POT)

    This qualitative study examined how life narratives affected the experience of therapy. The study revealed how clients assigned meaning to therapy as an episode within their larger occupational narrative.

35. Helfrich, C., Kielhofner, G., & Mattingly, C. (1994). Volition as narrative: An understanding of motivation in chronic illness. *American Journal of Occupational Therapy, 48* (4), 311–317. (QET)

    This qualitative study examined how narratives shaped clients' motives. Detailed investigation of the life histories of two persons with psychiatric illness indicated that they actively narrated their lives and sought to enact these narratives in their everyday lives.

36. Hemmingsson, H., & Borell, L. (1996). The development of an assessment of adjustment needs in the school setting for use with physically disabled students. *Scandinavian Journal of Occupational Therapy, 3* (4), 156–162. (PSU)

    This psychometric study examined the reliability and validity of the School System Interview (SSI) with 45 severely disabled students attending their first semester in one of the four Swedish upper secondary schools. Thirteen occupational therapists assessed the students using the SSI. The results showed that the SSI is highly sensitive. Inter-rater reliability for the content areas was good or very good. The 11 content areas appeared to be adequate.

37. Hemmingsson, H., & Borell, L. (2000) Accommodation needs and student-environment fit in upper secondary school for students with severe physical disabilities. *Canadian Journal of Occupational Therapy, 67* (3), 162–173. (POT)

    This study used the School Setting Interview (SSI) to identify, from the perspective of 45 students with disability, their needs for physical and social accommodations in upper secondary schools. The study indicated that the schools generally were able to meet the students' accommodation needs in the physical environment. However, accommodations in occupations requiring reading, remembering, and speaking were unsatisfactory.

38. Hemmingsson, H., Borell, L., & Gustavsson, A. (1999). Temporal aspects of teaching and learning – Implications for pupils with physical disabilities. *Scandinavian Journal of Disability Research, 1*, 26–43. (QET)

    This qualitative study examined how the organization of time in the social group and occupational forms of a classroom affected seven physically disabled students. The study revealed how teachers' classroom style and other factors affected students' ability to perform and participate in the classroom.

39. Henry, A. D., Baron, K. B., Mouradian, L., & Curtin, C. (1999). Reliability and validity of the self-assessment of occupational functioning. *American Journal of Occupational Therapy, 53* (5), 482–488. (PSU)

    Two studies examined psychometric properties of the Self Assessment of Occupational Functioning (SAOF) and tested the ability of the SAOF to discriminate subjects. Study 1 included 37 college students who completed the SAOF twice. Study 2 included 39 adolescents and young adults having their first psychiatric hospitalization. The SAOF showed acceptable levels of test-retest reliability and internal validity for the subscale and total scores of the SAOF. The SAOF classified 76.6% of persons in both the groups from the two studies correctly. (Note: SAOF is the predecessor to the Occupational Self Assessment.)

40. Jacobshagen, I. (1990). The effect of interruption of activity on affect. *Occupational Therapy in Mental Health, 10* (2), 35–45. (GC)

    This group comparison study examined what happens in the process of doing an occupational form. Thirty female students participated in a stenciling activity. They were randomly assigned into two groups: an interrupted group who completed the form and a noninterrupted group who, were unable to finish the product. The results indicated that the interrupted group had significantly lower scores on factors of "power" and "action" than the noninterrupted group.

41. Jonsson, H., Josephsson, S., & Kielhofner, G. (2000). Evolving narratives in the course of retirement: A longitudinal study. *American Journal of Occupational Therapy, 54* (5), 463–470. (QET)

    This qualitative study was the second phase of a longitudinal study of retirement. Data were gathered through interviews with 29 participants (ages 65 to 66 years). Their current narratives were compared to narratives they told 2 years earlier. The findings suggest that although narratives play a role in shaping the direction of a person's life, they also interweave with and change directions as a result of ongoing life events and experiences.

42. Jonsson, H., Josephsson, S., & Kielhofner, G. (2001). Narratives and experience in an occupational transition: A longitudinal study of the retirement process. *American Journal of Occupational Therapy, 55* (4), 424–432. (QET)

This qualitative study examined the process of transition into retirement. Data were gathered through collecting narratives with 12 Swedish participants over a period of 7 years beginning when they were still working and continuing through the early years of their retirement. The findings showed that while some participants managed a transition into a satisfying pattern of retirement, others found it an ongoing process of frustration and dissatisfaction. Central to a positive narrative was the establishment of an engaging occupation.

43. Jonsson, H., Kielhofner, G., & Borell, L. (1997). Anticipating retirement: The formation of narratives concerning an occupational transition. *American Journal of Occupational Therapy, 51* (1), 49–56. (QET)
This qualitative study investigated how 32 persons (63 years and older) anticipated their retirement. The findings demonstrated the process by which persons anticipate and make choices about life change. The findings also demonstrated how people anticipate retirement through volitional narratives in which they link together the past, present, and future.

44. Josephsson, S., Backman, L., Borell, L., Nygård, L. & Bernspång, B. (1995). Effectiveness of an intervention to improve occupational performance among persons with dementia. *Occupational Therapy Journal of Research, 15* (1), 36–49. (OR)
This outcome study examined the effectiveness of a MOHO-based intervention program to improve occupational performance among four persons with dementia. Three of four clients showed intervention gains with a decrease in amount of support required for task performance.

45. Kaplan, K. (1984). Short term assessments: The need and a response. *Occupational Therapy in Mental Health, 4* (3), 29–45. (PSU)
This psychometric study examined the content and inter-rater reliability of the OCAIRS. A panel of experts was polled to examine the content validity of the instrument. Four occupational therapists then rated nine videotaped interviews of adult psychiatric inpatients with diagnoses of depression or dementia. The results supported the content validity of the OCAIRS and indicated that it had acceptable inter-rater reliability.

46. Katz, N., Giladi, N., & Peretz, C. (1988). Cross-cultural application of occupational therapy assessments: Human occupation with psychiatric inpatients and controls in Israel. *Occupational Therapy in Mental Health, 8* (1), 7–30. (GC)
This group comparison study examined the applicabil-

ity and generalizability of MOHO beyond the United States. A battery of 6 assessments representing volition and habituation were given to 50 patients admitted to psychiatric hospitals in Israel and 30 adults without disabilities. Different patterns of volition and habituation differentiated psychiatric clients from the nondisabled subjects. The results supported the cross-cultural relevance of MOHO.

47. Katz, N., Josman, N. & Steinmetz, N. (1988). Relationship between cognitive disability theory and the model of human occupation in the assessment of psychiatric and nonpsychiatric adolescents. *Occupational Therapy in Mental Health, 8* (1), 31–43. (PSU)
This study of assessment utility administered an assessment battery of instruments derived from MOHO and another model to 20 adolescents with psychiatric impairments and 20 matched control subjects who participated in the study. The instruments from MOHO and the cognitive disabilities model were found to measure different domains.

48. Kielhofner, G., & Barrett, L. (1997). Meaning and misunderstanding in occupational forms: A study of therapeutic goal-setting. *American Journal of Occupational Therapy, 52* (5), 345–353. (QET)
This qualitative study examined occupational therapists' use of occupational forms as therapy and its impact on clients. The study focused on one client, Barbara, and the therapists who worked with her. The findings illustrate that therapists work both to give substance to the occupational form and to create the context of an implied narrative, which imbues it with particular meanings. Simultaneously, a client's experience of meaning is influenced by a personal volitional narrative. When the two narratives do not coincide, therapists' efforts to maintain the occupational form intensify as they encourage clients toward attitudes and performances, which do not resonate with their experience of reality.

49. Kielhofner, G., & Brinson, M. (1989). Development and evaluation of an aftercare program for young and chronic psychiatrically disabled adults. *Occupational Therapy in Mental Health, 9* (2), 1–25. (OR)
This study examined the effectiveness of an aftercare program based on MOHO. Twenty clients who participated in the 12-week program were compared to 14 control subjects. Trends in the data and program evaluation information suggested that the program positively influenced recidivism and quality of life. However, the differences were not statistically significant because of the small sample size.

50. Kielhofner, G., & Forsyth, G. (2001). Measurement prop-

erties of a client self-report for treatment planning and documenting therapy outcomes. *Scandinavian Journal of Occupational Therapy, 8 (3),* 131–139. (PSU)

This psychometric study examined the validity and reliability of the OSA. Data were collected from 302 clients who included physically disabled, psychiatrically disabled, and nondisabled adults from 6 countries. Results supported the preliminary validity and reliability of the OSA.

51. Kielhofner, G., Harlan, B., Bauer, D., & Maurer, P. (1986). The reliability of a historical interview with physically disabled respondents. *American Journal of Occupational Therapy, 40 (8),* 551–556. (PSU)

This psychometric study examined the reliability of a historical interview. Data were collected from 20 clients with physical disabilities using a modified Occupational Role History. The instrument demonstrated acceptable inter-rater and test-retest reliability.

52. Kielhofner, G., & Henry, A. D. (1988). Development and investigation of the Occupational Performance History Interview. *American Journal of Occupational Therapy, 42 (8),* 489–498. (PSU)

This psychometric study examined test-retest and inter-rater reliability of the Occupational Performance History Interview with 153 therapists and 153 clients from adult psychiatry, physical disability, gerontology, and adolescent psychiatry. The OPHI was found to have less than desirable levels of test-retest and interrater reliability. The findings also suggested that theory should be made more explicit in the OPHI.

53. Kielhofner, G., Henry, A., Walens, D., & Rogers E. S. (1991). A generalizability study of the Occupational Performance History Interview. *Occupational Therapy Journal of Research, 11,* 292–306. (PSU)

This psychometric study examined the reliability of the OPHI when used by therapists using two or more different frames of reference: MOHO and eclectic. Videotapes of 20 psychiatry patients were rated by 2 sets of 3 raters selected from a pool of 13 MOHO and 8 eclectic therapists. Results indicated that the interview was only moderately stable under both conditions.

54. Kielhofner, G., Lai, J. S., Olson, L., Haglund, L., Ekbadh, E., & Hedlund, M. (1999). Psychometric properties of the work environment impact scale: a cross-cultural study. *Work: A Journal of Prevention, Assessment & Rehabilitation, 12 (1),* 71–77. (PSU, CV)

This psychometric and concept validation study examined the WEIS with 11 American and 10 Swedish subjects and with both American and Swedish raters. There was evidence that the WEIS items effectively constituted a unidimensional construct and work environment impact; it was also found to be culture free. It was effective in discriminating different levels of work environments among subjects. There was no evidence of any rater bias.

55. Kielhofner, G., Mallinson, T., Forsyth, K., & Lai, J-S. (2001). Psychometric properties of the second version of the Occupational Performance History Interview. *American Journal of Occupational Therapy, 55 (3),* 260–267. (PSU, CV)

This psychometric and concept validation study examined the validity of the occupational identity, occupational competency, and occupational behavior settings scales of the OPHI-II. Data were collected from 151 raters on 249 subjects from 8 countries and in 6 languages. Each of the scale's items was appropriately targeted to the subjects, and all three scales distinguished subjects into approximately three different levels. The three scales of the OPHI-II were shown to be valid across ages, diagnoses, cultures, and languages and effectively measured a wide range of persons.

56. Lai, J-S., Haglund, L., & Kielhofner, G. (1999). The Occupational Case Analysis Interview and Rating Scale: Construct validity and directions for future development. *Scandinavian Journal of Caring Sciences, 13 (4),* 267–273. (PSU)

This psychometric study examined the validity and reliability of the OCAIRS. Six raters and 145 clients participated in the study, resulting in 290 ratings. The results suggested minimal rater bias, and the OCAIRS was shown to be a valid measure of occupational adaptation. However, problems with the scale properties suggested a need for some revisions.

57. Lederer, J., Kielhofner, G., & Watts, J. (1985). Values, personal causation and skills of delinquents and non delinquents. *Occupational Therapy in Mental Health, 5 (2),* 59–77. (GC)

This group comparison study contrasted 15 delinquent males with 15 nondelinquent males. The results indicated that fewer delinquents valued the student and worker roles highly, more delinquents assigned no value to the volunteer and home maintainer role, and valued hobbyist/amateur roles. There was no difference in personal values, locus of control, or perceptual motor skills.

58. Lycett, R. (1992). Evaluating the use of an occupational assessment with elderly rehabilitation patients. *British Journal of Occupational Therapy, 55 (3),* 343–346. (PSU)

This study investigated the relevance of an occupational assessment based on MOHO with elderly patients in rehabilitation wards. Participants were 16 inpatients from elderly care rehabilitation wards at three hospitals. All participants were older than 65 years of age, had no receptive or expressive communication problems, and had no signs of dementia. A questionnaire was used to evaluate the subjects. The questionnaire collected important information about patient values and attitudes.

59. Lynch, K., & Bridle, M. (1993). Construct validity of the Occupational Performance Interview. *Occupational Therapy Journal of Research, 13* (4), 231–240. (PSU)
This study examined the psychometric properties of the Occupational Performance History Interview (OPHI) with 143 persons with spinal cord injury. Scores on the OPHI were correlated with scores on the Multidimensional Pain Inventory (MPI) and the Center for Epidemiologic Studies Depression Scale (CES-D). As expected, results provided evidence of construct validity.

60. Mallinson, T., Kielhofner, G., & Mattingly, C. (1996). Metaphor and meaning in a clinical interview. *American Journal of Occupational Therapy, 50* (5), 338–346. (QET)
This qualitative study aimed to identify narrative features present in interviews and illustrate how these features can be identified. Data collected previously from 20 Occupational Performance History Interviews were analyzed. Metaphors were identified as the main feature assigning meaning to client narratives. Findings suggested that metaphors provide possibilities or impediments to therapy and therapy could build on the metaphors to help patients improve.

61. Mallinson, T., Mahaffey, L., & Kielhofner, G. (1998). The Occupational Performance History Interview: Evidence for three underlying constructs of occupational adaptation. *Canadian Journal of Occupational Therapy, 65* (4), 219–228. (PSU)
This psychometric study aimed to establish the construct validity of a modified version of the Occupational Performance History Interview (OPHI-R). Data previously gathered on 20 clients in a psychiatric setting were analyzed. The results indicated that the items of the OPHI-R do not effectively measure a single construct of occupational adaptation. The OPHI-R items measured three underlying constructs: occupational competence, identity, and environment.

62. Muñoz, J., Lawlor, M., & Kielhofner, G. (1993). Use of the model of human occupation in psychiatric practice: A survey of skilled therapists. *Occupational Therapy Journal of Research, 13* (2), 117–139. (TR)
This study sought to examine how occupational therapists used MOHO concepts to describe the occupational functioning of their clients. Fifty occupational therapists who identified MOHO as their primary practice model completed a survey and an interview. The findings suggested that therapists valued the holistic approach of this model and found major concepts of the model (personal causation, values, interests, role, habits, and environment) useful for conceptualizing their clients' occupational functioning.

63. Neville-Jan, A. (1994). The relationship of volition to adaptive occupational behavior among individuals with varying degrees of depression. *Occupational Therapy in Mental Health, 12* (4), 1–18. (COR)
This correlation study examined the relation between volition and adaptation among 100 persons with varying levels of depression. The results indicated a significant positive correlation between volition and adaptive occupational functioning.

64. Oakley, F., Kielhofner, G., & Barris, R. (1985). An occupational therapy approach to assessing psychiatric patients' adaptive functioning. *American Journal of Occupational Therapy, 39* (3), 147–154. (PSU)
This study examined the utility of MOHO for assessment of 30 persons with mental disorders. A therapist blindly rated the adaptiveness of clients from results from MOHO-based assessments. This MOHO rating was highly correlated with adaptive behavior of the clients as observed by nursing staff. Symptomatology was only moderately correlated with adaptive behavior, and diagnosis was unrelated.

65. Oakley, F., Kielhofner, G., Barris, R., & Reichler, R. K. (1986). The Role Checklist: Development and empirical assessment of reliability. *Occupational Therapy Journal of Research, 6,* 157–170. (PSU)
This psychometric study examined the test-retest reliability of the Role Checklist. The assessment was administered to 124 normal volunteers on 2 occasions. The Checklist showed satisfactory test-retest reliability.

66. Peterson, E., Howland, J., Kielhofner, G., Lachman, M. E., Assmann, S., Cote, J., & Jette, A. (1999). Falls self-efficacy and occupational adaptation among elders. *Physical & Occupational Therapy in Geriatrics, 16* (1/2), 1–16. (COR)
This correlational study examined the relationship between personal causation (feelings of efficacy related to falling) and pattern of occupational engagement in 270 older adults. They found, as expected, that lower falls self-efficacy was related to reduced leisure and social occupations, mediated by the elders' choices to restrict what they did.

67. Restall, G., & Magill-Evans, J. (1994). Play and preschool children with autism. *American Journal of Occupational Therapy, 48* (2), 113–120. (GC)

This comparative study sought to understand how the play of nine children with autism differed from that of nine normally developing children matched by mental age, gender, and socioeconomic status. The results indicated the need to evaluate and develop the interpersonal skills and habits of preschool children with autism.

68. Rosenfeld, M. S. (1989). Occupational disruption and adaptation: A study of house fire victims. *American Journal of Occupational Therapy, 4,* 89–96. (QET)
This qualitative study examined the disruption to daily living routines caused by house fires and of the adaptation processes victims undertook to reestablish effective patterns of purposeful activity. Data were gathered by observation on scenes of 15 house or tenement fires and in-depth interviews with members of 10 families displaced by fires. The findings suggested that roles of tasks and activities were important in recovery. Occupational disruption and adaptation were identified as a valuable perspective from which to view the victims of house fires.

69. Rust, K., Barris, R., & Hooper, F. (1987). Use of the model of human occupation to predict women's exercise behavior. *Occupational Therapy Journal of Research, 7,* 23–35. (PR)
This study used MOHO as a framework for predicting engagement in exercise by 140 adult women. Number of roles and leisure values predicted levels of physical activity. However, exercise-specific measures of MOHO variables were found to be a better model for predicting women's exercise behavior.

70. Smith, N., Kielhofner, G., & Watts, J. (1986). The relationship between volition, activity pattern and life satisfaction in the elderly. *American Journal of Occupational Therapy, 40* (4), 278–283. (COR, CV)
This study examined the relationship between volition, activity pattern, and life satisfaction of 60 elderly subjects. Life satisfaction was correlated with time spent in work, daily living tasks, recreation and rest in a day, amount of value, and personal causation in a typical day. Interests, values, personal causation, recreation, and work positively correlated with life satisfaction. Time in work and leisure correlated with life satisfaction.

71. Smyntek, L., Barris, R., & Kielhofner, G. (1985). The model of human occupation applied to psychosocially functional and dysfunctional adolescents. *Occupational Therapy in Mental Health, 5* (1), 21–40. (GC)
This group comparison study investigated differences between adolescents with psychosocial problems and nondisabled adolescents by using MOHO as a framework. The groups differed on personal causation.

72. Spadone, R. A. (1992). Internal-external control and temporal orientation among southeast Asians and white Americans. *American Journal of Occupational Therapy, 16* (0), 713–719. (GC)
This group comparison study examined ethnic group differences between immigrants from Thailand, immigrants from Vietnam, and white Americans by using MOHO as a framework. There was no difference between the groups in internal versus external locus of control. The Thai and white Americans showed significant differences on time orientation.

73. Tham, K., & Borell, L. (1996). Motivation for training: A case study of four persons with unilateral neglect. *Occupational Therapy in Health Care, 10* (3), 65–79. (QET)
This qualitative study sought to explore and describe the influence of volition on four persons with unilateral neglect who participated in an intervention to improve sustained attention. The findings suggested that the four persons' awareness of their own disabilities influenced their motivation toward training and that they sometimes overestimated their own capacities, especially concerning activities they had not practiced in since before the stroke. The findings indicated that motivation for training is related to how persons view the future and if the person has goals.

74. Viik, M. K., Watts, J. H., Madigan, M. J., & Bauer, D. (1990). Preliminary validation of the Assessment of Occupational Functioning with an alcoholic population. *Occupational Therapy in Mental Health, 10* (2), 19–33. (PSU)
This psychometric study examined the utility of the Assessment of Occupational Functioning (AOF). Twenty-four adults who were inpatients being treated for alcoholism and 24 adults with 1 year of alcohol abstinence who were attending Alcoholics Anonymous (AA) were given the Alcohol Dependence Scale (ADS) and the AOF. The rater was unaware of the group to which subjects belonged. The AOF was found to discriminate between the two groups successfully. Habits and role competence scores were the important variables for discriminating between the two groups.

75. Velozo, C., Kielhofner, G., Gern, A., Lin, F-L., Azhar, F., Lai, J-S., & Fisher, G. (1999). Worker Role Interview: Validation of a psychosocial work-related measure. *Journal of Occupational Rehabilitation, 9* (3), 153–168. (PSU)
Three studies examined the validity of the WRI. The first study of 119 work-hardening clients with low back pain showed that the scale items worked together to measure a unidimensional construct. The second study applied to 55 work-hardening clients in-

dicated that the ordering of items was similar to that in the previous study and similar across two different diagnostic groups, indicating that scale was sample invariant. The third study of 42 work-hardening clients examined the predictive validity of the WRI. The results indicated that none of the variables in the WRI successfully predicted return to work.

76. Watts, J. H., Brollier, C., Bauer, D., Schmidt, W. (1988). A concurrent validity study of two occupational therapy evaluation instruments: The AOF and OCAIRS. Occupational Therapy in Mental Health, 8(4), 49–60. (PSU)

     This psychometric study compared the Assessment of Occupational Functioning (AOF) and the Occupational Case Analysis Interview and Rating Scale (OCAIRS) when used with 41 persons diagnosed with schizophrenia. Correlations of the AOF and OCAIRS and qualitative feedback from practicing therapists were analyzed. The two assessments appeared to measure persons similarly.

77. Watts, J. H., Brollier, C., Bauer, D., & Schmidt, W. (1988). A comparison of two evaluation instruments used with psychiatric patients in occupational therapy. Occupational Therapy in Mental Health, 8 (4), 7–27. (COR)

     This correlation and qualitative study compared two MOHO instruments, the Assessment of Occupational Functioning (AOF) and the Occupational Case Analysis Interview and Rating Scale (OCAIRS). Data on the AOF and OCAIRS were collected from 41 clients with schizophrenia. Five occupational therapists with MOHO experience completed qualitative evaluation forms about the AOF and OCAIRS. The total AOF score was highly correlated with the total OCAIRS score. The therapists reported belief in the potential clinical value of both assessments.

78. Watts, J. H., Kielhofner, G., Bauer, D., Gregory, M., & Valentine, D. (1986). The Assessment of Occupational Functioning: A screening tool for use in long-term care. American Journal of Occupational Therapy, 40 (4), 231–240. (PSU)

     This study examined the psychometric properties of the Assessment of Occupational Functioning (AOF)

with 83 subjects, 60 years or older. They were evaluated using the AOF, the Geriatric Rating Scale (GRS), and the Life Satisfaction Index-Z (LSI-Z). The AOF was also readministered after 14 to 21 days. The AOF showed acceptable test-retest and inter-rater reliability. There was positive correlation between scores on the LSI-Z and the AOF.

79. Weeder, T. (1986). Comparison of temporal patterns and meaningfulness of the daily activities of schizophrenic and normal adults. Occupational Therapy in Mental Health, 6 (4), 27–45. (GC)

     This group comparison study compared 20 adults with schizophrenia and 20 normal adult volunteers to look for differences in temporal patterns of daily activities, meaningfulness of daily activities, amount of time spent in each daily activity, and the meaningfulness of that daily activity. The results indicated that the temporal patterns of schizophrenic adults were different concerning the amounts of time spent in activities of sleep, work, passive leisure, and socialization. No significant differences were found in the meaningfulness of daily activities. There was significant correlation between external locus of control and active leisure, suggesting that schizophrenics were experiencing a serious lack of control considering the amount of time they spent in that activity.

80. Zimmerer-Branum, S., & Nelson, D. (1994). Occupationally embedded exercise versus rote exercise: A choice between occupational forms by elderly nursing home residents. American Journal of Occupational Therapy, 49 (5), 397–402. (GC)

     This study examined the preferences of elderly nursing home residents when presented with an occupationally embedded exercise (i.e., a true occupational form) versus a rote exercise. Fifty-two nursing home residents were presented with a choice between an occupationally embedded exercise that involved unilateral dunking of a small, spongy ball into a basketball hoop and a rote exercise that involved moving the arm above the head in a simulation of the dunking exercise. Subjects preferred the occupationally embedded exercise.

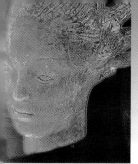

Appendix A: MOHO Bibliography

A

Adelstein, L. A., Barnes, M. A., Murray-Jensen, F., & Skaggs, C. B. (1989). A broadening frontier: Occupational therapy in mental health programs for children and adolescents. *Mental Health Special Interest Section Newsletter, 12,* 2–4.

Affleck, A., Bianchi, E., Cleckley, M., Donaldson, K., McCormack, G., & Polon, J. (1984). Stress management as a component of occupational therapy in acute care settings. *Occupational Therapy in Health Care, 1* (3), 17–41.

Arnsten, S. M. (1990). Intrinsic motivation. *American Journal of Occupational Therapy, 44* (5), 462–463.

Aubin, G., Hachey, R., & Mercier, C. (1999). Meaning of daily activities and subjective quality of life in people with severe mental illness. *Scandinavian Journal of Occupational Therapy, 6* (2), 53–62.

B

Baron, K. (1987). The model of human occupation: A newspaper treatment group for adolescents with a diagnosis of conduct disorder. *Occupational Therapy in Mental Health, 7* (2), 89–104.

Baron, K. (1989). Occupational therapy: A program for child psychiatry. *Mental Health Special Interest Section Newsletter, 12,* 6–7.

Baron, K. B. (1991). The use of play in child psychiatry: Reframing the therapeutic environment. *Occupational Therapy in Mental Health, 11* (2/3), 37–56.

Baron, K. B., & Littleton, M. J. (1999). The model of human occupation: A return to work case study. *Work: A Journal of Prevention, Assessment & Rehabilitation, 12*(1), 37–46.

Barrett, L., Beer, D., & Kielhofner, G. (1999). The importance of volitional narrative in treatment: An ethnographic case study in a work program. *Work: A Journal of Prevention, Assessment & Rehabilitation, 12* (1), 79–92.

Barris, R. (1982). Environmental interactions: An extension of the model of human occupation. *American Journal of Occupational Therapy, 36* (10), 637–644.

Barris, R. (1986a). Activity: The interface between person and environment. *Physical and Occupational Therapy in Geriatrics, 5* (2), 39–49.

Barris, R. (1986b). Occupational dysfunction and eating disorders: Theory and approach to treatment. *Occupational Therapy in Mental Health, 6* (1), 27–45.

Barris, R., Dickie, V., & Baron, K. (1988). A comparison of psychiatric patients and normal subjects based on the model of human occupation. *Occupational Therapy Journal of Research, 8,* 3–37.

Barris, R., Kielhofner, G., Burch, R. M., Gelinas, I., Klement, M., & Schultz, B. (1986). Occupational function and dysfunction in three groups of adolescents. *Occupational Therapy Journal of Research, 6,* 301–317.

Barris, R., Oakley, F., & Kielhofner, G. (1988). The Role Checklist. In *Mental health assessment in occupational therapy* (pp. 73–91). Thorofare, NJ: Slack.

Barrows, C. (1996). Clinical interpretation of "predictors of functional outcome among adolescents and young adults with psychotic disorders." *American Journal of Occupational Therapy, 50,* 182–183.

Bavaro, S. M. (1991). Occupational therapy and obsessive-compulsive disorder. *American Journal of Occupational Therapy, 45* (5), 456–458.

Bernspang, B., & Fisher, A. (1995). Differences between persons with right or left cerebral vascular accident on the assessment of motor and process skills. *Archives of Physical Medicine and Rehabilitation, 76,* 1144–1151.

Biernacki, S. D. (1993). Reliability of the Worker Role Interview. *American Journal of Occupational Therapy, 47* (9), 797–803.

Blakeney, A. (1985). Adolescent development: An application to the model of human occupation. *Occupational Therapy in Health Care, 2* (3), 19–40.

Borell, L., Gustavsson, A., Sandman, P., & Kielhofner, G. (1994). Occupational programming in a day hospital for patients with dementia. *Occupational Therapy Journal of Research, 14* (4), 219–238.

Borell, L., Sandman, P., & Kielhofner, G. (1991). Clinical decision making in Alzheimer's disease. *Occupational Therapy in Mental Health, 11* (4), 111–124.

Branholm, I., & Fugl-Meyer, A. R. (1992). Occupational role preferences and life satisfaction. *American Journal of Occupational Therapy, 12* (3), 159–171.

Braveman, B. (1999). The model of human occupation and prediction of return to work: A review of related empirical research. *Work: A Journal of Prevention, Assessment & Rehabilitation, 12* (1), 13–23.

Braveman, B. H., Sen, S., & Kielhofner, G. (2001). Community-based vocational rehabilitation programs. In M. Scaffa (Ed.), *Occupational therapy in community-based practice settings* (pp 139–162). Philadelphia: FA Davis.

Bridgett, B. (1993). Occupational therapy evaluation for patients with eating disorders. *Occupational Therapy in Mental Health, 12* (2), 79–89.

Bridle, M. J., Lynch, K. B., & Quesenberry, C. M. (1990). Long term function following the central cord syndrome. *Paraplegia, 28,* 178–185.

Broadley, H. (1991). Assessment guidelines based on the model of human occupation. *World Federation of Occupational Therapists: Bulletin, 23,* 34–35.

Brollier, C., Watts, J. H., Bauer, D., & Schmidt, W. (1988a). A concurrent validity study of two occupational therapy evaluation instruments: The AOF and OCAIRS. *Occupational Therapy in Mental Health, 8* (4), 49–60.

Brollier, C., Watts, J. H., Bauer, D., & Schmidt, W. (1988b). A content validity study of the Assessment of Occupational Functioning. *Occupational Therapy in Mental Health, 8* (4), 29–47.

Brown, T., & Carmichael, K. (1992). Assertiveness training for clients with psychiatric illness: A pilot study. *British Journal of Occupational Therapy, 55* (4), 137–140.

Bruce, M., & Borg, B. (1993). Psychosocial occupational therapy: Frames of reference for intervention. Chapter: The model of human occupation (p. 146–175). Thorofare, NJ: Slack.

Burke, J. P. (1988). Commentary: Combining the model of human occupation with cognitive disability theory. *Occupational Therapy in Mental Health, 8* (2), xi–xiii.

Burke, J. P., Clark, F., Hamilton-Dodd, C., & Kawamoto, T. (1987). Maternal role preparation: A program using sensory integration, infant-mother attachment, and occupational behavior perspectives. *Occupational Therapy in Health Care, 4* (2), 9–21.

Burrows, E. (1989). Clinical practice: An approach to the assessment of clinical competencies. *British Journal of Occupational Therapy, 52* (6), 222–226.

Burton, J. E. (1989a). The model of human occupation and occupational therapy practice with elderly patients, part 1: Characteristics of ageing. *British Journal of Occupational Therapy, 52* (6), 215–218.

Burton, J. E. (1989b). The model of human occupation and occupational therapy practice with elderly patients, part 2: Application. *British Journal of Occupational Therapy, 52* (6), 219–221.

C

Cermak, S. A., & Murray, E. (1992). Nonverbal learning disabilities in the adult framed in the model of human occupation. In Katz, N. (Ed.), *Cognitive rehabilitation: Models for intervention in occupational therapy* (pp. 258–291). Stoneham, MA: Butterworth Heinemann.

Chen, C., Neufeld, P. S., Feely, C. A., & Skinner, C. S. (1999). Factors influencing compliance with home exercise programs among patients with upper-extremity impairment. *American Journal of Occupational Therapy, 53* (2), 171–180.

Chern, J., Kielhofner, G., de las Heras, C., & Magalhaes, L. (1996). The volitional questionnaire: Psychometric development and practical use. *American Journal of Occupational Therapy, 50* (7), 516–525.

Cole, M. (1998). Group dynamics in occupational therapy: The theoretical basis and practice application of group treatment (2nd Ed.) Chapter: a model of human occupation approach (p. 268–290). Thorofare, NJ: Slack.

Corner, R., Kielhofner, G., & Lin, F. L. (1997). Construct validity of a work environment impact scale. *Work, 9* (1), 21–34.

Coster, W. J., & Jaffe, L. E. (1991). Current concepts of children's perceptions of control. *American Journal of Occupational Therapy, 45* (1), 19–25.

Cubie, S., & Kaplan, K. (1982). A case analysis method for the model of human occupation. *American Journal of Occupational Therapy, 36* (10), 645–656.

Cull, G. (1989). Anorexia nervosa: A review of theory approaches to treatment. *Journal of New Zealand Association of Occupational Therapists, 40* (2), 3–6.

Curtin, C. (1990). Research on the model of human occupation. *Mental Health-Special Interest Section Newsletter, 13* (2), 3–5.

Curtin, C. (1991). Psychosocial intervention with an adolescent with diabetes using the model of human occupation. *Occupational Therapy in Mental Health, 11* (2/3), 23–36.

D

Davies Hallet, J., Zasler, N., Maurer, P., & Cash, S. (1994). Role change after traumatic brain injury in adults. *American Journal of Occupational Therapy, 48* (3), 241–246.

DeForest, D., Watts, J. H., & Madigan, M. J. (1991). Resonation in the model of human occupation: A pilot study. *Occupational Therapy in Mental Health, 11* (2/3), 57–71.

de las Heras, C. G., Dion, G. L., & Walsh, D. (1993). Application of rehabilitation models in a state psychiatric hospital. *Occupational Therapy in Mental Health, 12* (3), 1–32.

DePoy, E. (1990). The TBIIM: An intervention for the treatment of individuals with traumatic brain injury. *Occupational Therapy in Health Care, 7* (1), 55–67.

DePoy, E., & Burke, J. P. (1992). Viewing cognition through the lens of the model of human occupation. In N. Katz (Ed.), *Cognitive rehabilitation: Models for intervention in occupational therapy* (pp. 240–257). Stoneham, MA: Butterworth-Heinemann.

Dickerson, A. E., & Oakley, F. (1995). Comparing the roles of community-living persons and patient populations. *American Journal of Occupational Therapy, 49* (3), 221–228.

Dion, G. L., Lovely, S., & Skerry, M. (1996). A comprehensive psychiatric rehabilitation approach to severe and persistent mental illness in the public sector. In S. M. Soreff (Ed.), *Handbook for the Treatment of the Mentally Ill.* Seattle, WA: Hogrefe & Huber Pub.

Doble, S. (1988). Intrinsic motivation and clinical practice: The key to understanding the unmotivated client. *Canadian Journal of Occupational Therapy, 55* (2), 75–81.

Doble, S. E. (1991). Test-retest and inter-rater reliability of a process skills assessment. *Occupational Therapy Journal of Research, 11* (1), 8–23.

Doughton, K. J. (1996). Hidden talents. *O.T. Week, 10* (26), 19–20.

Duellman, M. K., Barris, R., & Kielhofner, G. (1986). Organized activity and the adaptive status of nursing home residents. *American Journal of Occupational Therapy, 40* (9), 618–622.

Dyck, I. (1992). The daily routines of mothers with young children: Using a socio-political model in research. *Occupational Therapy Journal of Research, 12* (1), 17–34.

E

Early, M., & Pedretti, L. (1998). A frame of reference and practice models for physical dysfunction. In M. Early (Ed.), *Physical dysfunction practice skills for the occupational therapy assistant* (pp.17–30). St. Louis, MO: Mosby.

Ebb, E. W., Coster, W., & Duncombe, L. (1989). Comparison of normal and psychosocially dysfunctional male adolescents. *Occupational Therapy in Mental Health, 9* (2), 53–74.

Ecklund, M. (1996). Working relationship, participation, and outcome in a psychiatric care unit based on occupational therapy. *Scandinavian Journal of Occupational Therapy, 3* (3), 106–113.

Egan, M., Warren, S. A., Hessel, P. A., & Gilewich, G. (1992). Activities of daily living after hip fracture: Pre- and post discharge. *Occupational Therapy Journal of Research, 12* (6), 342–356.

Elliott, M., & Barris, R. (1987). Occupational role performance and life satisfaction in elderly persons. *Occupational Therapy Journal of Research, 7*, 215–224.

Esdaile, S. A. (1996). A play-focused intervention involving mothers of preschoolers. *American Journal of Occupational Therapy, 50* (2), 113–123.

Esdaile, S. A., & Madill, H. M. (1993). Causal attributions: Theoretical considerations and their relevance to occupational therapy practice and education. *British Journal of Occupational Therapy, 56* (9), 330–334.

Evans, J., & Salim, A. A. (1992). A cross-cultural test of the validity of occupational therapy assessments with patients with schizophrenia. *American Journal of Occupational Therapy, 46* (8), 685–695.

F

Fisher, G. S. (1999). Administration and application of the worker role interview: Looking beyond functional capacity. *Work: A Journal of Prevention, Assessment & Rehabilitation, 12* (1), 25–36.

Forsyth, K., Lai, J., & Kielhofner, G. (1999). The assessment of communication and interaction skills (ACIS): Measurement properties. *British Journal of Occupational Therapy, 62* (2), 69–74.

Fossey, E. (1996). Using the occupational performance history interview (OPHI): Therapists' reflections. *British Journal of Occupational Therapy, 59* (5), 223–228.

Froehlich, J. (1992). Occupational therapy interventions with survivors of sexual abuse. *Occupational Therapy in Health Care, 8* (2/3), 1–25.

Furst, G., Gerber, L., Smith, C., Fisher, S., & Shulman, B. (1987). A program for improving energy conservation behaviors in adults with rheumatoid arthritis. *American Journal of Occupational Therapy, 41* (2), 102–111.

G

Gerber, L., & Furst, G. (1992a). Scoring methods and application of the Activity Record (ACTRE) for patients with musculoskeletal disorders. *Arthritis Care and Research, 5* (3), 151–156.

Gerber, L., & Furst, G. (1992b). Validation of the NIH Activity Record: A quantitative measure of life activities. *Arthritis Care and Research, 5* (2), 81–86.

Gregory, M. (1983). Occupational behavior and life satisfaction among retirees. *American Journal of Occupational Therapy, 37* (8), 548–553.

Grogan, G. (1991a). Anger management: A perspective for occupational therapy (part 1). *Occupational Therapy in Mental Health, 11* (2/3), 135–148.

Grogan, G. (1991b). Anger management: A perspective for occupational therapy (part 2). *Occupational Therapy in Mental Health, 11*(2/3), 149–171.

Gusich, R. (1984). Occupational therapy for chronic pain: A clinical application of the model of human occupation. *Occupational Therapy in Mental Health, 4* (3), 59–73.

Gusich, R. L., & Silverman, A. L. (1991). Basava day clinic: The model of human occupation as applied to psychiatric day hospitalization. *Occupational Therapy in Mental Health, 11* (2/3), 113–134.

H

Hachey, R., Jumoorty, J., & Mercier, C. (1995). Methodology for validating the translation of test measurements applied to occupational therapy. *Occupational Therapy International, 2* (3), 190–203.

Haglund, L. (1996). Occupational therapists' agreement in screening patients in general psychiatric care for occupational therapy. *Scandinavian Journal of Occupational Therapy, 3* (2), 62–68.

Haglund, L., & Henriksson, C. (1994). Testing a Swedish version of OCAIRS on two different patient groups. *Scandinavian Journal of Caring Sciences, 8* (4), 223–230.

Haglund, L., Karlsson, G., Kielhofner, G., & Lai, J. S. (1997). Validity of the Swedish version of the Worker Role Interview. *Scandinavian Journal of Occupational Therapy, 4* (1–4), 23–29.

Haglund, L., & Kjellberg, A. (1999). A critical analysis of the model of human occupation. *Canadian Journal of Occupational Therapy, 66* (2), 102–108.

Haglund, L., Thorell, L., & Walinder, J. (1998a). Assessment of occupational functioning for screening of patients to occupational therapy in general psychiatric care. *Occupational Therapy Journal of Research, 18* (4), 193–206.

Haglund, L., Thorell, L., & Walinder, J. (1998b). Occupational functioning in relation to psychiatric diagnoses: Schizophrenia and mood disorders. *Nordic Journal of Psychiatry, 52* (3), 223–229.

Hammel, J. (1999). The life rope: A transactional approach to exploring worker and life role development. *Work: A Journal of Prevention, Assessment & Rehabilitation, 12* (1), 47–60.

Harrison, H., & Kielhofner, G. (1986). Examining reliability and validity of the Preschool Play Scale with handicapped children. *American Journal of Occupational Therapy, 40* (3), 167–173.

Helfrich, C., & Aviles, A. (2001). Occupational therapy's role with domestic violence: Assessment and intervention. *Occupational Therapy in Mental Health, 16* (3/4), 53–70.

Helfrich, C., & Kielhofner, G. (1994). Volitional narratives and the meaning of occupational therapy. *American Journal of Occupational Therapy, 48* (4), 319–326.

Helfrich, C., Kielhofner, G., & Mattingly, C. (1994). Volition as narrative: Understanding motivation in chronic illness. *American Journal of Occupational Therapy, 48* (4), 311–317.

Hemmingsson, H., & Borell, L. (1996). The development of an assessment of adjustment needs in the school setting for use with physically disabled students. *Scandinavian Journal of Occupational Therapy, 3*, 156–162.

Hemmingsson, H., & Borell, L. (2000). Accommodation needs and student-environment fit in upper secondary schools for students with severe physical disabilities. *Canadian Journal of Occupational Therapy, 67* (3), 162–173.

Hemmingsson, H., Borell, L., & Gustavsson, A. (1999). Temporal aspects of teaching and learning: Implications for pupils with physical disabilities. *Scandinavian Journal of Disability Research, 1* (2), 26–43.

Henry, A. D., Baron, K. B., Mouradian, L., & Curtin, C. (1999). Reliability and validity of the self-assessment of occupational functioning. *American Journal of Occupational Therapy, 53* (5), 482–488.

Henry, A. D., & Coster, W. J. (1996). Predictors of functional outcome among adolescents and young adults with psychotic disorders. *American Journal of Occupational Therapy, 50* (3), 171–181.

Henry, A. D., & Coster, W. J. (1997). Competency beliefs and occupational role behavior among adolescents: Explication of the personal causation construct. *American Journal of Occupational Therapy, 51* (4), 267–276.

Hocking, C. (1989). Anger management. *Journal of the New Zealand Association of Occupational Therapists, 40* (2), 12–17.

Hubbard, S. (1991). Towards a truly holistic approach to occupational therapy. *British Journal of Occupational Therapy, 54* (11), 415–418.

Hurff, J. M. (1984). Visualization: A decision-making tool for assessment and treatment planning. *Occupational Therapy in Health Care, 1* (2), 3–23.

J

Jackoway, I., Rogers, J., & Snow, T. (1987). The role change assessment: An interview tool for evaluating older adults. *Occupational Therapy in Mental Health, 7* (1), 17–37.

Jacobshagen, I. (1990). The effect of interruption of activity on affect. *Occupational Therapy in Mental Health, 10* (2), 35–45.

Jongbloed, L. (1994). Adaptation to a stroke: The experience of one couple. *American Journal of Occupational Therapy, 48* (11), 1006–1013.

Jonsson, H. (1993). The retirement process in an occupational perspective: a review of literature and theories. *Physical and Occupational Therapy in Geriatrics, 11* (4), 15–34.

Jonsson, H., Borell, L., & Sadlo, G. (2000). Retirement: An occupational transition with consequences of temporality, balance, and meaning of occupations. *Journal of Occupational Science, 7* (1), 29–37.

Jonsson, H., Josephsson, S., & Kielhofner, G. (2000). Evolving narratives in the course of retirement: A longitudinal study. *American Journal of Occupational Therapy, 54* (5), 463–470.

Jonsson, H., Josephsson, S., & Kielhofner, G. (2001). Narratives and experience in an occupational transition: A longitudinal study of the retirement process. *American Journal of Occupational Therapy, 55* (4), 424–432.

Jonsson, H., Kielhofner, G., & Borell, L. (1997). Anticipating retirement: The formation of narratives concerning an occupational transition. *American Journal of Occupational Therapy, 51* (1), 49–56.

Josephsson, S., Bäckman, L., Borell, L., Bernspång, B., Nygård, L., & Rönnberg, L. (1993). Supporting everyday activities in dementia: An intervention study. *International Journal of Geriatric Psychiatry, 8,* 395–400.

Josephsson, S., Bäckman, L., Borell, L., Nygård, L., & Bernspång, B. (1995). Effectiveness of an intervention to improve occupational performance in dementia. *Occupational Therapy Journal of Research, 15* (1), 36–49.

Jungersen, K. (1992). Culture, theory, and the practice of occupational therapy in New Zealand/Aotearoa. *American Journal of Occupational Therapy, 46* (8), 745–750.

K

Kaplan, K. (1984). Short-term assessment: The need and a response. *Occupational Therapy in Mental Health, 4* (3), 29–45.

Kaplan, K. (1986). The directive group: Short term treatment for psychiatric patients with a minimal level of functioning. *American Journal of Occupational Therapy, 40* (7), 474–481.

Kaplan, K. (1988). *Directive group therapy: Innovative mental health treatment.* Thorofare, NJ: Slack.

Kaplan, K. L., & Eskow, K. G. (1987). Teaching psychosocial theory and practice: The model of human occupation as the medium and the message. *Mental Health Special Interest Section Newsletter, 10* (1), 1–5.

Kaplan, K., & Kielhofner, G. (1989). *Occupational case analysis interview and rating scale.* Thorofare, NJ: Slack.

Katz, N. (1985). Occupational therapy's domain of concern: Reconsidered. *American Journal of Occupational Therapy, 39* (8), 518–524.

Katz, N. (1988a). Interest checklist: A factor analytical study. *Occupational Therapy in Mental Health, 8* (1), 45–56.

Katz, N. (1988b). Introduction to the collection (MOHO). *Occupational Therapy in Mental Health, 8* (1), 1–6.

Katz, N., Giladi, N., & Peretz, C. (1988). Cross-cultural application of occupational therapy assessments: Human occupation with psychiatric inpatients and controls in Israel. *Occupational Therapy in Mental Health, 8* (1), 7–30.

Katz, N., Josman, N., & Steinmetz, N. (1988). Relationship between cognitive disability theory and the model of human occupation in the assessment of psychiatric and non-psychiatric adolescents. *Occupational Therapy in Mental Health, 8* (1), 31–44.

Kavanagh, M. R. (1990). Way station: A model community support program for persons with serious mental illness. *Mental Health Special Interest Section Newsletter, 13*(1), 6–8.

Kavanaugh, J., & Fares, J. (1995). Using the model of human occupation with homeless mentally ill patients. *British Journal of Occupational Therapy, 58* (10), 419–422.

Kelly, L. (1995). What occupational therapists can learn from traditional healers. *British Journal of Occupational Therapy, 58* (3), 111–114.

Khoo, S. W., & Renwick, R. M. (1989). A model of human occupation perspective on the mental health of immigrant women in Canada. *Occupational Therapy in Mental Health, 9* (3), 31–49.

Kielhofner, G. (1980a). A model of human occupation, part two. Ontogenesis from the perspective of temporal adaptation. *American Journal of Occupational Therapy, 34* (10), 657–663.

Kielhofner, G. (1980b). A model of human occupation, part three. Benign and vicious cycles. *American Journal of Occupational Therapy, 34* (11), 731–737.

Kielhofner, G. (1984). An overview of research on the model of human occupation. *Canadian Journal of Occupational Therapy, 51* (2), 59–67.

Kielhofner, G. (1986a). A review of research on the model of human occupation: Part one. *Canadian Journal of Occupational Therapy, 53* (2), 69–74.

Kielhofner, G. (1986b). A review of research on the model of human occupation: Part two. *Canadian Journal of Occupational Therapy, 53* (3), 129–134.

Kielhofner, G. (1992). The future of the profession of occupational therapy: Requirements for developing the field's knowledge base. *Journal of Japanese Association of Occupational Therapists, 11,* 112–129.

Kielhofner, G. (Ed.) (1995). *A model of human occupation: Theory and application* (2nd ed.). Baltimore: Williams & Wilkins.

Kielhofner, G. (1999a). From doing in to doing with: The role of environment in performance and disability. *Toimintaterapeutti, 1,* 3–9.

Kielhofner, G. (1999b). Guest-editorial. *Work: A Journal of Prevention, Assessment & Rehabilitation, 12* (1), 1.

Kielhofner, G., & Barrett, L. (1998a). Meaning and misunderstanding in occupational forms: A study of therapeutic goal setting. *American Journal of Occupational Therapy, 52* (5), 345–353.

Kielhofner, G., & Barrett, L. (1998b). Theories derived from occupational behavior perspectives. In *Willard & Spackman's occupational therapy* (9th ed., pp. 525–535). Philadelphia: Lippincott.

Kielhofner, G., Barris, R., & Watts, J. (1982). Habits and habit dysfunction: A clinical perspective for psychosocial occupational therapy. *Occupational Therapy in Mental Health, 2* (2), 1–21.

Kielhofner, G., Braveman, B., Baron, K., Fisher, G., Hammel, J., & Littleton, M. (1999). The model of human occupation: Understanding the worker who is injured or disabled. *Work: A Journal of Prevention, Assessment & Rehabilitation, 12* (1), 3–11.

Kielhofner, G., & Brinson, M. (1989). Development and evaluation of an aftercare program for young and chronic psychiatrically disabled adults. *Occupational Therapy in Mental Health, 9* (2), 1–25.

Kielhofner, G., & Burke, J. (1980). A model of human occupation, part one. Conceptual framework and content. *American Journal of Occupational Therapy, 34,* 572–581.

Kielhofner, G., Burke, J., & Heard Igi, C. (1980). A model of human occupation, part four. Assessment and intervention. *American Journal of Occupational Therapy, 34* (12), 777–788.

Kielhofner, G., & Fisher, A. (1991). Mind-brain-body relationships. In A. G. Fisher, E. A. Murray, & A. C. Bundy (Eds.), *Sensory integration: Theory and practice* (pp. 27–45). Philadelphia: FA Davis.

Kielhofner, G., & Forsyth, K. (1997). The model of human occupation: An overview of current concepts. *British Journal of Occupational Therapy, 60* (3), 103–110.

Kielhofner, G. & Forsyth, G. (2001). Measurement properties of a client self-report for treatment planning and documenting therapy outcomes. *Scandinavian Journal of Occupational Therapy, 8* (3), 131–139.

Kielhofner, G., Harlan, B., Bauer, D., & Maurer, P. (1986). The reliability of a historical interview with physically disabled respondents. *American Journal of Occupational Therapy, 40* (8), 551–556.

Kielhofner, G., & Henry, A. D. (1988). Development and investigation of the Occupational Performance History Interview. *American Journal of Occupational Therapy, 42* (8), 489–498.

Kielhofner, G., Henry, A., Walens, D., & Rogers E. S. (1991). A generalizability study of the Occupational Performance History Interview. *Occupational Therapy Journal of Research, 11* (5), 292–306.

Kielhofner, G., Lai, J. S., Olson, L., Haglund, L., Ekbadh, E., & Hedlund, M. (1999). Psychometric properties of the work environment impact scale: A cross-cultural study. *Work: A Journal of Prevention, Assessment & Rehabilitation, 12* (1), 71–77.

Kielhofner, G., Mallinson, T., Forsyth, K., & Lai, J. S. (2001). Psychometric properties of the second version of the Occupational Performance History Interview (OPHI-II). *American Journal of Occupational Therapy, 55* (3), 260–267.

Kielhofner, G., & Nicol, M. (1989). The model of human occupation: A developing conceptual tool for clinicians. *British Journal of Occupational Therapy, 52* (6), 210–214.

Krefting, L. (1985). The use of conceptual models in clinical practice. *Canadian Journal of Occupational Therapy, 52* (4), 173–178.

Kyle, T., & Wright, S. (1996). Reflecting the model of human occupation in occupational therapy documentation. *Canadian Journal of Occupational Therapy, 63* (3), 192–196.

L

Lai, J-S., Haglund, L., & Kielhofner, G. (1999). The Occupational Case Analysis Interview and Rating Scale: Construct validity and directions for future development. *Scandinavian Journal of Caring Sciences, 13* (4), 267–273.

Lancaster, J., & Mitchell, M. (1991). Occupational therapy treatment goals, objectives, and activities for improving low self-esteem in adolescents with behavioral disorders. *Occupational Therapy in Mental Health, 11* (2/3), 3–22.

Larsson, M., & Braholm, I. B. (1996). An approach to goal-planning in occupational therapy and rehabilitation. *Scandinavian Journal of Occupational Therapy, 3* (1), 14–19.

Law, M., Cooper, B., Strong, S., Stewart, D., Rigby, P., & Letts, L. (1997). Theoretical contexts for the practice of occupational therapy. In C. Christiansen & C. Baum (Eds.), *Occupational therapy: Enabling function and well-being* (pp.74–102). Thorofare, NJ: Slack.

Lederer, J., Kielhofner, G., & Watts, J. (1985). Values, personal causation and skills of delinquents and non-delinquents. *Occupational Therapy in Mental Health, 5* (2), 59–77.

Levine, R. (1984). The cultural aspects of home care delivery. *American Journal of Occupational Therapy, 38* (11), 734–738.

Levine, R. E., & Gitlin, L. N. (1990). Home adaptations for persons with chronic disabilities: An educational model. *American Journal of Occupational Therapy, 44* (10), 923–929.

Levine, R. E., & Gitlin, L. N. (1993). A model to promote activity competence in elders. *American Journal of Occupational Therapy, 47* (2), 147–153.

Lycett, R. (1992). Evaluating the use of an occupational assessment with elderly rehabilitation patients. *British Journal of Occupational Therapy, 55* (9), 343–346.

Lynch, K., & Bridle, M. (1993). Construct validity of the Occupational Performance Interview. *Occupational Therapy Journal of Research, 13* (4), 231–240.

Lyons, M. (1984). Shaping up: The model of human occupation as a guide to practice. *Proceedings of the 13th Federal Conference of the Australian Association of Occupational Therapists, 2*, 95–100.

M

Mallinson, T., Kielhofner, G., & Mattingly, C. (1996). Metaphor and meaning in a clinical interview. *American Journal of Occupational Therapy, 50* (5), 338–346.

Mallinson, T., Mahaffey, L., & Kielhofner, G. (1998). The occupational performance history interview: Evidence for three underlying constructs of occupational adaptation. *Canadian Journal of Occupational Therapy, 65* (4), 219–228.

Maynard, M. (1986). An experiential learning approach: Utilizing historical interview and an occupational inventory. *Physical & Occupational Therapy in Geriatrics, 5* (2), 51–69.

Mentrup, C., Niehaus, A., & Kielhofner, G. (1999). Applying the model of human occupation in work-focused rehabilitation: A case illustration. *Work: A Journal of Prevention, Assessment & Rehabilitation, 12* (1), 61–70.

Michael, P. S. (1991). Occupational therapy in a prison? You must be kidding! *Mental Health Special Interest Section Newsletter, 14*, 3–4.

Mocellin, G. (1992a). An overview of occupational therapy in the context of the American influence on the profession: Part 1. *British Journal of Occupational Therapy, 55* (1), 7–12.

Mocellin, G. (1992b). An overview of occupational therapy in the context of the American influence on the profession: Part 2. *British Journal of Occupational Therapy, 55* (2), 55–60.

Muñoz, J. P., & Schweikert, P. (1988). A program for acute inpatient psychiatry. *Mental Health Special Interest Section Newsletter, 11*, 3–4.

Muñoz, J. P., Lawlor, M., & Kielhofner, G. (1993). Use of the model of human occupation: A survey of therapists in psychiatric practice. *Occupational Therapy Journal of Research, 13* (2), 117–139.

N

Nave, J., Helfrich, C., & Aviles, A. (2001). Child witnesses of domestic violence: A case study using the OT PAL. *Occupational Therapy in Mental Health, 16* (3/4), 121–135.

Neville, A. (1985). The model of human occupation and depression. *Mental Health Special Interest Section Newsletter, 8* (1), 1–4.

Neville, A., Kriesberg, A., & Kielhofner, G. (1985). Temporal dysfunction in schizophrenia. *Occupational Therapy Mental Health, 5* (1), 1–19.

Neville-Jan, A. (1994). The relationship of volition to adaptive occupational behavior among individuals with varying degrees of depression. *Occupational Therapy in Mental Health, 12* (4), 1–18.

Neville-Jan, A., Bradley, M., Bunn, C., & Gehri, B. (1991). The model of human occupation and individuals with co-dependency problems. *Occupational Therapy in Mental Health, 11* (2/3), 73–97.

O

Oakley, F. (1987). Clinical application of the model of human occupation in dementia of the Alzheimer's type. *Occupational Therapy in Mental Health, 7* (4), 37–50.

Oakley, F., Kielhofner, G., & Barris, R. (1985). An occupational therapy approach to assessing psychiatric patients' adaptive functioning. *American Journal of Occupational Therapy, 39* (3), 147–154.

Oakley, F., Kielhofner, G., Barris, R., & Reichler, R. K. (1986). The Role Checklist: Development and empirical assessment of reliability. *Occupational Therapy Journal of Research, 6* (3), 157–170.

Olin, D. (1984). Assessing and assisting the persons with dementia: An occupational behavior perspective. *Physical & Occupational Therapy in Geriatrics, 3* (4), 25–32.

P

Padilla, R. (1998). Application of occupational therapy theories with elders. In H. Lohman, R. Padilla, & S. Byers-Connon (Eds.), *Occupational therapy with elders: Strategies for the certified occupational therapist assistant* (pp. 63–79). St. Louis, MO: Mosby.

Padilla, R., & Bianchi, E. M. (1990). Occupational therapy for chronic pain: Applying the model of human occupation to clinical practice. *Occupational Therapy Practice, 1* (3), 47–52.

Peterson, E., Howland, J., Kielhofner, G., Lachman, M. E., Assman, S., Cote, J., & Jette, A. (1999). Falls self-efficacy and occupational adaptation among elders. *Physical and Occupational Therapy in Geriatrics, 16* (1/2), 1–16.

Pizzi, M. (1989). Occupational therapy: Creating possibilities for adults with HIV infection, ARC and AIDS. *AIDS Patient Care, 3,* 18–23.

Pizzi, M. (1990a). The model of human occupation and adults with HIV infection and AIDS. *American Journal of Occupational Therapy, 44* (3), 257–264.

Pizzi, M. (1990b). Occupational therapy: Creating possibilities for adults with human immunodeficiency virus infection, AIDS related complex, and acquired immunodeficiency syndrome. *Occupational Therapy in Health Care, 7* (2/3/4), 125–137.

Pizzi, M. A. (1984). Occupational therapy in hospice care. *American Journal of Occupational Therapy, 38* (4), 252–257.

Platts, L. (1993). Social role valorisation and the model of human occupation: A comparative analysis for work with people with a learning disability in the community. *British Journal of Occupational Therapy, 56* (8), 278–282.

R

Reid, C. L,. & Reid, J. K. (2000). Care giving as an occupational role in the dying process. *Occupational Therapy in Health Care, 12* (2/3), 87–93.

Restall, G., & Magill-Evans, J. (1994). Play and preschool children with autism. *American Journal of Occupational Therapy, 48* (2), 113–120.

Rosenfeld, M. S. (1989). Occupational disruption and adaptation: A study of house fire victims. *American Journal of Occupational Therapy, 43* (2), 89–96.

Rust, K., Barris, R., & Hooper, F. (1987). Use of the model of human occupation to predict women's exercise behavior. *Occupational Therapy Journal of Research, 7* (1), 23–35.

S

Salz, C. (1983). A theoretical approach to the treatment of work difficulties in borderline personalities. *Occupational Therapy in Mental Health, 2* (3), 33–46.

Scarth, P. P. (1990). Services for chemically dependent adolescents. *Mental Health Special Interest Section Newsletter, 13,* 7–8.

Schaaf, R. C., & Mulrooney, L. L. (1989). Occupational therapy in early intervention: A family centered approach. *American Journal of Occupational Therapy, 43* (11), 745–754.

Schindler, V. J. (1988). Psychosocial occupational therapy intervention with AIDS patients. *American Journal of Occupational Therapy, 42* (8), 507–512.

Schindler, V. P. (1990). AIDS in a correctional setting. *Occupational Therapy in Health Care, 7* (2/3/4), 171–183.

Sepiol, J. M., & Froehlich, J. (1990). Use of the Role Checklist with the patient with multiple personality disorder. *American Journal of Occupational Therapy, 44* (11), 1008–1012.

Series, C. (1992). The long-term needs of people with head injury: A role for the community occupational therapist? *British Journal of Occupational Therapy, 55* (3), 94–98.

Shimp, S. L. (1989). A family-style meal group: Short-term treatment for eating disorder patients with a high level of functioning. *Mental Health Special Interest Section Newsletter, 12* (3), 1–3.

Shimp, S. L. (1990). Debunking the myths of ageing. *Occupational Therapy in Mental Health, 10* (3), 101–111.

Sholle-Martin, S. (1987). Application of the model of human occupation: Assessment in child and adolescent psychiatry. *Occupational Therapy in Mental Health, 7* (2), 3–22.

Sholle-Martin, S., & Alessi, N. E. (1990). Formulating a role for occupational therapy in child psychiatry: A clinical application. *American Journal of Occupational Therapy, 44* (10), 871–882.

Simons, D. (1999). The psychological system in adolescence. In *Pediatric therapy: A systems approach* (pp. 430–432). Philadelphia: FA Davis.

Smith, H. (1987). Mastery and achievement: Guidelines using clinical problem solving with depressed elderly clients. *Physical & Occupational Therapy in Geriatrics, 5,* 35–46.

Smith, N., Kielhofner, G., & Watts, J. (1986). The relationship between volition, activity pattern and life satisfaction in the elderly. *American Journal of Occupational Therapy, 40* (4), 278–283.

Smith, R. O. (1992). The science of occupational therapy assessment. *Occupational Therapy Journal of Research, 12* (1), 3–15.

Smyntek, L., Barris, R., & Kielhofner, G. (1985). The model of human occupation applied to psychosocially functional and dysfunctional adolescents. *Occupational Therapy in Mental Health, 5* (1), 21–39.

Spadone, R. A. (1992). Internal-external control and temporal orientation among Southeast Asians and White Americans. *American Journal of Occupational Therapy, 46* (8), 713–719.

Stein, F., & Cutler, S. (1998). Theoretical models underlying the clinical practice of psychosocial occupational therapy. In *Psychosocial occupational therapy: A holistic approach* (pp. 150–152). San Diego, CA: Singular Publishing.

Stofell, V. (1992). The Americans with Disabilities Act of 1990 as applied to an adult with alcohol dependence. *American Journal of Occupational Therapy, 46* (7), 640–644.

T

Tatham, M., & McCree, S. (1992). Leisure facilitator: The role of the occupational therapist in senior housing. *Journal of Housing for the Elderly, 10* (1/2), 125–138.

Tham, K., & Borell, L. (1996). Motivation for training: A case study of four persons with unilateral neglect. *Occupational Therapy in Health Care, 10* (3), 65–79.

V

Velozo, C., Kielhofner, G., Gern, A., Lin, F-L., Azhar, F., Lai, J-S., & Fisher, G. (1999). Worker Role Interview: Validation of a psychosocial work-related measure. *Journal of Occupational Rehabilitation, 9* (3), 153–168.

Velozo, C. A. (1993). Work evaluations: Critique of the state of the art of functional assessment of work. *American Journal of Occupational Therapy, 47* (3), 203–209.

Viik, M. K., Watts, J. H., Madigan, M. J., & Bauer, D. (1990). Preliminary validation of the Assessment of Occupational Functioning with an alcoholic population. *Occupational Therapy in Mental Health, 10* (2), 19–33.

W

Watts, J. H., Bauer, D., & Schmidt, W. (1986). A concurrent validity study of two occupational therapy evaluation instruments: The AOF and OCAIRS. *Occupational Therapy in Mental Health, 8* (4), 49–60.

Watts, J. H., Brollier, C., Bauer, D., & Schmidt, W. (1989a).

The Assessment of Occupational Functioning: The second revision. *Occupational Therapy in Mental Health, 8* (4), 61–88.

Watts, J. H., Brollier, C., Bauer, D., & Schmidt, W. (1989b). A comparison of two evaluation instruments used with psychiatric patients in occupational therapy. *Occupational Therapy in Mental Health, 8* (4), 7–27.

Watts, J. H., Kielhofner, G., Bauer, D., Gregory, M., & Valentine, D. (1986). The Assessment of Occupational Functioning: A screening tool for use in long-term care. *American Journal of Occupational Therapy, 40* (4), 231–240.

Weeder, T. (1986). Comparison of temporal patterns and meaningfulness of the daily activities of schizophrenic and normal adults. *Occupational Therapy in Mental Health, 6* (4), 27–45.

Weissenberg, R., & Giladi, N. (1989). Home economics day: A program for disturbed adolescents to promote acquisition of habits and skills. *Occupational Therapy in Mental Health, 9* (2), 89–103.

Wieringa, N., & McColl, M. (1987). Implications of the model of human occupation for intervention with native Canadians. *Occupational Therapy in Health Care, 4* (1), 73–91.

Woodrum, S. C. (1993). A treatment approach for attention deficit hyperactivity disorder using the model of human occupation. *Developmental Disabilities Special Interest Section Newsletter, 16* (1), 1–2.

Y

Yelton, D., & Nielson, C. (1991). Understanding Appalachian values: Implications for occupational therapists. *Occupational Therapy in Mental Health, 11* (2/3), 173–195.

Z

Zimmerer-Branum, S., & Nelson, D. (1995). Occupationally embedded exercise versus rote exercise: A choice between occupational forms by elderly nursing home residents. *American Journal of Occupational Therapy, 49* (5), 397–402.

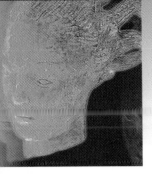

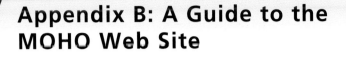

Appendix B: A Guide to the MOHO Web Site

Model of Human Occupation (MOHO) Clearinghouse Web Site

Information regarding MOHO is disseminated through the MOHO Clearinghouse web site at www.uic.edu/ahp/ot/mohoc.

The web site provides a range of information and resources related to MOHO inception and development. For example, the web site maintains a bibliography of all the literature that has been published on MOHO. This bibliography is updated on a monthly basis. The web site also includes information regarding ongoing MOHO-related projects throughout the world. It also has several links to related sites.

Finally, it has information and resources on manuals and videotapes developed using the theoretical constructs from MOHO. Products include assessment tools, clinical program descriptions, and clinical issues such as implementation of the Americans with Disabilities Act (ADA). Product information includes:

- A brief outline of each product
- Information on how to obtain the product (in a few cases the assessments can be downloaded directly; in other cases, links or downloadable order forms for purchasing assessments are provided)
- Cost of the product.

MOHO Listserv

The web site also provides an opportunity for persons who are learning MOHO, using it in practice, or conducting research on MOHO to join a listserv to engage in dialogue with others. The MOHO listserv acts as a forum for discussion and participation in issues related to MOHO theory, research, and application. Therapists and other professionals from around the world are part of the listserv, thus providing international involvement in further development of the model.

The procedure to become a listserv member is as follows:

- To subscribe to the MOHO listserv, send an e-mail to listserv@uic.edu with the following command in the message area:
  subscribe MOHO [your name]
  (e.g. subscribe MOHO John Doe)
- You will receive a confirmation reply from the listserv (please read this e-mail and follow any further instructions it gives). Please be sure to file this message for future reference as it contains useful information on setting options for your subscription
- Send your posting to:
  moho@listserv.uic.edu
  The posting will be automatically distributed to all subscribers to the MOHO list
- To remove yourself from the MOHO listserv, send an e-mail to listserv@uic.edu with the following command in the message area:
  signoff MOHO.

MOHO E-mail

Technical inquiries such as manual distribution, information on becoming a collaborator for an ongoing research project, or problems joining the Listserv can be addressed by sending an e-mail to mohoc@uic.edu.

INDEX

In this index, page numbers in *italics* designate figures; page numbers followed by the letter "t" designate tables; (*see also*) cross-references designate related topics or detailed topic breakdowns.